Nutrition
for Life

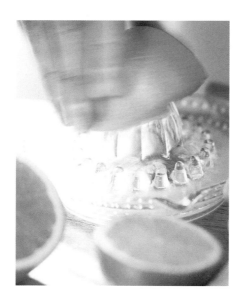

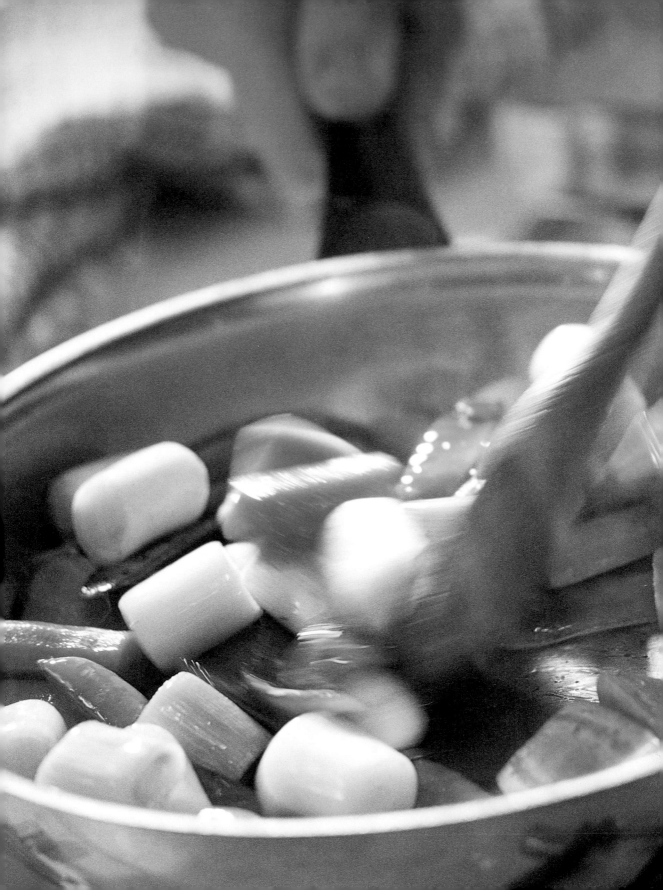

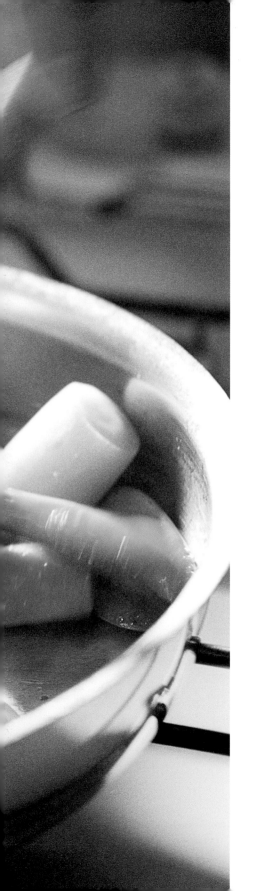

Nutrition
for Life

Lisa Hark, Ph.D, RD
and Darwin Deen, MD

LONDON, NEW YORK, MUNICH, MELBOURNE, DELHI

Senior Editors Irene Lyford, Liz Coghill
Project Art Editor Sara Kimmins
Editor Becky Alexander
Designer Isabel De Cordova
Design Assistant Iona Hoyle
DTP Designer Julian Dams
Production Controller Wendy Penn
Senior Managing Editor Jemima Dunne
Managing Art Editor Marianne Markham
Category Publishers Mary Thompson, Corinne Roberts
Art Director Bryn Walls

First published in the United States in 2005 by DK Publishing, Inc.
375 Hudson Street, New York, New York 10014

00 01 02 03 04 05 06 07 08 09 10 9 8 7 6 5 4 3 2 1

Copyright © 2005 Dorling Kindersley
Text copyright © 2005 Lisa Hark and Darwin Deen

A CIP catalog record for this book is available from the Library of Congress.
ISBN 0-7566-0522-9

Publishers Note

Every effort has been made to ensure that the information in this book is accurate. The information in this book will be relevant to the majority of people but may not be applicable in each individual case so you are therefore advised to obtain expert medical advice for specific information on personal health matters. Never disregard expert medical advice or delay in receiving treatment due to information obtained from this book. The naming of any product, treatment, or organization in this book does not imply endorsement by the authors or the publisher, nor does the omission of any such names indicate disapproval. Neither the publisher nor the authors accept any legal responsibility for any personal injury or other damage or loss arising from any use or misuse of the information and advice in this book.

Note: Any recipes in this book are intended for people of generally good health, without specific food allergies

Color reproduction by Colourscan, Singapore
Printed and bound by Tien Wah Press, Singapore

See our complete product line at
www.dk.com

Contents

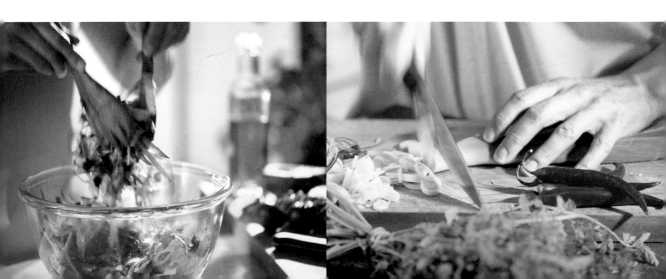

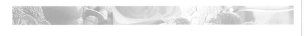

Eating for the time of your life 104

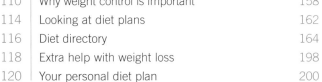

The truth about weight control 156

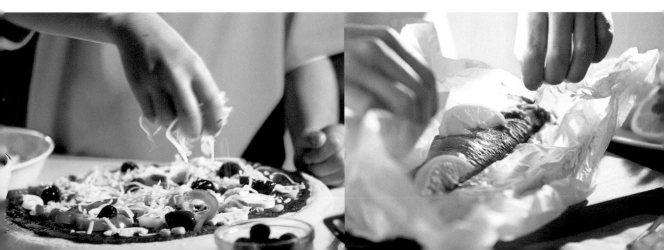

The food you buy   272

Food as medicine   210

Food analysis   294

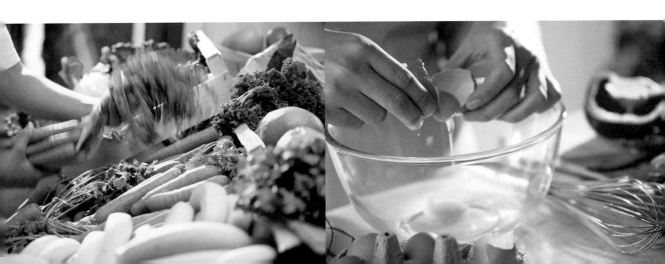

Introduction

The publication of our book, *Nutrition for Life*, could not be more relevant today, with obesity at epidemic proportions both here, in North America, and throughout the industrialized and the developing world. The World Health Organization estimates that there are now over 300 million obese adults worldwide, with more than 115 million suffering from obesity-related problems such as cardiovascular disease, cancer, and diabetes. These health problems are overtaking more traditional public health concerns such as undernutrition and infectious disease.

But what does this mean to you? Nutrition and lifestyle play a critical role at all stages of life, from infancy to old age; in *Nutrition for Life*, we show you how you can improve your health throughout your life, from many different perspectives. This is where our book is particularly relevant, since it addresses all the questions you may raise about taking care of your health and your family's health.

In the first part of the book we help you to analyze your eating and lifestyle habits, and identify any areas where changes would be beneficial to your health. This section includes a look at your family medical history, since diet and exercise can play a crucial role in minimizing your risks of developing many diseases, even those with an inherited component. Making changes is challenging, so we also include tips on behavior-modification strategies.

In the chapters that follow, we look at why our bodies need food, why each nutrient—including protein, fat, and carbohydrate—is essential, and why certain types of food are better for us than others. We include a comprehensive directory of vitamins and minerals, in which we look at the role of each of them, our daily requirements, signs and symptoms of deficiency, and lists of good sources for each vitamin and mineral listed. Subsequent chapters describe the basic food groups, with recommendations for healthier choices from each; changing nutritional needs through the various life stages; the major topic of weight control, with a detailed look at 45 popular weight-loss programs. We look at major medical conditions in which nutrition plays a crucial role, in both prevention and management—including diseases of the cardiovascular and digestive systems, cancer, diabetes, and allergies. And we look at the food that is available in supermarkets and stores, with advice on how to make better-informed food choices, coupled with suggestions for healthier preparation and cooking methods.

The book is completed by a comprehensive food-analysis section, in which we list the most common foods and give a breakdown of the nutrients each one provides, such as protein, carbohydrate, different types of fats, vitamins, and minerals. Throughout the book, we have included case studies, questionnaires, recipes, and nutritional analyses, designed to illustrate and enhance your understanding of the key nutritional points being covered.

Nutrition for Life has been designed to help you to think seriously about your diet and lifestyle in an easy and enjoyable way. Whether you are single, married, have young or older children, are healthy, or suffer from a chronic medical condition, you will gain short-term and long-term health benefits from reading this book and by putting into effect the advice it contains.

LISA A. HARK, PhD, RD
University of Pennsylvania
School of Medicine, Philadelphia

DARWIN DEEN, MD, MS
Albert Einstein College
of Medicine, New York

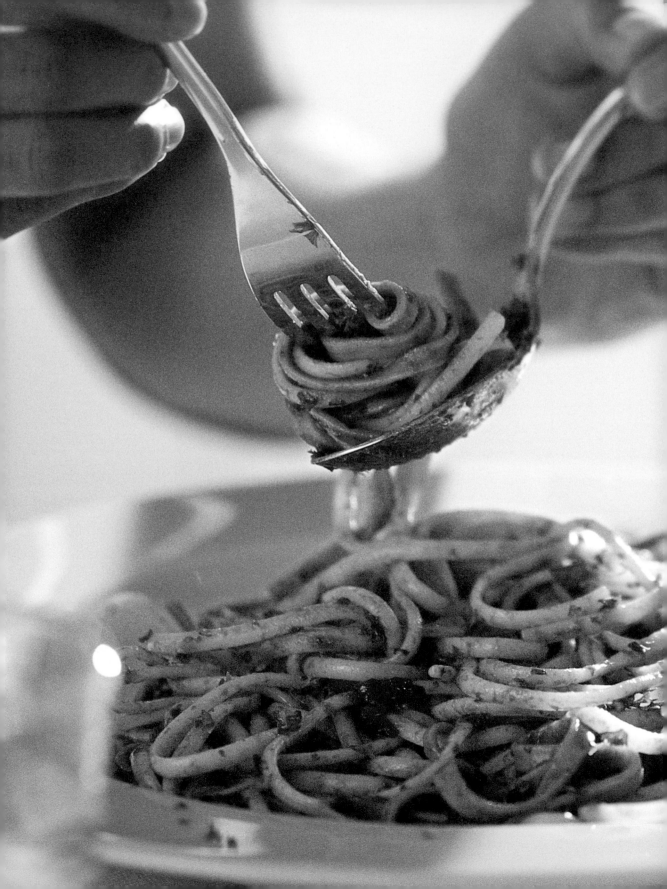

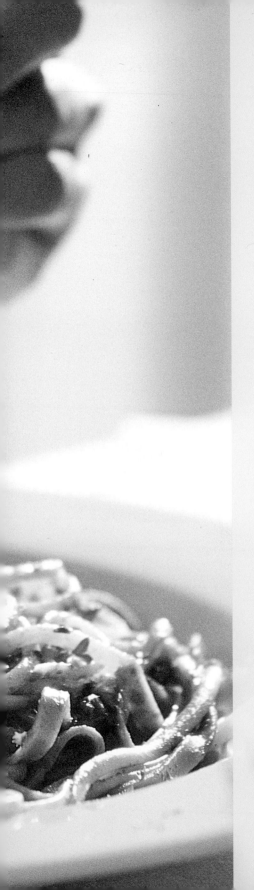

Assess your health and lifestyle

As you think about improving your health, you will most likely start by making dietary and lifestyle changes. It is important to think about why you want to make these changes. Are they right for you, and will they help you achieve your goals? This chapter will help you identify key areas for change.

The nutrition–energy balance

Good nutrition and regular exercise help you stay healthy and live longer.

You are what you eat. Everything that you eat and drink affects how your body functions. And, as your body's needs vary at different stages of your life and according to how you live your life, your nutritional needs vary also.

Know your body's needs

The connection between diet and health is clear: to grow properly and function normally, you need a complete range of nutrients, including carbohydrates, proteins, fats, fiber, and water, as well as a variety of vitamins and minerals (*see Food for Life, pp.32–67*).

Many of these nutrients are not just essential for normal body functioning, but they can actually improve your state of health and protect you against a number of diseases. Eating well makes you feel well, which improves your mood and enables you to cope better with stress.

Is your diet healthy?

If your diet lacks any nutrients or provides too much of certain factors, you will not function at an optimum level. At the same time, you may be creating future

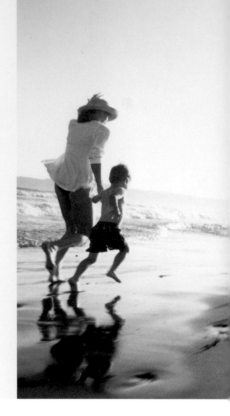

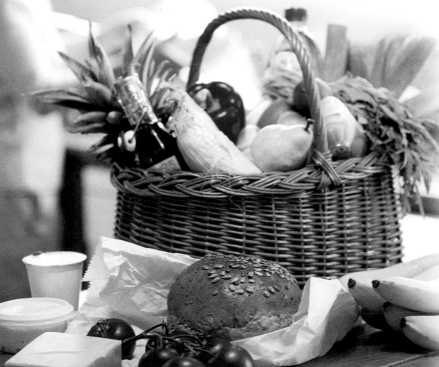

Five-a-day Include a minimum of five servings of fruits and vegetables each day to ensure that you have a health-giving range of vitamins and nutrients in your diet.

The elements of good nutrition

To function properly, your body needs a daily intake of a full range of essential nutrients, including a variety of fruits, vegetables, legumes, whole grains, low-fat dairy products, lean meats, fish and shellfish, and healthy oils, such as olive.

The foods we eat contain two main categories of nutrients: macronutrients and micronutrients. Macronutrients are needed in large quantities every day and form the foundation of any diet. They include proteins, carbohydrates, and fats, and provide energy.

Vitamins and minerals are found in small amounts in foods and make up the micronutrients. They play a critical role in maintaining the body's normal processes and functions.

Most foods contain both macro- and micronutrients in varying proportions. The key to achieving a healthy, well-balanced diet is to eat a wide variety of different foods.

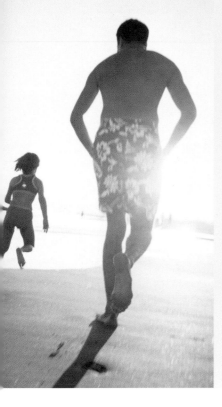

problems. For example, there is strong evidence that eating too much animal fat can lead to cardiovascular disease (*see p.214*), while skipping calcium-rich foods in your teens may lead to osteoporosis later (*see p.240*).

The food–energy balance

To maintain a healthy weight, you need to balance the energy you take in from the food you eat with the energy you expend in the course of your daily life.

Because of our lifestyles or the type of work that we do, many of us do not get as much exercise as we need. Excess food intake is stored in the body as fat, leading to weight gain and possibly to

Vibrant good health A nutritious diet that meets your body's nutritional and energy needs, coupled with an active lifestyle, is the key to optimum health and well-being.

obesity. This, in turn, can lead to various medical conditions, such as diabetes, cardiovascular disease, cancer, and joint problems.

Of course, the reverse is also true: if we expend more energy than we take in, we will lose weight—and this is the rationale behind many weight-loss diets (*see pp.162–197*). However, being underweight brings its own health problems and a reduced life expectancy (*see pp.208–209*).

Is your lifestyle healthy?

In this chapter, we shall look at various aspects of diet, exercise, physical health, and weight, and invite you to review your status in those areas. If you already recognize the importance of diet and exercise, congratulations! If not, this information will help you identify any areas that are preventing you from achieving optimum health and fitness.

Food and energy

The body gets energy, which is essential for life, from food. Our bodies expend the energy in various ways: some energy is used to maintain the critical day-to-day bodily functions that help us survive, such as breathing, heart rate, and other unconscious—also known as involuntary—activities. We also expend energy through our conscious daily activities, which can range from the sedentary—such as sitting, reading, or watching television—to participating in strenuous exercise and sports. Even activities such as thinking and sleeping require energy to occur.

During some stages of our lives and in certain circumstances, including childhood, pregnancy and breast-feeding, athletic training, and when we are sick, or recovering from an illness,

Energy equation For optimum health, all of the energy we expend in activities must be balanced by the energy we obtain from food.

our bodies require extra energy to cope with the additional demands that are made. Similarly, people recovering from surgery or trauma have extremely high energy requirements for their bodies'

repair mechanisms to function properly. If these extra energy requirements are not met by the food we eat, wounds may fail to heal and a full recovery will take a longer time to occur.

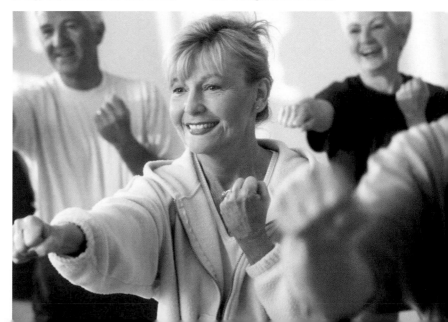

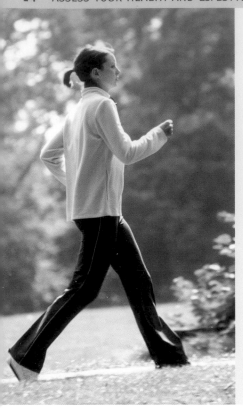

Look at your lifestyle

Take the first move toward optimizing your health.

Our aim in this book is to explain the link between what you eat and how you feel, whatever your lifestyle or dietary habits. We will also suggest ways of achieving optimum health and well-being for yourself and your family.

As a first step, we invite you to consider some simple questions about your diet and other lifestyle factors. First, we examine every aspect of your eating habits,

Stepping up activity Exercise is essential for health and well-being, so try to incorporate regular activity into your daily routine.

including how many times a day you eat, as well as what and how much you eat.

Then we look at other aspects of your lifestyle. For example, how active are you? Do you take part in any sports or exercise programs or do you get plenty of exercise walking the children to and from school or in your daily work? Finally, we look at any other factors that could affect your nutritional health, such as your use of alcohol and tobacco.

Assess your status

Once you have considered these questions, complete the quiz on page 21. Your score will identify what you are doing right as well as pinpoint any areas where changes could be made.

The optimum number of meals a day

Do you eat three meals a day? There is no right or wrong answer to this question. Everyone's biological clock is different, and we all have different demands on our schedules. However, your body and mind need a steady supply of energy and nutrients throughout the day, so eating three balanced meals is the optimum way to achieve a healthy diet.

Studies show that people who eat less frequently than three times a day are more likely, when they do sit down to eat or have a snack, to indulge in foods that are higher in fat and calories. If you prefer to have just two meals a day, be sure that one of those is breakfast (*right*), and avoid eating big meals late at night. Children in particular need regular meals and snacks throughout the day.

Regular meals Eating three well-balanced meals every day gives your body a steady supply of vital nutrients.

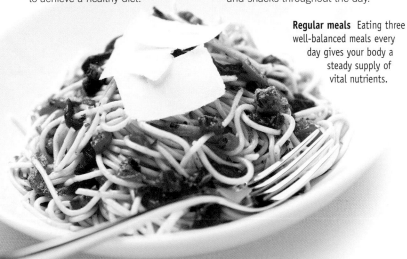

Don't skip breakfast

Breakfast is an important meal. It breaks the long overnight fast, helping you wake up and get going; it stops you from feeling hungry later; and it helps you be more alert at school or work. If you eat before you leave home, you'll be less likely to grab a high-fat snack on the way to work.

- For a quick and healthy breakfast, have a bowl of fortified cereal with fresh or dried fruit and low-fat or fat-free regular milk or soymilk.
- If you have time, make an omelet with two egg whites and one egg yolk. Serve with whole-wheat toast and low-sugar jam.
- Try whole-wheat or oat-bran waffles with low-sugar syrup. These waffles are low in fat and calories and contain some fiber.
- If you must eat on the run, grab a piece of fresh fruit, such as a banana or apple, some nuts and seeds, or a low-fat yogurt.

Snacking

Some people can get by on just three meals a day but, for most, snacking is a regular and enjoyable part of their daily routine. If you do snack, the key issues are what you snack on, and why you do it. Are you really hungry, eating out of habit, or just craving food (*right*)?

If you really are hungry, then eat a healthy snack, rather than wait for the next mealtime. This will prevent you from becoming over-hungry, which in turn reduces the temptation to eat a nutrient-poor convenience food. A good choice for a snack includes fresh or dried fruit, raw vegetables, low-fat yogurt, rice cakes with peanut butter, and nuts and seeds. Stock up on healthy snacks for home, travel, and work so that you always have what you need to hand.

Snacks are particularly important for children, who are unlikely to eat enough to meet their nutritional requirements at three meals a day as they have small stomachs. Regular healthy snacks are important for maintaining energy levels.

Many popular snacks, such as chips, candy bars, and cookies, contain high levels of sugar, fat, and salt, with little nutritional value, and should be once in a while rather than an everyday habit.

The key to regulating your dietary intake is to eat only when you are hungry and to stop when you are full. When you have the urge to snack, try to decide whether you really are hungry. Are you thirsty? Have a glass of water, and see if you still need food.

Think about what is triggering your urge to eat—is it boredom or was it brought on by something you saw? Try to pinpoint exactly what it is that you are craving—and satisfy it. For example, if you want chocolate, have just one piece—and enjoy it.

Hunger and cravings

When it comes to snacking, it is important to distinguish between real hunger and cravings.

Hunger This is a physiological response by which the body alerts the brain that nourishment is needed. If hungry, you may experience stomach discomfort or intestinal rumbling.

Appetite This is an instinctive, physical desire to eat that occurs when you are hungry. It can be stimulated by outside influences.

Cravings This is a psychological state affected by outside influences, such as the sight or smell of food, and by emotions, habits, moods, and imagination, rather than by hunger.

Eating fruits and vegetables

Fruits and vegetables should form the basis of every diet. Every meal should contain them, and they should be your first choice for snacks.

Vegetarians (*see pp.100–101*) will already be reaping the benefits of these nutritious foods, but many people are not eating enough. Fruits and vegetables are fat-free, low in sodium, and provide essential nutrients, such as vitamins A, C, and folate, fiber, and phytochemicals. Evidence shows that eating at least five servings of fruits and vegetables a day may help prevent the development of cardiovascular disease (*see pp.214–221*) and cancer (*see pp.258–263*).

According to the National Health and Nutrition Examination Surveys, the risk of cardiovascular disease is reduced in people who eat more than three servings of vegetables and fruits a day. There is also mounting evidence that eating at least five servings of fruits and vegetables daily halves the risk of developing cancer of the digestive and respiratory tracts. In addition, eating plenty of vegetables can help with weight control as they are high in fiber, which creates a feeling of fullness.

The American Heart Association, the National Cancer Institute, and the American Cancer Society all recommend eating at least five servings of fruits and vegetables daily. Meeting the five-a-day target is not difficult, yet few North Americans currently do so. You may be unsure what a serving comprises. The following examples will give you an idea:
● 1 medium-sized fruit, such as a banana, apple, or peach
● 6floz (180ml) fruit or vegetable juice
● 1 cup cooked vegetables.
If you have cereal topped with a banana for breakfast, a small bag of carrots as a snack, and a side dish of green beans and a salad with dinner, you will easily be getting what you need.

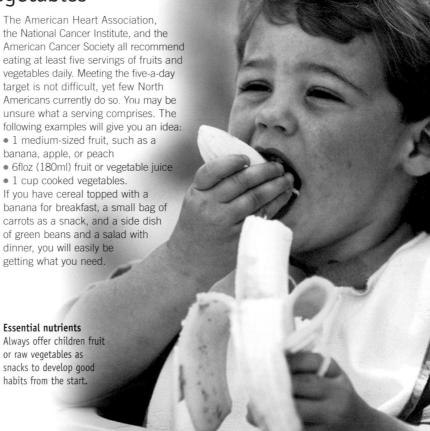

Essential nutrients
Always offer children fruit or raw vegetables as snacks to develop good habits from the start.

Dairy products and calcium

Milk, yogurt, cheese, and other dairy products are a prime source of calcium (*see p.62*) and are also fortified with vitamin D. Calcium is the most abundant mineral in the body, but it is also the one most likely to be inadequately supplied in the diet. Most North Americans do not consume enough calcium, with older adults and teenagers particularly at risk for low intake.

HEALTHY BONES AND TEETH
Calcium is essential for the normal growth and maintenance of bones and teeth, and calcium requirements must be met throughout life. Requirements are greatest during periods of growth, such as childhood, during pregnancy, and when breast-feeding. Long-term calcium deficiency can lead to

osteoporosis, in which the bone deteriorates and there is an increased risk of fractures (*see p.241*). You can meet your calcium needs by eating or drinking at least three or four servings of dairy products daily.

Some dairy products, such as hard cheese and whole milk, do contain a significant amount of saturated fat (*see right*), which can contribute to cardiovascular disease. Therefore, you should choose low-fat or fat-free dairy products (*see pp.82–83*) that will meet your calcium requirements.

Cheese is the most common source of saturated fat in the North American diet. If you cannot imagine giving it up, try substituting a low-fat variety made with part-skim milk, such as mozzarella, ricotta, cottage, or farmer's cheese.

Jargon buster

Saturated fats Mainly of animal origin, these fats have chemical bonds "saturated" with hydrogen. A diet high in these fats is linked to raised blood cholesterol levels and cardiovascular disease.

Unsaturated fats With chemical bonds not fully "saturated" with hydrogen, unsaturated fats occur mainly in vegetable and fish oils. Monounsaturated fats occur in olive, canola, and sesame oil and help protect against cardiovascular disease. Polyunsaturated fats, found in sunflower, corn, peanut, soy, and fish oils, are needed for growth, cell structure, and a healthy immune system (*see p.38*).

Fish and shellfish are healthy choices

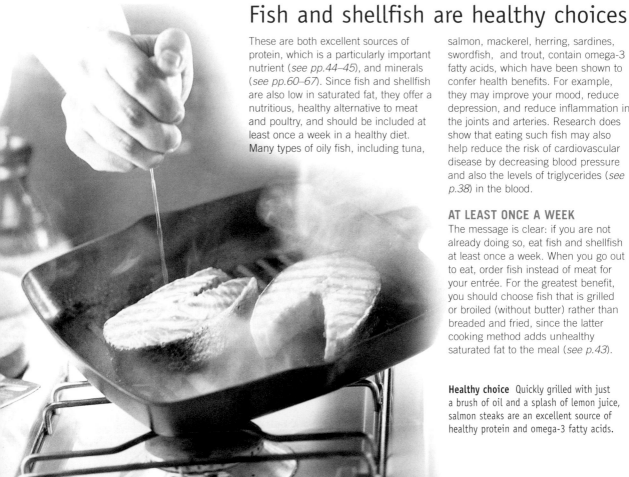

These are both excellent sources of protein, which is a particularly important nutrient (*see pp.44–45*), and minerals (*see pp.60–67*). Since fish and shellfish are also low in saturated fat, they offer a nutritious, healthy alternative to meat and poultry, and should be included at least once a week in a healthy diet. Many types of oily fish, including tuna,

salmon, mackerel, herring, sardines, swordfish, and trout, contain omega-3 fatty acids, which have been shown to confer health benefits. For example, they may improve your mood, reduce depression, and reduce inflammation in the joints and arteries. Research does show that eating such fish may also help reduce the risk of cardiovascular disease by decreasing blood pressure and also the levels of triglycerides (*see p.38*) in the blood.

AT LEAST ONCE A WEEK
The message is clear: if you are not already doing so, eat fish and shellfish at least once a week. When you go out to eat, order fish instead of meat for your entrée. For the greatest benefit, you should choose fish that is grilled or broiled (without butter) rather than breaded and fried, since the latter cooking method adds unhealthy saturated fat to the meal (*see p.43*).

Healthy choice Quickly grilled with just a brush of oil and a splash of lemon juice, salmon steaks are an excellent source of healthy protein and omega-3 fatty acids.

Benefits of turkey and chicken

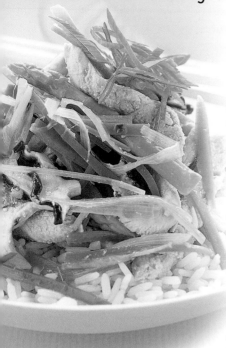

In addition to being excellent sources of protein, vitamins, and minerals, white-meat turkey and chicken are lower in both total and saturated fat than red meat and should be substituted for red meat wherever possible.

However, the fat and calorie content of both turkey and chicken increase significantly when the skin or dark meat (wings and legs) is eaten. Fat content is also higher in poultry products such as turkey hot dogs or ground turkey. For example, turkey or chicken hot dogs contain around 70 percent fat, but this is still a lower fat content than a regular beef hot dog, which contains about 80 percent fat.

If you really enjoy hot dogs, try tofu and soy varieties, which are excellent alternatives to meat hot dogs.

Asian-style chicken Unhealthy saturated fat is kept to a minimum in this appealing dish of lightly steamed white-meat chicken and vegetables, served with plain, steamed rice.

Eating red meat

Red meat includes beef, lamb, veal, and pork, and is a major source of protein. However, it is also high in saturated fat and cholesterol.

People who eat red meat daily have higher rates of cardiovascular disease than those who eat it less often. This is probably related to the saturated fat and cholesterol content. A high intake may also increase your risk of colon cancer. Studies have shown that people who replace red meat with chicken and fish have a lower risk of cardiovascular disease and colon cancer. Nutritionists now encourage you to eat more fish, healthy fats, and whole grains instead of red meat, saturated fat, and refined carbohydrates (see pp.72–73).

However, meat is an important source of protein, vitamin B_{12}, iron, and zinc. If you really like red meat, make a point of choosing lean cuts, such as pork loin or filet mignon, and eat them only occasionally rather than every day. In addition, trim off excess fat and use low-fat cooking methods (see p.43).

Using fats and oils

Fats are found not only in foods, but are also added during preparation, cooking, and serving. They are essential to your health, but one of the most interesting nutritional discoveries of the past decade has been that not all fats have the same effect on your health.

Saturated fats, such as butter, lard, and drippings, have been identified as having the potential to increase the risk of cardiovascular disease. This is because they raise the levels of cholesterol in the bloodstream. However, we now know that other fats, such as monounsaturated and polyunsaturated fats, found in plant-based oils and fish, are healthy and may protect against disease (see p.40).

As a first step in modifying your diet, substitute olive or canola oil for animal fats in your cooking (see p.41). Bear in mind that whichever oil you choose, fat is a concentrated source of energy, providing 100 calories per tablespoon, and should be used in moderation.

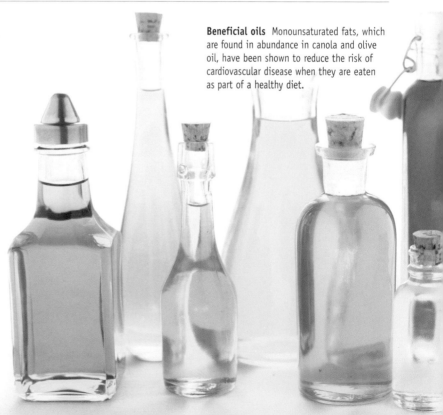

Beneficial oils Monounsaturated fats, which are found in abundance in canola and olive oil, have been shown to reduce the risk of cardiovascular disease when they are eaten as part of a healthy diet.

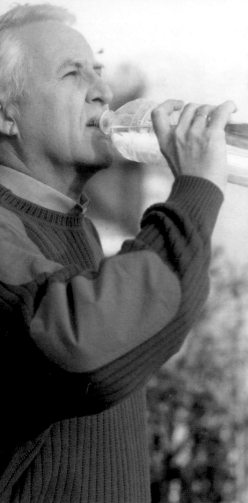

Drinking water

Water is an essential part of the diet. Humans are able to survive for several weeks without food, but for only a few days without water. Since the body has no means of storing water, you need a constant supply to replenish the fluid that is lost through sweating and urination. This means that you need to drink at least six to eight glasses of water every day, and more when it is hot or when playing sports or taking exercise. Do not wait until you are thirsty, since thirst may indicate that you are already lacking the water you need (*see pp.96–97*).

LIMIT SODAS AND JUICE

North Americans drink an average of 50 gallons (200 liters) of soda and 8 gallons (32 liters) of uncarbonated fruit drinks per person each year. Soda, sweetened iced tea, lemonade, sports drinks, fruitade, and fruit juices, while providing fluids, also contribute a large amount of calories and sugars to the diet. The huge increase in soda and juice consumption over the past 30 years is a major factor in the increased number of overweight children.

Water of life To help you get into the habit of drinking more water, carry a bottle with you or have one on your desk at work.

MAKING CHANGES

You can save hundreds of calories each day by paying attention to what you drink during the day, and by trying to substitute plain or sparkling water or other low-calorie beverages for drinks with a high sugar content. If you make only one dietary change after reading this book, this may be the most realistic and the most effective one that anyone can do. If you currently drink soft drinks with lunch and dinner and soda with snacks, wean yourself gradually by substituting water with one meal for about a week then slowly, over time, introduce more water or diet beverages. Try to introduce a glass of fat-free milk with snacks for a boost to your fluid levels and calcium intake.

We are urged from all sides to drink six to eight glasses of water a day for better health. For many years, it was believed that caffeinated beverages did not count toward this fluid intake because of their dehydrating effect. However, a recent study found no evidence to substantiate this belief, so beverages such as coffee, tea, and soft drinks, which consist mainly of water, do count toward your daily fluid needs.

Adequate fluid intake is vital for everyone, but especially for the elderly, who are prone to dehydration because of a decline in their thirst sensation.

Eating away from home

The number of meals eaten away from home in North America continues to rise. According to recent research, this trend is most likely due to the increase in the number of two-career families, who have very little time for shopping, preparing, and cooking meals at home during the week.

It may be that you have to eat away from home on a regular basis because of your work schedule, lifestyle, or family life but, if you are aware of the pitfalls, you can still make healthy choices. For example, you could choose a grilled-chicken sandwich instead of a cheese-topped burger, and order small portions or share larger ones. Instead of having french fries, choose a side salad, which is nutritious and low in fat.

Restaurant meals usually contain more fat and therefore more calories than food prepared at home. Since portions in restaurants are also considerably larger than those served at home, it is a good idea to share an entrée when eating out,

or to eat only part and take the rest home with you. Try to control portion sizes by not feeling obliged to eat everything on your plate, and stop eating when you feel full.

Fast-food restaurants and pizza parlors are the most frequent sources of food consumed away from home. Beware of the "super-sized" portions and special-value meals that are often offered at such establishments—for example, double cheeseburger, extra large fries, and a large soda. Deals such as this are marketed together to seem like a bargain, and therefore offer a financial incentive to consume more food than you would otherwise have purchased or eaten.

Wherever possible, select grilled, poached, baked, or broiled entrées, rather than fried, which are high in calories and saturated fat content. Order sauces and salad dressings on the side—or, if you can, avoid them altogether—and choose fruit or sherbet for dessert, or better still, skip it.

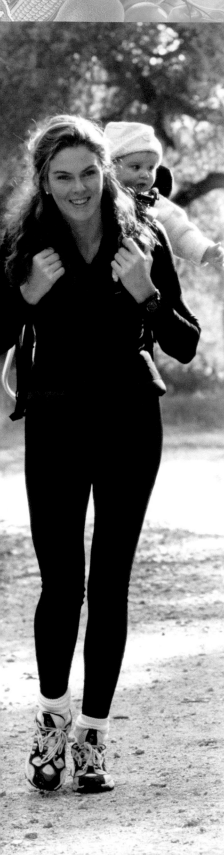

Starting young Walking is a healthy, cost-free activity that everyone can enjoy, so get children into the habit from an early age.

Maintaining an active lifestyle

Your level of activity depends on your lifestyle and how you regularly spend your days. For example, if your work involves standing or moving around for most of the day, or lifting, moving, and carrying heavy objects, then you have an active lifestyle. If you have young children, you may be walking a long distance daily, taking them to and from school. Alternatively, you may expend a great deal of energy on the physical aspects of caring for babies and toddlers. Domestic and leisure pursuits may also involve you in a high level of physical activity—for example, you may regularly spend time doing housework, gardening, or carrying out home maintenance and repair work.

On the other hand, your lifestyle may be predominantly sedentary: you may drive to work, sit at a desk all day, then come home and watch television or work on a computer in the evenings.

HEALTH BENEFITS
Keeping active will help you stay healthy and feel good. Health is more than just the absence of disease: it is a state of physical, mental, and spiritual well-being. On a physical level, your health reflects how well your body functions in terms of allowing you to carry out your daily activities. But it is also a reflection of your state of mind. No matter how physically fit you are, if you do not feel good about yourself, then you are not healthy.

It is important to be as active as possible, incorporating activities into your life that keep you moving in an enjoyable and rewarding way. This is particularly important if you have a sedentary job, such as sitting at a computer for eight hours a day.

INACTIVE CHILDREN
Children are born with a desire to be active; toddlers love to run around, climb, and explore, and this energy and love of exercise should be continued into later life. It is important for long-term health that parents encourage their children to be active, and provide the opportunity for children to fulfill this need.

Most North American children today are less active than those in previous generations. This coincides with an increase in the number of overweight children in North America (*see p.206*). Decreased opportunities for exercise, and increased interest in sedentary activities for children of all ages, especially teenagers, have led to an increase in weight problems.

Overweight children are at risk for many of the same problems as overweight adults (*see p.206*), and statistics show that these problems continue into adult life. Leading an active life as a family can help your child attain long-term good health.

TV and weight gain

It is well documented that the more television you watch, the more likely you are to be overweight, with all the negative implications for health that this involves.

Excessive television watching and computer use has been linked to the increase in numbers of overweight children and adolescents in North America. It is now recommended that television and video viewing and the use of computers for children should be limited to two hours per day.

Therefore, it is advisable that you limit the time you and your family spend watching television or using the computer, and find more active ways of using your leisure time.

You can also try to be more active while you watch the television. For example, you could buy an exercise bike or a treadmill and use it while you view. If that sounds a little too strenuous, you could do the ironing, do light cleaning, or lift light weights as you sit on the sofa.

Health and exercise

Recent figures indicate that 70 percent of North American adults do not get enough exercise. The combination of more sedentary behaviors and increased caloric intake is believed to be the major reason for the current epidemic of obesity in North America.

Regular physical exercise provides many health benefits. It reduces your risk of cardiovascular disease and osteoporosis, helps with weight control, improves flexibility, reduces stress, and improves your overall quality of life. Many studies state that brisk walking for 30 minutes each day can reduce the risk of developing both cardiovascular disease and diabetes by at least 30 percent. Even if you do not want to take up a new exercise program, you can improve your level of physical activity by making simple modifications in your daily life. For example, take the stairs instead of the elevator, park your car farther away than usual from your destination, and take a walk after dinner.

Regular exercise Whether you visit the gym, go swimming, or have a daily stroll, regular exercise is essential for good health.

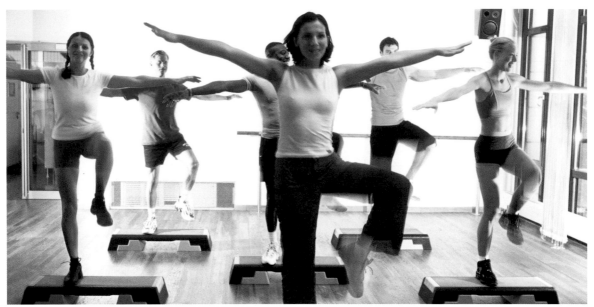

Drinking alcohol

Alcohol has very little nutritional value, and excess consumption can lead to a number of medical problems, including certain vitamin deficiencies (see pp.52–58). Alcohol also adds a significant amount of empty calories to the diet, with consequent weight gain. Beer and ale are particularly high in calories, as are cordials and liqueurs.

However, moderate drinkers have lower rates of cardiovascular disease than either abstainers or excessive drinkers. Drinking alcohol in moderation may even offset some of the harmful effects of a high-fat diet. This is exemplified by the French, who tend to eat a diet that is moderately high in saturated fat, but suffer less cardiovascular disease than would be expected. This "French paradox" may be due to the antioxidants in red wine, which may protect against the harmful effects of saturated fats.

Jargon buster

Antioxidants These are substances that help neutralize the damaging effect on cells and tissues of by-products known as free radicals. Sources of antioxidants available from the diet include vitamins A, C, and E and the minerals copper, selenium, and zinc.

Smoking

Quitting smoking is the best lifestyle change you can ever make. Smoking increases your risk of cardiovascular disease, chronic lung disease, and many cancers; passive smoking—inhaling "secondhand" smoke—can cause pneumonia and asthma; and pregnant smokers put their babies at risk of prematurity, low birth weight, and even fetal death.

Within months of cutting down on the amount you smoke, your health will improve. Many smokers are concerned about gaining weight if they quit, but from a health standpoint, smoking is much more risky than carrying a few extra pounds in weight.

Questionnaire How healthy is your lifestyle?

Circle the letter corresponding to the answer that best describes your habits. Then find your score by adding the points associated with the circled letters.

1 How many meals do you usually eat each day ?
a   3 meals and 1 snack
b   3 meals with no snacks
c   2 meals, skipping breakfast or lunch
d   I usually eat only 1 meal each day

2 What types of snacks do you eat?
a   Fruits, vegetables, nuts, and/or yogurt
b   Pretzels, nuts, popcorn, fruit, and/or yogurt
c   Chips, pretzels, popcorn, and/or other "junk" food
d   Sweets, such as candy, pastries, and/or cookies

3 How many servings of fruits and vegetables do you eat each day?
a   I always eat 5 or more servings of fruits and vegetables a day
b   I usually eat 3–4 servings
c   I usually eat about 1 serving
d   I usually eat fruits and vegetables only a few times per week

4 Which dairy products, if any, do you usually eat or drink?
a   Fat-free dairy products, such as yogurt and milk
b   1 percent milk, 1 percent yogurt, and part-skim cheeses
c   2 percent milk, low-fat cream cheese, and low-fat ice cream
d   Regular fat dairy products, such as whole milk and ice cream

5 How often do you usually eat fish or shellfish?
a   I eat fish or shellfish at least twice a week
b   I usually eat fish or shellfish once a week
c   I usually eat fish or shellfish a few times a month
d   I rarely or never eat fish or shellfish

6 Which types of poultry do you eat?
a   Chicken or turkey breast with the skin removed
b   Chicken or turkey breast with the skin on
c   I occasionally eat breaded, fried chicken or turkey breast
d   I frequently choose dark-meat chicken, duck, goose, etc.

7 How often do you eat red meat?
a   I never eat red meat
b   I eat red meat 1–2 times a month
c   Several times a week
d   I eat red meat every day

8 Which fats and oils do you use?
a   I try to limit my use of any fat or oil when cooking
b   I usually use olive or canola oil
c   I usually use butter when cooking
d   I frequently use bacon fat, fat back, lard, or chicken fat when cooking

9 Apart from coffee, what do you usually drink during the day?
a   I usually drink water exclusively
b   100 percent fruit juice, water, and diet beverages
c   Soda, sports drinks, fruit drinks, and sugar-sweetened iced teas
d   Soda and sugar-sweetened beverages

10 When eating out, which of the following would you usually choose?
a   Grilled, broiled, baked, or steamed entrées
b   Pasta with seafood in marinara or red sauce
c   Prime rib, steak, veal, lamb, or pasta in a cream sauce
d   Pizza, sausage, hoagies, fried foods, or hot dogs

11 How much exercise do you get?
a   I usually exercise for at least 30–60 minutes on most days
b   I usually exercise for 30 minutes a few days a week
c   I exercise for 30 minutes a few times a month
d   I rarely participate in any physical activity

12 How much TV do you watch?
a   I rarely watch television
b   I watch a few hours of television every week
c   I watch less than 2 hours daily
d   I usually watch 3 or more hours of television daily

13 How often do you drink alcohol and how much?
a   I usually have 1–2 drinks of alcohol a week
b   I usually have 1–2 drinks of alcohol daily
c   I rarely drink alcohol
d   I usually have at least 3 alcoholic drinks daily

14 Do you smoke? If so how many cigarettes do you smoke per day?
a   I have never smoked, or I quit more than 8 years ago
b   I smoke fewer than 5 cigarettes a day
c   I smoke 5–10 cigarettes a day or up to 5 cigars
d   I smoke more than 10 cigarettes a day

Score a 1 **b** 2 **c** 3 **d** 4

11–20 points Congratulations! Your diet is healthy and you should be proud of yourself. Keep up the good work. Read on to learn more.

21–29 points You are making good choices, but are you ready for the next step? This book will give you the information you need to improve your health now and for the future. Set realistic goals that you can achieve and maintain.

30–52 points Your diet may be too high in fat and too low in fruits and vegetables. You are risking your future health by selecting high-fat foods and not getting enough exercise. Use the information in this book to help you understand your barriers to making changes and how you can really improve your health and the health of your family.

Check your physical health

Understanding your own health status helps you take control.

Once you begin to understand your health status in the context of both your lifestyle behaviors and your medical history, you will be in the best possible position to work with your doctor and dietitian to take charge of your health. Being able to understand why changes in diet and exercise will improve your health, longevity, and mental well-being will make it easier for you to achieve any changes necessary.

Get a checkup

As part of the assessment of your current physical health, you may visit your doctor for a checkup. Many of the exams that he or she

Family traits To help you assess your risks of developing certain diseases, it is useful to look at your family medical history.

carries out, such as measuring weight, height, pulse, and blood pressure, relate to your risk of developing cardiovascular disease, which is the leading cause of death in North America.

Some of the risks, such as your age, gender, and family history, cannot be altered (*below right*), but other risk factors can be modified by making changes to your diet and lifestyle. If you are in a high-risk category for cardiovascular disease because of nonmodifiable risk factors, then it is vital that you tackle the areas where changes are possible to improve your overall health and long-term wellness.

Look at your family

You should consider your family medical history to become aware of the medical conditions from which your parents, grandparents, and other blood relatives suffered. This will provide you with an opportunity to identify potential health issues in your own life and

to take the appropriate action to modify your risks of developing those conditions yourself.

The risks of asthma, diabetes, migraines, and cardiovascular disease, for example, high blood pressure, tend to run in families or have a genetic component.

If you are reading this book because you currently suffer from a health problem, there is much that you can do yourself to control and improve matters with diet and lifestyle changes. This is covered in detail in the chapter Food as Medicine (*see pp.210–263*). It is a good idea to discuss any changes you wish to make with your doctor or a registered dietitian.

Risk factors for cardiovascular disease

Many factors are known to increase your risk of developing cardiovascular disease; some you cannot control, others you can.

Nonmodifiable high risk factors

Factors such as age, gender, and family history, are predetermined, but you can reduce their impact with nutrition and exercise:
- Age: men over the age of 45 and women over the age of 55.
- Gender: cardiovascular disease is more common in men than in premenopausal women.
- Heredity: the risk of heart attack is greater if there is a family history of cardiovascular disease before 60.

Modifiable high risk factors

You can change the following by adopting a healthier lifestyle:
- High cholesterol or LDL level
- Current cigarette smoking
- High blood pressure
- Diabetes
- Overweight or obesity
- Physical inactivity

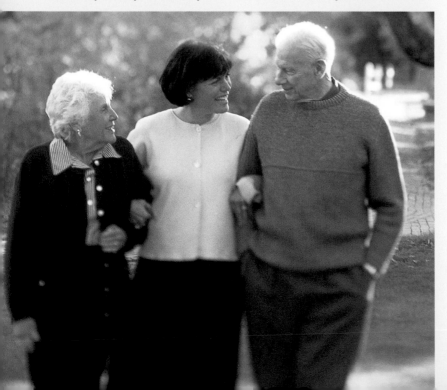

Having a medical checkup

When you visit your doctor for a medical checkup, he or she will take a number of measurements all of which will help assess your current state of health. These could include taking your temperature and pulse, listening to your heart and lungs with a stethoscope, measuring your blood pressure, and checking your weight and height.

Depending on your personal and family medical history, your doctor may also take a blood sample that will be tested in the laboratory for specific conditions (*below*).

CHECKING YOUR PULSE
Pulse is a measure of heart rate and can be felt where an artery (a blood vessel carrying blood away from the heart) runs close to the skin. In adults, the pulse rate is usually felt at the wrist.

A low resting pulse rate is a good indicator of physical fitness: the stronger your heart, the less frequently it needs to pump to provide oxygen to your tissues. Babies have a high pulse rate but, as we age, the pulse rate decreases. The normal pulse rate for adults is 60–80

beats per minute. Know your figures, and how these compare to others of your age and gender.

MEASURING BLOOD PRESSURE
This is a measure of the pressure of the blood in your arteries as your heart pumps. The value depends on the strength of your heart muscle, the elasticity of the arterial walls, and the volume and viscosity of your blood. The blood pressure of a healthy young adult should be no more than 120/80mmHg. High blood pressure is diagnosed when the reading taken is persistently higher than 140/90mmHg.

LIFESTYLE CHANGES
If you are diagnosed with high blood pressure, make lifestyle changes, such as losing weight, increasing the amount of exercise you take, and limiting your use of salt and alcohol (*see p.220*). If these are not enough to normalize your blood pressure, your doctor may prescribe medication, since high blood pressure is a risk factor for other cardiovascular diseases, such as heart attack.

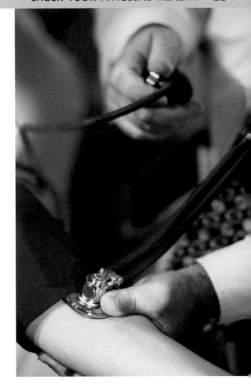

Blood pressure Persistently high blood-pressure levels are associated with an increased risk of cardiovascular disease, so regular checks are essential.

Blood tests and health

Depending on the reason for your medical checkup, the symptoms that you have described, or your family medical history, your doctor may take a blood sample to be sent for laboratory testing. These tests help to assess your health and diagnose certain diseases.

Cholesterol A waxy substance in the blood that is necessary for the normal functioning of the body (*see p.40*). Excess amounts of cholesterol can form deposits on the inside of blood vessels, leading to narrowing of the arteries and cardiovascular disease.

An elevated blood cholesterol level (more than 200mg/dL) may be hereditary and/or due to a diet that is high in saturated fat (*see p.38*). For information on how to lower your blood cholesterol, see page 217.

Low density lipoprotein (LDL) Often called the "bad" cholesterol, LDL carries cholesterol from the liver to tissues. Levels more than 130mg/dL are linked with increased risk of cardiovascular disease (*see p.214*).

High density lipoprotein (HDL) Carries cholesterol from the tissues back to the liver. It is often referred to as the "good cholesterol," since high levels (more than 60mg/dL) are associated with a reduced risk of cardiovascular disease (*see p.214*).

Triglycerides Fatty substances in the blood that are absorbed from the diet or synthesized from excess calories. High triglyceride levels (more than 150mg/dL) may be a risk factor for cardiovascular disease. Eating fish regularly can help to reduce levels.

Glucose The predominant sugar in the blood and may be measured at different times during the day—for example, first thing in the morning, before eating, or two hours after meals. Interpreting the results depends on when the glucose was measured. Raised levels (more than 126mg/dL) indicate diabetes (*see p.246*).

Hemoglobin The protein in red blood cells that carries iron. Anemia occurs when hemoglobin levels are lower than 13.5g/dL for men or 12g/dL for women (*see p.66*).

Hematocrit The measure of the volume percentage of red blood cells in whole blood. Levels lower than 41 percent for men and 36 percent for women indicate anemia. Eat foods rich in iron to boost hematocrit.

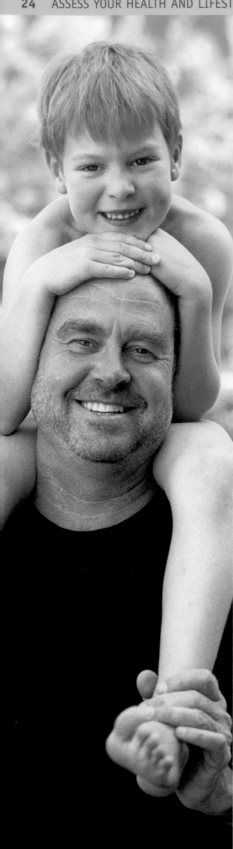

Family likeness Body shape and weight are associated with various health risks but, although our basic body type is inherited, this can be modified by diet and exercise.

Assess your shape and weight

Body shape and weight provide vital clues to health.

Most of us will wind up looking like one of our parents. Just as the color of our hair and eyes is transmitted through our genes, so too is our height and weight distribution, though these can be influenced by diet and exercise.

Weight distribution
Studies show that in overweight people, the distribution of excess body fat can affect their risk of developing cardiovascular disease and diabetes. Compared to "pear-shaped" individuals, who store fat around their hips and thighs, "apple-shaped" people are at an increased risk. Having a "beer belly" is no joke: those extra few inches around your waist may be a signal of bad things to come.

Assessing healthy weight
Healthy weight is now defined according to body mass index (BMI), which is calculated as a ratio of weight to height (*see pp.26–27*). This index provides a more accurate measure of body fat than weight alone. Along with body shape, BMI assesses the risk of developing diabetes, cancer, and cardiovascular disease.

US national guidelines define overweight people as those with a BMI of 25–29.9 and obese people as those with a BMI of 30 and above. Those people with a BMI over 40 are classified as being extremely obese. These definitions are based on evidence that many people with a BMI of 25 or greater begin to develop an increase in LDL, total cholesterol, and blood-sugar levels, in addition to high blood pressure or prehypertension.

Risks of excess weight
It is estimated that two out of three Americans are overweight, and one in three is obese. Obesity is becoming more common among both adults and children, and this is having an impact on national health. About 300,000 deaths each year in the US are associated with being overweight, and obesity is the country's second leading cause of preventable death (after smoking).

If your BMI is above 25, we suggest you read the information and advice on weight control and weight reduction (*see pp.156–207*).

Health risks of obesity
If your BMI is 30 or above, you are considered "obese," and your health may be at risk. It is advisable to see your doctor and make every effort to lose weight.

Statistics show that being obese greatly increases your chance of diabetes and cardiovascular diseases such as hyperlipidemia, high blood pressure, and stroke.

Being obese also increases your chance of gallbladder disease, sleep apnea, osteoarthritis, and respiratory problems. You are also more at risk of certain types of cancers, including breast, colon, prostate, and endometrial.

If you need surgery of any kind, you may be required to lose some weight first to minimize risk; this could lead to a lengthy delay.

Where is your fat located?

Men and women store fat in different areas of the body. In men, it is deposited mostly in the upper arms, shoulders, and abdomen; in women, it is mainly deposited in the breasts, hips, buttocks, and thighs. For both sexes, measuring your waist is a good indication of whether you are carrying excess weight:

• In your underwear, find the mid-point between the uppermost part of your hip bone and your lowest rib.

• Mark this point and measure around your abdomen with a tape measure.

• Ensure that the tape is parallel to the floor all the way round and is snug, but not tight, around your waist.

• Make sure you breathe normally as you take the measurement.

A waist circumference above 40in (102cm) in men and 35in (88cm) for women indicates that you are carrying excess weight around your middle (near your heart), which increases your risk of developing high blood pressure, raised cholesterol levels, diabetes, and cardiovascular disease.

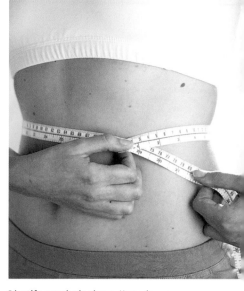

Identify your body shape Measuring your waist is a simple way of checking whether you are an apple or a pear and if you are at increased risk of certain diseases.

Are you an apple or a pear?

People who tend to gain weight mainly in the abdominal region (a paunch or "beer belly") are said to have an apple shape. If you tend to gain weight mostly on your hips, buttocks, and thighs, you are said to have a pear shape. The location of your body fat affects your health. If you are apple shaped, you are at increased risk for the health problems associated with obesity, including cardiovascular diseases, such as high blood pressure, and diabetes (*opposite*). You cannot do anything to change being an apple or a pear—it is an inherited characteristic. However, you can limit its extent by controlling your weight and keeping fit.

How to weigh yourself

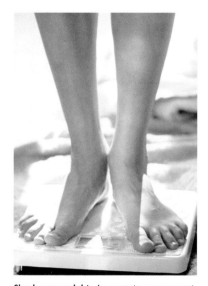

Check your weight An accurate measurement of your weight is an essential part of your assessment. Consistently weigh yourself in the same clothes, in your underwear, or naked and always at the same time of day, ideally in the morning before breakfast.

There are several dos and don'ts to be aware of if you want to get the most accurate measurement of your weight from your bathroom scale, especially if you are trying to lose weight.

• For accuracy, make sure that the scale you use is from a reputable company. Don't buy the cheapest one that you can find because it may not be very accurate.

• Each time you weigh yourself, do it wearing the same clothes, in your underwear, or naked.

• Make sure that you use the same scale in the same place each time you weigh yourself. If possible, get yourself a bathroom scale that only you use. Because different scales vary in their accuracy and how they are calibrated, it is likely that you will get slightly different results if you change the scale that you use. For example, you might find that you are heavier on a different scale just because it is not very accurate. Beware of using the scale in the gym—it may look as though it is accurate, but hundreds of people use it and it is prone to wear and tear.

• Always weigh yourself at the same time of day, ideally with an empty bladder and bowels and nothing in your stomach. First thing in the morning after visiting the bathroom and before breakfast is the best time of day.

• Don't weigh yourself more than once a week. We all have normal fluctuations in body weight—especially for women during their menstrual cycle—and you may be disheartened if you weigh more than on the previous day.

• If you are trying to lose weight through an exercise regime, you should be aware that muscle weighs more than fat tissue. There may be a point in your regime when you look slimmer and more toned but you stay the same weight or even weigh more because you are more muscular. Don't get discouraged.

Are you a healthy weight for your height?

Body mass index (BMI) is based on a ratio of your weight to your height. Use the chart below to find out whether or not your weight is within the normal range for your height.

If you find that you are overweight, it is advisable that you consult your doctor, dietitian, or nurse to discuss how to begin a weight-control program (*see also pp.156–207*).

While BMI is a more useful indicator of body fat than the gender-specific height–weight tables that were used previously, it does have limitations. For example, it may overestimate body fat in very muscular people, because muscle weighs more than fat. It may underestimate the amount of body fat in some underweight people who have lost lean tissue, such as older adults. Also, people who are tall but have a small frame might have excess fat around their waist, yet show a normal BMI. If

you are puzzled or concerned by your BMI result, talk to your doctor, who will explain the implications to you and give you advice on modifying your diet and lifestyle. If you have not had your height measured for many years, get it measured again, because height can change with age.

There are other devices for measuring the proportion of fat in the body, and your doctor may double-check your findings. The most widely used device uses a harmless electric current that passes through the body. It identifies areas of muscle and fat.

Using the BMI table Find your height in the left-hand column of the body mass index (BMI) table (*below*), then move across that row until you find the column that corresponds with your weight. The number shown where these two measures converge is your BMI score. The color coding shown in the

key below will indicate whether your weight is underweight, normal, overweight, or obese.

For example, if your height is 66in (168cm), and your weight is 140lb (64kg), your BMI is 23. This means that your weight is in the "normal" range. If your height is 66in (168cm) and your weight is 155lb (70kg), your BMI is 25, which means that you are classified as being overweight.

For a more detailed interpretation of BMI scores, and advice on nutritional or lifestyle changes that may be beneficial to your health, see opposite.

Key

Underweight: BMI 19.0 or below
Normal: BMI 19.0–24.9
Overweight: BMI 25–29.9
Obese: BMI above 30

BODY MASS INDEX (BMI) TABLE

Weight / Height	100lb /45kg	105lb /48kg	110lb /50kg	115lb /52kg	120lb /55kg	125lb /57kg	130lb /59kg	135lb /61kg	140lb /64kg	145lb /66kg	150lb /68kg	155lb /70kg	160lb /73kg	165lb /75kg	170lb /77kg
								BMI							
60in/153cm	20	21	21	22	23	24	25	26	27	28	29	30	31	32	33
61in/155cm	19	20	21	22	23	24	25	26	26	27	28	29	30	31	32
62in/158cm	18	19	21	22	22	23	24	25	26	27	27	28	29	30	31
63in/160cm	18	19	20	21	21	22	23	24	25	26	27	27	28	29	30
64in/163cm	17	18	20	21	21	21	22	23	24	25	26	27	27	28	29
65in/165cm	17	17	19	20	20	21	22	22	23	24	25	26	27	27	28
66in/168cm	16	17	19	19	19	20	21	22	23	23	24	25	26	27	27
67in/171cm	16	16	18	19	19	20	20	21	22	23	23	24	25	26	27
68in/173cm	15	16	17	18	18	19	20	21	21	22	23	24	24	25	26
69in/176cm	15	16	17	18	18	18	19	20	21	21	22	23	24	24	25
70in/178cm	14	15	17	17	17	18	19	19	20	21	22	22	23	24	24
71in/181cm	14	15	16	17	17	17	18	19	20	20	21	22	22	23	24
72in/183cm	14	14	16	16	16	17	18	18	19	20	20	21	22	22	23
73in/186cm	13	14	15	16	16	16	17	18	18	19	20	20	21	22	22
74in/188cm	13	13	15	15	15	16	17	17	18	19	19	20	21	21	22
75in/191cm	12	13	14	14	15	16	16	17	17	18	19	19	20	21	21
76in/193cm	12	13	13	14	15	15	16	16	17	18	18	19	19	20	21

What does my result mean?

Once you have found out what your BMI (Body Mass Index) is, check below to see whether it indicates that you are underweight, a normal, healthy weight, overweight, or obese and what you should then do about your weight.

BMI 19.0 or below: Underweight You need to eat more food to provide your body with the fuel it needs. You may need to eat more at each meal and have more snacks during the day. Be sure to choose nutritious foods from a range of food groups (*see pp.208–209*).

BMI 19.0–24.9: Normal weight You are eating the right amount to keep your weight at a healthy level, but you still need to make sure that your diet is balanced, healthy, and nutritious.

BMI 25–29.9: Overweight It would be beneficial to your health if you lose some weight and avoid gaining any additional weight. Follow the advice in this book about healthy eating and regular exercise to help manage your weight long-term. Making just one or two adjustments to your diet each day, for example, cutting out high-fat or high-sugar snacks, should result in a healthy, gradual weight loss.

BMI 30–34.9: Obesity (Class 1) Your health may be at risk at your current weight. Look for healthy ways of losing the excess weight; do not be tempted to try any "crash" diets, which could place more strain on your health.

BMI 35–39.9: Obesity (Class 2) Your health is at risk at your current weight. You should use this book to find ways of changing your eating habits. You are advised to seek advice from your doctor or dietitian.

BMI 40 or higher: Obesity (Class 3) Being this overweight poses a serious risk to your health. You are advised to seek advice from your doctor or dietitian for a weight-loss plan.

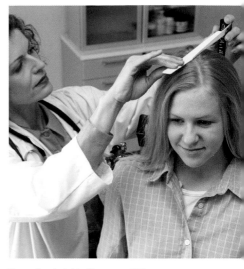

Measuring height Since your BMI score is based on your height and your weight, accurate measurements are essential.

175lb /79kg	180lb /82kg	185lb /84kg	190lb /86kg	195lb /89kg	200lb /91kg	205lb /93kg	210lb /95kg	215lb /98kg	220lb /100kg	225lb /102kg	230lb /104kg	235lb /107kg	240lb /109kg	245lb /111kg	Weight
						BMI									Height
34	35	36	37	38	39	40	41	42	43	44	45	46	47	48	60in/153cm
33	34	35	36	37	38	39	40	41	42	43	43	44	45	46	61in/155cm
32	33	34	35	36	37	37	38	39	40	41	42	43	44	45	62in/158cm
31	32	33	34	35	35	36	37	38	39	40	41	42	43	43	63in/160cm
30	31	32	33	33	34	35	36	37	38	39	39	40	41	42	64in/163cm
29	30	31	32	32	33	34	35	36	37	37	38	39	40	41	65in/165cm
28	29	30	31	31	32	33	34	35	36	36	37	38	39	40	66in/168cm
27	28	29	30	31	31	32	33	34	34	35	36	37	38	38	67in/171cm
27	27	28	29	30	30	31	32	33	33	34	35	36	36	37	68in/173cm
26	27	27	28	29	30	30	31	32	32	33	34	35	35	36	69in/176cm
25	26	27	27	28	29	29	30	31	32	32	33	34	34	35	70in/178cm
24	25	26	26	27	28	29	29	30	31	31	32	33	33	34	71in/181cm
24	24	25	26	26	27	28	28	29	30	31	31	32	33	33	72in/183cm
23	24	24	25	26	26	27	28	28	29	30	30	31	32	32	73in/186cm
22	23	24	24	25	26	26	27	28	28	29	30	30	31	31	74in/188cm
22	22	23	24	24	25	26	26	27	27	28	29	29	30	31	75in/191cm
21	22	23	23	24	24	25	26	26	27	27	28	29	29	30	76in/193cm

Do you need to change?

Take charge of your health by evaluating your diet and lifestyle.

The purpose of this chapter is to help you identify any dietary and lifestyle habits that you could change to improve your health. The fact that you are now reading this book shows that you are interested in making changes.

Putting health in context
The results of the questionnaire on page 21 have to be interpreted in the context of both your current health and your family history.

If you are aware of a medical condition that runs in your family, you may be able to reduce your risk of developing the condition by following the advice that we offer in this book.

Minimizing risk
This is not a "diet" book in the usual sense. Our goal is to translate the best medical research available into a sensible lifestyle program that will help you maintain and improve your health in the long-term. Evidence shows that "crash" diets do not work and that very rarely do they help people change their eating habits or lifestyle. This

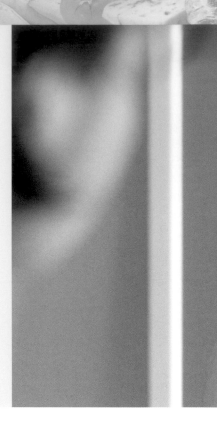

Assess yourself

Now it is time to review your findings about your current nutritional and lifestyle status. When you understand the connection between these and your health, you will be ready to move on to making the necessary changes.

REVIEW YOUR STATUS
In the first part of this chapter, we looked at various nutritional and lifestyle factors that have an important bearing on your health. We invited you to think about what you eat and drink and how active or inactive your lifestyle is, as well as other important factors.

Whatever your final score in the quiz, look back over your answers now and think about those questions where you scored three or four points. These pinpoint the areas where making changes will improve your long-term health. For example, you would have scored three or four points if you eat red meat more than twice a week. Make replacing red meat with other sources of protein, such as chicken, fish, or legumes, one of your goals.

This book will help you understand why your current habits are likely to create health risks and offers you advice on how to make changes.

MINIMIZING RISKS
The second section of the chapter invited you to look at your current state of health and to understand it in the context of your family medical history. When you visit your doctor for a checkup, he or she will carry out various tests (for example, blood pressure) to assess your health and look at the results of the tests in the context of your family history. Many medical conditions have a hereditary component, but you can minimize your risk of developing many of these diseases by tackling the associated risk factors that can be modified by alterations in diet, exercise, and lifestyle.

In this book, we explain in detail why these modifiable risk factors are significant, and help you find ways of making the changes that will benefit your long-term health and well-being.

CONTROLLING YOUR WEIGHT
Finally, we looked at the issue of weight, body shape, and body mass index (BMI) and their implications for health. With obesity the second leading cause of preventable death in North America today, the importance of this issue cannot be overstated. In a later chapter, The Truth about Weight Control (*see pp.156–207*), we look in detail at the risks associated with being overweight and provide comprehensive information and advice on how to control and reduce weight.

MAKING CHANGES
Use this book to help you identify areas of your health that need improvement and to find ways of making the changes (*see pp.30–31*). Don't try to be perfect right from the start, or all the time: no one is. Do as well as you can and remember that your journey to health is as important as your final destination. Each small change you make can have a long-term benefit. You need to accept the choices you make, and give yourself permission to do the best you can.

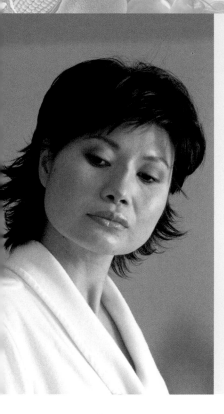

book will help you make these long-term changes.

There are no guarantees in life. You may exercise regularly, eat the right foods, and still develop a medical problem. But we know, from all the research evidence available, that those who eat a nutritious diet, exercise, and maintain a healthy weight are less likely to develop serious health problems.

Use the knowledge you have gained throughout this chapter to determine the most important areas of nutrition, exercise, and lifestyle for you to work on—and get started right now.

Taking stock Take time to reflect in detail on your current health status, your diet, and your lifestyle. Consider what changes you need to make, and draw up a list.

Checklist for change

In this chapter we have looked at various aspects of diet and lifestyle that can affect your health and well-being. Before moving on to the next section, check whether you have understood these clearly:
- Have you completed the questionnaire on page 21 and checked your score?
- Are you familiar with your family medical history (*see p.22*)?
- Have you checked your body mass index (*see pp.26–27*) and looked at how to interpret it?
- Have you identified your body shape (*see p.25*) and considered whether it places you at risk of ill health or disease?
- Are you aware of the health risks associated with being overweight and obesity (*see p.24*)?

Case study Lawyer with fatigue and weight gain

Name Richard

Age 30 years

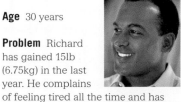

Problem Richard has gained 15lb (6.75kg) in the last year. He complains of feeling tired all the time and has been drinking more and more coffee to stay alert. However, this keeps him awake at night so he is not getting enough sleep. He has sought advice from a nutritionist for his fatigue and to help him lose some weight. He also suffers from constipation but has no other serious medical problems.

Lifestyle Richard is a lawyer who eats most of his meals on the run. He skips breakfast, snacks on doughnuts at work, and drinks at least four 24floz (720ml) cups of coffee with cream and sugar every day. On work days, Richard mostly eats lunch in a fast-food restaurant where he orders a double cheeseburger, large fries, and a large soda. On Fridays, he has two slices of pepperoni pizza with a large soda. Since he works late, he often orders take-out for dinner from local Chinese and Italian restaurants.

On weekends, Richard eats cereal and milk for breakfast, skips lunch, and eats out with friends in the evening, choosing appetizers such as chicken wings or mozzarella sticks, and entrées such as prime rib, London broil, or fried chicken, and French fries. He rarely eats any vegetables and does not take a multivitamin supplement. He usually drinks two beers on Friday and Saturday nights in the restaurant. He does not smoke and does not have time to exercise.

Advice Richard's main complaints are most likely related to his diet and sedentary lifestyle. He does not eat fruits and vegetables, so his diet is low in fiber as well as in vitamins and minerals. He has gained weight because he takes in more calories than he burns, and this is not helped by the fact that he eats most of his meals away from home, where larger portions are served.

Richard's constipation and fatigue can be corrected by incorporating more fiber and water into his diet and decreasing his coffee and soda intake. He can increase his fiber intake by eating a bowl of bran cereal for breakfast, having fresh or dried fruit as an alternative to doughnuts, and including some vegetables in his lunch and dinner.

Richard's diet is high in saturated fat and calories. If he ordered grilled chicken instead of high-fat burgers and fries a few days a week, this would be a good start. He could opt for a vegetable topping or a slice of tomato pie with a salad instead of the Friday pepperoni pizza. For dinner, he could choose lean proteins, such as broiled or grilled fish or chicken, and order a salad.

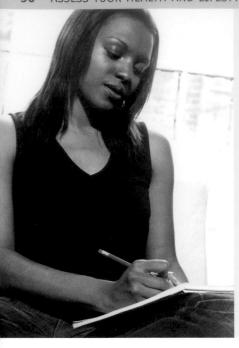

Making changes

Forge new habits in diet and lifestyle for optimum health.

Confidence and conviction are prime requisites for any behavior change. Confidence reflects your attitude about your ability to change: if you don't believe you will succeed, chances are you

won't. Boost your confidence with self-talk and enlist the aid of family, friends, and health professionals if necessary. Conviction, on the other hand, reflects your determination to accomplish change. If you don't believe a change is important, you are unlikely to make it; so be sure to select a change that you firmly believe will make a difference to your future health—and go for it.

Planning for change Thinking about which behavior change—dietary or lifestyle—will best benefit your health is a vital step. Find ways to begin making that change.

Don't give up
When it comes to changing your behavior, your motto should be: "If at first I don't succeed, try, try, try again." Studies of former smokers

Key stages in behavior change

Therapists who specialize in helping people change their behavior recognize that most people pass through certain key stages as they proceed. Developed by two psychologists, Prochaska and DeClemente, the following six stages are often used to assess an individual's readiness for change.

PRECONTEMPLATION
This refers to the time before you are aware that you need to change. As you are reading this book, it is likely that you have already passed this stage.

CONTEMPLATING CHANGE
Now you are thinking about making changes but haven't done anything yet. It may be that in reading this book you are seeking expert advice on what changes are most important.

It is important to select a specific dietary behavior to target for change. The questionnaire on page 21 should have helped you identify areas that could be improved. We suggest that you select the change you think would be easiest for you to make, and start there. Why choose an easy goal? Simply because if you try and succeed, you will feel much better than if you try and fail; and once

you have achieved the first target, you are more likely to go on to set another one. Base your initial target on your current diet: for example, if you eat fruit only a few times a week, set as your goal the intention to eat at least one piece of fruit every day.

PREPARING FOR ACTION
This is the stage when you think about the best way of bringing about whatever changes are necessary to establish your new habit. For example, if your goal is to eat at least one piece of fruit each day, it is a good idea to decide exactly how you will achieve this goal. Try to be as specific as possible. For example, you may need to change your shopping habits—you may need to shop more often in order to have a supply of fresh fruit.

You must think about how you can have fresh or dried fruit available all the time and how to include it in your daily life, whether you eat it as a dessert, as a snack in the car when traveling, or to take with you to work.

If you do not do your homework and fail to prepare a realistic plan of action, your new habit will not stick, and you will soon revert to your old ways.

INITIATING CHANGES
Now is the time to put your plans into action. Remember that small changes are easier to make than large ones, and that you must give yourself enough time for new habits and tastes to be established before moving on to the next change. For example, make sure you always take your piece of fruit in the car to work and eat it. And if you forget to eat your fruit in the car, eat it as soon as you can.

Bear in mind, too, that eating one unhealthy meal won't undermine an otherwise healthy diet. If you overeat at lunch, just have a salad and a serving of vegetables for dinner. And, if you are going out to dinner in the evening, be sure to exercise during the day.

MAINTAINING NEW HABITS
New behaviors take about six weeks to become established. Once you are confident that your first change is well established, then you can move on to the next one. This stage is about ensuring that all the effort you put into making a change doesn't go to waste. Don't worry about occasional lapses— you are aiming to improve your eating habits for the long-term and, so long as you keep trying, you are succeeding.

show that most of them tried and failed several times before finally succeeding in quitting. However, changing your dietary habits is more difficult than successfully quitting smoking. At some point after stopping smoking, you lose the desire to smoke and are then at very little risk of taking it up again. But this is not the same for your diet: you must eat and drink, day in and day out, making decisions about what to eat or drink several times a day, every day, for the rest of your life.

How to change your diet

Throughout the book we will make suggestions for ways of improving your diet. We also include tips on how to make changes. If one way doesn't work, try another and, if you slip up, just remember that no one needs to be perfect when it comes to how they eat—better is good enough.

If you think you might find it difficult to make a radical change in your diet or lifestyle, you can begin by selecting just one simple modification that should be easy for you to achieve, so you get off to a successful start. For example, you may choose to drink more water each day, instead of high-calorie fruit drinks or soda. Then use more of our strategies to help you move toward your goal of achieving optimum health through improved diet and nutrition.

Are you ready to change?

Your answers to the following questions will provide insights that may help you achieve your goals:
● What one change would bring the most significant improvement in your health?
● What other changes would you like to make?
● What would help you change?
● If you have tried to change your diet or exercise recently, did you encounter any problems?
● Are you able to deal with the occasional failure?
● Do you think you can maintain any of the changes that you have made over the past few months?

WHAT IF I RELAPSE?

Failing is just another part of the cycle—each time you fail, you learn something that will help you the next time you try to make a change. Reviewing barriers to change, or what has impeded progress, provides useful insights. So, too, does thinking about motivations that have helped in the past and analyzing the circumstances of previous successful behavior change or relapse. Above all, do not think of one lapse as relapse—look through the reasons why you did not succeed and start again.

Tips for changing

The following key strategies will help when you try to change your lifestyle habits:
● Break down each change you want to make into manageable, small stages; be sure that each stage is firmly established before moving on to the next one.
● Always include your favorite foods, but look for healthier ways of preparing and cooking them. For example, brush French fries with olive oil and bake in the oven.

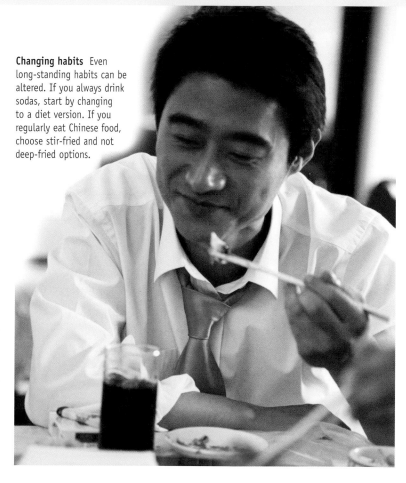

Changing habits Even long-standing habits can be altered. If you always drink sodas, start by changing to a diet version. If you regularly eat Chinese food, choose stir-fried and not deep-fried options.

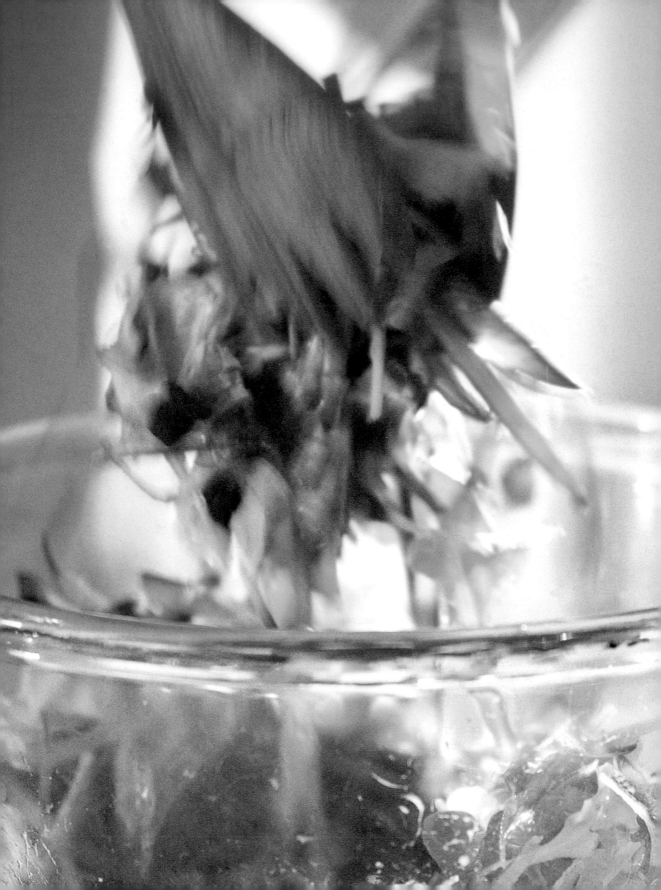

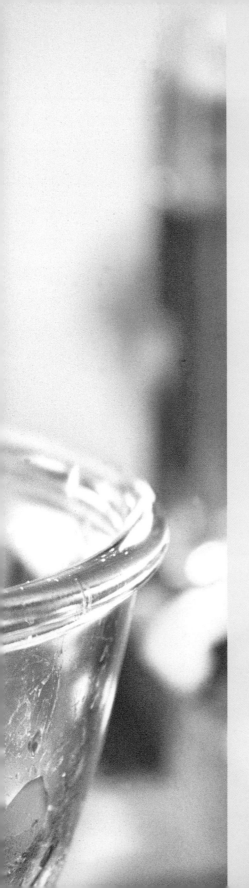

Food for life

Every food we eat provides the body with a range of nutrients, each with its own role to play. Eating a balanced, varied diet every day will ensure that you have everything you need for good health, including foods that provide energy, fiber, protein, carbohydrates, fats, vitamins, and minerals.

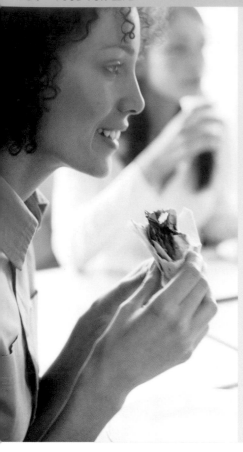

Why we need food

The foods we eat are the essential building blocks of life.

All foodstuffs, from apples to whole-wheat bread or ice cream, contain two main categories of nutrients: macro- and micronutrients. Macronutrients are required in large amounts for healthy growth and development; they form the basis of every diet and provide energy for all the body's everyday functions and activities. Macronutrients are usually further categorized as being either primarily fats (see pp.38–43), proteins (see pp.44–45), carbohydrates (see pp.46–47), or fiber (see pp.48–49)—though most foods contain all of these in varying proportions (see p.37).

Vitamins and minerals, which make up the micronutrients, are chemical compounds found in tiny amounts in foods (see pp.50–67). Unlike macronutrients, vitamins and minerals do not provide energy and are needed in only minute amounts, but they do play a critical role in the normal functioning of the body and in digestive processes.

How we get nutrients
Take a look at what you eat in an average day: the chances are that your diet includes a wide variety of foods from all the basic food groups, and that it provides a range of essential nutrients. Your breakfast, for example, may be rich in carbohydrates and fiber

Nutritious snack A simple tortilla wrap, filled with lettuce, tomato, and slices of chicken breast, is a healthy snack, containing many of the nutrients that your body needs.

Calculating energy requirements

Your energy requirements depend on various factors, including age, gender, physical activity, muscle mass, body temperature, and whether you are still growing. Pregnancy, breast-feeding, menstruation, illness, infection, how much you eat or sleep, and hormone levels are additional factors.

Basal metabolic rate (BMR) is a measure of how much energy you need for essential functions such as breathing and heart rate. BMR is highest in the young and decreases after the age of ten. Because of their greater muscle mass, men generally have a higher BMR (and therefore require more calories) than women. Due to declining muscle mass, older adults generally have a lower BMR and require fewer calories.

Examples of the maintenance calorie requirements for different activities in adults are listed below.
- Sedentary or bedbound people: 11.5cal per lb (0.45kg) of body weight per day.
- People who only do light or routine activities: 13.5cal per lb (0.45kg) of body weight per day.
- People doing moderate activities and a regular exercise program: 16cal per lb (0.45kg) of body weight per day.
- Those doing vigorous exercises, such as athletes, manual laborers, or patients recovering from serious trauma: 18cal per lb (0.45kg) of body weight per day.

Jargon buster

Metabolism A collective term for all the chemical processes constantly occurring within the body, including those in which the nutrients from food are converted into substances that the body uses or excretes as waste.

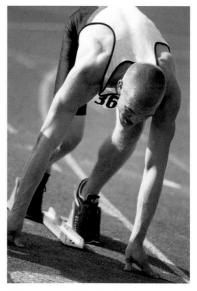

High-energy activity Physical activity accounts for 15–30 percent of total energy expenditure. An athlete expends more energy than someone who sits at a desk.

from cereal or toast; you may have a mixed salad for lunch and grilled fish and vegetables for dinner, providing protein and a variety of vitamins and minerals. Whatever you eat at individual meals, your diet is made up of foods from the five basic food groups (see pp.70–73).

The energy yield of food

In addition to supplying nutrients, food provides your body with energy (right). About half to two-thirds of the energy that we obtain from food goes to support the body's basic, involuntary functions —these are the activities that are performed without any conscious control, such as maintaining breathing, heart rate, and body temperature. The minimum energy needed to carry out these functions is determined by your basal metabolic rate (BMR), which is your baseline rate of metabolism (opposite below), measured when the body is at rest.

You also expend energy through conscious, voluntary activities, which range from the sedentary to the strenuous. All your body's energy needs are met from the foods that you eat or from your body's energy stores.

Nutrition and health

In the following pages of this book, we examine in detail the various elements of nutrition—proteins, fats, carbohydrates, fiber, and micronutrients such as vitamins and minerals—and how your body utilizes them. For example, you need protein for growth and repair, carbohydrates for energy, and fiber for effective digestion. We shall also suggest ways of improving your general health and reducing your risks of developing certain diseases by making healthier food choices.

Calories and energy

The energy you obtain from food is measured in calories. However, since one calorie represents a tiny amount of energy, kilocalorie units are used in nutritional analysis. 1 kilocalorie (kcal) equals 1,000 calories, and this is the amount of energy required to raise the temperature of 1 kilogram of water 1° Celsius. However, the term "calorie" has come to be used as a shorthand reference to kilocalorie, and we have used this convention (1cal represents 1kcal) in this book. Each type of nutrient generates a specific amount of energy:

- 3½oz (100g) protein: 400cal
- 3½oz (100g) carbohydrate: 400cal
- 3½oz (100g) fat: 900cal

Kilojoules Energy is sometimes measured in kilojoules (kJ), and you may find this information on food labels alongside the caloric value. 1cal (1kcal) equals 4.184kJ.

Guidelines for nutritional requirements

In addition to identifying the types of nutrients that we must include in our diets on a daily basis, we also need to know how much of each element is required for optimum health. Official guidelines have been established that provide us with this information.

in guidelines for nutritional needs reflects a shift in focus toward the prevention of long-term, or chronic, disease.

The nutrition labels on food products show a breakdown of the product into its component parts and displays the percentage of protein, carbohydrate, and fat in a particular food, as well as the amounts of certain vitamins and minerals it contains. Each percentage refers to the Dietary Reference Intake. In addition, the nutrition label indicates the number of calories the product provides (see p.277).

DIETARY REFERENCE INTAKES

Until fairly recently, the dietary standards in North America were published as the Recommended Dietary Allowances (RDA). Since 1997, however, this advice has been extended by the introduction of the Dietary Reference Intakes (DRI; right). These intakes are considered to better address the changing nutritional needs of North Americans.

DRIs not only provide a range of safe and appropriate intakes for nutrients, but they also include advice on Tolerable Upper Intake Levels (right), which are based on current research. The change

Dietary Reference Intake (DRI) Values

There are four nutrient-based dietary reference values for every life stage and gender group:

- Recommended Dietary Allowance (RDA) is the intake level that meets the daily requirements of 97–98 percent of the people in a specific life-stage and gender group.
- Estimated Average Requirement (EAR) is the intake estimated to meet the needs of 50 percent of people in a defined group.

- Adequate Intake (AI) is used when no EAR has been established.
- Tolerable Upper Intake Level (UL) is the maximum intake that poses little risk of adverse effects for most people in a defined group (see pp.268–271).

In the Vitamin and Mineral Directories that follow (see pp.50–67), we provide the DRI for healthy men and women, wherever this is available. If the DRI has not yet been established, the RDA is given.

How do we process food?

Before the nutrients in food can be used, they must be broken down into components that the body can absorb. This process, which starts in the mouth and ends with the expulsion of waste products, can take between one and three days. Food is subjected to chemical changes, as digestive juices break it down into its smallest components. Proteins are broken into amino acids, fats into fatty acids and glycerol, and carbohydrates into simple sugars, such as glucose. The vitamins and minerals consist of tiny molecules that the body can absorb without breaking them down first. In the small intestine, bile produced by the liver helps digest fats, while pancreatic secretions break down carbohydrates and continue the digestion of proteins and fats. Nutrients are absorbed into the bloodstream through the intestinal walls. The food that is not digested and absorbed is passed out of the anus.

Mouth The process begins here as food is broken down by the mechanical action of the teeth, tongue, and jaws.

Epiglottis Swallowing food triggers this flap of cartilage to seal off the windpipe. At the same time the soft palate closes off the nasal cavity.

Esophagus Food is propelled down this muscular tube from the throat to the stomach by rhythmic contractions known as peristalsis.

Stomach In the stomach, food spends up to five hours being churned to a pulp and mixed with gastric juices. These consist of acid, which kills bacteria in food, and enzymes that help break down protein into amino acids. The resulting fluid, called chyme, is squirted into the small intestine. Vitamin B_{12} is released from food in the stomach.

Gallbladder This saclike organ stores bile produced by the liver and releases it into the small intestine to help break down food molecules.

Pancreas This organ secretes digestive juice into the small intestine.

Rectum Stools collect here before being expelled from the anus.

Digestive system This is made up of the digestive tract—a long, muscular tube that extends from mouth to anus and includes the esophagus, stomach, intestines, and rectum. Also part of this system are various organs such as the liver, pancreas, and gallbladder.

Salivary glands In the mouth, there are three pairs of salivary glands, which secrete saliva. The digestive enzyme amylase in saliva moistens the chewed food and helps break it down further.

Liver The largest internal organ, the liver produces up to 2 pints (1 liter) of the digestive juice bile each day. Vitamins A, D, E, and K are stored here.

Small intestine Food passes from the stomach into the small intestine, a long tube consisting of the duodenum, jejunum, and ileum. Here, food mixes with more digestive juices and nutrients, including many vitamins and minerals, are absorbed into the bloodstream.

Large intestine The food mass moves from the small intestine into the large intestine, which is populated by bacteria that digest whatever has been left behind after small intestinal absorption. Water and nutrients released by bacteria are absorbed.

Anus The digestive tract opens out of the body here and stools are expelled.

What is in the food we eat?

Foods are usually categorized as being primarily carbohydrate, protein, fat, or fiber. However, most foods contain all or most of these elements, in varying proportions, as well as traces of various vitamins and minerals.

For example, grain-based products, such as bread or pasta, are typically thought of as carbohydrate foods, but they may also contain significant amounts of protein, fat, vitamins, and minerals. Animal foods, such as meat, poultry, or fish, are rich in protein—and often in fat—and most have very low levels of carbohydrate. Even ice cream, which you may think of as just a treat or a dairy product, contains protein, carbohydrate, minerals, and vitamins, as well as fat.

Everything you eat contributes to your overall nutritional intake, but no single group of foods will provide all your nutritional needs. It is therefore important to eat a varied diet, choosing foods from all the main food groups. Combining certain foods can improve the nutrient quality of your diet. For example, eating foods rich in vitamin C with iron-rich foods can improve your absorption of the iron. Food also contains water, in various amounts. Some fruits and vegetables contain a large quantity

of water, and they can provide a useful supply of liquids. The chart below shows the percentages of nutrients in various foods (dry weight). See page 296 for a key to the abbreviations used for vitamins and minerals in the chart.

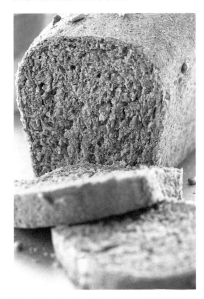

Complete foods Although you might think of bread primarily as a carbohydrate source, it also contains useful amounts of protein, fat, fiber, and many vitamins and minerals.

Macronutrients and micronutrients

Most food contains both macro- and micronutrients. When we try to plan a balanced diet, we tend to think of the macronutrient groups first: carbohydrates, proteins, and fats, and the quantities required (*see p.73*) for good health and weight management. These foods provide the fuel the body needs for all its key functions.

Food labels show the amount of each of these key macronutrients, to help you make the best choice for your diet.

All foods also contain a variety of micronutrients, otherwise known as vitamins and minerals. Each food contains a different selection of micronutrients, in different quantities. Micronutrients play an important role in many processes in the body including:
• Driving metabolic processes in the body, such as enzyme reactions and manufacture of red blood cells.
• Proper functioning of the heart and nervous system.
• Helping to manufacture the antibodies that fight infection.

FOOD	FAT	PROTEIN	CARBS	FIBER	GOOD SOURCE VITAMINS/MINERALS
Whole-grain bread	14%	12%	74%	4.1%	B_1, Nia, Fol / Mg, P, K, Fe, Zn
Brown rice	9%	10%	81%	1.7%	B_1, Nia / Mg, P, Zn
Green beans	0%	9%	91%	4%	A, Fol, Vit K / K
Apple	0%	0%	100%	3%	K
Low-fat fruited yogurt	9%	17%	74%	0%	B_2 / Ca, P, K
White-meat chicken	27%	73%	0%	0.1%	B_2, Nia, B_6, B_{12} / P, K, Zn
Filet mignon	36%	64%	0%	0%	B_1, B_2, Nia, B_{12} / P, K, Fe, Zn
Salmon	54%	46%	0%	0%	B_1, B_2, Nia, Pant, B_{12}, Fol / P, K, Fe, Zn
Lentils	3%	30%	67%	15.6%	B_2, Nia, Pant, B_{12}, Fol / P, K
Almonds	78%	12%	10%	0%	B_2 E / Mg, P, K, Fe, Zn
Eggs	61%	38%	1%	0%	A, B_2, B_{12}, D / Ca, P, Zn

The need for fats

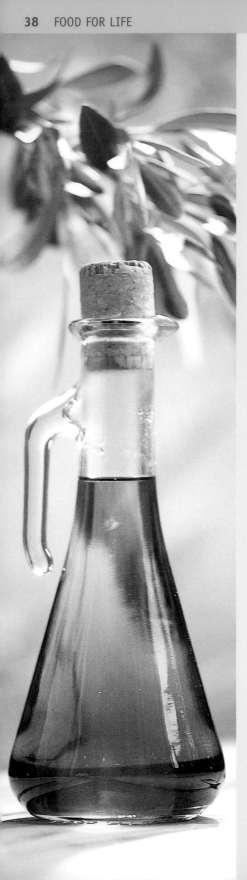

Some fats are vital for healthy body functioning.

Part of a group of compounds known as lipids, and composed of the elements carbon, oxygen, and hydrogen, fats are found mainly in plants, fish, and meats. They form a major part of all cell membranes in the body and play a vital role in the absorption of the fat-soluble vitamins A, D, E, and K (*see pp.52–58*) from foods.

Fat gives the body insulation, helping to maintain a constant temperature against extremes of hot and cold. It is also serves as an important source of energy.

Lipids and lipoproteins

In addition to fats, lipids include phospholipids, triglycerides, waxes, and sterols. The most well-known sterol is cholesterol (*see p.40*), which circulates in the blood attached to compounds known as lipoproteins. Low-density lipoproteins (LDL), which carry cholesterol to tissues and organs, are often called "bad cholesterol," since high levels in the blood are associated with an increased risk of cardiovascular disease (*see p.216*).

High-density lipoproteins (HDL), which carry cholesterol away from the tissues and back to the liver, are known as "good cholesterol," since high levels decrease the risk of cardiovascular disease.

Fats are also referred to as good or bad, depending on whether their chemical bonds are "saturated" with hydrogen. Unsaturated fats are further classified into mono- and polyunsaturates, which differ in their nutritional makeup.

Beneficial oil Olive oil is a rich source of monounsaturated fat, which is now known to confer important health benefits.

Avoid saturated fats

With the exception of palm and coconut oil, most saturated fats are derived from animal and dairy products. Red meat and meat products, such as hot dogs, are major sources of saturated fat in the diet, along with whole milk and its products, including cheese, cream, and ice cream.

Excessive intake of saturated fats and trans fatty acids (*below*) are now believed to increase the risk of cardiovascular disease by raising unhealthy LDL levels, and they should be restricted in the diet.

Unsaturated fats

A diet high in monounsaturated fats, found in plant oils, avocados, peanuts, and pecans, helps lower levels of LDL and triglycerides in the blood, without lowering healthy HDL levels.

Polyunsaturated fats consist of two major types—omega-3 fatty acids, found in fish oils (*opposite*) and omega-6 fatty acids, found in vegetable oils such as sunflower, canola, and corn (*see p.41*). Your diet should include both types.

Trans fatty acids

These substances are created when liquid oils are heated to very high temperatures in a process known as hydrogenation, which turns them into a solid tub or stick margarine. The process essentially turns an unsaturated fat into a saturated one—and trans fatty acids (also known as hydrogenated fats) act like saturated fats in the diet (*above*). A similar effect occurs when liquid oils are heated beyond smoking point, such as when deep-frying, or with repeated re-heating.

Hydrogenated fats are used in many manufactured products, such as crackers and cookies, as well as in margarine and spreads.

Choosing healthier meats

Meat and meat products are one of the major sources of fat, especially saturated fat, in the diet but, as the chart on the right shows, there is a wide variation in the amount of total fat and saturated fat in different types of meat.

Manufactured products such as hot dogs and salami contain the most fat, so if you are trying to lose weight or improve your diet, you could begin by replacing these with healthier choices. In a supermarket, choose products without visible white fat or marbling.

An easy way to reduce the fat content of chicken or turkey is to avoid eating the skin. If you cook poultry with the skin on to retain moisture, remove it and discard after cooking. Also, eat the white meat of poultry rather than the dark meat, which contains more fat.

FOOD TYPE	FAT	% SATURATED FAT
Sausage or hot dog (beef)	80%	33%
Bacon	77%	27%
Salami or corned beef	72%	32%
Hot dog (chicken or turkey)	70%	19%
Ground beef (extra lean)	58%	23%
Chicken wing (with skin)	56%	16%
Chicken thigh (with skin)	56%	16%
Spare ribs	52%	22%
Filet mignon	42%	16%
Chicken breast (no skin)	27%	7%
Pork loin	26%	9%
Ground turkey breast	20%	7%
Turkey breast (no skin)	18%	6%

Eat more fish and shellfish

Fish and shellfish are a good source of protein (*see pp.44–45*), polyunsaturated fats, and B vitamins (*see pp.53–56*). Many types of oily fish are high in omega-3 fatty acids, which are essential for health. It was once advised that all shellfish contained levels of cholesterol too high to be healthy for those on low-cholesterol diets. Recent studies show that although shrimp contains more cholesterol than other shellfish, it is still very low in saturated fat, as long as it is not breaded or fried. As a rule, all fish—including shellfish—are beneficial due to the heart-healthy oils that they contain. Therefore, fish and shellfish provide a healthy alternative to red meat and you should eat them at least once a week.

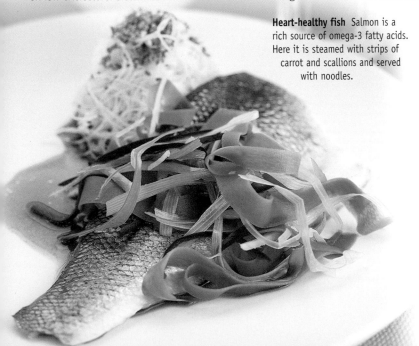

Heart-healthy fish Salmon is a rich source of omega-3 fatty acids. Here it is steamed with strips of carrot and scallions and served with noodles.

Good sources

Most fish contain less than five percent fat, and this fat is mainly polyunsaturated. "Oily" fish contain five to 15 percent fat—a few have more. This list ranks fish by their relative fat content (oily to lean):
- Herring
- Mackerel
- Sardines
- Anchovies
- Salmon
- Tuna
- Halibut
- Cod
- Crab
- Scallops
- Shrimp
- Lobster

Good fats, bad fats

Some types of fat confer important health benefits.

In recent years, countless words have been written about fat, how much we need, and which types are "good" or "bad" fats. It is not enough to know which foods are high or low in fat; now we also need to identify the different kind of fats contained in various foods, and to understand why some are good for us while others pose serious health risks.

Healthy fats
Scientific studies have shown that a diet high in monounsaturated fat reduces the levels of "bad" low-density lipoprotein (LDL) and triglycerides without decreasing levels of "good" high-density lipoprotein (HDL). This is doubly advantageous, since very low HDL levels, like high LDL levels, increase the risk of cardiovascular disease. Oils high in monounsaturates (*opposite above*) are also especially good for cooking since they develop fewer free radicals (*see p.58*) than polyunsaturated oils when they are heated.

The two major categories of polyunsaturated fats—omega-3 and omega-6—are known as essential fatty acids since they cannot be synthesized by the body. Omega-3 fatty acids are found in oils from cold-water fish such as tuna, herring, and sardines. They are involved in regulating blood pressure, blood clotting, and immune responses, as well as for the normal functioning of the brain, spinal cord, and the retina of the eye.

Omega-6 fatty acids are found in vegetable oils, such as sunflower and corn oil. These fatty acids are essential for growth, cell structure, and the maintenance of a healthy immune system.

Avoid animal fats
Unlike unsaturated fats, which have an essential role to play in the diet, saturated fats are known to increase the risk of cardiovascular disease (*see pp.214–221*). These fats come mainly from animal sources, such as meat and dairy products, and from certain plant oils (*opposite above*). Due to their damaging effects on health, you should limit the amount of saturated fat you consume in your diet.

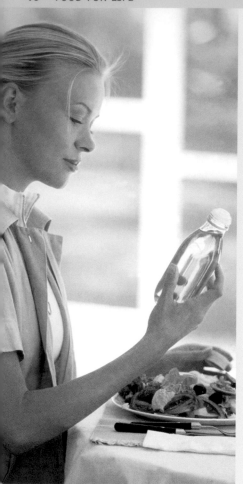

Salad dressing High in monounsaturated fat and low in saturates, olive oil is the perfect accompaniment to a fresh salad. Serve it separately or as the basis of a vinaigrette.

What is cholesterol?

Cholesterol is a waxy substance in your blood that is a major component of every cell wall in your body and is required for the production of some hormones, such as the sex hormones estrogen and testosterone.

Cholesterol occurs in very high concentrations in the cells that protect the brain and nervous system. It is particularly important, therefore, that cholesterol intake is not restricted in children under the age of two years, whose brain and nervous system are still developing.

Cholesterol is also required to make bile acid and in the manufacture of vitamin D by the skin (*see p.57*). Bile acids assist with the absorption of fat from the diet.

Most of your body's cholesterol needs are met by the cholesterol your body makes for itself, but high levels of dietary cholesterol are found in egg yolks and organ meats, such as liver and kidneys.

Excessive amounts of cholesterol in the blood can cause cardiovascular disease (*see pp.214–221*). Cholesterol forms fatty deposits in the arteries, which may lead to narrowing of the arteries, restricted blood flow, and eventually to heart attack or stroke.

An elevated blood cholesterol level (*see p.23*) may be hereditary or influenced by dietary factors—specifically by a diet that is high in cholesterol, total fat, and saturated fat. However, studies have found that dietary intake of saturated fat has a greater impact on cholesterol levels and associated health risks than the intake of dietary cholesterol alone.

Choosing the best oils

Advice to limit your intake of saturated fat is unequivocal, but it may not be immediately obvious which oils should be chosen for cooking, since they all contain a combination of saturated, monounsaturated, and polyunsaturated fats. The graph (*right*) ranks vegetable oils according to their monounsaturated fat content and will help you make the healthiest choices.

Whichever one you choose, remember that oil is 100 percent fat, and one tablespoon equals 100 calories. If you are trying to control your weight, you should limit all fat intake.

When choosing oil for cooking, look for one with a high smoking point to minimize the risk of unpleasant odors, impaired flavor, and reduced vitamin content. Some oils, such as corn and peanut oils, are suitable for heating to high temperatures, but olive oil is not.

Which oil? It is easy to see from this graph that coconut oil is particularly high in saturated fat. It should be avoided in favor of healthier oils such as olive and canola, which are high in beneficial monounsaturated and polyunsaturated fats.

Key

■ **Saturated fat**
■ **Polyunsaturated fat**
■ **Monounsaturated fat**

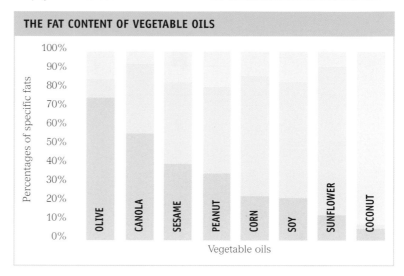

THE FAT CONTENT OF VEGETABLE OILS

Percentages of specific fats — Vegetable oils: OLIVE, CANOLA, SESAME, PEANUT, CORN, SOY, SUNFLOWER, COCONUT

Questionnaire: How much fat do you add to food?

Circle the letters that accompany your answers to these questions, then check your score.

1 How often do you fry food in either shallow or deep fat?
a 3 or more times a week
b About once a week
c Less than twice a month

2 What type of fat do you generally use for cooking?
a Butter, lard, or vegetable shortening
b Margarine or vegetable oil
c Olive or canola oil

3 What type of milk do you generally use in sauces or soups?
a Whole milk or cream
b Reduced-fat or low-fat
c Fat-free milk

4 Do you add butter to vegetables?
a I always add butter

b I occasionally add butter
c I never add butter

5 Which method do you generally use when cooking meat, fish, or poultry?
a Roasting or frying
b Baking or sautéing
c Broiling or grilling

6 What fat do you usually have with bread?
a I always have butter on my bread
b I usually have low-fat margarine or spread
c I dip bread in olive oil

7 What fat do you use when you make gravy?
a Dripping from the roasted meat
b Dripping with the fat removed
c None; I use vegetable stock

8 What topping do you usually serve with desserts such as apple pie?
a Heavy whipping cream
b Ice cream
c Low-fat or fat-free yogurt

Score a 1 **b** 2 **c** 3

20–24 points Well done! You are aware of the health benefits of low-fat cooking. Aim to continue with your healthy ways.

13–19 points You are making some good choices. Now look for even more ways of reducing the fat content in your cooking.

8–12 points You are using too much fat and your health could be at risk. Experiment with the low-fat cooking methods described on page 43 and learn how easy it is to reduce fat levels in your diet.

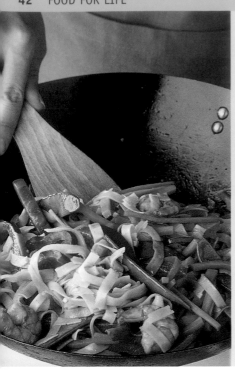

Reducing saturated fat

Lessen your risks of developing disease by modifying your dietary fat intake.

From the previous few pages, you will now be familiar with two key factors that should be considered in relation to fats in the diet. First, you need to know which fats should be included in your diet because of their health benefits, and which fats should be avoided because they increase your risk of developing certain diseases.

The other important factor is the need to regulate the intake of all fats in your diet to avoid unhealthy weight gain. This is important since being overweight and obesity are associated with an increased risk of developing certain diseases, especially diabetes and cancer.

Making healthy choices

You should aim to reduce the saturated-fat sources in your diet by choosing healthy ingredients, and by preparing, cooking, and serving these in ways that do not add unhealthy fat. This means

Asian technique Stir-frying finely cut ingredients in a wok is a quick and healthy cooking method derived from Chinese cuisine.

Same food, less fat

Unhealthy high-fat meals are easily converted to tasty low-fat alternatives. For example, the meals shown here are similar in many respects: chicken is the main ingredient of both, and preparation and cooking times are roughly the same. However, the total fat and saturated fat content of the meal below is about one-fifth that of the meal above, and the total calorie content is nearly halved (see captions).

The reduction in fat and calorie content was achieved by choosing chicken breast rather than thighs or wings, which are much higher in fat content (see p.39); removing the skin before cooking; grilling with just a light brushing of oil instead of coating in crumbs and deep-frying; and serving with a salad and boiled potatoes rather than with fat-laden fries. Other healthy substitutions include:
- Lean ham instead of bacon.
- Sliced white-meat turkey instead of corned beef or pastrami.
- Garden-vegetable burger instead of meat or sausage pattie.

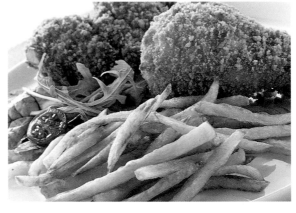

Deep-fried chicken This meal is loaded with 492 calories and 26g of fat, of which 5.8g is saturated. Dark chicken meat has been coated in crumbs and with the fries has been deep-fried in oil then served with minimum vegetables.

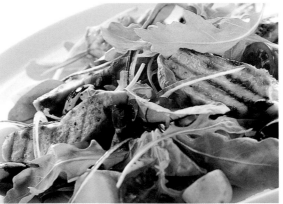

Pan-grilled chicken breast Served with a fresh salad (no dressing) and boiled new potatoes, this is an appealing, healthy variation on the meal above. The result provides only 264 calories and 6g of fat (of which only 1.4g is saturated).

eating more fish, shellfish, white-meat poultry, and plant proteins instead of red meat; choosing low-fat or fat-free dairy products; avoiding cream- and butter-based sauces; and using low-fat cooking methods (*below*).

Recommended fat limits

Fat intake should be 25–35 percent of total calories, with saturated fat making less than seven percent of your total caloric intake. If we take an average of 30 percent fat and 2,000 calories per day for women and older adults and 2,500 calories for men, the recommended daily limit for women and older adults is then 67g of fat, with no more than 16g of saturated fat; and for men, 83g of fat, with no more than 19g of saturated fat.

Butter versus margarine

The controversy over butter and margarine regarding which should be used as a spread or for cooking rests on how much cholesterol, saturated fats, and trans fatty acids each has.

Butter has no trans fatty acids, but it does have high levels of cholesterol and saturated fat. Healthy people should not consume more than 200mg of cholesterol each day, and butter has 33mg of cholesterol in each tablespoon. A healthy range of saturated fat intake is 10–15g each day. One tablespoon contains over 7g of saturated fat. For this reason, limit butter in your diet.

Vegetable shortenings do not contain any cholesterol and have only 3g of saturated fat per tablespoon, but they are high in trans fatty acids. Vegetable oil is better for baking or frying.

Margarine contains no cholesterol and has low levels of saturated fat, but some products have high trans fat levels. Stick margarine contains the most trans fat, while tub or liquid margarine has about two-thirds less. Trans-fat-free varieties of margarine in a tub form are available, and they are the best choice for use as a spread. As you cannot cook with trans-fat-free or light margarine, use tub or liquid margarine, keeping your trans fat intake to no more than 3g per day. By 2006, all food companies will have to include weight of trans fatty acids on food labels.

Low-fat cooking

Frying—and particularly deep-frying—is a method of cooking that greatly increases fat content and should be used rarely if you are trying to reduce the fat content in your diet.

Instead, look for methods that help keep fat levels to a minimum, such as those illustrated here. These are all simple to use and allow you to cook meat, fish, vegetables, and fruit in quick and healthy ways, retaining essential nutrients without adding unhealthy fat. Other low-fat cooking tips include:
• Add water, wine, and lemon juice if the ingredients require extra moisture.
• Choose lean cuts of meat and poultry and remove visible fat before cooking.
• Use a rack to cook so the fat drops down, and use a gravy separator to de-fat the gravy from roast meat or poultry before serving.
• Instead of cooking in oil or fat, use nonstick cookware or vegetable spray.
• Stir-fry in stock rather than in oil.
• Consider using the microwave or steaming food.
• Instead of deep-frying, brush food with a little oil and broil, roast, or grill for the same crispy effect.

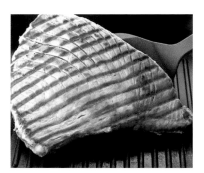

Pan grilling Very little additional oil is needed to prevent food from sticking, and excess fat drains into the grooves of the skillet.

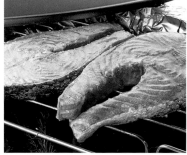

Hot-smoking Fish, meat, and poultry can be quickly and healthily cooked on a wok rack over a layer of tea leaves and flavorings.

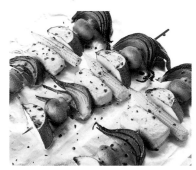

Broiling This method browns foods quickly on the outside, while sealing flavor inside. Marinating ingredients first prevents sticking.

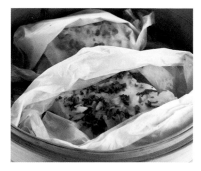

En papillote Seal in the flavor, nutrients, and juices by cooking food in the oven or in a steamer in parchment or foil parcels.

Proteins for growth

These are a major component of every cell in our bodies.

Like fats (see pp.38–43) and carbohydrates (see pp.46–47), proteins are complex compounds that contain the elements carbon, hydrogen, and oxygen. They are also rich in the element nitrogen, which makes up about 16 percent of their total weight. The building blocks of proteins are called amino acids (opposite).

How we use protein

Every type of tissue in the body, including bones, skin, muscles, and organs, has its own set of proteins that help it perform its characteristic functions. Proteins help give structure to our cells and are important in cell growth, repair, and maintenance. Like carbohydrates and fats, they can also serve as an energy source. In addition, enzymes, hormones, and antibodies are all different types of proteins.

The protein that we eat has to be broken down, or digested, into amino acids and peptides (chains of amino acids) and absorbed into the bloodstream. This pool of amino acids provides most of the elements that are needed to build new proteins.

Good sources

When we think of dietary protein, we tend to think of animal meats. While these are rich sources of this vital dietary element, protein is also found in plant foods, such as grains and legumes, and in eggs and dairy products, such as milk and yogurt. In order to obtain the full range of essential amino acids (opposite), you should eat a variety of protein foods. Many people choose red meat (beef, pork, lamb, and veal) as their main source of protein, and eat it regularly through the week. However, we suggest that you eat no more than one serving of red meat a week (see pp.86–87). Examples of one serving of red meat include a small burger, steak, or cutlet.

Studies have shown that people who eat less red meat and eat more fish and chicken lower their risk of developing cardiovascular disease (see pp.214–221) and colorectal cancer (see p.259). In addition, fish provides a range of key nutrients (see pp.90–91) that can help boost health, and legumes and grains are a useful source of fiber.

Changing requirements Protein needs are greatest during periods of growth, such as childhood, pregnancy, and convalescence.

How much protein do you need?

According to the recently updated Dietary Reference Intakes guidelines, the recommended daily consumption of protein for adult men and women is the following:
• Women aged 19–70 need to consume 46g of protein per day.
• Men aged 19–70 need to consume 56g of protein per day.
The difference is due to the fact that, in general, men's bodies have more muscle mass than those of women.

How much protein you need in your daily diet is determined, in large part, by your overall energy intake, as well as by your body's need for nitrogen and essential amino acids. Physical activity and exertion increase your need for protein (see p.147). Requirements are also greater during childhood for growth and development, during pregnancy or when breast-feeding in order to nourish your baby, or when your body needs to recover from malnutrition or trauma or after an operation.

Because the body is continually breaking down protein from tissues, even adults who do not fall into the above categories need to include adequate protein in their diet every day. If you do not take in enough energy from your diet, your body will use protein from the muscle mass to meet its energy needs, and this can lead to muscle wasting over time.

IS DEFICIENCY COMMON?

Protein deficiency is rare in developed countries, but it can occur in people who are dieting to lose weight, or in older adults, who may have a poor diet. Convalescent people recovering from surgery, trauma, or illness may become protein deficient if they do not increase their intake to support their increased needs. A deficiency can also occur if the protein you eat is incomplete and fails to supply all the essential amino acids (opposite above).

CAN YOU EAT TOO MUCH?

Since the body cannot store protein, it has to break down and dispose of any excess obtained from the diet. The liver removes nitrogen from amino acids, so that they can be burned as fuel, and the nitrogen is incorporated into urea, the substance that is excreted by the kidneys. These organs can normally cope with any extra workload but if kidney disease occurs, a decrease in protein will often be prescribed.

Excessive protein intake may also cause the body to lose calcium, which could lead to bone loss in the long-term. Foods that are high in protein (such as red meat) are often high in saturated fat, so excessive protein intake may also contribute to increased saturated fat.

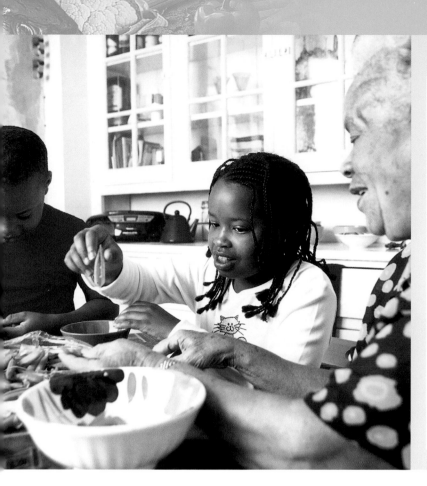

What are amino acids?

Just as the letters of the alphabet can be combined in different ways to form an endless variety of words, amino acids can be linked together in varying sequences to form a huge variety of proteins. The unique shape of each protein determines its function in the body.

Essential amino acids Our bodies require about 20 amino acids for normal functioning. Nine of these are considered essential—that is, your body cannot make them by itself and must get them from food. The essential amino acids are lysine, histidine, isoleucine, phenylalanine, leucine, methionine, tryptophan, threonine, and valine.

Nonessential amino acids The remaining 11 amino acids are nonessential; although you can obtain them from food, the body can also synthesize them as needed.

Good protein sources

Meat, poultry, fish, eggs, milk, and milk products such as cheese are excellent sources of protein, providing all the amino acids that your body needs (*above*). However, the nutritional advantage of these animal foods must be set against their undesirable fat content (*see pp.40–43*) and lack of carbohydrates and dietary fiber.

Protein is also available from plants, in the form of legumes, nuts, seeds, and grains. With the exception of soy and soy products, plant proteins do not provide the full complement of amino acids, and must be combined with other foods if they are the sole source of dietary protein (*see p.100*). Plant foods also contain useful amounts of dietary fiber (*see pp.48–49*) and carbohydrates (*see pp.46–47*), which are essential in a healthy diet.

FOOD	SERVING SIZE	PROTEIN	CALORIES
Pork loin	3½oz (100g)	30g	166
Turkey breast (no skin)	3½oz (100g)	30g	157
Beef (sirloin)	3½oz (100g)	29g	194
Chicken breast (no skin)	3½oz (100g)	27g	142
Salmon (sockeye)	3½oz (100g)	21g	216
Tofu	½ cup	20g	180
Almonds	3 tbsp	19g	167
Soybeans, cooked	½ cup	14g	149
Low-fat cottage cheese	½ cup	14g	82
Shrimp	3½oz (100g)	12g	99
Low-fat fruited yogurt	8floz (240ml)	10g	231
Eggs	2 medium	10g	122
Lentils, cooked	½ cup	9g	116

Carbohydrates for energy

Carbohydrates form the foundation of a healthy diet, providing a readily available source of energy.

Carbohydrates are compounds composed of carbon, hydrogen, and oxygen and are generally classified as simple or complex, depending on their structure. Carbohydrates are obtained from grains, bread, and pasta, as well as from fruits, vegetables, legumes, and dairy products.

Variable complexity

All carbohydrates are composed of chains of sugar molecules. Those composed of just one or two sugar molecules are known as simple carbohydrates, and are divided into monosaccharides and disaccharides. Monosaccharides include glucose, which is present in the blood; fructose, which is found in fruits; and galactose, which is found in dairy products. Disaccharides include sucrose (table sugar) and lactose (the primary sugar present in milk).

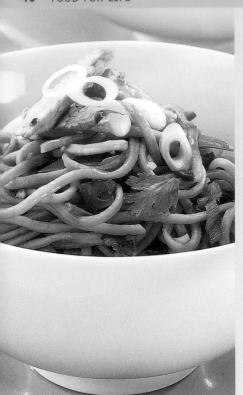

Soba noodles Quick to prepare and made from buckwheat, soba noodles are high in fiber and very versatile.

Choose the right carbohydrates

Some carbohydrates are wonderful sources of energy and nutrients, but others are a waste of calories. So which are the best carbohydrates, and how should you choose them?

The health benefits of complex carbohydrates are well established. These are found in nearly all foods of plant origin—grains, vegetables, and legumes—and are high in nutritional value, containing vitamins, minerals, phytochemicals, protein, and fiber, in addition to providing a good source of energy for the body. However, once grains are refined, they lose their natural goodness, leaving them nutritionally deficient (*see p.75*).

• Choose whole-grain bread and pasta and whole, unrefined grains and cereals to form the foundation of your diet.

• Eat plenty of fruits and vegetables (skin on when possible), raw or cooked for a minimum time (*see p.288*).

• Limit your consumption of refined products such as cakes, cookies, candies, and sweetened beverages.

POOR CARBOHYDRATE SOURCE	GOOD CARBOHYDRATE SOURCE
White bread	7-grain or whole-wheat bread
White rice	Brown rice
Croissant	Whole-wheat English muffin
Carrot cake	Angel food cake with fresh fruit
Doughnut	Whole-wheat waffle
Chocolate-chip cookies	Oatmeal cookies
Apple juice (presweetened)	Apple (with skin)
White potato	Sweet potato
Corn	Lentils
Fried tortilla or corn chips	Baked tortilla or corn chips
Cornflake cereal	Raisin bran cereal
Instant oatmeal cereal	Oatmeal (rolled oats)
White pasta	Couscous
Egg noodles	Barley

Complex carbohydrates, also called polysaccharides, are composed of many simple-sugar molecules that are linked together. Examples of complex carbohydrates include starch, which gives potatoes and grains their hearty character; glycogen, which the body stores as a source of energy; and dietary fiber (see pp.48–49).

Why do we need them?

Carbohydrates provide energy for all the body's activities. As they are digested, carbohydrates are broken down into simple sugars, such as glucose. Glucose supplies energy for most of the body's activities and, in some cells and tissues such as red blood cells and the brain, it is the sole source of energy.

Carbohydrates are needed for building the nonessential amino acids that the body uses to create proteins (see p.45). They also help in the processing of fat and in the building of cartilage, bone, and tissues of the nervous system.

Choosing carbohydrates

As the major source of energy, carbohydrates must form a large part of your diet, but you should choose the best types to optimize your health. This means eating a wide variety of different types of

Jargon buster

Insulin resistance A reduced sensitivity in the tissues of the body to the action of the hormone insulin (see p.246). As a result of this sensitivity, blood glucose does not enter those tissues to be used as a source of energy, so blood glucose levels remain abnormally high. The condition is found frequently in overweight and obese people.

grains, fruits, and vegetables. As far as possible, try to eat whole grains and products made from unrefined grains in preference to refined varieties. In this way, you will benefit from the nutrients and fiber that are removed during the refining process (see p.75).

Some researchers believe that the glycemic index (GI; below) provides a useful guide to the best carbohydrates, and that low-GI foods, which release sugar more slowly into the blood, are of particular benefit to people with diabetes (see p.246) and insulin resistance (left). However, we believe that while the concept of the glycemic index is interesting, it should not be relied on as the sole indicator of a carbohydrate's healthfulness. Nutritional content and fiber are also important and these should be borne in mind when choosing carbohydrates.

Understanding the glycemic index

The glycemic index (GI) classifies foods according to how fast they release sugar (glucose) into the bloodstream. High-GI foods release glucose quickly, causing a rapid rise in blood-glucose levels, to which the body reacts with insulin, which turns on fat storage. Low-GI foods, in contrast, release glucose steadily over several hours, so less insulin is required. Diets based on low-GI foods are therefore recommended for those with diabetes (see p.246) and insulin resistance (above), as well as for people with cardiovascular disease (see p.214) and certain digestive disorders (see p.226).

GI value This figure depends on various factors, including the type of carbohydrate the food contains, how it has been processed, and the presence of fat and dietary fiber. In general, low-GI foods contain

more fiber, are less processed, and do not contain as much glucose as high-GI foods. However, there is not a simple correlation between complex carbohydrates and low-GI values. For example, whole-grain oat cereal is a healthy carbohydrate, but it has a high-GI value, whereas fructose— the type of sugar found in fruits and frequently added to soft drinks in the form of corn syrup—has a low-GI value. However, this does not mean that products sweetened with corn syrup are healthy.

Glycemic loading This is a concept that has been developed to deal with anomalies thrown up by the glycemic index, which cast doubt on its usefulness as a nutritional tool. For example, a well-known brand of chocolate fudge cake has a relatively low GI of 41, while a 100 percent whole-grain loaf has a GI of 62—

though common sense tells us that the latter is healthier. To deal with such paradoxes, glycemic load is calculated by multiplying the GI value of a food by the amount of carbohydrate in one serving. This gives a figure that reflects both the time the food takes to be broken down into glucose and its carbohydrate content.

Conclusion Our view is that while glycemic loading is a better indicator of glycemic response than glycemic index alone, this is still only part of the story. Other aspects of the nutritional value of foods must also be considered, including vitamin and mineral content, phytochemicals, fiber, and protein. In terms of health benefits, the evidence is clear that eating refined grain products increases the risk of a variety of diseases, while eating whole grains has beneficial health effects.

Facts about fiber

Fiber is essential for maintaining a healthy digestive system.

Dietary fiber, which is obtained solely from foods of plant origin, plays a vital role in the digestive process. There are two types of dietary fiber: soluble fiber, which can dissolve in water; and insoluble fiber, which does not have the ability to dissolve in water.

Soluble fiber
The inclusion of soluble fiber in the diet slows the breakdown of complex carbohydrates, such as starch, into simple sugars, such as glucose, thereby slowing the absorption of sugar and possibly leading to reduced levels of sugar in the blood. During digestion, soluble fiber forms a gel-like mass that binds cholesterol to the stool; if eaten in sufficient quantities, soluble fiber can also help reduce the levels of cholesterol in your blood. Good sources of soluble fiber include grains, such as oats, barley, and rye, vegetables, fruits, and legumes.

Insoluble fiber
This type of fiber occurs naturally in brown rice, whole-wheat breads and cereals, seeds, legumes, and in the skins of fruits and vegetables. It is not easily dissolved in water and is not digested or absorbed by the body. However, insoluble fiber's inclusion in the diet helps keep the gastrointestinal tract clean and promotes regular bowel movements. It does this by drawing water into the stools, making them larger, softer, and easier to pass.

The benefits of fiber
Foods that are high in dietary fiber often take longer to eat, and they increase the feeling of fullness after a meal because they slow down the passage of food through the intestine. This improves the body's blood-sugar response because fiber slows the rate at which glucose is released from food. This, in turn, slows the rise of blood-sugar levels so that less insulin (see p.246) is released into the bloodstream. In addition, because fiber-rich foods increase the feeling of fullness, they can help with weight control.

Fighting disease
By promoting bowel regularity and keeping the gastrointestinal tract clean, inclusion of insoluble fiber in the diet may also reduce the risk of developing conditions such as diverticular disease (see p.234) and constipation (see p.229). Studies have also shown that a high-fiber diet helps prevent diabetes (see p.246) and, as a result of the activity of gut flora, reduces the risk of developing colorectal cancer (see p.259). This cancer is rare in countries where the traditional diet consists mainly of cereals, fruits, and vegetables.

Gut flora
The bacteria in the large intestine, which are referred to as gut flora, can break down some of the chemical bonds in fiber that are resistant to the digestive enzymes. People who eat plenty of fiber have healthy colons teeming with millions of these bacteria.

Researchers have suggested that the action of gut flora on fiber creates an acidic environment in the colon that decreases the risk of developing colorectal cancer (see p.259), which is currently the second most common cause of cancer death in North America.

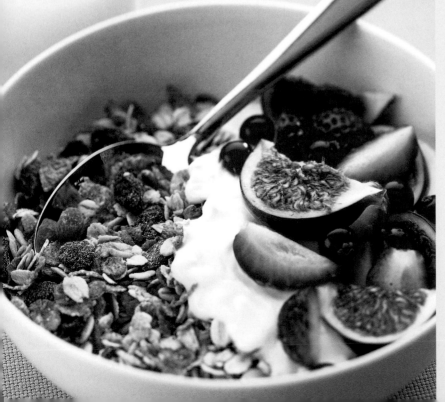

High-fiber breakfast Get your day off to a healthy start with a bowl of mixed-grain muesli, topped with fresh fruit (skin on), and a serving of fat-free or low-fat yogurt.

How much fiber do I need?

According to the latest government guidelines, your total fiber intake should be 20–40g per day, depending on your age and gender (*see p.136 and p.151*). Most adults in North America, however, get less than 20g of fiber each day. In order to ensure an adequate intake of both soluble and insoluble fiber, you should include a wide variety of fruits, vegetables, and whole grains in your daily diet.

FOOD	SERVING SIZE	FIBER
Lima beans, boiled	1 cup	13.5g
Oatmeal, dry	½ cup	8.4g
Lentils, boiled	1 cup	7.9g
Black beans, boiled	1 cup	7.2g
Prunes, cooked	½ cup	7.0g
Kidney beans, boiled	1 cup	6.4g
Peas, boiled	1 cup	4.4g
Brown rice, boiled	1 cup	3.3g
Apple (with skin)	1 medium	3.0g
Whole-wheat bread	1 slice	1.6g

Increasing fiber intake

If you plan to increase your fiber intake, do so gradually to give your system time to adjust. As you increase your intake, drink plenty of water to balance that absorbed by the fiber. The tips below can help you meet the recommended intake:

• Eat more vegetables, either raw or steamed. Cruciferous vegetables, such as cabbage and broccoli, are particularly high in fiber.
• Eat more fruit with skin and seeds, such as apples, pears, and berries.
• Choose high-fiber breakfast cereals, cold or hot.
• Add bran or whole oats to casseroles and other dishes, or use them for crumbs and stuffing.
• Eat whole-grain products, such as whole-wheat bread, brown rice, and crackers made from whole-wheat flour rather than white flour.
• Add bran or oats to pancakes, meatballs, or burgers.
• Use cereal in place of nuts or in place of flour when making cookies.

Recipe Crunchy high-fiber apricot and apple bars

INGREDIENTS

1 cup dried apricots

2 apples

4floz (120ml) apple juice

1 cup margarine

½ cup soft brown sugar

1⅔ cups whole-wheat flour

1¼ cups oats

Makes 16 bars

1 Preheat the oven to 350°F (180°C). Lightly oil a shallow baking pan measuring 13 by 9in (32 by 22cm).

2 Chop the apricots, and peel, core, and finely chop the apples. Place in a pan with the apple juice and simmer for 10 minutes.

3 Let the mixture cool slightly, then blend in a food processor until smooth.

4 In a bowl, beat together the margarine and sugar until creamy, then fold in the flour and oats.

5 Spread half of the flour and oat mixture over the baking pan. Spoon the apricot and apple mixture on top and spread evenly. Cover with the remaining flour mixture and press down lightly.

6 Bake for 30 minutes, until light golden. Cut into 16 bars while in the tray, and let cool before removing. Store in an airtight container.

Each bar provides:
Calories 221, Total fat 10g (Sat. 2.0g, Poly. 0.5g, Mono. 0.3g), Cholesterol 0mg, Protein 3.6g, Carbohydrate 31g, Fiber 3.6g, Sodium 125mg. Good source of— Vits: A; Mins: Ca, Mg, P.

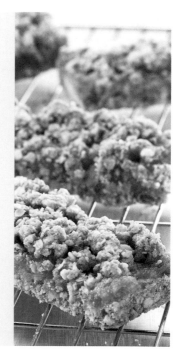

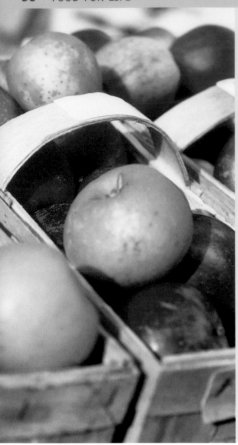

What are vitamins?

These are naturally occurring chemicals essential for health.

For many of us, the word "vitamin" conjures up the image of bottles of pills lining the shelves of the local drugstore, or perhaps the fortified cereals that we eat for breakfast each morning. But these chemical substances occur naturally, in minute quantities, in most of the foods that we eat and, for the most part, we rely on food sources to meet our vitamin needs. However, there are a few vitamins that we obtain by other means: for example, microorganisms in the intestine—

commonly known as gut flora— produce vitamin K and biotin, while one form of vitamin D is synthsized in the skin with the help of natural ultraviolet sunlight.

Why we need vitamins

Although vitamins contain no calories, they are essential for normal growth and development, and many chemical reactions in the body. Vitamins are necessary for the body to use the calories provided by the food that we eat and help process proteins, carbohydrates, and fats. Vitamins are also involved in building cells, tissues, and organs—vitamin C, for example, helps produce healthy skin.

Vitamins are classified as fat-soluble or water-soluble based on how they are absorbed by the body. Vitamins A, D, E, and K are fat-soluble, while the water-soluble

Getting vitamins Most of the foods we eat—either of plant or animal origin— contain some vitamins. Fruits such as apples and pears are a good source of vitamin C.

How do you get vitamins?

For the most part, we rely on food sources or supplements to meet our vitamin and mineral requirements. However, there are a few exceptions to this; for example, gut flora (the microorganisms in the intestinal tract) produce vitamin K. Vitamin D is also converted by the skin into a form that the body can use with the help of ultraviolet light in sunlight.

Because your body makes only a few vitamins itself, a balanced diet is very important since it ensures that your body receives the sufficient amount of vitamins, as well as minerals, that it requires each day.

EAT A VARIETY OF FOODS

The key to getting enough vitamins in your diet is to eat a variety of foods. This is because while some nutrients tend to be found in substantial amounts in certain groups of foods, such as

vitamin C in fruit and calcium in dairy products, other nutrients such as the B-complex vitamins are found in smaller amounts in a wide range of foods. No one food contains an adequate amount of all the vitamins that you require daily, but if you make healthy choices from a variety of foods, you are less likely to miss out any one particular nutrient.

Most people buy the same foods each week, which can result in a limited range of vitamins. If you think this applies to you, we suggest that you read the "Good sources" boxes on the following pages, and aim to try some different foods each week. For example, eat two apricots instead of one orange, for a boost of vitamin A. Or choose salmon on your bagel instead of your usual cream cheese for a good source of vitamin D. Buying vegetables and fruits in season helps vary your shopping choices.

What are enriched and fortified foods?

During processing, some foods have vitamins or minerals added. For example, in the US, it is now a requirement for folate (*see p.140*) to be added to all grain products.

Enriched foods Nutrients are replaced that were originally lost during processing. For example, some of the B-complex vitamins are added back to refined flour.

Fortified foods Nutrients are added that were never naturally a part of the food. For example, vitamins A and D are often added to milk, calcium to orange juice, and many vitamins and minerals are added to breakfast cereals in order to boost their nutritional value.

vitamins include vitamin C and the B-complex vitamins (thiamine (B_1), riboflavin (B_2), niacin (B_3), pantothenic acid (B_5), vitamin B_6, vitamin B_{12}, biotin, and folate).

Research has shown that foods rich in antioxidants are particularly beneficial for health. Antioxidants include vitamins A, C, and E, and they are found in a wide range of vegetables and fruits. Antioxidants neutralize free radicals (see p.58). A buildup of free radicals can damage body cells and tissues, resulting in disease. Studies have shown that diets rich in vegetables and fruits result in a lower incidence of some diseases, including certain cancers.

Vitamin deficiencies
Deficiencies of vitamins are either primary or secondary. A primary deficiency occurs because you do not get enough of the vitamin in the food you eat. A secondary deficiency may be due to a lifestyle factor, such as smoking, excessive alcohol consumption, or the use of certain medications that interfere with the absorption or the body's use of the vitamin. Prolonged use of antibiotics will kill off the useful gut flora that make vitamin K (see p.58). Vitamin deficiencies may also be due to an underlying problem, such as an intestinal disorder, that prevents or limits the absorption or use of the vitamin.

Well-known vitamin deficiencies (and the diseases they cause) are thiamine (beriberi), niacin (pellagra), vitamin C (scurvy), and vitamin D (rickets). In North America today, however, such deficiencies are rare due to an adequate food supply for most people, and food fortification programs that add vitamins and minerals to common foods.

Scientists now have shifted their focus to discovering ways in which vitamins can promote health, prevent disease, boost the body's protection against infection, and even slow down the aging process. At the same time, public interest in vitamins has heightened. This has been prompted by headlines in the media and widespread advertising by the manufacturers of nutrient supplements.

The definitions of the amounts of vitamins (and minerals) that you should receive daily, such as Dietary Reference Intakes (DRI), are discussed at the start of this chapter (see p.35).

Vitamin overdosing
The likelihood of consuming too much of any vitamin from food is remote, but overdosing from vitamin supplementation often occurs (see pp.266–271). For example, many people take large amounts of vitamin C, usually in the belief that this will relieve or "cure" a cold (see p.57). However, overdosing on vitamin C can lead to diarrhea or kidney stones. If you take vitamin supplements, you should always do so at the advice of your doctor or dietitian, and first consider whether your diet could be improved instead.

Preserving the vitamin content of food

Many vitamins are easily destroyed by the lengthy storage of food, processing, and cooking at high temperatures.
• Fruits and vegetables contain their highest level of nutrients when they are harvested at full ripeness and eaten soon thereafter, with minimum processing. The most nutritious produce consists of fresh fruits and vegetables picked at full maturity (avoid picking prematurely and allowing them to ripen off the vine) and eaten immediately.
• Frozen foods are a good choice for produce because they are generally picked at their peak freshness, quickly frozen, and stored at cold temperatures to preserve nutrients.
• Store foods properly to prevent nutrient losses. A cool, dark place is best since vitamin degradation accelerates at higher temperatures and several of the water-soluble vitamins, such as vitamin C and riboflavin (B_2) are very light sensitive.

• Cooking contributes to vitamin losses, and many water-soluble vitamins are destroyed by heat. Therefore, it is best to keep cooking times to a minimum. Avoid boiling vegetables in large amounts of water because the vitamins will leach into the water. Steam or even microwave vegetables in small amounts of water whenever possible in order to preserve the nutrient content.

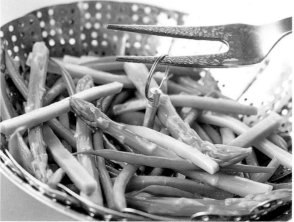

Keeping nutrients
Steam rather than boil vegetables to prevent vitamins, minerals, and other key nutrients from being leached out into the water.

Vitamin directory

Here, we look at the role of each vitamin, how much we need, the symptoms and signs of a deficiency, and which foods are good sources. The daily requirements (Dietary Reference Intakes) are for healthy adults (*see p.35*); needs do vary at different stages of life (*see Eating for the Time of your Life, pp.104–155*).

Vitamin A

DAILY REQUIREMENT
Men 900RE per day
Women 700RE per day

This vitamin plays an essential role in vision, particularly night vision, normal bone growth, reproduction, and the health of skin and mucous membranes (the mucus-secreting layer that lines body regions such as the respiratory tract). Vitamin A also acts in the body as an antioxidant (*see p.58*), a protective chemical that may reduce the risk of certain cancers.

There are two sources of dietary vitamin A. Active forms, which are immediately available to the body are obtained from animal products. These are known as retinoids and include retinal and retinol. Precursors, also known as provitamins, which must be converted to active forms by the body, are obtained from fruits and vegetables containing yellow, orange, and dark green pigments, known as carotenoids,

the most well-known being beta-carotene. For this reason, amounts of vitamin A are measured in Retinal Equivalents (RE). One RE is equivalent to 0.001mg of retinal, or 0.006mg of beta-carotene, or 3.3 International Units of vitamin A.

In the intestine, vitamin A is protected from being chemically changed by vitamin E. Vitamin A is fat-soluble and can be stored in the body. Most of the vitamin A you eat is stored in the liver. When required by a particular part of the body, the liver releases some vitamin A, which is carried by the blood and delivered to the target cells and tissues.

VITAMIN A DEFICIENCY

In developing countries, a dietary deficiency of vitamin A is common, with pregnant women and infants being the most often affected. In the West, it is rare but may occur in people who abuse alcohol or those with long-term conditions that affect their ability to absorb fats, such as cystic fibrosis or Crohn's disease (*see p.233*), because the vitamin is absorbed in fats. A common symptom of a severe

deficiency of vitamin A is the eye disorder xerophthalmia, in which the cornea, the transparent membrane at the front of the eye, hardens. This may progress to night blindness, corneal ulceration, and irreversible blindness.

Other signs and symptoms include growth problems in children, poor wound healing, and dry, bumpy skin rashes known as follicular hyperkeratosis. Vitamin A deficiency can also affect the health of the epidermis (skin) and the normal functioning of mucous membranes throughout the body.

Good sources

Vitamin A This is found naturally in all these foods, which contain at least 0.15mg of the vitamin or beta-carotene per 1¾–7oz (50–200g):
- Sweet potatoes (yams)
- Carrots
- Collard greens
- Kale
- Pumpkin
- Spinach
- Sweet peppers
- Winter squash
- Apricots
- Cantaloupe melon
- Mango
- Liver (beef, pork, chicken, or turkey)
- Eggs

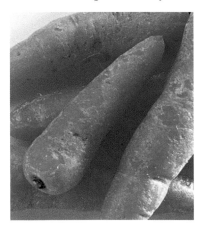

Carrots Rich in beta-carotene (a form of vitamin A), one medium carrot gives you all the vitamin A that you need for a whole day. Carrots also contain thiamine (B_1) and B_6.

Vitamin A helps night vision

Night blindness—the inability to see well in dim light—is associated with a deficiency of vitamin A. This vitamin is needed for the formation of rhodopsin. This is a pigment located in the eye's retina, which is the light-sensitive tissue lining in the back of the eye.

When stimulated by light, rhodopsin splits into two proteins: opsin and retinal (a form of vitamin

A); when it is dark, the reverse reaction occurs—the retinal and opsin combine to re-form rhodopsin, a reaction that requires extra retinal.

Without adequate amounts of retinal, regeneration of rhodopsin is incomplete and night blindness occurs. Since carrots are a good source of beta-carotene, there is truth in the old saying that carrots help you see better in the dark!

Thiamine

DAILY REQUIREMENT
Men 1.2mg per day
Women 1.1mg per day

Also known as vitamin B_1, thiamine plays an important role in helping the body convert carbohydrates and fats into energy. It is essential for normal growth and development and helps to maintain proper functioning of the heart and the nervous and digestive systems. Thiamine is water-soluble and cannot be stored in the body; however, once absorbed, the vitamin is concentrated in muscle tissue.

THIAMINE DEFICIENCY

Primary deficiency is rare because virtually all grain products in North America are fortified with this vitamin. However, deficiency sometimes occurs in people who abuse alcohol because excessive alcohol intake significantly decreases the body's ability to absorb thiamine and interferes with its chemical reactions in the body.

In the early stages of the deficiency, symptoms may include poor appetite, irritability, fatigue, and weight loss. As the deficiency becomes more advanced, weakness, nerve damage that may affect the hands and feet, headache, and a rapid heart rate may also develop.

A form of thiamine deficiency known as beriberi affects babies who are breast-fed by mothers with thiamine deficiency, people who abuse alcohol,

Good sources

Thiamine This is found naturally in all these foods, which contain at least 0.1mg of the vitamin per 1–3½oz (28–100g):
- Green peas
- Spinach
- Liver
- Beef
- Pork
- Navy beans
- Nuts
- Pinto beans
- Soybeans

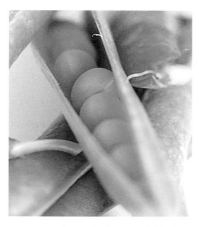

Green peas An excellent source of thiamine, peas also contain significant amounts of beta-carotene (a precursor of vitamin A), niacin (B_3), folate, vitamin C, and protein.

and those who eat a lot of carbohydrates, especially polished rice, from which the vitamin is removed during processing. In its advanced stages, beriberi causes problems with the nervous system and the heart, leading to an abnormal heart rhythm (arrhythmia) and heart failure (*see pp.216–221*).

Riboflavin

DAILY REQUIREMENT
Men 1.3mg per day
Women 1.1mg per day

This water-soluble vitamin, also known as vitamin B_2, is necessary for the release of energy from carbohydrates (*see p.46*). Riboflavin is needed for normal growth and development. It helps to build up glucose molecules into the complex carbohydrate glycogen, which is stored in the liver for future use; helps digest fats; is involved in changing the amino acid tryptophan into niacin (B_3); helps protect the nervous system; and also maintains mucous membranes—the mucus-secreting layer that lines body regions such as the respiratory tract.

RIBOFLAVIN DEFICIENCY

A deficiency of riboflavin can be primary—due to not getting enough of the vitamin from the diet—or

Good sources

Riboflavin This is found naturally in all these foods, which contain at least 0.1mg of the vitamin per 3–10½oz (85–300g):
- Asparagus
- Okra
- Cottage cheese
- Milk
- Yogurt
- Meat
- Eggs
- Fish

secondary, which may be a result of conditions that affect absorption in the intestine, the body not being able to use the vitamin, or an increase in the excretion of the vitamin from the body.

Signs and symptoms of riboflavin deficiency include cracked and red lips, inflammation of the lining of the mouth and tongue, mouth ulcers, cracks at the corners of the mouth, and a sore throat. A deficiency may also cause dry and scaling skin, fluid in the mucous membranes, and iron-deficiency anemia (*see p.55*). The eyes may also become bloodshot, itchy, watery, and sensitive to bright light.

Niacin

DAILY REQUIREMENT
Men 16mg per day
Women 14mg per day

Also known as vitamin B_3, nicotinic acid, or nicotinamide and abbreviated to Nia, niacin participates in at least 200 different chemical reactions involved in energy production. It is also necessary for the production and breakdown of glucose, fats, and amino acids; the development, maintenance, and function of the skin, intestine and stomach, and nervous system; and in manufacturing DNA (the substance that makes up our genes). This vitamin can also be made in the body from the amino acid tryptophan, provided that there is also sufficient vitamin B_6 (*see p.54*).

Although excessive amounts of the vitamin may be harmful to some people,

Good sources

Niacin This is found naturally in all these foods, which contain at least 1mg of niacin per 1–3½oz (28–100g):
- Green peas
- Liver
- Red meat
- Poultry
- Mackerel
- Mullet
- Salmon
- Swordfish
- Kidney beans
- Peanuts
- Soybeans

doses (1–3g per day) have been used successfully in the treatment of high blood-cholesterol levels (see p.216). Niacin has also been used to treat dizziness and ringing in the ears and to prevent premenstrual headaches.

NIACIN DEFICIENCY

Dietary deficiency of niacin is rare in North America because this vitamin is found primarily in protein-rich foods. However, it does affect people whose diet consists mainly of corn, which does not contain the essential amino acid tryptophan (see p.45).

Niacin deficiency can be caused by a deficiency of vitamin B_6 (right) since the manufacture of niacin from tryptophan

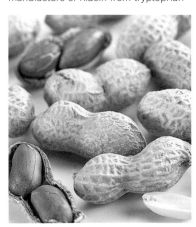

Peanuts Not only rich in niacin, peanuts—which are actually a legume, not a nut—are also a good source of vitamin D, magnesium, iron, zinc, and protein.

requires vitamin B_6. People who drink excessive amounts of alcohol (more than 20 units per week for men and more than 10 units for women) are also at increased risk of niacin deficiency because alcohol significantly reduces the body's ability to absorb this vitamin.

Early symptoms of niacin deficiency—which is known as pellagra—include fatigue, loss of appetite, weakness, mild diarrhea, anxiety, irritability, and sometimes depression. The lining of the mouth and the tongue may become inflamed and sore and have a burning sensation. If the pellagra becomes advanced, symptoms may then include severe diarrhea, skin rashes, delirium, and death if not treated.

Pantothenic acid

DAILY REQUIREMENT
Men 5mg per day
Women 5mg per day

This B-complex vitamin, also known as vitamin B_5 or abbreviated to Pant, helps to break down proteins and their amino acids, fats, and carbohydrates. It is also required for the manufacture of vitamin B_{12}, hemoglobin (the oxygen-carrying pigment in red blood cells), and cell membranes, which enclose the contents of body cells.

Good sources

Pantothenic acid This is found in all these foods, which contain at least 0.5mg of the vitamin per 3½–8½oz (100–245g):
- Sweet potatoes (yams)
- Avocado
- Mushrooms
- Yogurt
- Kidney
- Liver
- Red meat
- Mackerel
- Mullet
- Salmon
- Trout
- Lentils
- Lima beans
- Navy beans

PANTOTHENIC ACID DEFICIENCY

There is no evidence that a deficiency of pantothenic acid occurs naturally, because the vitamin is made by the body. However, it is thought that nerve inflammation seen in people who abuse alcohol may be due to a deficiency of this vitamin; although further evidence is needed to confirm this association.

Symptoms may include stomach pain, cramp, and fatigue, but this may mean a deficiency in all B-complex vitamins.

Vitamin B_6

DAILY REQUIREMENT
Men 1.3mg per day
Women 1.3mg per day

Also known as pyridoxine, vitamin B_6 is involved in the production and digestion of amino acids (see p.45). This vitamin helps the body manufacture the hormone insulin (see p.246); antibodies that fight infection; and certain chemicals that send messages between nerve cells. It is involved in the production of the chemical histamine, which is involved in allergic reactions. Vitamin B_6 also plays a key role in the production of hemoglobin (the oxygen-carrying molecule in red blood cells) and in the ability of oxygen to bind with the hemoglobin molecule.

A form of vitamin B_6 is used to treat or relieve the symptoms of a variety of disorders, including premenstrual syndrome, gestational diabetes, asthma, and depression. The vitamin may also help prevent cardiovascular disease in people who have high blood levels of the amino acid homocysteine—which may lead to cardiovascular disease (see pp.214–221).

VITAMIN B_6 DEFICIENCY

This can occur in babies fed infant formula that does not contain vitamin B_6. It can also affect people who abuse alcohol, cigarette smokers, and women who use oral contraceptives. Certain medications can lower the level of vitamin B_6 in the body. For example, isoniazid, which is used to treat or prevent the lung infection tuberculosis, makes vitamin B_6 inactive.

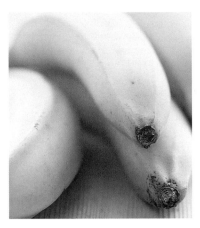

Bananas A particularly good source of vitamin B$_6$, bananas also provide folate, potassium, and soluble fiber. They are best eaten ripe—when the skin is speckled brown.

Medical conditions that are thought to decrease the levels of vitamin B$_6$ in the blood are asthma, kidney disease, Hodgkin's disease, sickle-cell anemia, and diabetes.

The symptoms of a mild vitamin B$_6$ deficiency include cracked lips, oily, flaky skin, nausea, and diarrhea. If the deficiency becomes more severe, loss of appetite, depression, and confusion may then develop.

Because vitamin B$_6$ is required to convert the amino acid tryptophan into niacin (B$_3$), there may also be signs and symptoms of a niacin deficiency (*opposite*), including fatigue, weakness, irritability, and anxiety.

Good sources

Vitamin B$_6$ This is found in these foods, which contain at least 0.5mg of vitamin B$_6$ per 3½–7oz (100–200g):

- Potatoes
- Sweet potatoes (yams)
- Bananas
- Chicken
- Turkey
- Mackerel
- Mullet
- Salmon
- Swordfish
- Trout
- Tuna

Vitamin B$_{12}$

DAILY REQUIREMENT
Men 0.0024mg per day
Women 0.0024mg per day

Also known as cyanocobalamin or cobalamin, vitamin B$_{12}$ is released from food in the stomach. In order for this vitamin to be absorbed into the blood, it has to bind with a protein called intrinsic factor, which is produced by the cells lining the stomach.

Vitamin B$_{12}$ is necessary for normal growth and development, especially in babies, young children, and teenagers, and, with the vitamin folate (*see p.56*), in the production of oxygen-carrying red blood cells. It is also required for the proper functioning of the nervous system; manufacturing DNA (the substance that makes up our genes); and the processing of fats and carbohydrates.

The vitamin is found naturally only in foods of animal origin, including seafood, although many other foods are now fortified with it. Vegetarians, especially vegans (*see p.100*), are therefore at risk of a vitamin B$_{12}$ deficiency and should take a supplement.

Anemia and deficiencies

This is any of various disorders in which hemoglobin (the oxygen-carrying pigment in red blood cells) is deficient or abnormal, resulting in body cells and tissues not getting enough oxygen. Symptoms include constant fatigue, pale skin, and shortness of breath on exertion. Some types result from vitamin or mineral deficiencies.

Iron-deficiency anemia This is caused by low levels of iron in the body. Iron is part of hemoglobin. This type of anemia is usually due to an insufficient intake of iron in the diet (*see p.66*) or blood loss.

Megaloblastic anemia This results from either low levels of vitamin B$_{12}$ (*above*) or folate (*see p.56*). These vitamins are essential for the

Good sources

Vitamin B$_{12}$ These foods naturally contain at least 0.0005mg of vitamin B$_{12}$ per 2–8½oz (55–250g):

- Dairy products
- Organ meat (liver, heart, kidneys)
- Eggs
- Beef
- Seafood

VITAMIN B$_{12}$ DEFICIENCY
A deficiency may also occur in people who cannot produce intrinsic factor, placing them at risk of pernicious anemia (*below*). Because vitamin B$_{12}$ is absorbed toward the end of the intestine (*see p.36*), people who have had their ileum surgically removed need injections of the vitamin.

Many older people lose their ability to produce sufficient gastric acid and pepsin, which is an enzyme necessary to separate vitamin B$_{12}$ from food, so that they absorb less vitamin B$_{12}$. As a result, they may need to take vitamin B$_{12}$ supplements (*see p.150*).

In addition, older people may have too many bacteria in the stomach that are normally killed by stomach acid.

formation of red blood cells, and a deficiency of either causes the formation of abnormally large red blood cells known as macrocytes, or megaloblasts, because the red blood cells do not divide properly and cannot carry oxygen effectively.

Pernicious anemia Megaloblastic anemia sometimes develops because of an autoimmune reaction in which the body's immune system attacks the lining of the stomach. This damage decreases the amount of intrinsic factor made by the stomach lining. This leads to vitamin B$_{12}$ deficiency because vitamin B$_{12}$ has to bind with intrinsic factor in order to be absorbed into the bloodstream and used by the body. When megaloblastic anemia is caused by this autoimmune reaction, it is known as pernicious anemia.

These bacteria use up dietary vitamin B_{12} for their own needs, leaving less available for the body to use.

Symptoms of vitamin B_{12} deficiency include megaloblastic anemia (*see p.55*), nerve damage (often felt as tingling in the hands and feet), and inflammation of the tongue and mouth. A long-term deficiency can cause irreversible nerve damage. Dementia has also been linked to B_{12} deficiency.

Biotin

DAILY REQUIREMENT
Men 0.03mg per day
Women 0.03mg per day

Another of the B-complex vitamins, biotin is essential for converting proteins, carbohydrates, and fats into forms that the body can use.

BIOTIN DEFICIENCY
Pregnant women, people who abuse alcohol, and those who do not produce sufficient amounts of stomach acid, such as older people, may have low levels of biotin. About 50 percent of pregnant women in North America have reduced levels of biotin.

Symptoms and signs of biotin deficiency include inflammation and increased sensitivity of the skin, hair loss, muscle pain, loss of appetite, nausea, mental problems, high blood levels of cholesterol, and reduced levels of hemoglobin, the oxygen-carrying pigment in red blood cells, leading to the symptoms of anemia (*see p.55*).

Good sources
Biotin This is found in these foods, which contain at least 0.001mg of biotin per 1–3½oz (28–100g):
- Cauliflower
- Mushrooms
- Liver
- Egg yolks
- Mackerel
- Sardines
- Black-eyed peas
- Peanuts
- Yeast

Folate

DAILY REQUIREMENT
Men 0.4mg per day
Women 0.4mg per day

Another of the B vitamins, also called folacin or folic acid and abbreviated to Fol, folate cannot be made by the body and must therefore come from food or supplements. Folate plays a vital role in making DNA (the substance that makes up our genes) and RNA (a substance needed to make proteins), in normal growth and development, and in the production of new cells. It works with vitamin B_{12} to form hemoglobin for red blood cells, and helps convert the amino acid homocysteine to methionine.

A good supply of folate prior to and in early pregnancy reduces the risk of the baby developing a neural tube defect such as spina bifida (*see p.140*).

FOLATE DEFICIENCY
A deficiency of folate is common today since many people consume diets high in fat and processed foods and eat less than the daily recommended five servings of fruits and vegetables. A folate deficiency occurs in people with an intestinal disorder in which they cannot absorb this and other vitamins, such as Crohn's disease (*see p. 233*). Folate deficiency in older people may be the

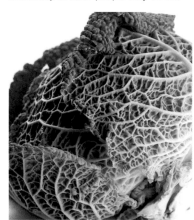

Cabbage This is a superfood. Rich in folate, cabbage is also a good source of beta-carotene (a precursor of vitamin A), vitamin C, fiber, and cancer-fighting phytochemicals.

Good sources
Folate This is found naturally in all these foods, which contain at least 0.03mg of folate per 3–7oz (85–200g):
- Corn
- Asparagus
- Brussels sprouts
- Cabbage
- Cauliflower
- Fresh green vegetables
- Green peas
- Spinach
- Oranges
- Liver
- Black-eyed peas
- Black beans
- Chickpeas
- Lentils
- Pinto beans
- Kidney beans

result of a poor diet and aging. In addition, older people produce lower amounts of the stomach acid necessary for the digestion of folate.

Certain medications, such as antacids, cimetidine, sulfasalazine, and phenytoin, and alcohol affect the body's ability to take up folate. In addition, the cancer drug methotrexate blocks the action of folate in the body.

Lack of folate causes a type of anemia called megaloblastic anemia (*see p.55*) with symptoms such as fatigue, pale skin, and shortness of breath on mild exertion. Other symptoms include sore mouth, diarrhea, weight loss, and heartburn. A deficiency also results in raised levels of homocysteine (an amino acid), which may lead to cardiovascular disease.

Vitamin C

DAILY REQUIREMENT
Men 90mg per day
Women 75mg per day

Also known as ascorbic acid, vitamin C cannot be manufactured by the body so it must be acquired from the diet. It is the least stable of the vitamins and is easily destroyed during cooking and food processing. If consumed in high quantities, excess vitamin C is excreted

Vitamin C and the common cold

The role of vitamin C in fighting infection has been controversial for decades. At present, research shows that vitamin C reduces histamine levels in the body, and it can be helpful in reducing the symptoms as well as the duration of a cold. However, there is no evidence to suggest that vitamin C can prevent or cure the common cold. It is advisable to try to get all your vitamin C from your diet. If you do take supplements, limit them to less than 500mg per day because higher doses may cause problems such as diarrhea and kidney stones.

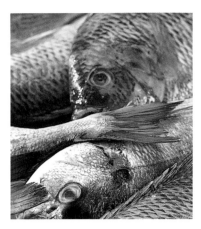

Mackerel A good source of vitamin D, this fish also contains vitamins niacin (B_3), B_6, and B_{12}, phosphorus, iodine, selenium, potassium, and heart-protecting omega-3 fatty acids.

in the urine. Vitamin C is essential for the formation of collagen, an important structural protein that strengthens bones and blood vessels and anchors teeth into the gums, in addition to being necessary for body growth, tissue repair, and wound healing. It also acts as an antioxidant (*see p.58*), protects against infection by enabling white blood cells to break down bacteria, is involved in the production of red blood cells and their oxygen-carrying pigment hemoglobin, and helps the body absorb iron from the intestine.

VITAMIN C DEFICIENCY

People who do not get enough fresh citrus fruits and juices may have insufficient vitamin C intake, as may those who are following a restricted diet. Regular drinkers and smokers are at risk of vitamin C deficiency since alcohol prevents the absorption of the vitamin and cigarette smoking depletes levels. People with wounds and burns, pneumonia, tuberculosis, and rheumatic fever, as well as those recovering from surgery, may need more vitamin C to help with the healing process.

Vitamin C deficiency causes scurvy, which is a condition that leads to muscle weakness, joint pain, problems with wound healing, loose teeth, bleeding and swollen gums, easily bruised skin or little red spots on the skin, fatigue, and sometimes depression.

Vitamin D

DAILY REQUIREMENT
Men 0.005mg per day
Women 0.005mg per day

This fat-soluble vitamin has an essential role in the absorption and use of calcium (*see p.62*) and phosphorus (*see p.63*), and therefore in the formation and health of bones, teeth, and cartilage (the tough, fibrous tissue that covers the ends of bones at joints). Vitamin D occurs in two forms: vitamin D_2, which is found in a small number of foods, and vitamin D_3, which is synthesized by the skin when it is exposed to sunlight. Both D_2 and D_3 are converted into a form that the body can use (active form) in the liver and kidneys.

When calcium levels in the blood are low, parathyroid hormone is released by the parathyroid glands, which are located in the neck. This hormone stimulates the kidneys to convert vitamin D into its active form, which in turn stimulates the intestine to increase the absorption of calcium and phosphorus. Vitamin D is also measured in International Units (IU), in which 40IU equals 0.001mg.

VITAMIN D DEFICIENCY

In countries where milk and dairy foods are enriched with vitamin D, deficiency is rare. Because sunlight is so important in the manufacture of vitamin D, people most at risk are older adults, especially those who are bed-ridden or unable to get out and about easily.

Deficiency may also occur in people who cover themselves for religious or cultural reasons or for necessity, such as in cold climates, and those living in urban areas with high air pollution who get little exposure to sunshine. Other groups at risk of vitamin D deficiency include those requiring long-term use of certain anticonvulsant medications, which interfere with the conversion of vitamin D into its active form. In addition, people with chronic kidney disease are at risk of a deficiency due to the kidney's

Good sources

Vitamin C This is found in these foods, which contain at least 10mg of the vitamin per 1¾–7oz (50–200g):
- Plantain
- Asparagus
- Broccoli
- Brussels sprouts
- Cabbage
- Bell peppers
- Tomatoes
- Blackberries
- Grapefruit
- Guava
- Kiwifruit
- Mango
- Melon
- Oranges
- Pineapples
- Strawberries

Good sources

Vitamin D This is found naturally in all these foods, which contain at least 0.003mg of the vitamin per 1¾–3½oz (50–100g):
- Egg yolk
- Cod and halibut liver oils
- Mackerel
- Salmon
- Sardines
- Tuna

inability to convert vitamin D into its active form. Deficiency of the vitamin is characterized by softening of the bones, a condition called osteomalacia in adults and rickets in children. Osteomalacia may lead to pain in the legs, ribs, hips, and muscles, easily broken bones, and difficulty in climbing stairs or getting up from a sitting position. Rickets leads to deformity of the bones, especially bowing of the legs and abnormal curvature of the spine.

Vitamin E

DAILY REQUIREMENT
Men 0.015mg per day
Women 0.015mg per day

This fat-soluble vitamin is considered to be one of nature's most effective antioxidants, which protect the body against free radicals (*right*). Vitamin E also protects vitamin A from becoming chemically changed, helps make red blood cells, and prevents blood from clotting. It is stored primarily in the liver, in fat, and in muscle tissue.

VITAMIN E DEFICIENCY
Dietary deficiency of vitamin E is very rare. The deficiency only really occurs in people with long-term conditions that prevent the absorption of fats from the intestine, such as cystic fibrosis or Crohn's disease (*see p.233*).

Signs and symptoms of vitamin E deficiency include problems with the nervous system and anemia (*see p.55*), which is due to the shortened lifespan of red blood cells.

Good sources
Vitamin E This is found in these foods, which contain at least 0.5mg of the vitamin per 1–2oz (28–55g):
- Wheat germ
- Shrimp
- Almonds
- Hazelnuts
- Peanuts
- Pistachio nuts
- Soybeans
- Sunflower seeds

Jargon buster

Free radicals These are chemical by-products generated during normal biochemical reactions in the body. They are highly reactive and are used by the body to kill bacteria, fight inflammation, and maintain the tone of smooth muscle. If allowed to build up, free radicals damage—by a process called oxidation—proteins, fats, DNA (the substance that makes up genes), and, if enough accumulate, body cells and tissues.

Antioxidants These are chemicals that occur in fruits and vegetables and are also made naturally in the body that can neutralize free radicals (*above*). Antioxidant sources include vitamins A, C, and E and the minerals copper, selenium, and zinc.

Vitamin K

DAILY REQUIREMENT
Men 0.12mg per day
Women 0.09mg per day

This fat-soluble vitamin is an essential component in the body's normal blood-clotting process. Most of the vitamin K that we require is produced by the gut flora, which are the microorganisms living naturally in the intestine, but it is also obtained from food. Vitamin K is stored mainly in the liver.

If you have been prescribed blood-thinning medication, consult your doctor or dietitian about your vitamin K intake because vitamin K may interfere with the effect of your medication.

Antibiotics and vitamin K
If you take antibiotics for more than a few weeks, it is likely that such treatment will kill off helpful gut flora (microorganisms in the intestine including the bacteria that make vitamin K) as well as the harmful bacteria targeted by the medication. This will therefore reduce the amount of vitamin K you absorb. To restore the gut flora, you can eat yogurt with active cultures; otherwise, you should discuss taking a vitamin K supplement with your doctor or dietitian.

Good sources
Vitamin K This is found in these foods, which contain at least 0.01mg of the vitamin per 1¾–7oz (50–200g):
- Asparagus
- Broccoli
- Brussels sprouts
- Cabbage
- Carrots
- Cauliflower
- Celery
- Green peas
- Spinach
- Apricots
- Grapes
- Pears
- Plums

VITAMIN K DEFICIENCY
A dietary deficiency of this vitamin is rare because we get almost all our requirements of this vitamin from the gut flora. However, a deficiency may occur in people with any condition that affects the absorption of fats from the intestine, such as cystic fibrosis. In addition, long-term use of antibiotic medication can lead to vitamin K deficiency because of the effect of the antibiotics on gut flora (*below*).

Because vitamin K deficiency reduces the ability of blood to clot, symptoms may include bleeding from the mouth, genital and urinary tracts, stomach, intestine, and skin. The skin may also bruise easily.

In newborn infants, the manufacture of vitamin K in the intestine takes about a week to become established; therefore there is a risk of the bleeding disorder called hemorrhagic disease of the newborn. Infants now routinely receive a vitamin K injection at birth to help the blood clot if bleeding occurs.

Phytochemicals

Protective chemicals found in foods of plant origin.

Phytochemicals, also known as phytonutrients, are naturally occurring protective chemicals that are found in foods of plant origin (*phyto* is derived from the Greek word for plant). Studies show that there may be as many as 100 different phytochemicals in just one serving of vegetables.

Phytochemicals and health
Evidence has shown that people who consume a diet rich in fruits and vegetables, and therefore in phytochemicals, have a lower incidence of many disorders, including cardiovascular disease, diabetes, and certain types of cancer. Phytochemicals have an antioxidant effect (*opposite*) that protects cells from cancer and cardiovascular disease, as well as from urinary tract infections, rheumatoid arthritis, and reduced immunity. Make sure you eat at least five portions of fruits and vegetables a day to get plenty of phytochemicals.

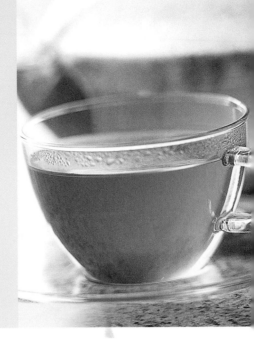

Green tea A potent phytochemical called polyphenol, thought to lower the risk of stomach cancer, is found in green tea.

What are the different types of phytochemicals?

There are hundreds of phytochemicals found in foods of plant origin. The key benefits of some of the most well-known phytochemicals are listed below:

Bioflavonoids These are helpful in the absorption of vitamin C and protect it from oxidation (damage). Citrus fruits, such as lemons, limes, grapefruit, and oranges, are particularly good sources of bioflavonoids.

Carotenoids These may protect against cardiovascular disease. Carotenoids are found in carrots, cantaloupe, sweet potatoes, and butternut squash.

Glucosinolates Found in vegetables, these help the liver in its detoxification function. They help regulate certain white blood cells involved in immunity. They may also help reduce tumor growth, particularly in the breast, liver, colon, lung, stomach, and esophagus.

Organosulfides These give onions and leeks their pungent odor. They stimulate anticancer enzymes, and slow the formation of blood clots. They are also known to boost the immune system.

Phytoestrogens These protect the body against cardiovascular disease and osteoporosis. Phytoestrogens may also slow the progression of cancer. They are found in soy products and flaxseeds.

Flavonoids These may protect the body from inflammation, allergic reactions, and viral infections.

Indoles These phytochemicals are thought to help against breast cancer.

Isoflavones These may inhibit estrogen-promoted cancers and lower high levels of blood cholesterol.

Limonoids Found in the peel of citrus fruits, these phytochemicals appear to protect lung tissue.

Lycopene Found in tomatoes, this may protect against cancers of the cervix, stomach, bladder, colon, and prostate, and cardiovascular disease.

Para-coumaric acid This phytochemical helps prevent cancer by interfering with the development of cancer-causing nitrosamines in the stomach.

Phenols and polyphenol These protect plants from chemical damage and perform the same function in humans. Found in green tea, polyphenol is thought to protect against stomach cancer.

Phytosterols These include stanols, which can reduce the absorption of cholesterol from the diet and therefore lower cholesterol levels in the blood. Stanols are found in soy products and fortified margarines.

Terpenes These may block action of cancer-causing factors (carcinogens) and may inhibit hormone-related cancers such as ovarian cancer.

Good sources
Phytochemicals These are found in all foods of plant origin. The following foods listed below are thought to contain particularly beneficial phytochemicals:
- Whole grains
- Broccoli
- Brussels sprouts
- Cauliflower
- Citrus fruits
- Dark-green leafy vegetables
- Garlic
- Green tea
- Herbs and spices
- Onions
- Tomatoes
- Soybeans
- Wine

What are minerals?

These are substances originating in rocks and metal ores.

Many minerals are essential for health. We obtain them by eating plants, which take up minerals from the soil, by eating animals that have eaten plants (or eaten other animals that have eaten plants), and, to some extent, by drinking water that contains minerals.

Minerals are needed by the body in only tiny quantities and are termed macrominerals or microminerals, according to the percentage of your total body weight they constitute and how much you need in your daily diet.

Macrominerals make up more than 0.005 percent of the body's weight and you need to be taking more than 100mg of these daily. They include calcium, magnesium, phosphorus, potassium, sodium, and sulfur. Microminerals, which are also known as trace elements, make up less than 0.005 percent of the body's weight and you need less than 100mg daily. Those microminerals with identified roles in health include chromium, copper, fluoride, iodine, iron, selenium, and zinc.

Why we need minerals

Minerals work together in making and breaking down body tissues and in regulating metabolism—the chemical reactions constantly occurring in the body. Bone, for example, consists of a framework of the protein collagen in which most of the body's calcium, phosphorus, and magnesium are deposited. Minerals are stored in your bones so that in the event of a dietary deficiency such as a calcium deficiency, some of the

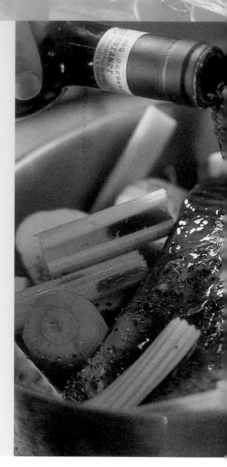

How do you get minerals?

No single food is the best source of all minerals, but eating a variety of foods usually ensures that you get enough. In addition, the body can store minerals for future use when intake might be low.

Animal foods are generally the best sources of minerals because they tend to contain minerals in the proportions we need. Fruits and vegetables are also good sources, especially organic produce, which is richer in minerals compared to produce grown nonorganically. Mineral water can be a source of minerals (right), including magnesium.

Minerals are often lost when a food is processed. For example, potassium, iron, and chromium are removed from whole grains during the refining process. US law now states that certain minerals lost during processing must be replaced. Refined grains described as "enriched" contain added iron to compensate for the amount lost. However, other lost nutrients are not replenished. Table salt often has iodine added to it. In addition, all breakfast cereals and milk are now fortified with a range of minerals that are essential for good health.

Minerals differ from vitamins in that they are not damaged by heat or light, but some can be lost in the water used for cooking. Avoid boiling vegetables so that you preserve the mineral content. Steam them using as little water as possible and/or keep the cooking time short by using the microwave. If you do boil, add the vegetables when the water is bubbling. If you put them in cold water and then bring it to a boil, many more nutrients are lost. Consider saving the water that you used for soup stock.

Sometimes, you may need to take mineral supplements: for example, if you do not eat enough calcium-rich foods you may need a supplement to prevent osteoporosis (see pp.268–271).

Minerals in water

We also get some minerals from tap water and commercially bottled mineral water, which has varying amounts of many minerals.

Fluoride is present naturally in many water sources, and in other areas, water supplies are often fluoridated since fluoride prevents tooth decay.

Hard water contains calcium and magnesium—leaving the evidence as scaly deposits in pipes and on kitchen utensils. These minerals can be neutralized with salt crystals in order to produce softer water that leaves less scaling.

Bottled mineral water has a unique mineral content dependent on the geographical area of origin. The water collects minerals as it percolates through rocks. It may contain calcium and iron.

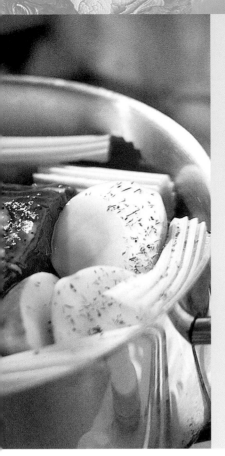

mineral can be released from the bones for the body's needs. The teeth also contain significant amounts of the minerals calcium and phosphorus.

Minerals are found in many key molecules in the body and are involved in essential chemical reactions. For example, sulfur is part of thiamine (B_1); calcium activates a digestive enzyme that breaks down fats; and copper is needed to incorporate iron into hemoglobin, the oxygen-carrying molecule present in red blood cells. The minerals calcium, magnesium, potassium, and sodium are especially important in cell functioning, particularly in the transmission of electrical impulses along nerve fibers and in muscle contractions.

Mineral-rich dish Minerals are present in most foods in varying quantities. Red meat is a particularly good source of iron, needed by the body to make red blood cells.

Mineral deficiencies

The most widespread mineral deficiencies in North America (and the diseases they cause) are iron (iron-deficiency anemia), calcium (osteoporosis), iodine (enlarged thyroid gland), and fluoride (tooth decay). Because the body stores and reuses minerals, it may be years before symptoms first occur.

Causes of a mineral deficiency can be primary or secondary. Primary deficiency occurs if you do not get enough of a mineral in your diet. Secondary deficiency occurs when the dietary intake is adequate but another factor results in the body not being able to absorb or use a mineral. Poor absorption may be caused by disorders of the intestine, such as Crohn's disease, the effects of medications, or because other substances in food bind to minerals and prevent them from being absorbed. Minerals can be lost from the body as a result of alcohol abuse, excessive sweating, or medications.

Case study Teenage girl who feels constantly cold and tired

Name Jennifer

Age 19

Problem Jennifer is constantly tired and in spite of doing regular exercise, she is not able to run a mile due to overwhelming fatigue.

Jennifer complains of "always being cold." Over the last year, her fatigue has gradually become worse. Jennifer has a history of heavy menstrual periods, which usually last for seven days.

Jennifer also has a history of iron-deficiency anemia, which was initially diagnosed two years ago. Her doctor prescribed iron supplements to treat this condition. Unfortunately, Jennifer found that the supplements caused

abdominal pain and constipation so she decided to stop taking them.

Lifestyle Jennifer is a college student who avoids red meat, but regularly eats chicken and fish. She usually has dairy products with each meal. Her vegetable intake comes mostly from salads. She does not eat much fruit. Jennifer used to be an avid runner.

Advice The fatigue is almost certainly caused by iron deficiency. Therefore, Jennifer needs to obtain more iron in her diet. Because she loses iron on a monthly basis from menstrual periods, her iron stores need to be continually replenished.

Good sources of iron in the diet are red meat, poultry, fish and shellfish, nuts and seeds, green leafy vegetables, dried fruits, whole grains,

and fortified cereals. In Jennifer's case, dietary factors contributing to her ongoing iron deficiency include her avoidance of red meat and her intake of dairy products, which may reduce the absorption of iron.

She should also take a separate iron supplement of 50–60mg per day. Vitamin C-rich foods, such as citrus fruits, or a vitamin C supplement taken with her iron supplement, will increase the absorption of iron.

Because Jennifer suffers from constipation and abdominal pain when she takes iron supplements, she should add fiber to her diet and drink plenty of water, which will help her avoid constipation. She could also consult a gynecologist about taking an oral contraceptive that can decrease the flow of her menstrual periods.

Mineral directory

Here we look at the role of each mineral, good sources, and what happens if there is a deficiency. Macrominerals are discussed first, followed by the microminerals. The daily requirement (Dietary Reference Intake) for adults is given, although needs do vary at different stages of life (*see Eating for the Time of your Life, pp.104–155*).

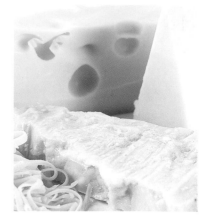

Cheese A small amount of cheese will give you your daily requirement of calcium. Available in many different tastes and textures, cheese is also a good source of protein and zinc.

Calcium

DAILY REQUIREMENT
Men 1,000mg per day
Women 1,000mg per day

This is the main mineral present in bones and teeth, which between them contain about 99 percent of the body's calcium (Ca); the remaining one percent is used for various functions in the body such as blood clotting, nerve signals, and muscle contraction. Calcium absorption in the intestine is regulated by vitamin D (*see p.57*). People who have problems absorbing vitamin D also have poor calcium absorption.

The absorption of calcium can be enhanced by lactose, which is the sugar found in dairy products; whereas the compounds oxalate and phytate, which are present in foods such as spinach, beets, celery, and parsley, can actually reduce the body's ability to absorb calcium. In addition, people who are following a high-protein diet excrete more calcium in the urine, and for this reason, people who have kidney stones may be advised to reduce their dietary intake of protein.

Adolescents—children aged between 9 and 18 years—need much more calcium in their diets than younger children or adults in order to fuel bone development during their growth spurt.

CALCIUM DEFICIENCY

A deficiency of calcium is likely to remain undetected for several years because the bones continue to release calcium into the blood to maintain normal blood levels if the dietary intake of the mineral is low.

Symptoms of calcium deficiency include bone pain, pins and needles in the hands and feet, muscle cramps and twitching, convulsions, and osteoporosis (*see p.242*), which is characterized by weakened bones that may fracture and crumble, leading to loss of height.

If you do not get enough calcium in your diet during childhood, it will result in reduced bone mass, which increases your risk of osteoporosis later in life. The signs and symptoms of calcium deficiency in childhood include stunted growth, muscle weakness, irritability, and muscle cramps and twitching. Untreated, a childhood deficiency of calcium may be fatal.

Calcium and body fat

The mineral calcium has been found to help weight loss. Studies have shown that when your dietary intake of calcium is increased, there is also an increase in the breakdown of fat and a decrease in the production of fat, and, as a result, body fat is lost.

This relationship was discovered when studies of children and adults who consumed higher levels of calcium and dairy products were shown to have less body fat. Obese adults who were following a reduced-calorie diet high in calcium, lost more weight and fat than those on a reduced-calorie diet that had a low intake of calcium.

Researchers believe that each 300mg increase in calcium intake is associated with approximately 2lb (1kg) less body fat in children and 5–6lb (2.25–2.7kg) lower body weight in adults.

When calcium intake is low, levels of a hormone called calcitriol, which is involved in calcium metabolism, increase in order to help conserve calcium in the body. Calcitriol also causes fat cells to expand and increase fat stores in the body. Conversely, by maintaining your calcium levels, you can suppress the calcitriol and therefore help your body increase the breakdown of fat.

Good sources

Calcium This is found naturally in all the foods listed below, which contain at least 150mg of calcium per 3½oz (100g):
● Bok choy
● Collard greens
● Mustard greens
● Spinach
● Turnip greens
● Dairy products
● Canned salmon
● Sardines
● Almonds
● Tofu

Magnesium

DAILY REQUIREMENT
Men 420mg per day
Women 320mg per day

This mineral plays a vital role in the formation of bones and teeth and, with the minerals calcium, sodium, and potassium, is involved in transmitting nerve signals and causing muscle contractions. Magnesium (Mg) also helps the body process fat and protein and make proteins and is necessary for the secretion of parathyroid hormone, which helps control the levels of calcium in the blood. Vitamin D increases the absorption of potassium in the intestine. Once absorbed, magnesium is stored in bone, muscles, cells, and the fluid that surrounds cells.

Because of magnesium's role in muscle contraction, it is used medically to reduce irregular heart rhythms (arrhythmias) or contractions of the uterus in pregnant women.

MAGNESIUM DEFICIENCY
A dietary, or primary, deficiency of magnesium is rare. However, it can result from problems with the absorption of nutrients from the intestine, long-term use of diuretic medications, excessive vomiting, kidney disease, chronic alcohol abuse, hyperparathyroidism,

Good sources
Magnesium This is found naturally in all the foods below, which contain at least 50mg of magnesium per 3½oz (100g):
- Whole grains
- Artichokes
- Okra
- Spinach
- Swiss chard
- Turnip greens
- Lamb kidney
- Red meat
- Legumes
- Nuts such as Brazils, almonds, cashews, and peanuts
- Sunflower seeds
- Tofu

and liver cirrhosis. Because magnesium is also needed for the normal functioning of the parathyroid glands, which secrete parathyroid hormone, low magnesium levels may adversely decrease the levels of calcium in the blood.

A magnesium deficiency leads to low levels of calcium and potassium in the blood, as well as changes to the digestive system, nervous and muscular systems, heart and circulatory systems, and the development of blood cells.

People who develop a magnesium deficiency may have the following signs and symptoms: fatigue, weakness, poor appetite, impaired speech, anemia, irregular heart rhythms, and tremors. Affected babies and young children may fail to thrive. Advanced signs of the deficiency include abnormally rapid heart rate and convulsions, and it may be fatal if not treated.

Phosphorus

DAILY REQUIREMENT
Men 700mg per day
Women 700mg per day

Essential for bones and teeth, phosphorus (P) is also found in lipids (fats and fatlike compounds), proteins, carbohydrates, enzymes, and DNA (the substance that makes up our genes). It is also a part of ATP (adenosine triphosphate)—a

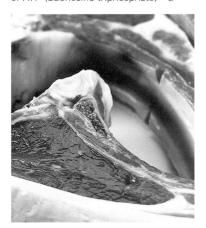

Red meat Not only a reliable source of protein, red meat is rich in phosphorus and other micronutrients, including B vitamins, magnesium, potassium, chromium, and iron.

Good sources
Phosphorus This is found naturally in all the following foods, which contain at least 150mg of phosphorus per 1oz (28g):
- Whole grains, especially oats
- Dairy products
- Red meat
- Poultry
- Seafood
- Legumes, especially lentils
- Nuts such as almonds, Brazils, peanuts, and pine nuts
- Sunflower seeds

compound that stores energy needed by all cells. The amount of phosphorus absorbed from food varies depending on your need for the mineral. Vitamin D (*see p.57*) is essential for the absorption of phosphorus.

PHOSPHORUS DEFICIENCY
People who take excessive amounts of antacid indigestion medication for a prolonged period may develop a phosphorus deficiency. Antacids bind with dietary phosphorus and prevent its absorption into the bloodstream.

Symptoms of phosphorus deficiency include muscle weakness and bone pain. Anemia, impaired function of red and white blood cells, problems with the nervous system including psychological disorders, abnormal excretion of calcium in urine, and kidney stones (*see p.238*) may also result from phosphorus deficiency.

Potassium

DAILY REQUIREMENT
Men 3,500mg per day
Women 3,500mg per day

Together with sodium and chloride, potassium (K) is involved in controlling the amount of water and maintaining the correct acid–alkali balance in the body.

Potassium also helps the body store blood sugar in the form of glycogen, which is the principal source of energy required by all muscles in the body, in order to work properly.

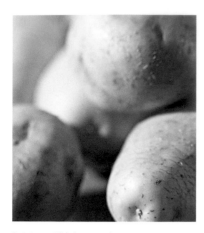

Potatoes Rich in potassium, potatoes are also a good source of folate, iron, protein, and fiber. If boiled or baked rather than fried, potatoes are filling and not fattening.

Potassium is also essential for the normal functioning of muscles, nerve cells, the heart and heart valves, the kidneys, and the adrenal glands.

According to the most recent studies, regular consumption of high-potassium foods can help to lower and control blood pressure, so it is especially important for people with heart failure (*see p.221*) or high blood pressure (*see p.220*) to eat enough of this mineral. Good sources of potassium include avocados, bananas, and potatoes (*below*). A high potassium intake has also been linked to decreasing the risk of stroke (*see p.216*), the bone

Good sources

Potassium This is found naturally in all the foods below, which contain at least 160mg of the mineral per 3½oz (100g):
- Whole grains
- Potatoes
- Asparagus
- Avocados
- Spinach
- Tomatoes
- Bananas
- Cantaloupe
- Oranges
- Dairy products
- Red meat
- Lima beans

disease osteoporosis, and calcium-containing kidney stones (*see p.238*). In addition, you may need to eat more potassium-rich foods in warm weather as the mineral is lost from the body through sweating.

POTASSIUM DEFICIENCY
A dietary deficiency of potassium is rare. Low levels of potassium in the blood, known as hypokalemia, are usually caused by loss of potassium through excessive vomiting or diarrhea, or as a result of kidney disease or a metabolic disorder, in which the body chemistry is affected in some way. A potassium deficiency may also be due to taking too many laxatives or eating disorders such as anorexia and bulimia that may involve vomiting (*see p.207*).

Symptoms include fatigue, muscle weakness, constipation, cramps, and reduced kidney function. Severely low levels can lead to heart problems such as abnormal heart rhythms.

Sodium

DAILY REQUIREMENT
Men 500mg per day
Women 500mg per day

Best known as a component of table salt (sodium chloride), sodium (Na) is vital for controlling the amount of water in the body, maintaining the normal pH (degree of acidity or alkalinity) of blood, transmitting nerve signals, and helping muscular contraction. It is present in all foods in varying degrees, and almost all processed foods also have added salt.

Unlike all other minerals, sodium is, on the whole, overconsumed. Dietary intake is very high in North America—averaging about twenty times the recommended daily requirement of 500mg. Symptoms of increased salt intake include nausea, vomiting, diarrhea, and abdominal cramps. High concentrations of sodium in the body can also result from excessive water or fluid loss. Persistently high levels of sodium in the blood can result in swelling, high blood pressure (*see p.220*), difficulty in breathing, heart failure (*see p.221*), and may be fatal.

SODIUM DEFICIENCY
A deficiency of this mineral is rare since our dietary intake is so high. However, the levels of sodium in the body can become too low as a result of prolonged vomiting or diarrhea, or during a period of prolonged illness. Levels of sodium in the body can also become low as a result of dehydration or excessive or persistent sweating, which may occur during very hot weather or affect marathon runners, athletes who participate in triathlons, or people who have certain forms of kidney disease, such as acute kidney failure.

Symptoms of sodium deficiency include headache, nausea, vomiting, muscle cramps, drowsiness, fainting, fatigue, and possibly coma.

Sulfur

DAILY REQUIREMENT
Men 800–1,000mg per day
Women 800–1,000mg per day

The macromineral sulfur plays a key role in the manufacture of amino acids (*see p.45*) and in the conversion of carbohydrates to a form that the body can use. Sulfur (S) occurs in insulin, the hormone secreted by the pancreas that helps regulate the levels of the sugar glucose in blood. It is also involved in the manufacture of connective tissue (which surrounds body structures and

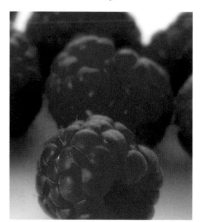

Raspberries An excellent source of sulfur, these fruit also contain vitamin C, calcium, magnesium, potassium, and iron, and are one of the best fruit sources of soluble fiber.

Good sources

Sulfur This is found naturally in all the foods listed below, which contain at least 100mg of the mineral per 3½oz (100g):
- Bean sprouts
- Leafy green vegetables such as cabbage, kale, and turnip greens
- Raspberries
- Dairy products
- Red meat, especially organ meats
- Egg yolks
- Chicken
- Seafood
- Legumes
- Nuts

holds them together), skin, hair, and nails, and in the manufacture of the vitamins thiamine (B$_1$; *see p.53*) and biotin (*see p.56*) in the body.

As yet, a deficiency of sulfur has not been diagnosed in humans because it occurs naturally in all foods.

Chromium

DAILY REQUIREMENT
Men 0.035mg per day
Women 0.025mg per day

This micromineral works with insulin, the hormone that regulates the levels of the sugar glucose in blood. Chromium (Cr) helps insulin bind to its receptors on the membrane of body cells, which

Good sources

Chromium This is found naturally in these foods, which contain at least 1mg of the mineral per 1¾oz (50g):
- Potatoes
- Broccoli
- Green beans
- Tomatoes
- Apples
- Bananas
- Grapes
- Oranges
- Red meat, especially beef, pork, and ham
- Turkey

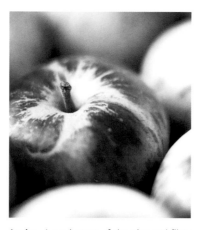

Apples A good source of chromium and fiber, all apples also contain quercetin, a flavonoid phytochemical that can help lower the levels of cholesterol in the blood.

then allows for the sugar glucose to move into the cell where it is used to produce energy for the cell's needs.

CHROMIUM DEFICIENCY
A deficiency of chromium is very rare and is most likely to occur in people who have had long-term intravenous feeding. Some studies of male runners have shown that urinary chromium loss was increased by endurance exercise. This finding suggests that your need for chromium is greater if you exercise on a regular basis.

Copper

DAILY REQUIREMENT
Men 0.9mg per day
Women 0.9mg per day

Copper (Cu) plays a key role in several body functions. These include the production of pigment in skin, hair, and eyes; the development of healthy bones, teeth, and heart; the protection of body cells from chemical damage since it acts as an antioxidant (*see p.58*); the maintenance of the myelin sheath, which surrounds and protects nerve fibers; and the functioning of the nervous system. It is also involved in the processing of iron in the body and the formation of red blood cells.

Good sources

Copper This is found naturally in all the foods listed below, which contain at least 1mg of the mineral per 1¾oz (50g):
- Whole grains, especially barley
- Liver
- Seafood such as crab, lobster, and oysters
- Nuts such as almonds, Brazils, and pistachios
- Sesame seeds

COPPER DEFICIENCY
A deficiency of copper is rare, though it can occur in malnourished infants. The deficiency results in anemia (*see p.55*) and its related symptoms.

Left untreated, a deficiency can lead to lung damage and excessive bleeding due to reduced production of red blood cells and damage to the connective tissues (which surround body structures and hold them together).

Fluoride

DAILY REQUIREMENT
Men 4mg per day
Women 3mg per day

This micromineral is found at varying concentrations in drinking water—it is often added by public water suppliers—and in soil; fluoride (F) is also present in very small amounts in the body. About 99 percent of the fluoride in the body is in the teeth and bones; it helps increase tooth mineralization and bone density and reduce the risk of tooth decay. It also promotes enamel remineralization throughout life.

Fluoridation of public water supplies has been endorsed by more than 90 professional health organizations as the most effective dental public health measure in existence. However, about half of the people in North America still fails to receive the maximum benefits from community water fluoridation and the use of products that have had fluoride added to them.

Fluoride can be obtained from any food that is prepared in or with water

Water fluoridation

By definition, water fluoridation is the adjustment of fluoride in a water supply to an optimum concentration of 0.7–1.2 parts per million in order to prevent tooth decay in the people who use the supply. The value of fluoridation has been demonstrated beyond question. Schoolchildren living in an optimally fluoridated community were shown to be at much lower risk of tooth decay compared with those children who do not live in such an area.

There is evidence that fluoridation reduces tooth decay in children by 20–40 percent, and helps to prevent tooth decay and loss in adults. Water fluoridation is beneficial for those living in poor communities, who are at greater risk of tooth decay and have less access to dental care and alternative fluoride resources.

that has been fluoridated. You can also obtain the mineral from fluoridated mouth rinses and toothpastes.

FLUORIDE DEFICIENCY

A deficiency of this mineral can lead to tooth decay. If you live in an area where fluoride is not added to the water supply, you would benefit from a fluoride supplement (p.270).

Iodine

DAILY REQUIREMENT
Men 0.15mg per day
Women 0.15mg per day

Although iodine (I) is found in all body cells, about 40 percent of the body's iodine is stored in the thyroid gland. Here, it is used for making thyroid hormones, which are required for normal body metabolism and growth. Iodine occurs naturally in the sea; our dietary iodine has to come from seafood or from plants grown in soil near to the sea. However, most table salt is now fortified with iodine. Excess iodine is secreted in the urine.

IODINE DEFICIENCY

If the body does not get enough iodine, there is a decrease in the production of the thyroid hormones. To compensate, the thyroid gland becomes enlarged.

A deficiency of iodine is a common worldwide cause of goiter (swelling in the neck due to a enlarged thyroid gland) and cretinism (dwarfism and learning difficulties) in those who do not get enough iodized salt or live in regions where iodine is not found.

Signs and symptoms of low iodine levels include slow metabolism and possibly weight gain. The signs and symptoms of cretinism include reduced growth of the muscles and skeleton and learning difficulties during childhood.

Iron

DAILY REQUIREMENT
Men 8mg per day
Women 18mg per day

This is an essential mineral in all cells of the body even though it is needed only in minute quantities. Iron (Fe) is a component of hemoglobin (the oxygen-carrying protein in red blood cells), and it plays a key role in transporting oxygen around the body. It is also part of myoglobin (a protein found in muscle cells) and is involved in the release of energy from glucose and fatty acids in the intestine.

Iron absorption requires gastric acid, which is secreted by the lining of the stomach, to convert it into a form that is best absorbed. Dietary iron from animal products—known as heme iron—is more easily absorbed by the body than the iron found in plants. However, the presence of vitamin C in the body is known to increase the absorption of iron from foods of plant origin.

A greater amount of iron is absorbed from food if the need is greater, such as during pregnancy, in adolescent girls, in people with anemia (see p.55), and in those who have suffered from bleeding, such as heavy menstruation or following childbirth, surgery, or trauma.

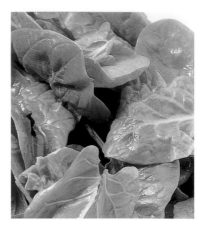

Spinach A useful source of iron, especially for vegetarians, spinach also contains beta-carotene (a precursor of vitamin A), vitamins C, E, and folate and calcium, and potassium.

IRON DEFICIENCY

This deficiency is most frequently caused by a poor intake of iron. It is one of the most widespread, and also most easily remedied, nutritional problems in the world. Pregnant women and breast-feeding and new mothers, infants and children, menstruating females, especially adolescents, and older adults are at greatest risk because of changes in their metabolic rate. Babies who are not breast-fed and not given iron-fortified formula or cereal may develop iron deficiency.

Vegetarians are also at risk of this deficiency since the amount of iron that the body can absorb from plants is lower than that from meats.

Good sources

Iron This is found naturally in all these foods, which contain at least 2mg of the mineral per 3½oz (100g):
- Spinach
- Dried fruit, especially prunes
- Organ meat (kidney and liver)
- Red meat
- Egg yolks
- Poultry
- Sardines
- Tuna
- Shrimp
- Legumes such as soy, lima, and kidney beans, and chickpeas

Iron deficiency is characterized by anemia (*see p.55*). Signs and symptoms of iron-deficiency anemia are common and include weakness, pale skin, fatigue and faintness, cold or numbness in the fingers and toes due to poor blood circulation, shortness of breath, greater susceptibility to infections, soft or brittle nails, poor work performance, and behavioral changes.

Young children with iron deficiency can become very tired and have low concentration. They may develop learning difficulties and behavioral problems that may be permanent.

Selenium

DAILY REQUIREMENT
Men 0.055mg per day
Women 0.055mg per day

This micromineral is an antioxidant (*see p.58*) and part of an enzyme that protects cells from the damaging effects of free radicals (*see p.58*), which can lead to cardiovascular disease. Selenium (Se) is vital for the normal functioning of the immune system and the thyroid gland. It is found naturally in fish, shellfish, poultry, and Brazil nuts.

Selenium is also thought to have anticancer properties, possibly from its antioxidant function, as well as from its ability to block the action of many

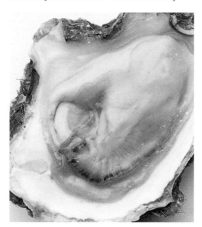

Oysters Shellfish such as oysters are a useful source of selenium and various other nutrients, including vitamins niacin (B₃), B₁₂, and the minerals potassium and zinc.

Good sources
Selenium This is found naturally in all the foods listed below, which contain at least 10mg of the mineral per 1oz (28g):
- Brown rice
- Wheat germ
- Whole-wheat bread
- Poultry
- Fish, especially tuna
- Shellfish, especially oysters
- Brazil nuts

enzymes that are involved in cell division and growth—which occur uncontrollably in cancer.

SELENIUM DEFICIENCY
A deficiency of selenium is rare. However, it has been seen in people who rely on intravenous nutrition, in people with intestinal problems that affect the body's ability to absorb nutrients, in severely malnourished infants and children, and in those with rheumatoid arthritis. A sign of selenium deficiency is an enlarged heart that is not able to pump blood efficiently.

Zinc

DAILY REQUIREMENT
Men 11mg per day
Women 8mg per day

Although needed in minute amounts, zinc (Zn) is essential for the breakdown of carbohydrates, fats, and proteins; in normal cell division, growth, and repair—especially during fetal growth; in the manufacture of DNA (the substance that makes up our genes) and RNA (a substance that is involved in making proteins); in the functioning of the immune system, including wound healing; in sexual maturation, fertility, and reproduction; and in the senses of taste and smell.

Zinc is also necessary to maintain normal levels of the male sex hormone testosterone in the blood and convert this hormone into the female sex hormone estrogen. This is why oysters have a reputation for increasing desire.

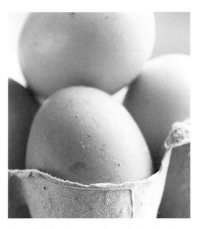

Eggs Rich in zinc, protein, and vitamins A, B₁₂, D, and E, eggs also contain, in their yolk, a substance called lecithin, which can protect against cardiovascular disease.

ZINC DEFICIENCY
This deficiency may be primary (due to insufficient zinc in the diet) or result from decreased absorption from the intestine or increased needs because of recovery from disease. Those most at risk include people who abuse alcohol, those with HIV infection or diabetes, people on protein-restricted diets, people with diseases that affect absorption from the intestine, and those with liver disease.

Symptoms of zinc deficiency include poor appetite, loss of sense of taste, digestive problems, diarrhea, vomiting, night blindness, hair loss, skin problems, poor wound healing, problems with growth in children, and delayed onset of puberty and sexual maturation.

Good sources
Zinc This is found naturally in all these foods, which contain at least 1mg of the mineral per 1oz (28g):
- Oat bran
- Dairy products
- Red meat
- Eggs
- Poultry
- Crab
- Lobster
- Brazil nuts
- Navy beans
- Soybeans

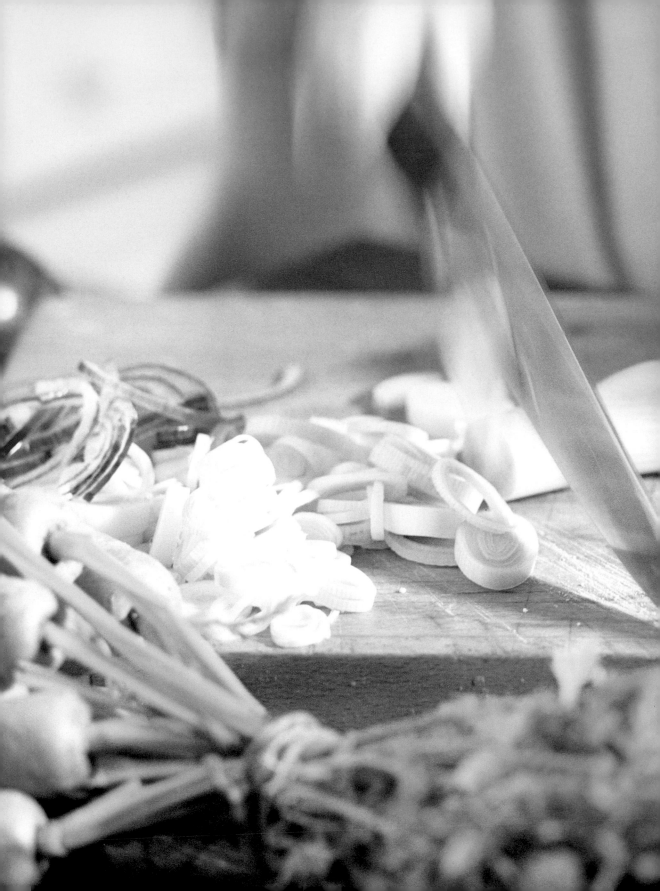

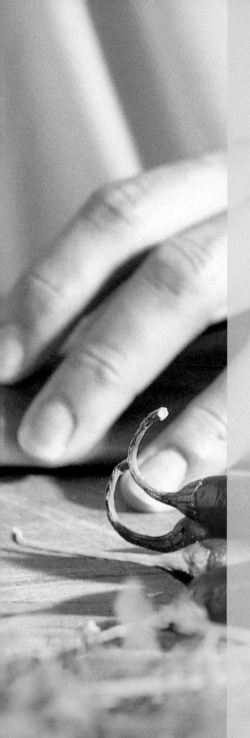

Elements of a healthy diet

The choices you make each time you buy food have an impact on your health, vitality, and well-being, as well as your weight. Eating foods from all the food groups, and in the right quantities, as outlined in this chapter, will help you achieve the maximum benefits from your diet.

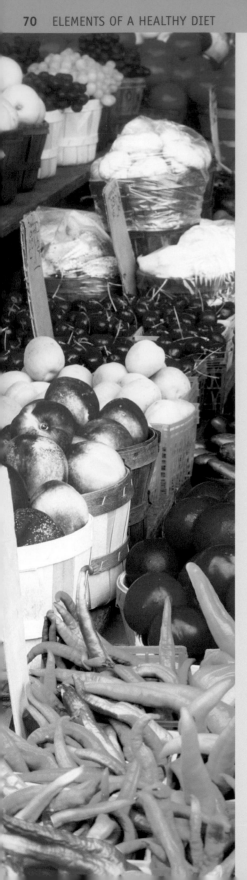

Making the best dietary choices

Choose your foods carefully to achieve optimum health.

In the first two chapters, we looked at why our bodies need food and how it is digested and used, and discussed the different types of nutrients that are needed in the diet—carbohydrates, proteins, fats, vitamins, and minerals.

Now we turn to the foods that supply these essential nutrients and the food groups from which they should be selected.

The main food groups

In the 1980s, the US Department of Agriculture (USDA) began to develop dietary guidelines aimed at encouraging the consumption of a nutritionally balanced diet and simplifying meal planning.

The official guidelines classify foods into six groups, of which five are highlighted as the "Basic Five." These five groups, which are recommended to form the basis of a healthy diet, include breads, cereals, and other grains (see pp.74–75); vegetables (see pp.76–77); fruits (see pp.78–79); milk and dairy products (see pp.80–83); and poultry, fish, meat, eggs, legumes, nuts, and seeds (see pp.84–95).

The sixth group includes fats, sweets, and alcohol: all of these items provide additional calories but few useful nutrients and are recommended to be eaten sparingly because of their harmful effects on health (see pp.98–99).

Choosing wisely Understanding the link between good nutrition and optimum health will help you to make the best choices from the vast array of available foods.

The need for water

Fluids are also a vital element of every diet: a man's body is about 60 percent water and a woman's about 50 percent, and every cell needs water to function properly. To remain healthy, you need to drink at least six to eight large glasses of fluids, preferably water, every day, and more when it is hot or when you are perspiring such as during exercise (see pp.96–97).

Beneficial compounds

In recent years, scientists have extended their understanding of the link between nutrition and health: it is now clear that eating particular foods contributes to good health and prevents disease. Thousands of potentially beneficial compounds in foods have now been identified, including vitamins, minerals, antioxidants, fiber, and phytochemicals. The list of foods that may help protect your health continues to grow—from many different vegetables and fruits to red wine, flaxseeds, and oily fish.

Making good choices

Any food can fit into a healthy way of eating. The key is to balance your choices over time so that your overall diet is sound. You can continue to eat your favorite foods, even if they are high in fat, salt, or sugars, but try to reduce your portion sizes.

Making good choices in your diet starts with educating yourself on sound nutritional guidelines and incorporating that knowledge into your eating habits. For example, by eating a variety of nutrient-rich foods, enjoying plenty of whole grains, vegetables, and fruits, and eating regular meals with moderate portions, you can manage your weight and stay healthy.

The basic food groups

Each of the food groups shown here provides some of the nutrients you need. No group is more important than another: you need them all for good health.

Foods from grains, such as bread, are necessary for fiber, vitamins, minerals, and complex carbohydrates, which are an important source of energy for the body. Vegetables and fruits are needed for vitamins and minerals. Naturally low in fat, they are also a source of fiber. Dairy products and protein sources provide protein and a range of important vitamins and minerals. Milk and dairy products also provide calcium.

Fats, oils, and sweet foods contain calories and little else of nutritional value, so eat them sparingly.

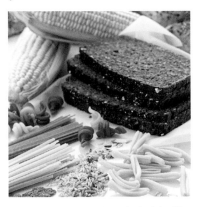

Breads, cereals, and grains The foods in this group are a valuable source of carbohydrates (*see pp.74–75*) and fiber.

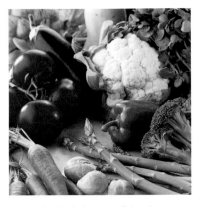

Vegetables A vital source of vitamins, minerals, and fiber, vegetables should form a major part of your diet (*see pp.76–77*).

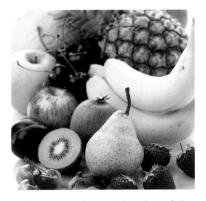

Fruits Packed with essential nutrients, fruits provide a good source of carbohydrates, fiber, vitamins, and phytochemicals (*see pp.78-79*).

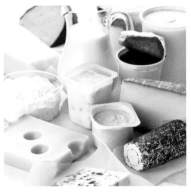

Milk and dairy products These are an important source of protein, vitamins, and minerals, especially calcium (*see pp.80–83*).

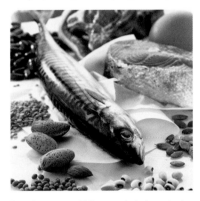

Protein sources This group includes animal products, such as meat, poultry, and fish, and plant proteins, such as legumes (*see pp.84–95*).

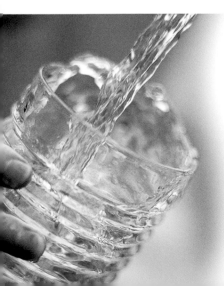

Water

Pure water is calorie-free, and the best drink to quench thirst. Your body cannot store water, so you must drink plenty of it to replenish losses and maintain healthy function of all your body cells. It is the most abundant substance in the body and is necessary for survival.

Essential element Although water has little nutritional content, it provides the perfect means of satisfying the body's vital need for fluid, since it contains no sugar, caffeine, or other unhealthy additives.

In many areas of North America, tap water is perfectly healthy, but if you suspect that your water is contaminated, have it tested and consider investing in a good filter to ensure that it is safe.

Bottled water is convenient to carry, making it easier for you to drink your six to eight glasses a day. Sparkling, still, and flavored water are all excellent, but watch out for "enhanced" water, which can contain unnecessary calories. Check the labels on bottled water if you are controlling your sodium intake, as most bottled water does contain sodium.

Dietary guidelines

The key message is to eat a variety of foods from the basic groups.

The US government's dietary guidelines are issued in the form of a Food Guide Pyramid, which provides a visual representation of the six food groups (*see p.71*) and the proportions they should form in your diet.

Food Guide Pyramid
Breads, cereals, rice, and other grains (*see pp.74–75*) should form the largest part of your diet, and are therefore shown at the base of the pyramid: six to 11 daily servings from this group are recommended. Next in quantity are vegetables (*see pp.76–77*), with three to five daily servings recommended, and fruits, with a daily recommendation of two to four servings (*see pp.78–79*).

Only two to three daily servings are recommended from the animal and plant protein group (*see pp.84–95*), which includes meat,

poultry, fish, legumes, eggs, and nuts. At the same level is the milk and dairy products group (*see pp.80–83*), with a recommendation of two to three daily servings. Sweet foods, fats, and alcohol (*see pp.98–99*) should be eaten sparingly, and are at the top of the pyramid.

Suggested modifications
These official guidelines may no longer accurately reflect the latest findings on nutrition and health. For example, there is evidence that eating too much red meat is harmful to your health because it is high in saturated fat (*see pp.86–87*).

On the other hand, since it has been shown that eating oily fish (*see p.39*) and certain plant oils (*see p.41*), such as canola and olive oil, reduces the risk of developing cardiovascular disease, current recommendations suggest that the consumption of these foods should be increased. The current Food Guide Pyramid has been criticized because it does not distinguish between whole- and refined-grain products, which

differ significantly in nutritional value (*see p.75*). Refined grains should be eaten sparingly, and whole grains should form the foundation of your diet.

The Mediterranean diet
Some dietary recommendations are based on studies of people living in Mediterranean countries who have lower cholesterol levels and rates of cardiovascular disease and cancer than people in North America. The Mediterranean diet, low in saturated fats and high in monounsaturated fats (*see p.38*), includes more grains, vegetables, fruits, legumes, nuts, and olive oil, while protein is supplied by fish, poultry, cheese, eggs, and yogurt.

A word of caution: a diet high in monounsaturated fats is also high in calories and leads to weight gain if you do not exercise enough.

Healthy lifestyle A diet of fresh, locally grown produce, rich in beneficial fats, and an active, outdoor lifestyle, contribute to the good health enjoyed in Mediterranean areas.

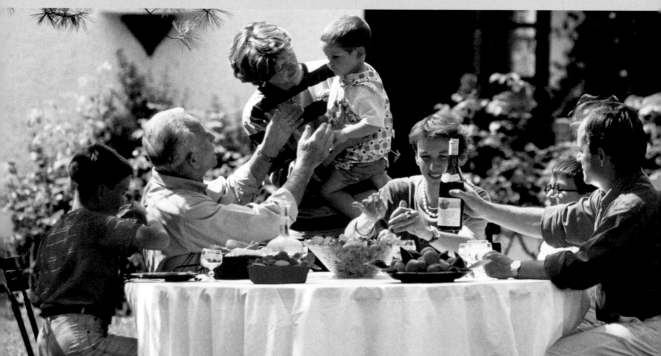

What is a serving?

Official guidelines indicate how many servings should be eaten daily from each food group. The recommendations are expressed as ranges, to cater for different energy needs (*see p.34*). For example, the lower number in each group applies to people with low energy requirements, such as older adults and sedentary people; the higher numbers are appropriate for teenage boys, active men, and very active women.

SERVINGS VS. PORTIONS

You may wonder whether these servings are the same size as the food portions served at home or in restaurants. They are not. Recommended servings are of a fixed, standard quantity (*right*), while portion sizes are variable. However, North Americans tend to eat particularly large portions of food and as a consequence have high rates of obesity.

It is a good idea to start thinking of food portions in terms of these standard serving sizes because this will help you maintain a healthy weight and eat less if you are trying to lose weight.

FOOD GROUP	DAILY SERVINGS	WHAT IS ONE SERVING?
Bread, cereal, rice, and pasta	6–11 servings	• 1 slice whole-wheat bread • ½ small whole-grain bagel • 1 cup ready-to-eat bran cereal • ½ cup cooked oatmeal, brown rice, or pasta
Vegetables	3–5 servings	• 1 cup raw, leaf vegetables • ½ cup cooked vegetables • 6floz (180ml) vegetable juice
Fruit	2–4 servings	• 1 medium whole fresh fruit • 1 cup berries • ½ cup canned fruit in own juice • 6floz (180ml) fruit juice
Milk, yogurt, and cheese	2–3 servings	• 8floz (240ml) low-fat milk • 8floz (240 ml) low-fat yogurt • 8floz (240ml) cottage cheese • 1oz (28g) or 1 slice of cheese
Meat, poultry, fish, legumes, nuts, seeds, and eggs	2–3 servings	• 2–3oz (55–85g) cooked poultry, fish, or lean red meat • ½ cup cooked dried beans • 2 medium eggs • 2 tbsp peanut butter • 3 tbsp nuts or seeds

Five-a-day campaign

The Five-a-day for Better Health Program, which encourages the consumption of at least five servings of vegetables and fruits every day, was launched in 1991 by the National Cancer Institute. This was in response to evidence that diets high in these foods reduce the risk of developing certain cancers.

While the program has helped raise public awareness of the need to eat more of these valuable foods, less than than half of all North Americans are meeting the five-a-day goal. In any event, five-a-day is only a minimum target: the official daily recommendation is for three to five servings of vegetables and two to four servings of fruits, which should be selected from a variety of different types and colors of vegetables and fruits in order to maximize the potential health benefits.

Take five servings One apple, a 6floz-(180ml-) glass of carrot juice, a handful of strawberries, and some broccoli and beans—that is all it takes to meet the five-a-day minimum target for fruit and vegetable intake.

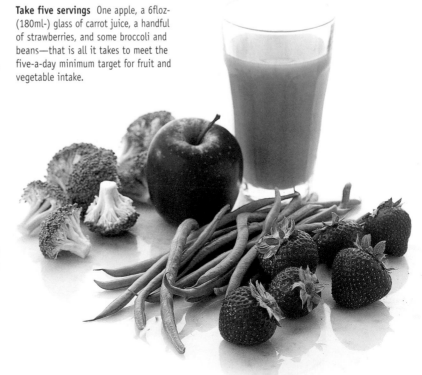

Wholesome grains

Choose whole rather than refined grains for optimum benefits.

Foods from the bread, cereal, rice, and pasta group are important sources of carbohydrates (*see pp.46–47*) and form the basis of your diet. Official guidelines recommend that you eat six to 11 servings from this group each day.

It is important to distinguish between whole and refined grains (*opposite*), and to make a point of choosing whole grains. Studies show that certain starchy foods may have a negative effect on

Whole-grain foods Rich in fiber, complex carbohydrates, and many other key nutrients, whole grains reduce the risk of many diseases.

health. For example, people whose diets consist primarily of potatoes, white rice, and foods made from refined (white) flour have higher rates of diabetes and cardiovascular disease than those who eat primarily from whole grains. Therefore, try to obtain most of your carbohydrates from whole-grain foods, such as whole-wheat bread, brown rice, and whole-wheat pasta, and limit the amount of refined products.

By including whole grains in your diet, you may lower your risk of cardiovascular disease because they are low in saturated fat and high in fiber, vitamins, minerals, and antioxidants. If you follow a vegetarian diet, whole grains are an important source of protein when they are combined with legumes or dairy products (*see p.100*).

The versatility of whole grains

Grains are a dietary staple in most cultures, and a look at other cuisines can provide inspiration for your own cooking. For example, long-grain rice is used as the basis of pilafs in Indian and Middle Eastern cuisine, while short-grain rice cooked in simmering broth produces the creamy risottos of Italy. These and other grains are now widely available, and you can be as creative as you like when cooking them.

WHICH GRAINS CAN I USE?

Grains can be eaten whole or processed into cold and hot cereals or flour for many food products, such as breads, muffins, and soups. In general, grains are a good source of vitamins and minerals, especially B vitamins and calcium, potassium, and phosphorus. Healthy grains to use include:

Whole wheat Used to make cereals and flour for bread, whole wheat can also be cooked as a cereal or used instead of rice. Whole wheat is packed

with B vitamins. Cracked wheat is wheat broken into small pieces for faster cooking. Bulgur wheat is partially cooked and dried before being cracked.

Oats These have more protein than most other grains. They are also high in soluble fiber, which helps eliminate cholesterol from the body. Whole oats (or groats) are the whole grain but with the hull removed. Rolled oats (or oatmeal) are whole oats steamed and then flattened between rollers.

Corn Rich in starch, corn can be eaten fresh, on or off the cob, or used as hominy—hulled and dried corn, which has neither the bran nor the germ. Ground hominy is known as grits, and cornmeal is made from dried kernels.

Barley Whole barley is nuttier and chewier than pearled barley (polished barley without the hull and bran) and must be soaked before cooking. In malted barley, the grain is allowed to begin sprouting; it is the main ingredient in beer and malt whisky.

Rye Similar to wheat in nutritional value, rye is frequently used with wheat in bread products. Rye is available in whole and cracked rye grains which can be cooked as cereal or ground into flour for baking.

Millet This grain contains nearly as much protein as wheat. It is available in whole and cracked forms and is usually stripped of its tough, inedible hull. It is used in cakes, cookies, bread puddings, and as a substitute for rice.

Quinoa An excellent source of protein, this grain can be substituted for, or added to, nearly any other grain and is particularly good in pilafs.

Brown rice Retaining both the bran and the germ of the rice kernel, brown rice is a source of protein, carbohydrates, and fiber. Brown rice may need to be cooked in more water than white rice and takes longer to cook (about twice as long).

Wild rice This has twice the protein of white rice and fewer calories. Use it in the same way as white or brown rice.

What are whole grains?

A whole grain is a grain that has not been processed. It consists of the bran, germ, and endosperm inside an inedible outer coating (hull). The bran forms a protective inner covering and is an excellent source of fiber (see pp.48–49). The germ is the embryo of a new plant, and is a source of protein, vitamins, and minerals; and it contains polyunsaturated fats.

The endosperm supplies most of the carbohydrates, mainly in the form of starch. When grains are processed, the hull, bran and germ are removed, leaving a product—such as white flour—that is deficient in protein, vitamins, and fiber. While some of these nutrients may be replaced and other important nutrients added to products, whole grains are undoubtedly the best choice.

Jargon buster

Refined grains These are whole grains that have been stripped of their outer coating, bran, and germ during the milling process, leaving only the endosperm to be ground into flour or other products.

Since 90 percent of the nutritional content of each grain is contained in the germ and bran, the refined product is deficient in many nutrients that are not only essential for good health but are known to provide protection against various diseases, including cardiovascular disease (see p.214), diabetes (see p.246), and some cancers (see p.258).

One of the most commonly used refined grains in North America is white flour, which is found in most commercially produced baked goods.

What is a serving?

Six to 11 daily servings are recommended from this food group, which includes bread, cereal, rice, and pasta. Suggested servings include:

- ½ cup cooked oatmeal
- 1 cup ready-to-eat cereal
- ½ whole-grain bagel
- 1 slice whole-wheat bread
- ½ English muffin
- 1 whole-wheat pancake
- ½ cup cooked brown rice
- ½ cup cooked wild rice
- ½ cup cooked pasta
- ½ cup cooked macaroni
- 1 medium tortilla
- ½ large baked sweet potato
- 1 cup mashed potatoes
- 1 cup cooked buckwheat noodles
- ½ cup cooked barley
- ½ cup cooked couscous
- ½ cup cooked quinoa
- 4 whole-grain crackers

Recipe Spicy whole-grain pilaf

INGREDIENTS

Serves 4

1 onion

2 garlic cloves

1 tsp cumin

1 tsp turmeric

1 cup whole-grain rice, uncooked

½ cup wild rice, uncooked

3 bell peppers

2 chili peppers

2 tbsp tomato purée

1 Slice the onion and crush the garlic. Sauté the cumin and turmeric for 2 minutes in a little vegetable oil. Add the onion and garlic and sauté for a further 2 minutes.

2 Add the two types of rice to the pan and mix with the onion and garlic. Add enough water or vegetable stock to cover the rice, and simmer for 20 minutes.

3 Remove the seeds from the peppers and slice lengthwise. Slice the chilis crosswise. Add to the pan with the tomato purée. Stir to combine then simmer for a further 5 minutes until the rice is tender and the peppers are softened.

4 Remove the pilaf to a serving dish. If you like, garnish with flaked almonds.

Variations Other grains may be substituted for the rice, and other vegetables, nuts, or diced chicken breast added.

Each serving provides

Calories 276, Total fat 1.7g (Sat. 0.3g, Poly. 0.7g, Mono. 0.5g), Cholesterol 0mg, Protein 7.6g, Carbohydrate 59g, Fiber 5.6g, Sodium 39mg; Good source of— Vits: A, Fol, C, K; Mins: Ca, Mg, P, K.

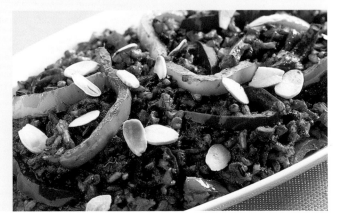

Vegetables for health

Improve your health by increasing your intake of vegetables.

According to official US dietary guidelines, you should eat three to five servings of vegetables daily. Very few people meet this target, and miss out on one of the most potent ways of improving health and preventing disease.

Vital nutrients
Vegetables are excellent sources of vitamins C (see p.56) and A (in the form of its precursor, beta-carotene, see p.52). Both vitamins help keep your skin and eyes healthy and your bones strong, and help fight infection. They work with other vitamins and minerals to keep muscles healthy.

In addition, vegetables are an excellent source of folate (see p.56), potassium (see p.63), and

fiber, which plays an important role in the diet: studies show a reduced incidence of cardiovascular disease in countries where a high-fiber diet is the norm.

Fiber also helps keep the intestinal tract in good working order and may help reduce the risk of colon cancer (see p.259). In addition, a high-fiber diet is often low in fat while providing a feeling of satiety, or fullness, without adding unnecessary calories. Because of this quality, fiber can play a vital role in weight control (see pp.48–49).

What is a serving?
Three to five servings each day are recommended from the vegetable group. Examples of vegetable servings include:
● 1 cup cooked carrots
● 1 cup cooked green beans
● 1 cup cooked spinach
● ½ cup cooked Brussels sprouts
● ½ cup cooked mushrooms
● 1 cup shredded lettuce
● ½ cup chopped tomatoes

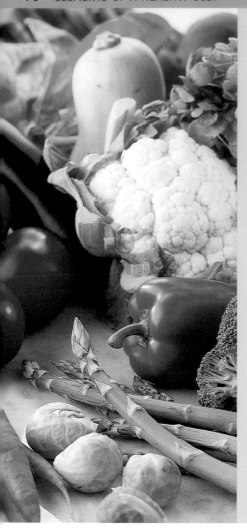

Naturally healthy Include a wide variety of vegetables in your daily diet to benefit from their potent, health-giving properties.

Increasing your vegetable intake

Vegetables are packed with vitamins and minerals and provide a great source of fiber (right), so try to eat at least three servings a day. This is not as hard as it may seem. Eat raw vegetables, such as bell peppers, celery, and lettuce, as often as possible, to benefit from their optimum nutritional content. Otherwise, you should use a cooking method that minimizes loss of nutrients (opposite above).

Always include a vegetable in your sandwich filling, and try dishes based on vegetables rather than meat. (See page 296 for a key to the abbreviations used for vitamins and minerals in the chart.)

VEGETABLE	SERVING	FIBER	VITAMINS/MINERALS
Artichoke	1 large	4.5	A, Fol / K
Broccoli	½ cup	2.8	A, Fol, C / Ca
Brussels sprouts	½ cup	3.8g	A, C / K
Carrots	½ cup	2.6g	A, Fol / K
Collard greens	½ cup	4.0g	A, Fol / Ca, Mg, K
Green beans	½ cup	0g	A, Fol / K
Green peas	½ cup	4.4g	A, Fol / K
Lima beans	½ cup	6.6g	Fol / Mg, K
Spinach	½ cup	2.7g	A, Fol / Ca, Mg, K, Fe
Zucchini squash	½ cup	3.0g	A / K

Super vegetables

Broccoli and other cruciferous vegetables, such as cauliflower, Brussels sprouts, and cabbage, are particularly beneficial for health. They contain phytochemicals (*see p.59*) and other nutrients that may help detoxify certain cancer-causing substances before they have a chance to cause harm in the body. These vegetables are also rich in fiber, beta-carotene, vitamins C and thiamine (B_1), calcium, potassium, and iron.

Tomatoes also have important health benefits. They are rich in lycopene, a carotenoid that helps to prevent cardiovascular disease and cancers. Lycopene is a fat-soluble substance that is absorbed best when cooked in oil. Tomatoes also contain the antioxidants beta-carotene, vitamin C, and vitamin E.

Carrots are a rich source of beta-carotene, which is a precursor of vitamin A. As an antioxidant, beta-carotene helps protect against cardiovascular disease and cancer.

Retaining the nutrients in vegetables

Vegetables are important sources of vitamins and minerals, but these delicate micronutrients are easily destroyed by heat. It is therefore best to eat at least some of your daily servings raw—for example, in salads or as snacks, such as baby carrots, celery sticks, or slices of cucumber or bell pepper.

When you do cook vegetables, the golden rule is to do so for the minimum amount of time and in as little liquid as possible, in order to retain their valuable nutrients. Suitable methods of cooking vegetables include steaming, stir-frying, sautéing, microwaving, and poaching (*see p.289*).

In addition to using healthy cooking methods, avoid adding saturated fat in the form of butter or cream sauces. If you think your vegetables need additional flavoring, add some fresh chopped herbs or freshly ground black pepper or lemon.

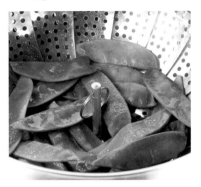

Steaming Since the vegetables are not immersed in water, this method retains the nutrients and taste of fresh vegetables.

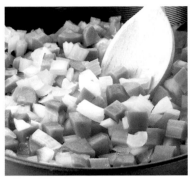

Sautéing Requiring very little oil, finely diced vegetables can be quickly fried in a large shallow pan over a high heat.

Recipe Crunchy vegetable stir-fry

INGREDIENTS

½ **cup basmati rice, uncooked**

1 **onion**

1 **garlic clove**

4 **stalks bok choy**

2 **bell peppers, one red, one yellow**

1½ **cups sliced mushrooms**

Serves 2

1 Steam the rice until the grains are tender.

2 Slice the onion, crush the garlic, and shred the bok choy. De-seed the bell peppers and cut them into strips that are ½in (1cm) wide.

3 Heat a little oil in a wok over high heat. Add the onion and garlic and stir-fry for 2 minutes. Add the peppers, mushrooms, and bok choy, and stir-fry for a further 4 minutes. Serve the stir-fried vegetables with the rice. If you like, accompany with ginger sauce (*right*).

Ginger Sauce In a small bowl, combine 2 tbsp cold water and 1 tbsp cornstarch. In a small pan, place 5½ tbsp white rice vinegar and 2 tbsp soy sauce. Bring to a boil. Reduce heat and add cornstarch mixture. Stir until mixture is clear and thickened. Remove from heat and stir in 1 tbsp minced ginger root. Set aside until required.

Each serving provides
Calories 246, Total fat 1.6g (Sat. 0.1g, Poly. 0.3g, Mono. 0g), Cholesterol 0mg, Protein 8.0g, Carbohydrate 54g, Fiber 7.0g, Sodium 27mg. Good source of— Vits: A, Fol, C, D; Mins: Ca, P, K.

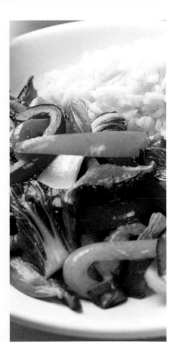

Fruits for health

These are easy to eat and packed with nutritional goodness.

Fruits—naturally sweet, colorful, high in vitamins and fiber, and low in calories and fat—are the ideal snack. Scientific research shows that a modest increase of one or two servings of fruit per day can dramatically reduce your susceptibility to many diseases.

Rich in antioxidants

Vitamin C and phytochemicals, including antioxidants, abound in fruit. Antioxidants destroy harmful substances in the body, called free radicals, which can build up and cause cancer. Of particular interest

are two types of phytochemicals—flavonoids and polyphenols—which together have a powerful antioxidant quality. In addition, other phytochemicals in fruit have been found to be antiallergenic, anticarcinogenic, antiviral, and anti-inflammatory (see p.59).

We truly do have a reason to say that an apple (or any fruit) a day keeps the doctor away.

What is a serving?

Two to four daily servings are recommended from the fruit group. Suggested servings include:
- 1 medium apple, pear, or orange.
- 1 cup raspberries or strawberries
- 15 grapes
- 2 dried figs or dates
- 6floz (180ml) 100 percent juice
- 2 tbsp raisins
- ½ grapefruit
- ½ large banana

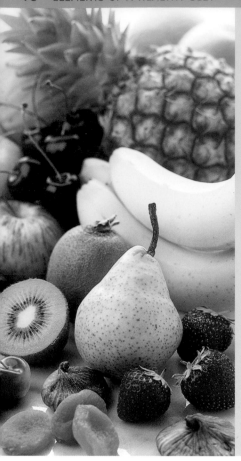

Nature's bounty Available in a huge array of colors, tastes, and textures, fruits are easy to eat and packed with healthy nutrients.

What is in fruits?

Packed with vitamins (see pp.52–58), beneficial phytochemicals (chemicals found in plants; see p.59), minerals (see pp.62–67), and fiber (see pp.48–49), fruits are an integral part of a healthy diet. They contain up to 80 percent water and are 100 percent cholesterol-free. Whether eaten with meals, as a snack, or on top of low-fat yogurt for dessert, eating fruits as often as possible throughout the day will help bolster the nutritive value of your diet.

The chart on the right gives several examples of the vitamin, mineral, and fiber content in commonly eaten fruits. Always bear in mind that it is better to eat fruit—preferably with the skin—rather than drink its juice in order to receive the maximum amount of fiber and nutritional benefits. (See page 296 for a key to the abbreviations used for vitamins and minerals in the chart.)

FRUIT	SERVING	FIBER	VITAMINS/MINERALS
Apple, with skin	1 medium	3.0g	A, Fol, C, Vit K / Ca, Mg, K, Na
Apricot, dried	4 halves	3.4g	A, Vit K / Ca, Mg, P
Blackberries	½ cup	4.0g	A, C, Vit K / Ca, Mg, P, Fe
Blueberries	½ cup	2.4g	A, Fol, C, Vit K / Ca, Mg, P, K
Dates	6 dates	3.6g	A / Ca, Mg, K
Figs	2 figs	4.6g	A / Ca, Mg, P
Peach	1 medium	2.0g	A, Fol, C / Ca, Mg, P, K
Orange	1 medium	3.0g	A, Fol, C, Vit K / K
Pear, with skin	1 medium	3.0g	A, Fol, C, Vit K / Ca, Mg, P, K
Prunes	3 pitted	2.0g	A, Vit K / Ca, Mg, P, Fe
Raisins	3 tbsp	3.0g	A, Fol, C / Mg, P
Raspberries	½ cup	4.2g	A, Fol, C, Vit K / Ca, Mg
Strawberries	1 cup	2.8g	A, C, Vit K / Ca, Mg, P

How to increase your fruit intake

Fruits are ideal snacks. They are delicious, healthy and require little or no preparation, and it is easy to take an apple, orange, or banana with you to work or when you go out for the day.

You should have no problem getting your daily two to four servings of fruits in this way, once you get into the habit of having a good selection available at home and at work. In addition to eating familiar types of fruits, be adventurous and try some of the more exotic and unusual varieties available from your supermarket, such as mangoes, loquats, figs, and lychees.

ADDING FRUITS TO YOUR MEALS

Fruits can be incorporated easily into your main meals of the day—breakfast, lunch, and dinner—in a variety of interesting ways. Try some of the following suggestions.

Breakfast In the morning, liven up your whole-grain cereal by topping it with a chopped apple, a sliced peach, or a handful of raisins. Or have a bowl of strawberries, raspberries, fresh pineapple, or melon chunks topped with low-fat yogurt. You can also drink a glass of 100 percent fruit juice, such as orange or grapefruit juice.

Lunch To spice up a garden salad, you can try adding fresh fruits, such as peaches and/or orange sections. Alternatively, instead of a sandwich with a meat or fish filling for your lunch, you can make a banana and walnut sandwich. You could make a fresh fruit smoothie (*see p.81*) or finish your lunch with a fruit salad.

Dinner Start with a slice of melon, then try an exotic combination, such as grilled chicken with mango and melon. Finish with a fruit dessert, such as mango sorbet or a baked apple.

Dried fruits

You can buy dried fruits from stores or dry them at home in special fruit dehydrators. During dehydration, most of the nutrients are concentrated in the remaining solids. In this way, dried fruits have more nutrients— and more calories—by weight than fresh fruits. Some light fruits, such as apples, apricots, peaches, pears, and golden raisins, are treated with sulfur dioxide to prevent discoloration and to help preserve nutrients. Some people with asthma (*see p.225*) or allergies (*see pp.252–255*) are sensitive to sulfur dioxide and should be cautious when eating treated dried fruit or choose nonsulfured fruits.

Dried fruits are good as snacks. Soaked or cooked, they can be used to top hot or cold breakfast cereals, make compotes and stuffings, or be added to baked goods.

Benefits of different fruits

Fruits are rich in vitamins and minerals, especially vitamins A and C, potassium, and fiber. Eat a variety to reap their individual nutritional benefits.

Apples The skin of this refreshing fruit is an excellent source of fiber. An apple has about 75 calories.

Apricots Due to a short life span once picked, most apricots are dried or canned. Half of an apricot has 9 calories.

Bananas Technically an herb and not a fruit, half of a banana has 60 calories and is loaded with vitamins and minerals.

Blueberries These delicious fruits are rich in antioxidants and help prevent urinary tract infections. One cup of blueberries has roughly 80 calories.

Cantaloupe This is incredibly rich in a form of carotene (vitamin A precursor) that is known to fight cancer. Half of a cantaloupe has 55 calories.

Grapes One cup has 90 calories with vitamins A and C and minerals.

Kiwifruit You can eat the skin of a kiwifruit, but you may prefer it without. 1oz (28g) of kiwi has 22 calories and a range of vitamins.

Peaches A medium-sized peach has about 40 calories and vitamins A, C, and D, and potassium.

Pears These should be picked unripe and allowed to ripen in a paper bag. One medium pear has about 100 calories.

Pineapple This fruit contains a potent enzyme, bromelain, that has been used to aid digestion, reduce inflammation, and help cardiovascular disease. One cup of chopped pineapple has 75 calories.

Plums An average-sized plum has 32 calories and is a good source of vitamins A and C, and potassium.

Raisins This dried fruit packs a nutritional punch. Raisins are a good source of energy but are rich in sugar.

Raspberries There are nearly 1,000 varieties of raspberries. They are very perishable and therefore expensive. They provide 60 calories per cup.

Watermelon One cup has 50 calories and a lot of vitamins and minerals.

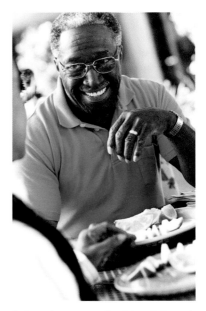

Fruits make great snacks Cut-up fruits, such as apples, oranges, melon, and pineapple, make a tasty, quick-to-prepare snack that is rich in fiber and beneficial nutrients, such as vitamins, minerals, and phytochemicals.

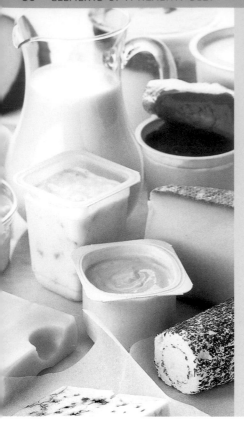

The benefits of dairy

Dairy products are nutritious—but avoid the full-fat options.

Milk and its products are excellent sources of protein, vitamins, and minerals—most particularly of calcium, which is essential for healthy bones and teeth (*see p.62*).

The varieties of milk
Although cow's milk is the most commonly used in North America, sheep and goat's is available too, as

Milk and milk products These are prime sources of calcium, and there are many low-fat and/or fat-free options to choose from.

are plant-based substitutes such as soymilk and oat milk. Cow's milk is processed in a variety of ways to create products that vary in their nutritional content and storage capability. Fat content is one of the most important distinctions, which varies from that of whole milk (containing no less than 3.25 percent milk fat) through low-fat, to fat-free forms.

Since products based on whole milk are high in saturated fat and cholesterol (*see p.40*), you should limit your intake. You can still reap their benefits, however, by choosing low-fat or fat-free varieties, which contain all the important nutrients of whole milk without its harmful saturated-fat content.

Tips on increasing your dairy intake

If you suspect that your diet does not include enough dairy products, here are some suggestions for increasing your intake. Remember to choose low-fat or fat-free varieties so that you do not increase your intake of unhealthy saturated fats.

Breakfast Get your day off to a good start with any of the following:
• Cereal served with low-fat milk.
• Fresh or dried fruit topped with low-fat yogurt.
• Oatmeal prepared with low-fat milk instead of water.
• Fruit smoothie, made with low-fat or fat-free milk or yogurt (*opposite*).

Lunch For a healthy addition to your midday meal:
• Have a glass of chocolate-flavored low-fat milk instead of a soda.
• Grab a whole-grain sandwich with low-fat Havarti cheese.
• Make a mini-pizza, topped with part-skim mozzarella, tomatoes, and fresh broccoli or mixed bell peppers.

• Eat low-fat or fat-free cottage cheese with sliced peaches or pears on top.
• Have a grilled-cheese sandwich made with fat-free American cheese slices.
• Try making a quesadilla with reduced-fat Monterey Jack or Jalapeno Jack cheese with grilled peppers and onions.

Dinner The main meal of the day provides an opportunity to add more dairy products to your diet:
• Sprinkle shredded, low-fat cheese over your salad or soup.
• Make macaroni and cheese, using low-fat or fat-free milk for the sauce.
• Have a baked sweet potato with cottage-cheese topping and broccoli.

Snack Try one of these nutritious options for a change:
• Low-fat yogurt with fresh or dried fruit.
• Low-fat frozen yogurt.
• Make your favorite pudding with low-fat or fat-free milk.
• Eat reduced-fat string cheese with a handful of dried fruit, such as raisins, prunes, or apricots.

Adapting to low-fat dairy products

If you are used to full-fat dairy products, make a gradual transition to low-fat or fat-free varieties.
• Start by mixing 50 percent whole milk and 50 percent low-fat milk. When you are used to this, gradually reduce the whole milk and increase the low-fat content.
• When you are used to low-fat milk, repeat the process with a low-fat and fat-free milk until you are drinking only fat-free milk.
• Use yogurt or evaporated fat-free milk instead of cream when making soups and sauces.
• Substitute fat-free yogurt or fat-free sour cream for regular sour cream in your favorite recipes.
• When cooking Italian dishes, such as lasagna, choose a low-fat or fat-free cheese for the sauce and for sprinkling on top.

Special milks are available for people with specific dietary needs, such as lactose intolerance (*see p.232*), while milk fortified with vitamins A and D ensures adequate intake of these important vitamins.

Milk is also available in dried, evaporated, and condensed forms, which are useful for cooking.

Milk products

Cheese is milk in concentrated form, which is why this is such a great source of the important nutrients found in milk. It is also the reason why cheese has such a high saturated-fat content. As with milk, the solution is to opt for reduced-fat varieties, which contain the vital nutrients while limiting unhealthy saturated fat.

Yogurt is another milk product. Made from milk that has been treated with a bacterial culture, it is available in many different types. Again, choose reduced-fat types.

Yogurt is also rich in protein and riboflavin (B_2) and contains active cultures that are very healthy for your intestines.

The importance of calcium

It is difficult to over-emphasize the need to maintain calcium levels throughout life. Each year in the US, 1.5 million bone fractures are attributed to osteoporosis (*see p.242*), a disease that may be caused by inadequate calcium intake. Women, particularly, are affected since they have less bone mass than men to begin with and lose it faster as they get older, especially after menopause. Restricting your intake of dairy products as part of a weight-loss program is therefore not advisable for women.

Remember that your body needs an adequate supply of calcium throughout life. If you do not get enough, your body will draw it from its reserves in your bones.

What is a serving?

One to three daily servings are recommended from this group, which includes milk, cheese, yogurt, and other milk products. The following are examples of individual servings:
- 8floz (240ml) reduced fat (2 percent), low-fat (1 percent), or fat free milk
- 8floz (240ml) lactose-reduced low-fat milk
- 1oz (28g) part-skim mozzarella
- 4floz (120ml) low-fat cottage cheese
- 8floz (240ml) enriched soymilk
- 1 cup vanilla ice cream
- 1 cup low-fat frozen yogurt
- 8floz (240ml) low-fat fruited yogurt
- 1 cup low-fat pudding made with low-fat milk
- 8floz (240ml) fruit smoothie
- 1oz (28g) low-fat farmer's cheese

Children's needs for calcium

Calcium is an essential nutrient for children. Official recommendations (Dietary Reference Intakes) are 500mg of calcium per day for 1–3 year olds; 800mg per day for 4–8 year olds; and 1,300mg per day for 9–18 year olds. Children also need 0.004mg of vitamin D per day to help the body process calcium. Many children in North America do not meet these targets, increasing their risk of osteoporosis when older.

Look for imaginative and appealing ways of offering low-fat dairy products to children and adolescents. For example:
- Encourage them to drink more milk, eat more yogurt, select milk over other drinks, and make their own milkshakes.
- Let them choose ice creams and yogurts when you go shopping, while you keep an eye on the fat content.
- Include individual cheese portions in their lunch boxes.
- Offer part-skim cheese sticks as snacks.

Recipe Calcium-rich fruit smoothie

INGREDIENTS
8 strawberries, hulled
1 cup orange sections
4floz (120ml) low-fat milk
4floz (120ml) low-fat yogurt
3 tbsp honey
2 tsp vanilla extract
6 ice cubes

Serves 2

1 Place the strawberries, orange, milk, yogurt, honey, vanilla, and ice cubes in a food processor or blender.

2 Blend until the mixture is smooth and creamy.

Variations Experiment with other fruits such as raspberries, melon, peaches, and bananas.

Each serving provides
Calories 225, Total fat 2.0g (Sat. 1.0g, Poly. 0.1g, Mono. 0.5g), Cholesterol 6.2mg, Protein 6g, Carbohydrate 47g, Fiber 3.0g, Sodium 76mg. Good source of— Vits: A, Fol, C, D; Mins: Ca, Mg, P, K.

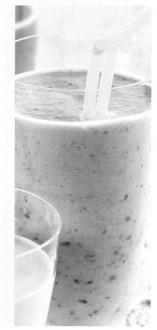

Choosing the right milk

Most milk consumed in North America is cow's milk. However, other milks are available as healthy alternatives.

Cow's milk Whole milk contains 8g of fat per 8floz (240ml) serving and 150 calories, compared to less than 0.5g and 86 calories in fat-free milk (*below right*). Calcium content is consistent in all varieties. All cow's milk is fortified with vitamins A and D.

Goat's milk With slightly less lactose than cow's milk, goats' milk also contains more vitamins A, niacin (B$_3$), and B$_6$, and calcium, potassium, copper, and selenium. However, goat's milk is higher in fat, and it is harder to find low-fat varieties and products.

Sheep's milk Rich in protein, fat, and minerals, sheep's milk is not available commercially for drinking. It is most often found in cheese and yogurt.

Soymilk Good for lactose-intolerant people as it does not contain any lactose or casein. One 8floz (240ml) serving contains almost 7g of protein, 5g of fat, no cholesterol, and has 80 calories. It is not a good source of calcium or vitamin B$_{12}$, so choose a fortified variety.

Rice milk This is a good substitute for low-fat and fat-free cow's milk, and is 100 percent lactose- and fat-free.

Oat milk Lactose- and cholesterol-free, and low in fat. Choose varieties fortified with calcium and vitamin D.

Almond milk Lactose-free and low in fat, this is also very low in sugar.

Complete food Milk is an ideal drink for children, providing protein, carbohydrate, and micronutrients—especially calcium. Cow's milk is fortified with vitamins A and D.

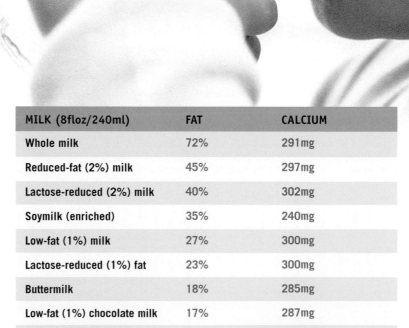

How milk is processed

To make milk safe for human consumption and more palatable, it is processed in various ways.

Pasteurization By heating milk, harmful bacteria and enzymes are destroyed, without affecting taste.

UHT After being sterilized by this ultra-high temperature process, milk can be stored unrefrigerated.

Homogenization This process breaks down and distributes cream (fat globules) throughout the milk.

Evaporation After removing 60 percent of the water, the milk concentrate is canned.

Condensation Up to half the water is removed and sugar is added to preserve the milk without heating.

MILK (8floz/240ml)	FAT	CALCIUM
Whole milk	72%	291mg
Reduced-fat (2%) milk	45%	297mg
Lactose-reduced (2%) milk	40%	302mg
Soymilk (enriched)	35%	240mg
Low-fat (1%) milk	27%	300mg
Lactose-reduced (1%) fat	23%	300mg
Buttermilk	18%	285mg
Low-fat (1%) chocolate milk	17%	287mg
Lactose-reduced fat-free milk	0%	312mg
Fat-free milk	0%	302mg

Which cheese?

Cheese is usually made from cow's, goat's, or sheep's milk. The milk is heated with the enzyme renin to separate the curds, which are collected, pressed, and may be salted or cured. Curing develops the flavor and texture of the cheese. The longer a cheese is cured, the harder the texture and the stronger the flavor. Since cheese is made from milk, they are similar in nutritive value. However, many cheeses are high in sodium and fat. Cheese made from fat-free (skim) milk is not always low in fats because extra cream may be added. The more water a cheese contains, the lower its percentage of fat. It is best to choose low-fat or fat-free varieties. The caloric, fat, and calcium content of several cheeses are shown below.

CHEESE (1oz/28g)	CALORIES	FAT	% SATURATED FAT	CALCIUM
Roquefort	105	75%	47%	188mg
Brie	95	75%	47%	52mg
Camembert	85	73%	46%	110mg
Feta (full-fat)	75	72%	51%	172mg
Goat	128	71%	49%	254mg
Ricotta (full-fat)	49	68%	43%	64mg
Parmesan	129	59%	38%	336mg
Mozzarella (part-skim)	72	56%	36%	183mg
Ricotta (part-skim)	40	50%	32%	84mg

Other dairy products

There are several other dairy products widely available in supermarkets. Common products include:

Buttermilk Made from pasteurized or partially skimmed milk, buttermilk is cultured with bacteria to make it thicker. It has about the same nutritive value and fat content as low-fat milk.

Sweet creams About 90–100 percent of the calories in sweet creams are from fat. If you use half-and-half or "lite" cream in coffee, try low-fat or fat-free milk instead, to reduce your fat intake. Heavy cream contains 50 calories per tablespoon and 61 percent of them are saturated fat. A healthier option is low-fat, nondairy whipped cream.

Sour cream This cream is cultured with bacteria and may contain enzymes and additives. It contains 26 calories per tablespoon with 50 percent from saturated fat. Choose fat-free varieties.

Yogurt With all the nutritive value of milk, yogurt is easier to digest and beneficial for the digestive tract. It may be made from whole, low-fat, or fat-free milk that is cultured with bacteria. It may have sugar, artificial sweeteners, flavorings, or fruit added. Try to choose "sugar-free" varieties.

Frozen desserts 30–50 percent of the calories of ice cream are from saturated fat. Frozen yogurt has less saturated fat but more sugar, so they have about the same amount of calories. Water ice and sorbet (or sherbet) tend to be lower in calories than ice cream, and are therefore the best choice for dessert, but some have milk powder added.

Jargon buster

Lactose intolerance This is the inability to digest lactose, the sugar naturally found in animal milk. The symptoms, which develop after consuming milk products, include abdominal bloating and cramping, diarrhea, and vomiting (*see p.232*).

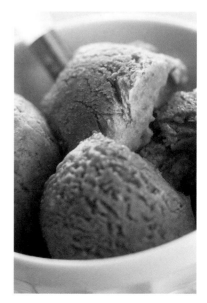

Frozen yogurt A refreshing alternative to ice cream, frozen yogurt is available in low-fat and fat-free varieties as well as in many flavors.

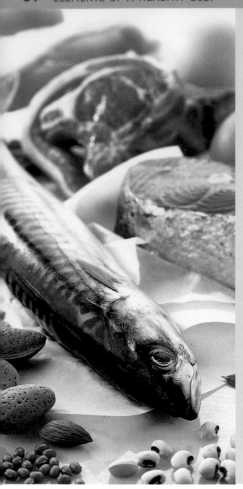

Healthy protein sources

Protein deficiency is rare, so the focus is now on fat content.

Protein is an essential nutrient that we must obtain from food every day, as it is not stored by the body. Deficiency is rare in North America, since protein is readily available.

For most Americans, protein is regarded as the basis of at least one meal a day, and this is usually more than enough to meet the recommended daily requirements.

For vegetarians, meat is not an option and they look to plant sources for their daily protein. Here, too, there is a wide variety

to choose from, including all the different types of legumes (peas, beans, and lentils), as well as a huge variety of nuts and seeds. Unlike animal protein, most plant sources do not contain all the amino acids that make up protein, and they have to be combined to form complete protein (see p.45). One of the exceptions is soy, which not only contains twice as much protein as other legumes, but has nearly as many amino acids as animal proteins (see p.93).

Protein is also found in milk, cheese, and bread, as well as in the foods described here.

Choosing animal proteins

Animal sources of protein include meat, poultry, fish, and shellfish, as well as animal products such as eggs. Each of these can be further classified according to the type and amount of fat they contain.

Body-building essentials Your body needs protein for growth and repair: the healthiest sources include low-fat options such as fish, white-meat poultry, and legumes.

How much protein do you need?

Protein is essential for muscle and tissue repair, muscle growth, and regulation of metabolism. The amount you need to eat depends on your body weight (*right*) and your health.

When you are sick or under stress, your body needs more protein as it uses energy to fight off what ails you. Your immune system depends on a constant supply of amino acids—the building blocks of protein. If you do not take in enough calories and proteins, you risk malnutrition and muscle wasting.

During pregnancy, the Recommended Daily Allowance (RDA) increases by 30g per day and 20g per day when breast-feeding. Children need more protein than adults for growth. They need about 2.2g of protein per 2.2lb (1kg) of body weight every day in the first 6 months of

life, and 2g per 2.2lb (1kg) for the next 6 months. A child's RDA then gradually decreases throughout childhood and teenage years, until age 18, when it becomes 0.8g per 2.2lb (1kg) per day.

The protein needs for athletes vary according to body weight and the type of activity (*see p.147*). Most athletes eat more protein than they need, believing it will help increase their muscle mass. But protein consumed in excess is either used as energy when carbohydrate and calorie intake is low or converted to fat.

Most people in the West eat far more protein than they need; deficiency is very rare. Some diets suggest eating extra protein to aid weight loss. Excess protein, however, has been linked with osteoporosis, kidney disease, and calcium stones in the kidneys.

How to calculate your daily protein needs

The government Recommended Daily Allowance (RDA) for dietary protein is calculated on ideal body weight (the average for your height and gender).

Adults need to eat 0.8g of protein per 2.2lb (1kg) of body weight each day. Therefore, a man who weighs 180lb (82kg) needs to consume about 65g of protein each day; and a woman who weighs 150lb (68kg) needs an intake of about 55g of protein each day.

However, growing children and adolescents and pregnant women require an increased amount of protein in their diet, *see left*.

For example, red meats, such as beef, lamb, pork, and veal, are excellent sources of high-quality protein, but they also contain high levels of saturated fats and may raise blood levels of "bad" LDL-cholesterol (*see p.23*). Because of the link between high dietary intake of saturated fat and the increased risk of cardiovascular disease and other disorders, we strongly advise that you reduce your dietary intake of red meat in favor of fish, white-meat poultry, legumes, and other plant proteins.

Poultry is another good source of protein, but it varies in fat and cholesterol content depending on which parts of the bird are eaten and how it is prepared and served (*see pp.88–89*).

The benefits of eating fish
Fish is now regarded as one of the healthiest sources of animal protein (*see pp.90–91*). Oily fish, such as salmon and tuna, are highly recommended since they are rich in omega-3 fatty acids, which help reduce the risk of developing cardiovascular disease (*see p.214*).

Shellfish are also a good source of protein, in addition to being low in total fat.

Eggs and protein
These are a good source of complete protein as well as other essential nutrients (*see p.95*). Since one egg contains about 210mg of cholesterol (mainly in the yolk), the American Heart Association recommends keeping track of how many eggs you eat and limiting egg yolks.

Plant-based proteins
Collectively known as legumes, peas, beans, and lentils are an important source of protein (*see pp.92–94*). Legumes are low in sodium and saturated fat and contain no cholesterol.

Nuts and seeds are also good sources of protein, and supply a useful range of vitamins, minerals, and healthy monounsaturated and polyunsaturated fats (*see p.94*).

All plant proteins also have a high soluble-fiber content, which helps reduce blood cholesterol levels (*see p.217*) and prevent constipation (*see p.229*).

What is a serving?
Two to three servings of protein sources are recommended per day, from foods of both plant and animal origin. Suggested servings include (meat and fish weights given are uncooked):
- $3\frac{1}{2}$oz (100g) red meat
- $3\frac{1}{2}$oz (100g) pork loin
- $3\frac{1}{2}$oz (100g) chicken breast
- $\frac{1}{2}$ cup chopped tofu
- $3\frac{1}{2}$oz (100g) turkey breast
- $3\frac{1}{2}$oz (100g) salmon (sockeye)
- $3\frac{1}{2}$oz (100g) sardines
- $3\frac{1}{2}$oz (100g) sea trout
- $3\frac{1}{2}$oz (100g) tuna
- $3\frac{1}{2}$oz (100g) shrimp, peeled
- $3\frac{1}{2}$oz (100g) lobster tail
- $3\frac{1}{2}$oz (100g) crab
- 2 medium eggs
- $\frac{1}{2}$ cup soybeans, cooked
- $\frac{1}{2}$ cup lentils, cooked
- $\frac{1}{2}$ cup lima beans, cooked
- $\frac{1}{2}$ cup kidney beans, cooked
- 3 tbsp sunflower seeds
- 3 tbsp macadamia nuts
- 3 tbsp almonds
- 4floz (120ml) low-fat cottage cheese

Choosing low-fat proteins

There are two key benefits in choosing low-fat protein foods regularly instead of high-fat types:
- When you choose a lean, protein-rich animal protein (such as fish), you will get a higher concentration of protein, weight for weight, than its higher-fat counterpart such as beef steak.
- These choices are integral for a heart-healthy diet for the rest of your life. High-fat animal proteins are associated with an increase in blood cholesterol levels and the risk of cardiovascular diseases. They should be eaten only in limited quantities.

Low-fat protein sources include low-fat or fat-free dairy products, low-fat soy-protein foods, poultry without skin, egg whites instead of whole eggs, and plenty of fish and shellfish.

FOOD	FAT	% SATURATED FAT
Almonds	80%	8%
Eggs	60%	21%
Salmon	46%	8%
Soybeans	45%	7%
Beef (sirloin)	42%	16%
Pork loin	26%	9%
Turkey breast (no skin)	18%	6%
Low-fat (1%) cottage cheese	11%	8%
Shrimp	10%	2.7%
Lentils	4%	1%

Red meat: good or bad?

Protein-rich, but also high in saturated fat, red meat should be eaten sparingly.

Red meat, which includes beef, lamb, veal, and pork, is an excellent source of protein in the diet. It is also a major source of unhealthy saturated fat (see pp.40–41).

US official dietary guidelines recommend that you should eat at least two servings (2–3oz/55–85g each—cooked weight) from the protein group on a daily basis. Many people, however, eat a great deal more meat than this, and medical studies show that people who eat red meat on a daily basis have a higher incidence of cardiovascular disease than those who eat it less often.

The relationship between red meat and cardiovascular disease is believed to be due to the high saturated fat and cholesterol content of these meats. There is also evidence to suggest that a high intake of red meat may significantly increase your risk of colon cancer. Not surprisingly, people who replace red meat with fish and chicken have been found to have lowered their risk of cardiovascular disease and colon cancer. For these reasons, we strongly recommend that you choose to eat healthier sources of protein.

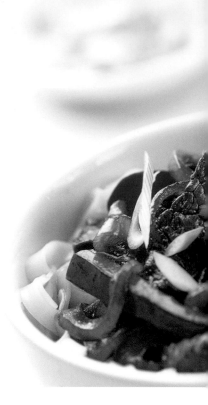

Which meat should I choose?

Whether it is a dinner at a steakhouse or a barbecue at home, when you are trying to cut back on calories and fat, red meat can pose difficult decisions. If you stick with traditional favorites like burgers or beef steak, start by choosing cuts that have a very low fat content (right), and reserve higher-fat cuts of meat (like most steak) for special occasions (once or twice a month). Remember to trim off the visible fat before eating the meat.

Be sure to read food labels in the supermarket and choose cuts with the lowest fat content as often as possible. The leanest types of red meat are round steak, super-lean ground beef (7–10 percent fat), pork tenderloin, buffalo (read label for fat content), and most wild game such as elk or venison. You do not have to avoid all red meat. In fact, 4oz (115g) of very lean red meat (such as filet mignon or flank steak), has a much lower fat and calorie content than the same quantity of roasted dark-meat chicken with skin.

MEAT	FAT	% SATURATED FAT
Sausage (beef)	80%	33%
Ground beef (extra lean)	58%	23%
Spare ribs	52%	22%
Lamb ribs	48%	22%
Flank steak (lean)	44%	19%
Sirloin steak	42%	16%
Filet mignon	42%	16%
Canadian bacon (ham)	41%	14%
Veal chop (lean)	39%	17%
Round steak	29%	11%
Liver (beef)	27%	11%
Pork loin	26%	9%
Venison	18%	8%

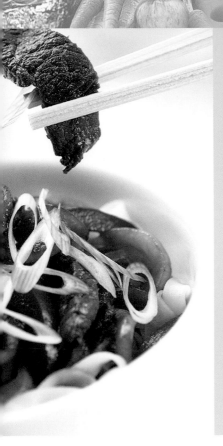

Other types of meats

Wild game such as buffalo, venison, elk, or boar, tend to have the same levels of cholesterol as other red meats, but, because these animals get more exercise, their meat is lower in fat and calories. As with all red meats, they, too, should be eaten in moderation.

Kidneys, liver, tongue, and tripe are high in cholesterol but are a good source of many B vitamins, in addition to vitamins A, D, and E, and the minerals copper, iron, and zinc. Liver, however, accumulates chemical residues from the animal, so we suggest that you eat the liver of only young animals, such as calves, and that you limit it to once a week.

Beef stir-fry Slivers of tender steak, quickly stir-fried with finely cut red bell peppers and scallions, offer a quick-and-easy, economical, and healthy low-fat meal.

You should try to avoid too many processed meat products such as pork and beef sausages, deli meats, and bacon because they contain preservatives that have been linked to cancer. Instead, you should choose soy alternatives or uncured varieties that are free of preservatives and lower in fat.

What is a serving?

While two to three servings from the protein group each day are recommended, we advise that red meat should be eaten no more than once a week and that you choose lean cuts. Servings include:

- 3½oz (100g) ground beef
- 3½oz (100g) pork loin
- 3½oz (100g) round steak
- 3½oz (100g) filet mignon
- 3½oz (100g) sirloin steak
- 3½oz (100g) flank steak
- 3½oz (100g) venison

Healthy ways with red meat

If you are reluctant to eliminate red meat from your diet completely, the solution is to eat it less often and to select lean cuts, such as filet mignon and pork loin.

You can also help minimize the fat content of meat by adopting healthy preparation and cooking methods (see p.289). For example:

- Trim off all visible fat from the meat, place it on a rack, then grill, bake, or broil it. Excess fat will drip down into the pan and can be discarded.
- Use only a light spray or brush of oil before cooking.
- Try stir-fried dishes with vegetables, where a small amount of meat, cut up into tiny strips, goes a long way.
- Cut down on portion sizes of meat, and fill up instead with extra helpings of vegetables and salads.
- When eating out, order small portions or share larger ones.

Recipe Low-fat game burgers

INGREDIENTS
1 onion
1 small carrot
12oz (340g) ground venison
¼ cup bulgar wheat, soaked then drained
4 tbsp chopped flat-leaf parsley
1 egg white
sprinkling of black pepper
sunflower oil

Makes 4

1 Chop the onion and grate the carrot. Mix all ingredients except oil in a large bowl. Cover and refrigerate for 1 hour.

2 Form mixture into four burgers, each 1in (2.5cm) thick. Heat broiler. Brush each burger with oil then broil for 5–8 minutes on each side until brown.

Each serving provides

Calories 477, Total fat 6.7g (Sat. 1.4g, Poly. 1.0g, Mono. 3.7g), Cholesterol 74mg, Protein 31g, Carbohydrate 75g, Fiber 15g, Sodium 79mg. Good source of—Vits: A, Fol, C, K; Mins: Ca, Mg, P, Se.

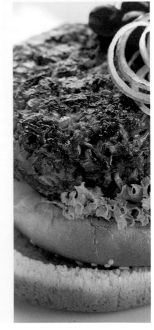

Poultry for protein

White-meat chicken and turkey are ideal protein sources.

While chicken, turkey, and other poultry are healthier than red meat in terms of saturated-fat content, there are significant differences according to which bird is chosen, which part is eaten, and how it is prepared and cooked. For example, turkey breast (no skin) contains 18 percent fat, while chicken breast (no skin) contains 24 percent fat.

The fat and calorie content of both turkey and chicken is much higher when the dark meat—the wings and thighs—and the skin are eaten (*opposite*).

To minimize the saturated fat content of poultry, grill, bake, or broil the meat and remove the skin before serving. There is no advantage in removing the skin before cooking: the skin helps the meat remain moist and does not add significantly to the saturated fat content of the finished dish. In terms of saturated fat content, manufactured turkey and chicken products, such as sausages, hot dogs, and burgers, are not much healthier than those made from red meat. However, if you are particularly fond of hot dogs and sausages, look for lower-fat and soy-based versions, which are good alternatives. If you like to make your own burgers, try using ground turkey breast instead of red meat: the result is much healthier (*opposite*).

Less common varieties

In addition to chicken and turkey, poultry includes other birds such as duck, goose, quail, pheasant, partridge, and guinea fowl, some of which are healthier than others depending on the parts of the bird and if you eat the skin.

Dark meat (including the wings, legs, and thighs) is higher in fat and cholesterol than white meat (the breast). It is important to cook game birds thoroughly to kill any bacteria such as salmonella.

What is a serving?

Two to three servings daily are recommended from the protein group. Poultry makes a good choice, particularly chicken and turkey breast, both of which are low in saturated fat.

- 3½oz (100g) chicken breast
- 3½oz (100g) chicken nuggets
- 3½oz (100g) dark-meat chicken
- 3½oz (100g) turkey hot dog
- 3½oz (100g) dark-meat turkey
- 3½oz (100g) turkey burger
- 3½oz (100g) white-meat turkey breast
- 3½oz (100g) duck breast, no skin
- 3½oz (100g) goose, no skin
- 3oz (88g) pheasant, no skin
- 3½oz (100g) guinea fowl
- 3½oz (100g) Cornish game hen

Choosing chicken White-meat chicken is an excellent source of low-fat protein. For a nutritious meal, broil skewered chicken breasts, stuffed with "lite" ricotta cheese.

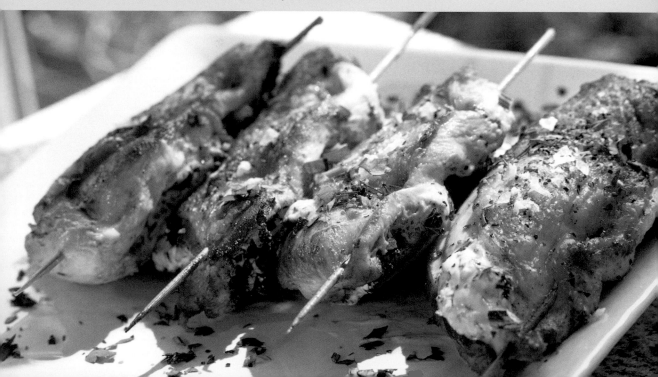

Which poultry should I choose?

Regarding fat content, it is important to keep in mind that all poultry are not created equal. White meat from chicken and turkey has a similar calorie and saturated fat content (*right*), but duck and goose meat are very fatty, one of the reasons they are so delicious when roasted. Ostrich, quail, and pheasant are lowest in fat, cholesterol, and calories, and they all have roughly an equivalent amount of protein per 3½oz (100g) serving.

Of concern to many people are the growth hormones and antibiotics given to birds to hasten their growth and immunize them against the diseases that come with being raised in close quarters. In response to public concern, the poultry industry has cut back on the amount of antibiotics used, but there is no scientific consensus on any harmful effects of eating treated birds. If you want to be cautious and avoid these chemicals, you may want to buy free-range or organic poultry.

POULTRY	FAT	% SATURATED FAT
Turkey hot dog	70%	19%
Cornish game meat (with skin)	63%	28%
Chicken dark meat (with skin)	56%	16%
Duck (with skin)`	50%	19%
Turkey sausage	50%	15%
Goose (no skin)	48%	17%
Turkey dark meat (with skin)	47%	14%
Chicken dark meat (no skin)	43%	12%
Turkey breast (with skin)	38%	5%
Chicken breast (with skin)	36%	10%
Chicken breast (no skin)	24%	7%
Guinea fowl (with skin)	21%	10%
Turkey breast (no skin)	18%	6%

Recipe Low-fat turkey wrap

INGREDIENTS

1lb (450g) turkey breast

1 tbsp dark soy sauce

1 tsp grated fresh root ginger

1 tbsp chopped fresh cilantro

½ tsp sea salt

sprinkling of black pepper

whole-wheat flour, seasoned

olive oil

Serves 4

1 Remove the skin from the turkey breast and mince or chop very finely.

2 In a large bowl, combine the turkey breast, soy sauce, ginger, cilantro, salt, and freshly ground black pepper. Mix thoroughly and then set aside for a few minutes.

3 Shape the mixture into four patties, each about 1in (2.5cm) thick. Toss each patty in the seasoned flour to coat.

4 Heat a little olive oil in a frying pan and fry the patties for 3–4 minutes on each side until they are cooked through. Alternatively, brush each patty

with olive oil and grill or broil, or bake in a moderately hot oven until they are well cooked through, turning them once.

5 To serve, wrap each patty in a soft tortilla, and serve with shredded lettuce, avocado slices, and low-fat mayonnaise. Or, serve in warm wholewheat

rolls and with fat-free sour cream instead of mayonnaise.

Each serving provides
Calories 243, Total fat 9.4g (Sat. 2.4g, Poly. 2.1g, Mono. 4.0g), Cholesterol 74mg, Protein 27g, Carbohydrate 12g, Fiber 2.0g, Sodium 506mg. Good source of— Vits: B_6, B_{12}; Mins: Ca, Mg, P, K.

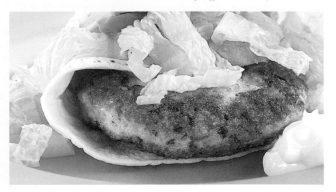

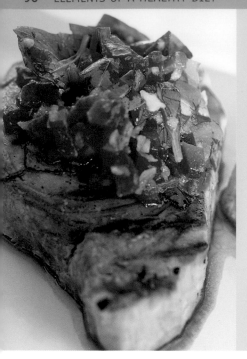

Fish and shellfish in a healthy diet

Eating fish once or twice a week reduces your risk of disease.

Low in both total and saturated fat content, fish and shellfish are excellent sources of protein and vitamins, so you should try to include them in your diet at least

Chargrilled swordfish Like other oily fish, swordfish are low in saturated fat but a good source of essential omega-3 fatty acids.

once or twice a week. They are high in important vitamins, such as thiamine (B_1), niacin (B_3), B_6, and D (*see pp.52–57*). Many fish are high in omega-3 fatty acids (*below*).

Benefits of fish
Ever since it was discovered that people such as Inuits, who eat a diet based on fish, have a low incidence of cardiovascular disease, the link between eating fish and reduced risk of heart attack has been a hot topic. Recent research confirms that eating fish, even a

Choosing fish for omega-3 fatty acids

Oily fish such as sardine, mackerel, and salmon contain a healthy fat called omega-3 fatty acids. This fat is believed to reduce the risk of developing cardiovascular disease by increasing the levels of "good" cholesterol and lowering the levels of "bad" cholesterol and triglycerides in the body.

Omega-3 fatty acids have also been found to prevent blood clots by making platelets less likely to clump together and stick to artery walls. Blood vessels are also less likely to constrict, making the heart less vulnerable to life-threatening irregular heart rates. There is evidence that omega-3 fatty acids help relieve the symptoms of arthritis (*see p.244*).

All fish and shellfish contain some omega-3 fatty acids, but the amount can vary. Generally, the fattier fish contain more than the leaner fish, but the proportion of omega-3 fatty acids can vary considerably between fish species (*right*).

The amount of omega-3 fatty acids in farm-raised products can also vary depending on the diet that the fish or shellfish are fed. Many companies now recognize this and provide a source of omega-3 fatty acids in their fish's diets.

FISH (3½oz/100g)	FAT	% SATURATED FAT	OMEGA-3
Mackerel	61%	14.0%	2.2g
Herring	51%	11.5%	1.7g
Sardine	50%	6.5%	1.7g
Bluefin tuna	3.2%	0.08%	1.6g
Anchovy	42%	9.4%	1.4g
Salmon	46%	8.0%	1.4g
Swordfish	30%	8.0%	1.1g
Halibut	19%	2.5%	0.9g
Mussel	24%	4.4%	0.8g
Oyster	32%	10.0%	0.6g
Sea trout	31%	9.0%	0.6g
Crab	14%	0.9%	0.4g
Sea bass	19%	5.0%	0.4g
Cod	7%	1.4%	0.3g
Haddock	7.5%	1.3%	0.1g

few times per month, can help to reduce your risk of developing cardiovascular disease.

Shellfish is healthy

This food source has acquired a bad reputation because some shellfish contain a high level of cholesterol. However, we now know that cholesterol levels are related to saturated fat intake rather than to cholesterol in the diet (*see p.40*). Since most shellfish are very low in fat, there is no reason to exclude them from your diet, particularly if you substitute them for high-fat animal proteins.

You should always use low-fat cooking methods, such as broiling, steaming, or grilling, to prepare fish rather than frying.

Fish and shellfish safety

When handled properly, fish and shellfish are as safe to eat as any other source of protein. Most harmful microbes found in fish are destroyed during cooking.

County Health Departments offer reports on contamination levels in local fishing waters. If you are healthy, however, you would have to be exposed to very large amounts of contaminants over a long period of time for them to have any harmful effects on your health.

Women who are pregnant or breast-feeding are advised to avoid eating any fish that are known to contain high levels of mercury. These fish include tuna, shark, and swordfish.

What is a serving?

Two to three servings from the protein group are recommended daily. Make sure you eat fish at least once and preferably twice a week because of its health benefits. Suggested servings include:
- 3½oz (100g) mussels, steamed (20 medium)
- 3½oz (100g) shrimp, steamed (7 medium)
- 3½oz (100g) lobster, steamed
- 3½oz (100g) clams, steamed
- 3½oz (100g) crab, steamed
- 3½oz (100g) oysters, steamed
- 3½oz (100g) salmon, grilled
- 3½oz (100g) sea bass, grilled
- 3½oz (100g) tuna, grilled
- 3½oz (100g) sardines, grilled

Tips for grilling fish

Grilling is a favorite activity across the land—and fresh grilled fish makes a great choice for those following a heart-healthy diet. Fish is easy to prepare and fast to cook, as well as being healthy and delicious. Almost any kind of fish can be cooked on a grill, but here are some useful tips:
- Choose the freshest fish available or use thawed frozen fish.
- Do not over-cook. Fish fillets require 4–5 minutes depending on thickness; fish steaks 1–2in (2.5–5cm) thick require 6–8 minutes on each side.
- Prevent fish from sticking to the grill by marinating it first in an olive-oil-based marinade or by spraying the grill with oil before heating.
- Always use a clean grill to avoid "off" flavors—fish picks up the flavor of foods previously cooked on the grill.
- For best results, use hardwood charcoal when grilling.
- Be creative: add interesting flavoring with hickory chips, grape vines, or other aromatic woods.
- Use herb aromatics—soak dried rosemary or thyme in water, squeeze them dry, and then sprinkle on the hot coals for a wonderful aroma.

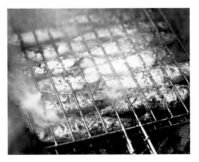

Fresh sardines High in beneficial omega-3 fatty acids, sardines are full of flavor and easy to grill with minimum preparation.

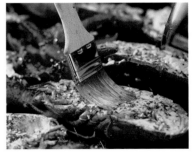

Brushing with oil Before grilling fish or shellfish, lightly brush with olive oil to prevent them from sticking to the grill.

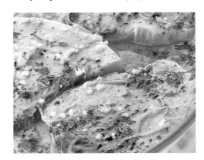

Marinating Prepare fish steaks and shellfish for grilling by marinating first in a wine- or oil-based marinade, flavored with fresh herbs.

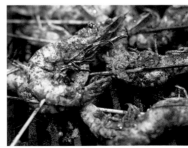

Herb aromatics Add flavor to grilled fish and shellfish by sprinkling fresh herbs, such as rosemary or thyme, over the hot coals.

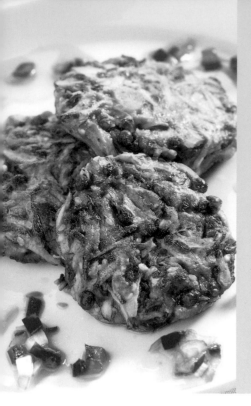

Legumes, seeds, and nuts

Inexpensive and versatile, these foods are nutritional gems.

Legumes, seeds, and nuts are all valuable sources of protein as well as being low in saturated fat and sodium and cholesterol-free. They are also good sources of fiber (*see pp.48–49*), complex carbohydrates (*see pp.46–47*), and vitamins and minerals, including thiamine (B_1),

Healthy proteins Lentils lend themselves to a variety of appetizing dishes. Here they are formed into patties with grated zucchini, almonds, and sesame seeds.

riboflavin (B_2), niacin (B_3), folate, calcium, potassium, iron, and phosphorus (*see pp.50–67*).

The term "legume" includes a huge range of peas, beans, and lentils (*below*). They are important foods and have the advantage over animal proteins of being both inexpensive and versatile in how they are cooked, as well as being packed with nutrients.

Due to their high soluble-fiber content, legumes are believed to help reduce blood cholesterol. They also have a very low glycemic index (*see p.47*), which means they are absorbed relatively slowly into the bloodstream and do not cause sudden increases in glucose blood

Choosing legumes

There is a myriad of legumes with a variety of colors, shapes, flavors, and uses. They are easy to prepare and can be eaten alone, combined with many other foods, or roasted to eat as a snack. Some legumes are available precooked, canned or frozen, but if you purchase them dry, soak them overnight and cook for 2–3 hours or until tender. Dried lentils do not require soaking and cook quickly.

FOOD (1 CUP COOKED)	CALORIES	PROTEIN
Black beans	132	8.9%
Black-eyed peas	109	7.4%
Chickpeas	171	9.4%
Fava beans	110	7.6%
Kidney beans	127	8.3%
Lentils	106	8.7%
Lima beans	110	7.7%
Peas	114	7.4%
Pinto beans	131	7.7%
Soybeans	149	14.0%
White beans	143	8.9%

Facts about soybeans

Soybeans supply nearly as many essential amino acids as animal proteins. They contain twice as much protein as other legumes and are a good source of vitamin A, the B vitamins, and the minerals calcium, phosphorus, potassium, and iron. They also contain large amounts of isoflavones, which are phytochemicals with beneficial health effects (*see p.59*). Soybeans are processed into a wide variety of products, including:

Soymilk Available in regular, low-fat, and flavored varieties.

Tofu Also known as soybean curd, this can be used in smoothies, stir-fry dishes, soups, and burgers.

Tempeh A chunky cake with a chewy texture and nutty flavor. It can be used instead of ground beef or chicken in a variety of recipes.

levels. This makes this group of foods particularly beneficial for anyone who has diabetes and those at risk of developing this disease, such as people who are overweight or have a family history of diabetes (*see p.246*).

Protein in seeds and nuts

Seeds are the embryo and food supply of new plants, whereas nuts are dried tree fruits, which are contained within hard shells. Both seeds and nuts contain 10–25 percent protein; they are high in mono- and polyunsaturated fat; and they are good sources of fiber, the vitamins thiamine (B_1), riboflavin (B_2), and E, and the minerals calcium, phosphorus, potassium, and iron.

Research shows that people who regularly eat nuts have a decreased risk of developing cardiovascular disease and diabetes. There are a number of possible explanations, in addition to the known benefits of unsaturated fat on cholesterol levels. For example, nuts are rich in arginine, an amino acid that boosts nitric oxide. This compound relaxes blood vessels and eases blood flow as well as making blood less likely to form clots.

Complementary proteins

Since the protein obtained from most plants lacks one or more of the amino acids that the body needs (essential amino acids), these sources of protein must be combined with a complementary plant-derived food or soybean product in order to form complete protein. This is not an issue when animal proteins are also included in the diet, but it is important for vegetarians who eliminate most animal products from their diets. (*see pp.100–101*).

What is a serving?

Two to three servings daily from the protein group are recommended. Legumes, seeds, and nuts are good sources of protein, and offer an alternative to red meat and dairy. The servings below are for cooked legumes and raw nuts and seeds:

- ½ cup soybeans
- ½ cup lentils
- ½ cup chickpeas
- ½ cup kidney beans
- 3 tbsp sunflower seeds
- 3 tbsp sesame seeds
- 3 tbsp alfalfa seeds
- 3 tbsp pumpkin seeds
- 3 tbsp flaxseeds
- 3 tbsp almonds
- 3 tbsp macadamia
- 3 tbsp Brazil nuts
- 3 tbsp pistachios
- 3 tbsp hazelnuts
- 3 tbsp cashew nuts

Ways of getting seeds into your diet

Seeds are ideal for snacking—they are nutritious, portable, and low in saturated fat. However, if you are trying to reduce the amount of fat in your diet, you should keep in mind that seeds are high in total fat and calories.

Pumpkin seeds Rich in protein, iron, zinc, and phosphorus, these seeds can be eaten raw, or cooked.

Sesame seeds A good source of protein and calcium, sesame seeds also contain iron and niacin (B_3). Mixed with sea salt, ground sesame seeds make a delicious condiment. You can also sprinkle the seeds over stir-fries.

Sunflower seeds These are rich in the minerals potassium and phosphorus and also contain protein, iron, and calcium. They make a great topping for salads.

Flaxseeds A good source of fiber and omega-3 fatty acids, crushed flaxseeds can be added to smoothies and baked goods. They are often used in energy bars.

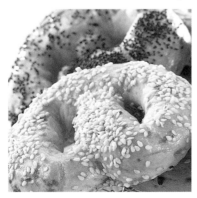

Seeded bread Poppy and sunflower seeds provide texture and increased nutritional value to these pretzels.

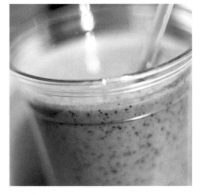

Healthy smoothie Crushed flaxseeds add fiber, omega-3 fatty acids, and a nutty flavor to a raspberry and yogurt smoothie.

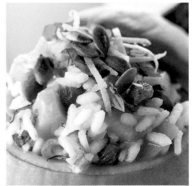

Pumpkin risotto Lightly roasted pumpkin seeds add texture, flavor, and a number of valuable nutrients to this savory dish.

Which nuts are the best?

Nuts are 10–25 percent protein, high in mono- and polyunsaturated fats, and a good source of dietary fiber and certain vitamins and minerals. Nuts are cholesterol-free—like other plant foods—but because all nuts are high in fat, and often salted, they should be eaten in moderation.

Almonds High in monounsaturated fat, almonds are also a good source of protein, riboflavin (B_2), vitamin E, calcium, iron, and zinc.

Brazil nuts Rich in protein, iron, calcium, and zinc, Brazil nuts also contain the highest natural source of selenium—one nut exceeds the Daily Recommended Intake (DRI).

Cashews High in fat (although lower than almonds, peanuts, pecans, and walnuts), cashews contain essential fatty acids, B vitamins, fiber, protein, carbohydrate, iron, and zinc.

Chestnuts Containing less fat than most other nuts, chestnuts do have microminerals and potassium, but are not a good source of protein.

Hazelnuts (filberts) Contain fiber, calcium, magnesium, and vitamin E, these are a good source of protein.

Peanuts Technically a legume, these contain more protein than most nuts (20–30 percent), and are a good source of fiber, folate, and vitamins.

Pecans These contain fiber, vitamin A, and thiamine (B_1), iron, calcium, copper, magnesium, potassium, and phosphorus. Pecans are also high in mono- and polyunsaturated fats.

Pine nuts The small edible seeds of pine trees. Pine nuts are high in protein, calcium, and magnesium.

Pistachios A very rich source of potassium, they contain calcium, magnesium, iron, fiber, and protein as well as vitamin A and folate.

Walnuts Rich in vitamins, especially folate, and magnesium, potassium, iron, and zinc, these are also high in antioxidants and omega-3 fatty acids.

Nuts and seeds and fat content

These foods have a high percentage of fat; however, being rich in fats does not mean that nuts and seeds are bad for our health. On the contrary, their fats are mostly mono- and polyunsaturated, which are beneficial in the prevention of cardiovascular disease and in lowering LDL cholesterol (*see p.40*). If you are following a low-fat diet, you should be aware that you will need to watch your intake of calorie-rich nuts and seeds.

Some nuts, such Brazil nuts, cashews, macadamias, and pine nuts, however, do contain significant amounts of unhealthy saturated fats and should therefore be eaten in moderation.

Brazil nuts, pine nuts, and walnuts contain two essential fatty acids that are particularly heart-healthy: linoleic and alpha-linolenic acids. Walnuts are especially rich in alpha-linolenic acid. The health benefits of nuts can be undermined if they are eaten salted.

High in polyunsaturated fats, seeds contain valuable nutrients. However, they are high in calories.

A small percentage of people are allergic to nuts (*see p.253*), which is why nuts must be listed on food labels.

Proportions of fats in nuts and seeds The chart shown below gives the breakdown of the proportions of saturated, polyunsaturated, and monounsaturated fats for some nuts and seeds. Nuts are generally high in healthy polyunsaturated and monounsaturated fats.

Key

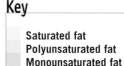

- Saturated fat
- Polyunsaturated fat
- Monounsaturated fat

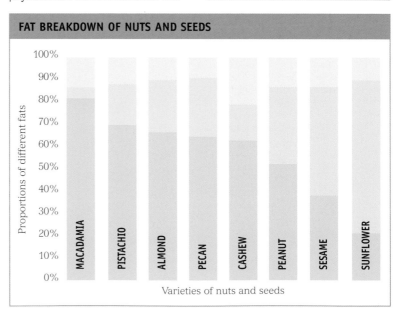

FAT BREAKDOWN OF NUTS AND SEEDS

Eggs and health

An excellent source of protein and other vital nutrients.

Eggs contain all the essential amino acids in the correct proportions (*see pp.44–45*) and are therefore a good source of complete protein. They are also a significant source of the vitamins riboflavin (B_2), folate, B_{12}, D, and E, in addition to iron (*see pp.50–67*). The iron in egg yolks, like that found in meat, is easily absorbed by the body.

Eggs contain other vitamins and minerals in smaller amounts, including thiamine (B_1), vitamin B_6, phosphorus, and zinc. Eggs are also one of the best sources of choline, a substance involved in the transport of fat in the body. Choline is also important for the manufacture of phospholipids, which are the major structural components of cell membranes. Most of the vitamins and minerals in eggs are found in the yolk, but the white is also a good source of protein and contains little fat and no cholesterol

Eggs and cholesterol

Of all the foods that are eaten in North America today, eggs are the main source of cholesterol. Yet, eggs are relatively low in calories and saturated fat—egg white does not contain any fat. However, the American Heart Association still recommends keeping track of the number of eggs you eat each day and limiting eggs yolks (*below*).

Ideal protein Low in saturated fat and calories, but an excellent source of complete protein, eggs provide an inexpensive and nutritious addition to your diet.

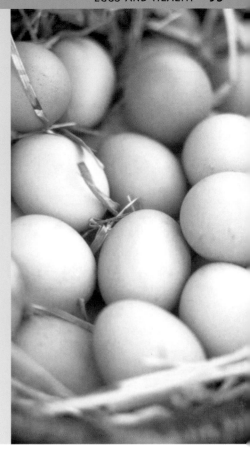

How many eggs can I eat?

Researchers have determined that saturated fat has more of an impact on blood-cholesterol levels than eating foods high in dietary cholesterol. However, your recommended total cholesterol intake should still be less than 200mg per day, especially if you have high blood cholesterol or a family history of cardiovascular disease. This is roughly the amount in one small egg. If you have eaten another source of saturated fat or cholesterol that day, you do not need to eat any more eggs. If you suffer from high blood cholesterol and/or your diet already includes large amounts of cholesterol and saturated fats from other sources, you may need to further cut back on eggs.

There is no limit to how many egg whites you can eat, so look at ways to use more egg whites in your cooking. When cooking eggs, avoid adding butter and cheese, which will add saturated fat.

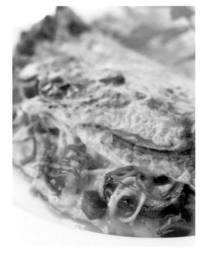

Low-fat omelet Made with two egg whites and only one yolk, the cholesterol level of this mushroom and tomato omelet is reduced, without changing the flavor.

Eggs and salmonella

According to the official figures, about 1 in 20,000 eggs in the US is contaminated with salmonella. This can cause an infection with symptoms that include abdominal pain, vomiting, and diarrhea.

In order to minimize your risk of this infection, always store your eggs in a refrigerator and cook them thoroughly. Scrambled, poached, and boiled eggs should be cooked until firm. Homemade salad dressings made with raw eggs could contain salmonella. Commercial mayonnaise contains pasteurized eggs and can be stored safely at room temperature.

Infants, children, pregnant women, elderly people, and those who are chronically ill should not eat raw or undercooked eggs due to the risk of salmonella.

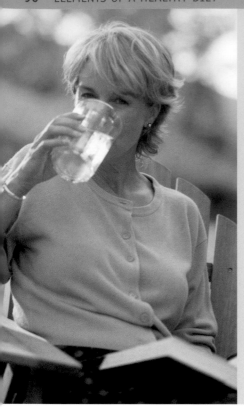

The need for fluids

Our bodies need fluids—and water is undoubtedly the best.

About 60 percent of a man's body and about 50 percent of a woman's body is made of water. Every cell in your body needs water to function properly, and if you do not drink enough, you may feel tired, develop a headache, suffer from dry eyes and a dry mouth, or find it difficult to concentrate. To stay healthy, you need to drink at least six to eight glasses of water each day. When it

is hot, when you are partaking in sports, or on any other occasions when you lose excessive fluid through perspiration, you will need to drink even more water or other water-based fluids.

People who drink plenty of water gain many positive health benefits. Studies have shown that they have fewer kidney stones (*see p.238*), are less likely to suffer from constipation (*see p.229*), and are at lower risk for developing cancer of the colon or the urinary tract.

Water power
Involved in every function of your body, water controls body temperature; gives you energy; assists in weight control; helps transport nutrients and waste products in and out of cells;

Thirst quencher Get into the habit of drinking water throughout the day: it is the best way of supplying your body with the fluid that it needs, without adding calories.

Increase your water intake

Many people believe they get enough water from coffee, tea, fruit juice, and soda, but these do not fully satisfy the need for water. If you exercise regularly and eat a healthy diet, yet you are not drinking enough water, you will not burn fat efficiently. This is because when the body perceives thirst, its processes slow, just as if you had skipped a meal. Whether you drink bottled, filtered, or tap water, with or without carbonation, any increase is beneficial to your health. Aim for six to eight 8floz (240ml) glasses of water a day.

Food can also supply your body with water, especially fruits and vegetables. For example, watermelon contains more than 90 percent water. On a warm day, eating plenty of salad leaves, tomatoes, and cucumber will boost your water intake.

Tips for drinking more water

Most people do not drink enough water. The recommended amount is six to eight 8floz (240ml) glasses a day. Here are some ways to improve your intake every day:
• While you are studying or working at your computer, keep a bottle or large glass of water on your desk and drink from it regularly.
• Drink water, sparkling water, or club soda with meals, instead of other carbonated drinks, coffee, or alcohol.

• When you go out for the day, pack a large water bottle in your car, briefcase, or backpack. Add some ice cubes to help keep it cool.
• Be sure to have a water bottle with you whenever you go to the gym, go out on your bicycle, or take part in sporting activities. Extra water is important when you are exercising.
• Buy a bottle of water instead of a can of soda from the vending machine when you are thirsty.

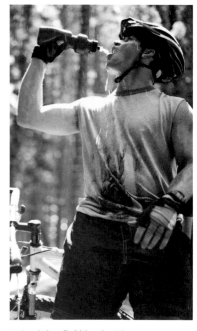

Maintaining fluid levels When you are exercising or taking part in sports, it is essential to replace fluids lost through perspiration by drinking lots of water.

helps prevent you from becoming dehydrated after sweating; and is needed for all digestive, absorptive, circulatory, and excretory functions.

Children adapt less efficiently than adults to hot weather and are more vulnerable to heat. They produce more body heat than adults but sweat less and therefore take longer to change their body temperature. In addition, children's thirst mechanism is not as fully developed as that of adults and they may not express the need to drink and should be encouraged to drink water before, during, and after exercise to prevent dehydration and heatstroke.

What about soft drinks?

Because soft drinks are composed largely of water, soda, lemonade, fruit juice, and other popular drinks do provide the body with essential fluids. However, they also contain large amounts of sugar, which, if consumed in excess, causes tooth decay and leads to an unhealthy increase in weight. Sweet drinks can also cause a sudden increase in blood sugar levels.

In North America, overweight and obesity in children is increasing and the excessive consumption of soft drinks is a major contributory factor to this problem. According to official figures, North American adolescents drink about twice as much carbonated soda as milk, contributing not only to excessive weight gain in this age group, but also to a poor intake of calcium, which has serious implications for bone health in later life (see p.81).

Studies also show that children who consume a lot of calorie-laden soft drinks eat less at their regular meals, causing them to miss out on essential nutrients. By substituting healthier drinks, such as low-fat milk or water, in place of soda, for all age groups, nutritional deficiencies and obesity may be prevented.

Caffeine and fluids

Coffee and tea are popular drinks, not least because of the stimulating effect of the caffeine content. While caffeine also acts as a mild diuretic and increases the amounts of fluid that the body loses in urine, this effect will not cause dehydration. For this reason, coffee and tea can count toward your daily intake of fluids. Caffeine is also present in hot chocolate, cocoa, and in carbonated drinks such as cola.

You should also be aware that caffeine can interact with certain medications: it diminishes the effect of some tranquilizers and reacts with some antidepressants. Consult your doctor or dietitian for more advice.

Fruit juice

Often a good source of vitamin C, many fruit juices are fortified with calcium, but that does not mean they should be unlimited, especially for children. The American Academy of Pediatrics (AAP) issued a policy statement regarding "The Use and Misuse of Fruit Juice in Pediatrics," but its concerns apply to adults as well.

According to the AAP, drinking too much juice can contribute to overweight and obesity, tooth decay, and digestive problems, such as diarrhea and bloating. Drinking too much juice is filling and will decrease your appetite for other more nutritious foods, including milk. The report recommends:
• Juice should be 100 percent fruit juice and not a "fruit drink."
• Infants should not be given juice. Children aged 1–6 years should have no more than 6floz (180ml) per day. Older children (6–12 years) should limit their intake to 12floz (360ml) per day.
• Instead of juice, children (and adults) should eat whole fruits for the fiber.

Check your caffeine intake

Moderate caffeine intake (250mg of caffeine or less per day) is not associated with any health risk. However, more than seven cups of coffee or tea may cause a health risk. The US Food and Drug Administration's recommendation is for pregnant women to reduce their caffeine intake. Also, regular caffeine consumption may increase urinary calcium excretion and the risk of osteoporosis (see p.242).

DRINK	SERVING SIZE	CAFFEINE
Filter coffee	8floz (240ml)	176–240mg
Espresso	2floz (60ml)	100mg
Leaf tea	8floz (240ml)	100mg
Instant coffee	8floz (240ml)	64–75mg
Cola	12floz (360ml)	31–55mg
Iced tea	8floz (240ml)	26–45mg
Instant tea	8floz (240ml)	30mg
Green tea	8floz (240ml)	15mg
Hot chocolate	8floz (240ml)	14mg
Decaffeinated coffee	8floz (240ml)	3mg

Foods to eat sparingly

If your overall diet is healthy, "junk foods" can be enjoyed as an occasional treat.

At the tip of the USDA food pyramid (see p.72) is a group of foods that are recommended to be eaten sparingly. These include cookies, candy, cake, canned fruit packed in heavy syrup, soft drinks, potato chips, and salad dressings—products that are sometimes categorized as junk foods. The reason for limiting their inclusion in the diet is that while they provide calories, they are either deficient in nutritive value, or they are high in unhealthy components such as saturated fat, trans fatty acids (see p38), and salt (see p.64)—all of which are associated with increased risk of developing certain diseases.

What your body needs

Following a healthy diet means choosing foods that give you the nourishment your body needs in addition to enough calories to fuel your daily activities. This does

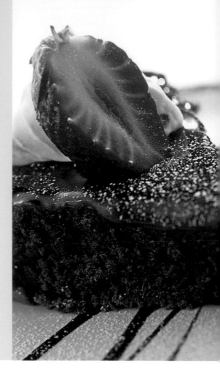

High in sugar and fat Although not totally devoid of nutritional value, this chocolate cake, and similar rich desserts, should be regarded as an occasional treat rather than a regular source of energy.

Is alcohol good for you?

Several studies have suggested that moderate drinkers have a longer life expectancy than both nondrinkers and heavy drinkers. The reason why moderate drinking may confer health benefits is not completely clear, but the serious health risks posed by excessive drinking are well known.

The health benefits of alcohol Many studies have shown that if you drink alcohol on a daily basis, you reduce your risk of developing cardiovascular disease (see pp.214–221). The precise reason why moderate alcohol drinking is good for you is not fully understood, but it is known that alcohol raises the levels of "good" HDL cholesterol in the bloodstream.

There are other health benefits attributed to moderate drinking. These benefits include:
• Lowering the risk of stroke
• Reducing levels of stress
• Increasing appetite—especially in older adults.

However, the same amount of alcohol that lowers the risk of developing cardiovascular disease may increase the risk of breast cancer (see p.259).

The risks of excessive drinking The risk factors associated with excessive drinking include high blood pressure, excessive weight gain and its related health risks (see p.158), increased risk of accidents, hemorrhagic strokes, and medication interactions.

In the US, alcohol abuse accounts for 75 percent of all cases of cirrhosis (liver disease) and is responsible for 250,000 deaths every year. Alcohol consumption by young drinkers is also a persistent public health problem that is associated with various social, emotional, and behavioral problems.

In addition, excessive intake of alcohol during pregnancy is linked with congenital birth defects, such as facial abnormalities, premature birth, low birthweight, and poor growth and development in babies.

Alcohol and nutrition There are 7 calories in each gram of alcohol, but, since most alcoholic beverages contain insignificant amounts of vitamins and minerals, these are "empty calories." Excessive use of alcohol may lead to nutritional deficiencies since heavy drinkers tend to eat poorly and suffer from impaired digestion of food and absorption of nutrients. They also suffer loss of nutrients (especially zinc) via urinary excretion.

Drink in moderation The official advice is that if you drink alcohol, do so in moderation. This means no more than one drink a day for women and over-65s, and two for men. One drink is: 12floz (360ml) beer, 5floz (150ml) wine, or 1½floz (45ml) of 80 percent proof liquor.

Alcohol should be avoided by women who are pregnant or planning to conceive and by people who are taking medication, driving cars, or operating machinery.

not mean that you have to give up delicious (but unhealthy) treats altogether, but rather that you should eat them less often. Every food group contains healthy and less healthy foods, and the healthy ones should form the basis of your diet. This means that you should choose whole-grain products over refined varieties; low-fat or fat-free sources of protein such as chicken, fish, and legumes, rather than meats high in saturated fat; and opting for low-fat and fat-free varieties of dairy products. If your overall diet is healthy, you can afford to include some junk foods without undue concern.

Why we like junk foods

Researchers have demonstrated that the worldwide popularity of junk foods is due to their ready availability, heavy advertising, and the fact that consumers find them highly palatable. Humans are born with a taste preference for sweets and fats, so sugar and fat are added to manufactured food products to make them more palatable and flavorful.

In recent years, because of growing health concerns, many foods have been reformulated to lower their fat content. However, some of these low-fat cookies and ice creams contain added sugar to improve their appeal to consumers and as a result they contain an even greater amount of calories. It is important to look at the food labels on such products to check their total nutritional content, rather than relying on the health claims that are made by the manufacturers (see p.277).

Why we love chocolate

Universally popular, chocolate combines a sweet taste with the texture of fat to create a palatable treat whose aroma is one of the most attractive to humans. It also contains substances that help us relax and improve mood—so there is a biological reason why eating chocolate makes you feel good.

Chocolate does provide some nutrients, and is a particularly good source of magnesium and calcium. It also has antioxidant and anti-inflammatory properties.

On the down side, chocolate's high fat content can contribute to weight gain and raised cholesterol levels, with their associated health risks. It also contains caffeine, which should be limited (see p.97).

Avoid empty calories

Eating too much of the foods at the top of the food pyramid is bad for your health in a number of ways: such foods tend to be high in fat and sugar, which means that they are also high in calories and are likely to lead to overweight and obesity. Secondly, the saturated fat and trans fatty acid content of many of these products, along with their reliance on refined flour, also has a detrimental effect on health. Moreover, many of these foods are devoid of nutritional value, hence the term "empty calories." This means that people who eat a lot of them may be overweight, yet suffer from malnutrition.

FOOD	SERVING	CALORIES	FAT	% SATURATED FAT
Apple pie	⅛ of 10in (25cm) pie	277	42%	14%
Vanilla ice cream	8floz (240ml)	266	47%	31%
Cheesecake	1/12 of 9in (23cm) pie	257	63%	28%
Milk shake (whole milk)	8floz (240ml)	255	23%	15%
Chocolate candy bar	1½oz (44g)	226	56%	32%
Soda	12floz (360ml)	152	0%	0%
Oatmeal raisin cookies	2 cookies	118	31%	8%
Potato chips	10 chips	107	7%	2.2%
Jelly beans	10 beans	104	0%	0%
Chocolate chip cookies	2 cookies	100	38%	13%
Popcorn (cooked in oil)	1 cup	55	3%	0.5%

Is a vegetarian diet healthier?

A carefully planned vegetarian diet has many health benefits.

Not all vegetarians follow the same dietary restrictions: lacto-vegetarians include dairy but no flesh, such as meat, chicken, or fish. Ovo-vegetarians include eggs in their diet and avoid all other animal sources. Lacto- and ovo-vegetarians include both dairy and/or eggs, while vegans don't eat any animal products at all.

Because of the limitations of vegetarian diets, careful planning is needed to avoid the nutritional deficiencies that can otherwise occur. Becoming a vegetarian, however, is not difficult and there is no question that well-designed vegetarian diets are healthy for most people, including pregnant women and children.

Benefits of vegetarianism

The diets of people who eat less animal protein and more plant-based protein tend also to contain less fat and cholesterol and more dietary fiber. This may explain why vegetarians have lower total and LDL cholesterol levels (see p.23) and lower rates of cardiovascular disorders, such as high blood pressure and heart attack, obesity, diabetes, and colon cancer than those who eat meat. It is not clear, however, whether these health benefits are due solely to the diet, or are linked to factors such as regular exercise, lack of smoking, or a low alcohol intake.

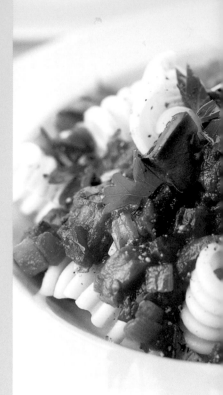

How to combine plant proteins

Plant-based foods are described as incomplete sources of protein, since (with the exception of soybeans and soybean products) they contain insufficient amounts of one or more essential amino acids (see p.45). They can be combined to form good-quality protein, however, because different essential amino acids are missing from each food source.

Legumes or soybeans and soybean products should form the basis of your main meal. Add a grain and/or a seed or nut to make a meal containing good-quality protein. Alternatively, make sure you eat something from each of these groups over each 12-hour period to ensure that all the amino acids have been included in your diet.

MEAL IDEA	LEGUMES	GRAIN	SEEDS AND NUTS
Lentil, zucchini, and sesame patties (see p.92)	Lentils	–	Sesame seeds
Macaroni and cheese with peas (see p.123)	Peas	Wheat	–
Hummous with pita bread (see p.127)	Chickpeas	Wheat	Sesame seeds
Spicy bean soup with corn bread (see p.155)	Mixed beans	Corn	–
Quinoa-stuffed peppers (see p.235)	Chickpeas	Quinoa	–
Vegetable and chickpea couscous (see p.250)	Chickpeas	Couscous	–
Tofu and vegetable stir-fry with nuts (see p.256)	Tofu	Rice	Cashew nuts
Crostini with canellini beans (see p.263)	Canellini beans	Wheat	–

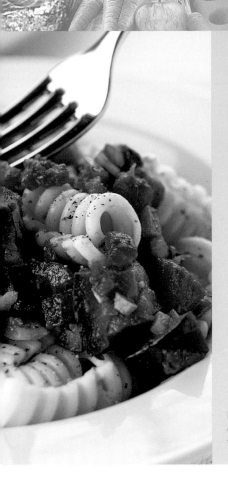

Nutritional issues

While vegetarian diets that include cheese and eggs are easier to balance nutritionally than those that exclude all animal products, vegetarians must still plan their diets carefully to obtain all the nutrients they need. For example, iron, which helps red blood cells carry oxygen to the tissues, is present in both plant and animal foods, but heme iron—which is obtained from animal products—is more readily absorbed in the intestine than the iron that is obtained from plants (*see p.66*).

Vitamin B_{12} is found only in animal and fortified soy products. Since this vitamin is necessary for the functioning of the nervous system, vegans may need to take a supplement in order to avoid deficiency (*see p.269*).

Pasta with vegetables Making one of your daily meals a vegetarian dish is an excellent way to improve your diet.

The macrobiotic diet

Based on ancient Eastern spiritual traditions that seek to balance the two opposing forces of Yin and Yang, this vegetarian diet claims to promote spiritual and physical well-being. By correcting what is perceived as energy imbalance, adherents of the diet claim it can prevent and cure disease.

The aim of the macrobiotic diet is to supply well-balanced meals that are composed of the essential components: grain, protein, sea vegetables, long-cooked vegetables, short-cooked (raw) vegetables, pickles, and dessert.

Strict adherence to this diet may cause health problems. Since no dairy or animal products are eaten, deficiencies in protein, vitamins B_{12} and D, zinc, calcium, and iron may occur. This is very significant for people with increased nutritional needs, such as children (*see p.265, and pp.268–271*).

Vegetarian tips

These tips will help ensure a nutritionally sound diet, high in nutrients and low in fat:
- Choose whole grains or foods with naturally occurring vitamins.
- Select fortified or whole-grain cereals, such as oatmeal.
- Eat egg whites; they are an excellent low-fat, low-cholesterol source of protein.
- If you eat dairy products, choose low-fat or fat free varieties.
- Eat foods containing vitamin C with meals in order to improve iron absorption.
- Have 1–2 servings of a good source of iron daily: for example eggs or red kidney beans.
- Strict vegans should include a good source of vitamin B_{12} daily, such as a fortified cereal, fortified soy beverage, or a supplement.

Recipe Protein-rich tofu and miso soup

INGREDIENTS

4 cups vegetable bouillon

2½oz (75g) tofu, diced

4 mushrooms, finely sliced

½ carrot, cut into julienne strips

3 tbsp miso

2 scallions, finely sliced crosswise

Serves 4

1 Place bouillon, tofu, mushrooms, and carrot in a pan. Bring to a boil and simmer for 3 minutes.

2 Dissolve miso in a little water. Remove pan from heat and stir in the miso.

Serve hot, garnished with sliced scallions.

Each serving provides
Calories 126, Total fat 2.6g (Sat. 0.7g, Poly. 1.0g, Mono. 0.7g) Cholesterol 0.7mg, Protein 6.0g, Carbohydrate 21g, Fiber 2.7g, Sodium 1,933mg. Good source of—Vits: A; Mins: Ca, Mg, K.

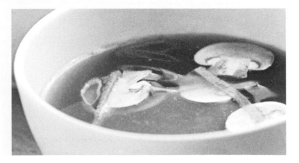

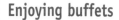

Eating away from home

Eating out does not have to wreck your healthy-eating plan.

Whether by choice or necessity, there are many occasions when you eat away from home—and these occasions will probably present a challenge to your healthy-eating program.

But eating is not just about satisfying nutritional needs. It is also a major focus of social activities—whether it is eating in restaurants with friends, taking part in office celebrations, or meeting family at parties and other events where hospitality, in the form of food and drink, is offered. There are ways to enjoy such occasions without losing sight of your long-term healthy diet goals: eating more fruits, vegetables, and whole grains; choosing lean meats and fish over red meats; limiting your intake of refined carbohydrates, saturated fat, and salt; and being careful with portion sizes and alcohol consumption.

Making healthy restaurant choices

There is no reason to avoid eating in restaurants, but, if you want to maintain your healthy-eating habits as well as preventing unwanted weight gain, you need to be very careful when ordering.

Whether you are making a quick stop at a fast-food outlet for lunch or enjoying a leisurely restaurant meal in the evening, it is possible to make healthy choices. Fast food and restaurant meals tend to be higher in calories and saturated fat than most of the meals that you prepare at home, so to enjoy a meal without sabotaging your weight-control program, balance restaurant meals with lighter meals at home. Do not be afraid to ask questions about how a dish on the menu is prepared—the same dish can usually be prepared in different ways, some healthier than others. And if you wish to order your entrée but without the rich sauce or other high-fat accompaniments, do so: the chef is unlikely to refuse your request.

Dinner-party strategies

Although you have no control over the food served when friends and family invite you to dinner, you can still limit how much you eat and drink. Fill up on salads and vegetables offered, and ask for a small portion of dessert.

You can offset any extra calories you are likely to eat by taking a walk or visiting the gym during the day: increasing your level of activity will help you burn the extra calories you are likely to take in. Exercise can also reduce your appetite and help you control how much you eat.

Enjoying buffets

An inviting array of buffet food is difficult to resist. Here are some tips to help you maintain control:
● Since going up to the buffet is the fun part, pace yourself.
● Start with a salad and skip the soup and bread.
● Avoid dressed vegetables, such as potato salad and coleslaw.
● Choose a low-calorie dressing rather than mayonnaise.
● For your entrée, pick low-fat foods such as turkey or fish.
● Choose fruit, sorbet, or low-fat yogurt for dessert.
● At a breakfast buffet, opt for the cold buffet, which includes fruits, breads, yogurts, and cereals.

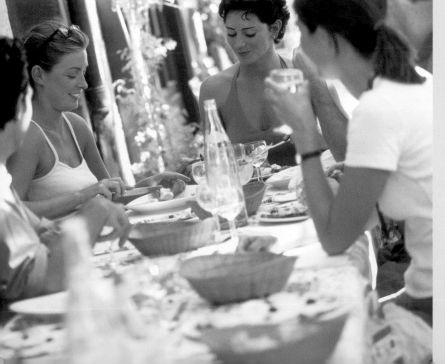

Dining out When eating out, don't lose sight of your long-term healthy-eating plan. Order carefully, stop eating when you are full, and, if you over-indulge, eat less the next day.

Choosing healthy restaurant options

Eating out is often arranged as a celebration or treat. It is possible to enjoy your experience without losing sight of your healthy eating habits.

ORDERING APPETIZERS

Think whether you need an appetizer; would you eat one at home? Consider skipping the first course, especially if you plan to have a full entrée.

- Consider ordering an appetizer and salad as your main meal, or share an appetizer or entrée.
- Choose low-fat, high-fiber soups such as vegetable or lentil soup. Avoid soups with added cream.
- Fried appetizers, such as potato skins, are high in fat and calories, so they are best avoided.
- If you have bread, eat it plain, or dip it in olive oil, rather than adding butter.
- When ordering salad, ask for the dressing on the side. Vinaigrette made with olive oil is the healthiest option. However, it is still high in calories.
- Choose a salad without shredded cheese, fried croutons, or a special dressing, such as Caesar dressing.

THE BEST ENTREES

Use eating out as an opportunity to eat a healthy meal, cooked well. You could also try something new.

- Grilled, baked, or broiled white meat poultry, fish, and shellfish are the best choices, since they are low in fat.
- Choose tomato-based pasta sauces rather than cheese- or meat-based.
- Order the smallest portion of meat, or share. If you are hungry, order extra vegetables and salad.
- Select barbecue sauce, horseradish, salsa, lemon or lime juice, mustard, or relish instead of condiments such as sour cream or mayonnaise.

ENJOYING DESSERTS

For a healthy, refreshing dessert, have a fruit salad or fresh berries that are packed with vitamins.

- Skip fruit pies or cobblers: the crusts may be made with unhealthy vegetable shortening and sugar.
- Sorbet is a good choice, especially if you share a portion. Ice cream and frozen yogurt served in restaurants can be high in fat and/or sugar.

Fast-food choices

The national fondness for fast food is a major factor in the increasing prevalence of obesity and associated diseases. This type of food is often high in saturated fat, calories, and sodium, lacking in fiber, vitamins, and minerals, and marketed to encourage the intake of unhealthily large portions. If you do not want to eliminate fast food from your diet, balance it out with what you eat the rest of the time, and try to make healthier choices when you do have it:

- Choose a small hamburger with lettuce and tomato (no cheese).
- Have salad or baked potato with your meal instead of fries.
- Eat broiled-chicken sandwiches with mustard instead of fried-chicken sandwiches.
- Use mustard or ketchup instead of mayonnaise or "special sauce."
- Order fat-free milk, water, or a small diet soda.
- Skip dessert, or try a yogurt and fruit parfait.

Chinese meal transformation

Most North Americans consider Chinese food to be a healthy option, and while this can be true, many of the most popular dishes are high in saturated fat and calories. Dishes that are batter-dipped, deep-fried, sweet and sour, or in a thick sauce are best avoided.

CHINESE CAN BE HEALTHY

Choose dishes based on authentic, everyday Chinese cooking, which are low in fat and protein and high in fiber. The cholesterol levels in China are far lower than in North America; this is because the diet is based mainly on grains and a wide variety of vegetables, with small amounts of protein and fat.

Stir-fried vegetables with tofu, chicken, or shrimp are healthy, low-fat Chinese options. Accompany any of these with plain steamed or boiled rice for a well-balanced, healthy meal.

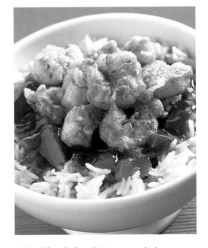

Unhealthy choice Batter-coated, deep-fried shrimp in sweet and sour sauce, with egg-fried rice. This meal provides 397 calories, 18g fat, and 122mg cholesterol.

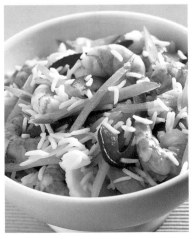

Low-fat option Lightly steamed shrimp and vegetables, with plain steamed or boiled rice. By contrast, this meal provides only 250 calories, 1g fat, and 65mg cholesterol.

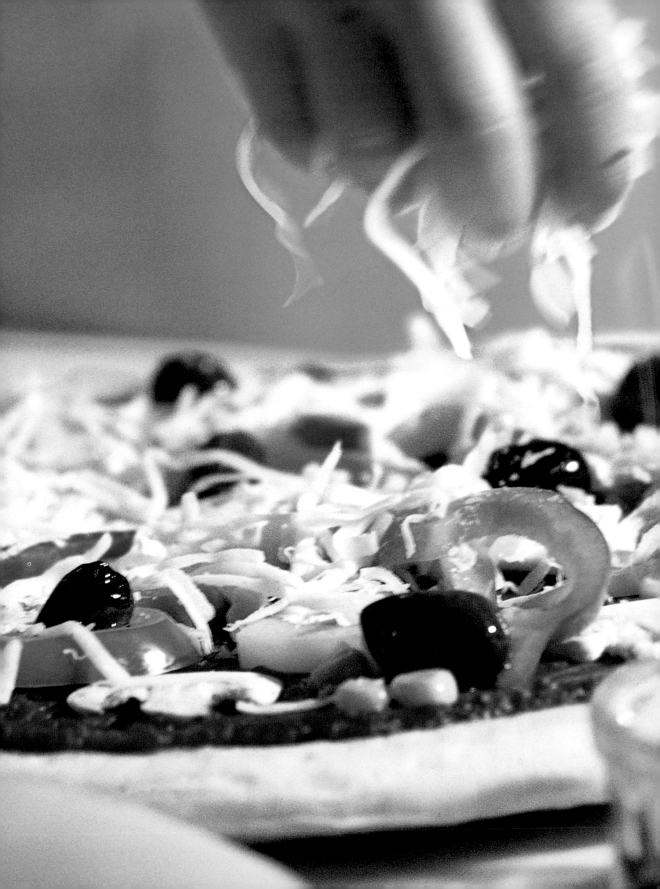

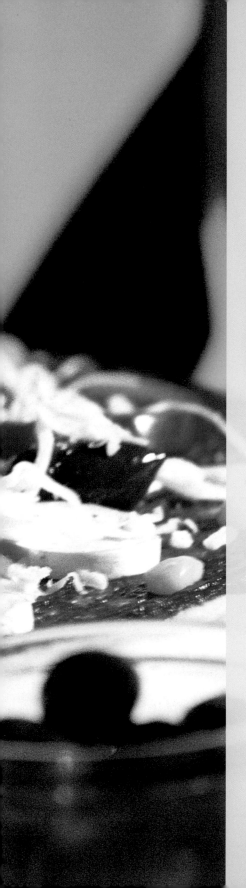

Eating for the time of your life

Healthy eating is the foundation of a healthy body. At every stage of your life—from early childhood to old age—good nutrition can make a difference in how you feel on a day-to-day basis and in the long-term. In this chapter, you will find helpful advice on how to achieve a healthy diet for yourself, your children, and your parents.

When our needs change

At different stages in life, we need to make sure our diet meets our body's needs.

So far in this book, we have looked at the nutritional needs of healthy adults. The focus has been on assessing your dietary habits and lifestyle and preventing disease. In this chapter, we will highlight different stages of life and show you key changes that need to be made at the different stages.

Nutrition for children
We start with nutrition for infants, children, and adolescents. Proper nutrition has an immediate impact on your children's health, well-being, and normal growth and development, and has long-term

consequences for their health as adults. Of particular importance is checking your child's growth throughout childhood to make sure he or she is getting enough calories and the right nutrients and to avoid the risk of becoming overweight or underweight.

We look at nutritional aspects of breast-feeding and bottle-feeding, when to introduce new foods during and after weaning, and the needs of preschool and school-age children, who may be picky eaters. Adolescents' needs, including calcium for strong bones and, in teenage girls, iron to replenish that lost during menstrual periods, are also described.

Nutrition for adults
In the second half of this chapter, the nutritional requirements for adults are covered. These include

the specific needs of men and women. Women's extra nutritional needs during pregnancy, after giving birth, and when breast-feeding are also covered. These topics are followed by dietary measures to lessen the symptoms and effects of menopause. We end the chapter with nutritional tips on staying healthy and feeling good into old age.

Nutrition for athletes
In this chapter we also address the nutritional needs of athletes, extremely active people who burn extra calories when they are performing, whether for short bursts or endurance exercises.

Eating as a family Make the time to eat together; encourage your children to taste new things and enjoy healthy food.

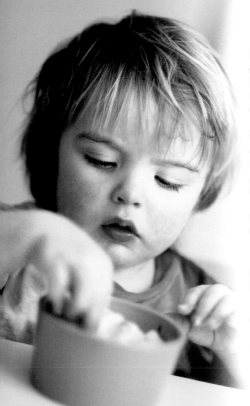

Establishing healthy eating habits

Encouraging good eating habits in your children significantly contributes to keeping them healthy and will help them maintain the right weight throughout childhood and into adulthood.

BE A GOOD ROLE MODEL
As a parent, you should be a good role model for your child's eating habits (*see p.126*). Introduce your child at a young age to a variety of healthy foods and be patient if he or she goes through a picky-eating phase (*see p.127*). Try to have sit-down meals as a family as much as possible (*opposite above*). Since children need plenty of snacks to keep them going through the day, make sure their snacks are healthy (*see p.129*). In

You are what you eat To help your child develop good eating habits that will last for life, offer him a variety of healthy foods during meals and snacks.

addition, if your child takes a packed lunch to school, make sure it is full of nutritious items (*see p.130*).

In order to prevent your children from becoming overweight, try to limit the amount of television they watch or video or computer games that they play and encourage them to be active. Also, limit junk food and sweetened drinks, such as soda and fruit drinks—these are high in calories and may lead to weight gain and obesity if not consumed in moderation (*see p.134*).

TEACH CHILDREN ABOUT FOOD
Stimulate your children's interest in food by cooking together, encouraging them to taste new foods, and planning healthy menus (*see p.131*). Making sure children know the difference between healthy and junk foods and that what they eat and drink is important for their growing body will help establish good eating habits that will stay with them for life.

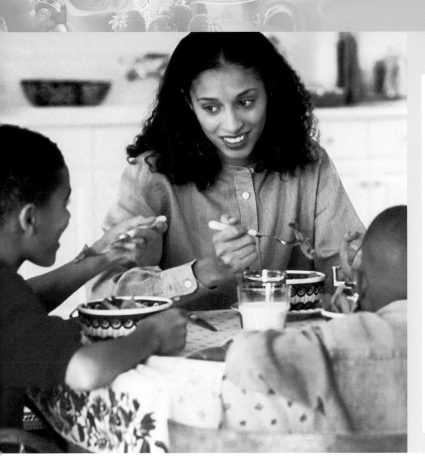

Eating together

It is important to eat together as a family at least once a day for many reasons. In today's busy society, with children and adolescents involved in lots of extracurricular activities, it may be the only time to actually catch up and talk about the day. Studies of children's diets have shown that family meals are an important way in which children develop healthy eating habits.

Eating together is an opportunity for children to learn about mealtimes and for you to provide a structured, nurturing environment where healthy foods can be served and good table manners established. It is a time to try new foods and for parents to serve as role models for good nutrition. For example, if everyone is drinking low-fat milk or water, rather than soda, your child is less likely to become a soda drinker as he or she gets older.

When do we need extra vitamins and minerals?

At certain times of life, or as a result of lifestyle factors, you may need extra vitamins (*see pp.50–59*) and minerals (*see pp.60–67*), either from your diet or by taking supplements (*see pp.268–271*).

INFANCY TO ADOLESCENCE

The extra needs of babies, children, and adolescents are discussed on pages 114–135. Extra calcium is vital during these years to help build strong bones and protect against the bone disorder osteoporosis in later life (*see p.242*).

ADULT NEEDS

When girls and women have menstrual periods, they lose iron in the blood. They may then need to eat iron-rich foods or take a supplement, especially if their periods are heavy, to reduce the risk of iron-deficiency anemia (*see p.55*).

During pregnancy (*see pp.138–141*), women have increased needs for vitamins riboflavin (B_2), B_{12}, C, and folate (which is also important for women planning to conceive). Some of these needs can be met through diet, but your doctor should prescribe a prenatal supplement (*see p.140*), to help you meet your increased needs for iron, magnesium, selenium, iodine, and zinc during pregnancy.

Mothers who are breast-feeding (*see pp.116–117*) need extra vitamins A, thiamine (B_1), riboflavin, E, and folate to produce enough breast milk. Extra vitamins niacin (B_3), C, and D are needed to replenish vitamins passed into breast milk. Extra zinc, iodine, and selenium are also needed.

Men may have extra vitamin and mineral needs depending on their activity level. For example, those involved in sports who tend to sweat a lot may need to replace sodium, potassium, and magnesium.

In addition, for the many peole who are following low-carbohydrate diets to lose weight, taking a multivitamin or a B-complex supplement is essential, since foods with carbohydrates contain important B vitamins.

THE OVER-FIFTIES

After the age of 50 (*see pp.150–153*), you may need to focus on foods rich in vitamins B_6, B_{12}, and folate because their absorption is reduced in older age. Extra calcium is vital to keep the bones strong, especially after menopause.

OTHER TIMES

Strict vegetarians will not get enough vitamins B_{12} and D, iron, and calcium if they do not eat fortified foods or take supplements. Cigarette smokers may need extra vitamin C, which neutralizes damaging free radicals (*see p.58*), that are created by inhaled smoke. If you are taking medication, it may interact with absorption of vitamins or minerals. Ask your doctor about possible interactions.

Fuel for children

Dietary needs vary in line with a child's stage of growth and development.

It is important to maintain a healthy diet throughout your life, but for children it is essential for their normal growth and development. Getting all the necessary nutrients from food and drinks such as milk, along with plenty of exercise, has an immediate impact on children's well-being, as well as long-term consequences for their health when they reach adulthood.

Good habits
Establishing good eating and exercise habits early in life will help your child achieve his or her growth potential and provide the foundation for a healthy life.

Children need the same basic proportions of foods from the different food groups (*see p.71*) as adults, but in smaller serving sizes. These calories and nutrients allow a child's brain to reach its full potential. Without sufficient nutrients, a child's brain may not grow properly, which can affect intellectual development.

Calcium for healthy bones
Although the height of a child's parents affects how tall he or she will eventually be as an adult, diet plays a key role too. Children who do not get enough calcium and vitamin D will be shorter than children of the same age and are also at greater risk for bone fractures compared to those who get enough of these nutrients.

Growing children Young children are active and curious about the world around them. Frequent snacks and meals are necessary to replenish the calories they burn.

Energy and nutrient needs
Body composition (the relative amount of body fat, muscle, and bone), the amount of physical activity that a child does, and his or her age determine the energy (*opposite*) and nutrient needs of the child. These requirements vary dramatically depending on the stage of a child's growth and development. For example, the more muscle an adolescent has, the greater his or her need for calorie requirements will be.

The changing body
Boys and girls have similar amounts of body fat until puberty. Babies and toddlers have a high amount of body fat, which decreases as they enter their elementary school years. During puberty, children's body fat increases again. At the end of adolescence boys lose some body fat, whereas girls maintain the extra body fat deposited during adolescence throughout their adult years.

There is also a difference in the proportion of muscle that boys and girls have. They have similar amounts until puberty, at which stage boys triple their muscle mass, but girls only double theirs. This difference helps explain the higher energy requirements of teenage boys and men compared to that of teenage girls and women.

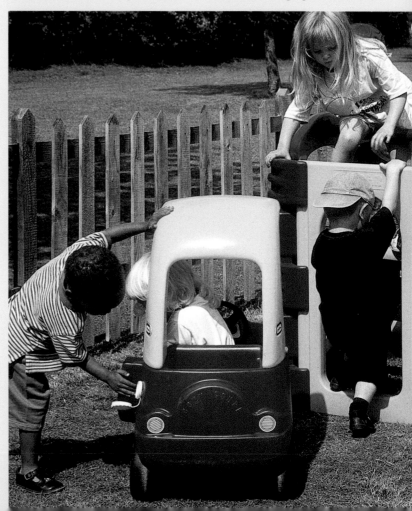

Energy requirements

The table below shows the recommended amounts of energy in calories (*see p.35*) that children from different age groups should be getting from food each day. It also shows the average amount of calories per lb (0.45kg) of body weight that each group needs for healthy growth. Although children of all ages grow rapidly, their energy needs vary; for example, the amount of energy needed, on a per lb/kg basis, for an 18-year-old teenager is much lower than that of an 18-month-old toddler. Babies double their body weight over a few months, whereas older children and adolescents may double their weight over 5–10 years.

Energy requirements vary in special cases. Physically active children use up more energy, so they need more calories than less active children. In addition, children who are ill or recovering from an injury need almost double their normal amount of calories to aid the healing process and continue growing.

AGE	CAL PER DAY	CAL PER LB (0.45kg)
0–6 months	650	49
7–12 months	850	45
1–3 years	1,300	46
4–6 years	1,800	41
7–10 years	2,000	32
11–14 years (girls)	2,200	21
11–14 years (boys)	2,500	25
15–18 years (girls)	2,200	18
15–18 years (boys)	3,000	20

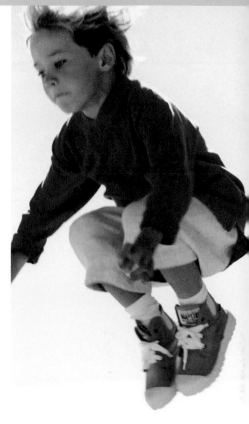

Spring-loaded Seven-year-olds are energetic and need about 2,000 calories per day, ideally from nutrient-dense foods, such as lean meat, whole grains, fruits, and vegetables.

Do children need vitamin and mineral supplements?

If children eat a varied diet, they should not need supplements. A very picky eater may need them. The most common vitamins and minerals that may be insufficient are listed below.

Calcium Most children get enough calcium as long as they drink milk and include yogurt and cheese in their diet. However, those who do not eat dairy products or do not drink milk may require a calcium supplement. Calcium needs are particularly high for adolescents because they gain more than 20 percent of their adult height and about 50 percent of their adult skeletal mass in this period.

Vitamin D Recent recommendations for all babies, including those who are exclusively breast-fed, now state that they should have a minimum intake of 0.005mg of vitamin D per day, beginning during the first two months of life. It is recommended that this intake level of vitamin D should be continued throughout childhood and adolescence to ensure strong and healthy bones.

Vitamin K Most newborn babies are given an injection of vitamin K immediately after delivery in order to prevent a bleeding disorder called hemorrhagic disease of the newborn.

Fluoride A supplement of fluoride is recommended for strong teeth development for babies 6 months or older who are exclusively breast-fed or living in an area without fluoridated water. Ask your doctor because too much fluoride can discolor the teeth.

Iron Newborn infants usually have enough iron stores from their mother for about four months. If they are not breast-fed, they should receive iron-fortified formula. Once babies begin to eat solid foods, they should be given iron-fortified cereal to prevent the risk of iron deficiency.

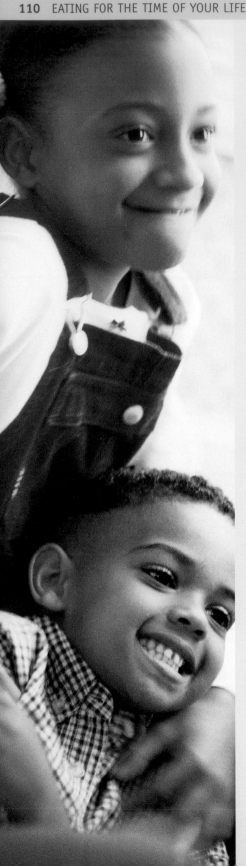

Your child's growth

Children's growth should be tracked to make sure they are eating enough.

Children need to be weighed and measured regularly to ensure that they are getting enough to eat for normal growth and development. This is especially important during their rapid growth spurts: the first in early childhood (first year of life), and the second, after a period of growth, in adolescence. These checkups can help detect any disorders that may be affecting their growth or development.

Regular wellness visits
Your child should have regular wellness visits during the first year, in which a nurse or doctor checks your child's length or height and weight. Head circumference is also checked for children under three years, since brain growth is reflected in the growth of the skull. These values are then plotted on growth charts appropriate for your child's age and gender (opposite and see p.112) to check that he or she is growing at a steady rate. Also assessed is your child's weight for his or her height by using body mass index (BMI; see p.26). BMI charts for boys and girls between 2 and 18 years are shown on page 113.

Growth spurts
Babies and adolescents require an increased amount of calories and nutrients in order to ensure normal development during rapid periods of growth.

Growing concerns A balanced diet with the appropriate amount of food allows children to grow and develop properly. It also helps keep them healthy and happy.

From birth to his or her third year, your child will grow rapidly and you will see huge changes as he or she develops. During this time you may worry that your toddler is eating too little or too much. Young children need a balanced diet to grow and flourish and each child burns calories differently, so do not be tempted to put your toddler on a weight-loss diet.

During puberty, children need extra calcium in the diet, which is vital for strong bone development. Teenage boys grow very quickly; at the height of their growth spurt, they may grow more than 2in (5cm) in a year. If your child does not get enough calories during puberty, it can have long-term effects on his or her growth and sexual development.

Plotting development
The growth charts opposite and on page 112 show the normal range of growth—weight and length or height for age—for 0–2 years olds and 2–18 years olds. These charts help you and your doctors see if your child's growth is normal.

The shaded band on each chart shows the normal range of growth. This area is made up of curves known as percentiles, based on what percentage of children of a certain age have a particular weight or length or height. These range from the 5th (95 percent of children are bigger than this) to the 95th percentile (95 percent of children are smaller than this) and show how your child compares with children across North America. The 50th percentile line is also shown, marking the middle of the range.

Your child's growth is considered normal if, over time, his or her measurements produce a steady upward curve within the shaded region of the chart.

Checking your baby's growth

At your child's wellness visits, a nurse or doctor will weigh and measure the length (from heel to crown) of your baby. These measurements are then plotted on growth charts: weight for age and length for age, with separate charts for boys and girls (*below*). The measurements can reassure breast-feeding mothers who do not know exactly how much their babies are getting.

Over time, a child's measurements should give a gradual upward curve, indicating normal growth. If growth is steady there is usually no cause for concern, even if a child stays within a low percentile. However, if your child's weight, length, or head circumference radically shifts or plateaus in a short period of time, your baby's doctor should further evaluate the cause. Most children are measured heel to crown until 24 months, although small or ill children may be measured in this way until 36 months.

Using the charts Find your baby's weight or length on the left of the chart and follow the horizontal line across until it meets the vertical line from your child's age. Mark a cross here. Plotting this at regular intervals will create a curve that lets you track your child's growth and development easily.

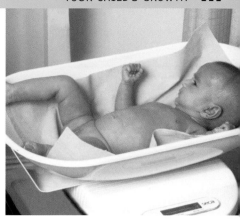

Weighing a baby A nurse or doctor will weigh and measure the length of your baby at each visit to ensure his or her growth is normal.

BOYS' WEIGHT (0–2 YEARS)

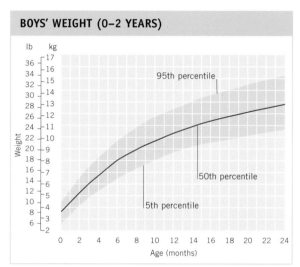

GIRLS' WEIGHT (0–2 YEARS)

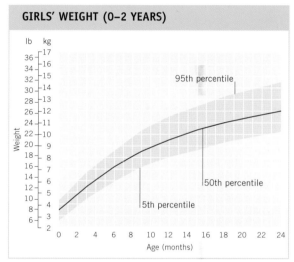

BOYS' LENGTH (0–2 YEARS)

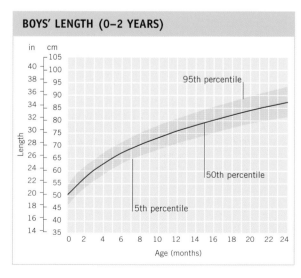

GIRLS' LENGTH (0–2 YEARS)

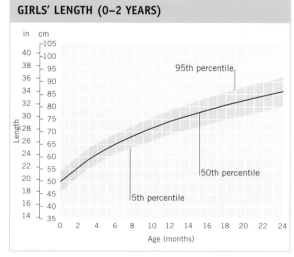

Checking your child's growth

To monitor your child's growth, you can weigh and measure him or her yourself. This will also be done at your doctor's office. The measurements can then be plotted on growth charts: weight and height for age, with separate charts for boys and girls (below).

Plotted over time, your child's weight and length should produce a gradual upward curve within the shaded gray band. This indicates that your child is growing normally. As long as the growth is steady there is usually no cause for concern, even if a child is consistently within a low percentile, such as the 5th.

However, If your child's weight or height changes, for example from the 85th to the 45th percentile (or vice versa) in a year, this change could indicate a problem, either medical or nutritional, that requires intervention.

Using the charts Find your child's weight or height on the left of the chart and follow the horizontal line across until it meets the vertical line from your child's age. Mark a cross at this point. By plotting this point at regular intervals, for example every six months, you will create a curve that clearly shows how your child is growing.

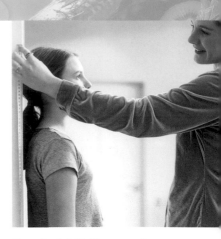

Measuring height When measuring your child's height, make sure she or he is barefoot and standing straight.

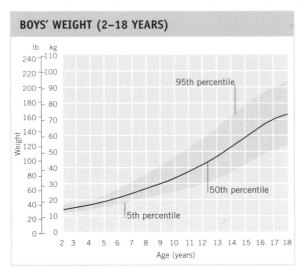

BOYS' WEIGHT (2–18 YEARS)

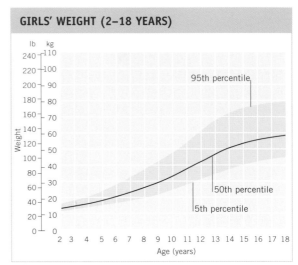

GIRLS' WEIGHT (2–18 YEARS)

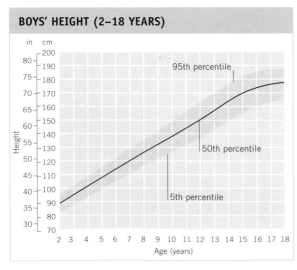

BOYS' HEIGHT (2–18 YEARS)

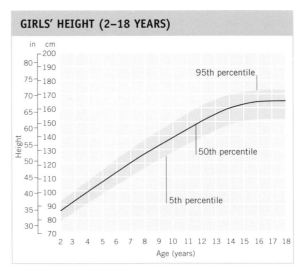

GIRLS' HEIGHT (2–18 YEARS)

Checking your child's weight for height

The BMI charts below show the range of body mass index (BMI) for North American boys and girls aged between 2 and 18 years. BMI is calculated as a ratio of weight to height, and gives a more accurate reflection of your child's body-fat content.

The charts have a shaded band made up of curves called percentiles. These range from the 5th percentile (95 percent of children of a particular age have a BMI greater than this) to the 95th percentile (95 percent of children have a BMI smaller than this). The gray band shows you how your child compares with other North American children and if he or she is underweight, normal weight, or overweight.

Regularly plotting BMI can also identify children who are at risk of becoming over- or underweight and who require nutritional or medical intervention.

Children may be diagnosed as being underweight if their BMI for their age and gender falls below the 5th percentile. Acceptable weight lies between the 5th and 85th percentile. A child with a BMI greater than the 85th percentile is at risk of being overweight. Greater than the 95th percentile indicates that your child is overweight.

Using the charts To use BMI charts, you will first need to calculate your child's BMI (*right*). Then find his or her BMI on the left of the chart and follow the horizontal line across until it meets the vertical line from your child's age. Mark a cross at this point. By plotting this value every 6 months, you can create a curve showing your child's BMI over time. Ask your doctor or medical advisor for a chart to fill in or visit the Centers for Disease Control and Prevention website (*see p.326*).

Working out BMI

To use the charts below, you need to work out your child's body mass index (BMI), for which you will need to know his or her height and weight in either English or metric measurements.

Using English measurements
1. Multiply your child's height (in inches) by itself.
2. Divide your child's weight (in pounds) by the result in step 1.
3. Multiply the result in step 2 by 703. This will tell you the BMI.

Using metric measurements
1. Multiply your child's height (in meters) by itself.
2. Divide your child's weight (in kilograms) by the result in step 1 to give you the BMI.

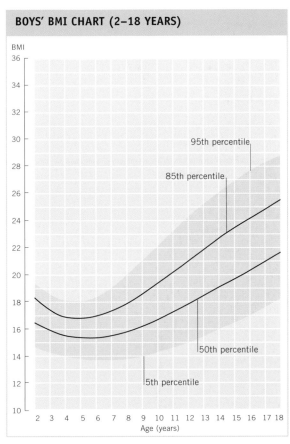

BOYS' BMI CHART (2–18 YEARS)

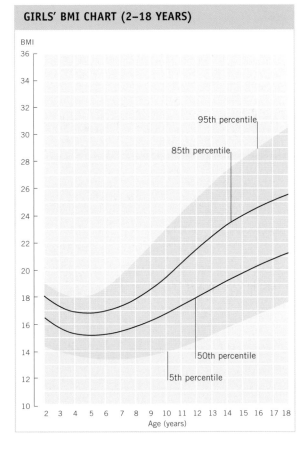

GIRLS' BMI CHART (2–18 YEARS)

Food in the first year

Breast milk and infant formula are the most important sources of nutrition for babies.

Feeding your new baby is one of the most rewarding things you do as a new parent. In the beginning, your breast-fed baby will eat every two to three hours (eight to 12 times a day) and formula-fed babies will eat every three to four hours.

You may have heard that breast-feeding is "best for your baby." and this chapter we help you understand the benefits for both you and your baby and teach you how to breast-feed. If you decide to give formula or introduce it while you are breast-feeding or when you return to work, you can follow the advice on choosing a formula and how to prepare and store it. We also outline how infant formula compares with breast milk nutritionally for health and for convenience.

Beginning solid foods

At about six months of age, your baby will sit up and hold his or her head up, and he or she will become much more interested in what you are eating. In the following pages, we outline why you should wait until your baby is ideally six months old before giving any solid food and why iron-fortified infant cereal is the ideal first food (*below*). We tell you how to make the transition from giving your baby infant cereal to baby foods during this critical first year, when your baby will triple his or her weight. New parents have many questions about nutrition during this time and we make an attempt to answer most of these.

Food allergies

Since food allergies have become increasingly common and may be life threatening, we discuss the issues involved and provide practical information for parents with children who have a history of food allergies.

Introducing a cup At six to eight months, you can start offering your child diluted 100 percent fruit juice or water in a sturdy cup with handles that she can hold herself.

Introducing first tastes

A question often asked by new mothers is, "When can I start feeding my baby table food?" Doctors now recommend waiting until at least four, but preferably six, months for breast-fed babies. There are three reasons for this. Firstly, at four months, the average baby needs about 24floz (720ml) of breast milk or formula each day, and early introduction of solid foods may result in babies drinking less milk, interfering with proper nutrition during this critical period. Secondly, young babies have a tongue reflex that pushes food out of the mouth. By four to six months, this reflex disappears, so they can accept food from a spoon. Thirdly, before the age of six months, a baby's digestive system cannot properly digest the nutrients in food.

In addition, if you introduce solid foods too early, it may result in the development of food allergies (*see p.120*) or cause your baby to choke or breathe food into his or her lungs.

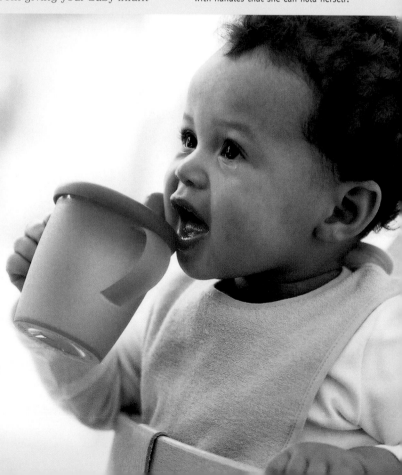

Breast milk versus infant formula

The perfect food for your baby is breast milk; it is convenient, ready-to-serve, sterile, and tailor-made to meet all the nutritional needs of a baby until six months of age. Already at the proper temperature, breast milk does not require heating.

Giving breast milk also benefits the mother—its production burns up calories, allowing you to return more quickly to your prepregnancy weight. It also confers some protection against developing certain disorders, including breast and ovarian cancer. However, for one reason or another, you may decide that breast-feeding is not for you and choose to give your infant formula instead. Most formulas are based on cow's milk or soymilk and have to be prepared with sterile water, such as chlorinated tap water, and then warmed. Your baby will still need the same amount of calories as a breast-fed baby, but since formula takes three to four hours to pass through your baby's digestive tract, compared to two hours for breast milk, he or she will need fewer feedings of formula a day.

Before you decide whether you want to breast-feed or bottle-feed with infant formula, consider the points below covering nutritional and health aspects and convenience.

BREAST MILK	INFANT FORMULA
The nutrient content of breast milk varies during the feeding, and the more your baby nurses, the more milk you produce.	Infant formula always has the same nutrients, and you can estimate your baby's needs.
Antibodies and living cells in breast milk help protect your baby against infections.	Infant formula does not contain protective antibodies and living cells.
Because breast milk contains antibodies, it is more protective against infections such as gastroenteritis.	Formula may introduce infection through contaminated water or dirty bottles, so ensure that everything is clean.
Breast milk contains the fatty acids docosahexanoic acid (DHA) and arachidonic acid (ALA), vital for brain and vision development.	Some formulas do contain these fatty acids. However, they all contain vitamin B_{12}, so if you are a vegetarian, your baby is much less likely to develop vitamin B_{12} deficiency, which is found naturally only in foods of animal origin.
The iron in breast milk is more easily absorbed than the iron in infant formula.	Formula contains more iron and more vitamin K, which is necessary for blood clotting, than breast milk.
A breast-fed baby is unlikely to be overfed because breast milk is supplied on demand.	It is easier to overfeed formula-fed babies because care-takers may try to get the baby to take more.
Your health, your diet, stress levels, any medications, or alcohol intake can affect breast milk.	Quality of infant formula is not affected by your diet or state of health.
Breast milk reduces the risk of your child developing asthma, eczema, other allergies, and intolerance to cow's milk later. There is a lower incidence of many other disorders from ear infections and colitis (inflammation of the colon) to diabetes, immune disorders, sudden infant death syndrome (SIDS), and the cancer lymphoma in breast-fed babies.	Formula has not been shown to reduce the risk of these disorders in babies.
Breast milk is always available wherever you are and is at the right temperature.	Formula needs to be prepared, refrigerated for storage, and warmed before giving it to your baby.
Breast-feeding does not require time to prepare the milk or special equipment (unless you express milk).	Formula requires equipment and time to prepare.
Breast-feeding is usually less expensive than formula.	You have to buy formula.
You are the only one who can feed the baby, unless you choose to express milk, in which case your partner or others can also help with feeding.	If others help with feeding, you can share feeding with your partner, have more time to yourself, get more sleep, and go back to work without expressing.

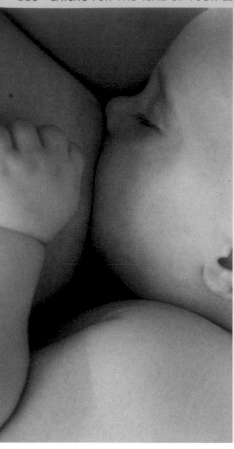

Benefits of breast milk

Breast milk is the perfect food for your baby in the first year.

Breast-feeding is recommended as the "gold standard" for feeding babies by all professional groups including the American Academy of Pediatrics and the World Health Organization. This is because of its health advantages for both the baby and mother. Breast milk is considered the ideal source of food to support optimum growth and development in your baby. Complemented by appropriate introduction of solid foods at around six months of age, breast

Breast-feeding This provides your baby with the ideal food, which can also protect against infection. In addition, breast-feeding can strengthen the bond between you.

milk is recommended for the entire first year of your baby's life, or longer if desired.

As a result of national efforts to promote breast-feeding, almost 60 percent of mothers are now breast-feeding when they leave the hospital after giving birth, which compares to only 20 percent in the 1970s. But many women stop breast-feeding within the first few weeks or months. It is hoped that by 2010, 75 percent of mothers will breast-feed for the first four to six weeks and 50 percent will still be breast-feeding six months later.

Protection against disease

Breast milk is not only the best source of nutrition for your baby, but it also contains antibodies (disease-fighting proteins) that are transferred from the mother to the baby during the first two weeks of breast-feeding. About

How do I breast-feed?

When you are breast-feeding, it is important to be comfortable with your back well supported with cushions. Have a snack and a glass of water by your side because you are likely to be feeding for a while. Over time, you and your baby will become more comfortable as you get to know each other, and both of you can relax and enjoy this bonding experience.

FEEDING POSITIONS

There is no right or wrong position in which to breast-feed your baby. The cradle position is the most popular, in which you and your baby are "tummy to tummy." You can put a pillow under your baby to raise him or her and to prevent you from leaning forward. Your baby's body will be in a straight line, with the neck in the proper position to feed. Lying on your side is another common position and can be very

relaxing. Again, you should be "tummy to tummy." The football-hold position is another position and recommended for mothers of twins who want to feed both babies at the same time. While sitting, place the twins, supported by cushions, on either side of you. Use your arms to support each head, with one arm for each baby.

LATCHING ON

No matter which position you choose, how your baby's mouth is positioned onto your nipple is very important and will help prevent you from getting sore nipples and improve your success at feeding. It will also ensure that your baby gets plenty of milk and that you produce enough.

To encourage your baby to latch on properly, you will need to touch your nipple to your baby's mouth, like tickling the lips at the corners of the

mouth. This action stimulates your baby to open his or her mouth wide. When your baby's mouth is open, bring him or her toward you and onto your breast to begin suckling. The entire areola—the pigmented area surrounding the nipple —should be in your baby's mouth while feeding to ensure that your nipple is in the right position. This is because the action of your baby's lips suckling on the areola stimulates milk production.

BREAKING THE SUCTION

When your baby has finished nursing, you may need to break the suction by inserting your finger into the corner of your baby's mouth. If your baby pulls away without breaking the suction, it can be painful and cause sore nipples.

Remember, during the first few days, breast-feeding may be painful, but as your breasts become accustomed to feeding, it will get easier.

80 percent of the cells in this early breast milk are macrophages, cells that kill viruses and bacteria, and even after these two weeks, breast milk remains full of antibodies.

Breast-feeding leads to fewer ear and gastrointestinal infections, and respiratory illnesses during the first year of a baby's life, and there is strong evidence that it can help prevent infections, such as bacterial meningitis, and colitis (inflammation of the colon). Breast milk may also protect your baby against immune system disorders, diabetes, allergies, and sudden infant death syndrome (SIDS).

Benefits for the mother

Breast-feeding strengthens the bond between mother and baby, helps you to lose the weight gained during pregnancy, and decreases your risk of breast cancer, ovarian cancer, and the bone disease osteoporosis later in life. All in all, breast-feeding is the best possible choice for both you and your baby.

Breast milk: the perfect food for babies

The human breast produces three types of breast milk: colostrum, transitional milk, and mature milk. Colostrum is made during late pregnancy and the first few days of breast-feeding and is high in protein, antibodies, some vitamins and minerals, and hormones. These nutrients encourage the growth of friendly bacteria in the intestine, also known as gut flora (see p.48), and the passage of the baby's first stools.

Transitional milk is produced in the second week, and it is higher in fat and the milk sugar lactose and lower in protein and minerals than colostrum. From day 15 onward, mature milk is produced—this is a blend of fat and sugary (lactose) water and is very nutritious.

Mature milk During each feeding, the composition of mature breast milk changes. Babies get 75 percent of the milk volume in the first 5–10

minutes, but only 50 percent of the calories. The milk produced after 5–10 minutes is richest in fat and is known as the "hind milk." It is therefore essential that your baby is allowed to nurse on each breast until satisfied in order to obtain enough calories for adequate growth.

Whey and casein Whey accounts for 60–80 percent of the total protein in mature breast milk, and it contains the proteins that help babies fight infections. Casein accounts for the remaining 20–40 percent of mature breast milk's total protein and forms compounds that increase your baby's ability to absorb minerals.

Lactose The main carbohydrate found in breast milk is the sugar lactose. Small amounts of other carbohydrates are also present in breast milk, some of which can help fight infection.

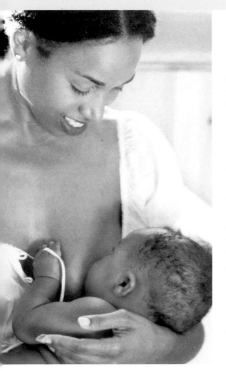

Feeding on demand

Breast-feeding should occur on demand, whenever your baby is hungry. It may take a few days to get used to your baby's feeding schedule; however, once you have both settled into a pattern, your milk supply will increase and you will be able to satisfy your baby's needs.

"LET-DOWN" REFLEX

It is best to begin breast-feeding within the first two hours after giving birth. Do not limit the time for each feeding in the early stages. You may find it takes two to three minutes of suckling to stimulate the release of oxytocin, a hormone that causes "let-down," a process in which milk begins to empty from the breasts.

Feeding properly Babies usually latch on to the breast very naturally. Make sure that you are sitting comfortably before you start, and have a drink and a snack at hand.

LET YOUR BABY DICTATE

When your baby stops suckling, he or she should be burped and then placed on the other breast for as long as he or she wants. Feeding should be dictated by the baby and not by the clock. If your baby falls asleep during breast-feeding, pause for a short time and resume when he or she is ready again.

FREQUENT FEEDINGS

A baby who suckles vigorously usually empties the breast in 10–20 minutes after let-down. It may take up to an hour to empty both breasts. Alternating the breast that your baby starts on each time will help ensure even milk production.

Babies will suckle until satisfied and in the first six weeks should feed eight to 12 times during 24 hours. Frequent feeding reduces the risk of breast engorgement, which can cause you discomfort and increase the risk of breast infection.

Feeding your baby formula

Infant formula provides a balanced food source for babies.

Infant formulas for babies have been developed as a substitute for breast milk when a woman is unable to breast-feed because of physical or medical reasons or because she chooses not to.

Infant formulas are made to meet babies' needs and to match the composition of breast milk as closely as possible. They also need to be friendly to your baby's immature intestine. For these reasons, the composition of infant formulas, including the vitamin and mineral content, is carefully controlled by the Food and Drug Administration (FDA), which sets strict standards.

Because breast milk contains living cells and other factors that cannot be reproduced artificially, it is impossible to produce a formula equal in all aspects to breast milk. However, formulas do meet the nutritional needs of most babies.

Types of formulas

Most infant formulas are derived from cow's milk or soymilk. These are known as standard formulas and are generally well tolerated by babies (*below*). However, special formulas are available for babies who are not able to digest, absorb, or process standard formulas properly (*below*).

Similar to breast milk

Cow's milk contains most of the nutrients necessary for growth and development, although not in the appropriate proportions that are suitable for human babies. However, cow's milk can be easily modified by formula manufacturers into the right proportions.

Once the milk has been modified, the formula has a similar amount of calories as breast milk and also similar amounts and proportions of proteins, fats, lactose (the sugar that is found naturally in milk), vitamins, and minerals.

Soymilk formulas are modified, too. For example, they have certain amino acids (building blocks of proteins) added to make them more like human milk.

Bottle-feeding If you do choose to bottle-feed your baby, other members of the family, especially dad, can help with the feedings and increase their bonding with the baby.

Choosing the right formula

Once you have decided to bottle-feed your baby, you will have to choose a suitable formula. If you are unsure of which type to opt for, your baby's doctor will be able to advise you. The most widely used formulas are made from cow's milk, although soymilk formulas are recommended for babies with milk allergy. Most cow's-milk and soymilk formulas are similar and will provide enough calories and nutrients to meet your baby's needs. However, the sources and kinds of nutrients differ between brands.

STANDARD FORMULAS

These are available in different forms: ready-to-feed liquid formulas do not need mixing with water and cost the most; concentrated liquid formulas require mixing with water in equal parts; and powdered formulas require mixing one scoop of powdered formula with 2floz (60ml) of water and are usually the least expensive.

SPECIAL FORMULAS

Your baby will need a special infant formula if he or she is diagnosed with a problem in which certain substances found in breast milk or formula cannot be digested or processed properly. In special formulas, one or more of the basic nutrients—usually the protein and/or carbohydrate—have been modified into an alternative form that your baby can tolerate better.

There are various types of special formulas. Examples include higher-calorie formulas for premature babies; hypoallergenic formulas for babies allergic to cow's milk or soymilk; and predigested formulas for babies who cannot digest proteins, fats, and other substances present in breast milk or standard formula.

There are also amino acid-modified, fat-modified, and carbohydrate-modified formulas for babies who have difficulty digesting, absorbing, or processing certain amino acids, fats, or sugars.

Essential fatty acids and docosahexanoic acid

Essential fatty acids (*see p.38*) are components of fats that we must get from our diet because our bodies are not capable of making them from other substances in food. They include linoleic acid and are necessary in the body to make cell membranes and many important hormones. They also make other chemical messengers, which "tell" our body how to function properly.

Docosahexanoic acid (DHA) is an important chemical that our body makes from essential fatty acids. It is essential from conception through infancy for the normal growth and development of the brain and vision. DHA is the most abundant fat in breast milk and certain infant formulas now contain this essential fatty acid.

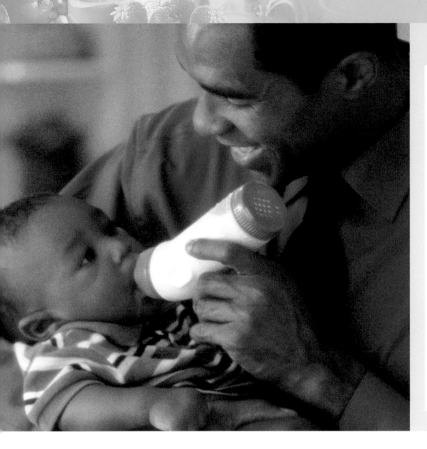

How much formula?

When preparing formula, always follow the manufacturer's directions carefully. Your baby's daily needs are 17–24floz (500–700ml) until six months then 24–32floz (700–1,000ml) until one year. Early on, your baby will only drink 1–2floz (30–60ml) at each feeding and gradually work up to 4–6floz (120–180ml). When starting solid foods, he or she may drink a 6–8floz (180–240ml) bottle after meals and one at bedtime.

Do not enlarge the hole in the nipple—this will lead to overfeeding and possibly rapid weight gain, or choking. When your baby refuses the bottle or drops it or stops sucking, he or she has most likely had enough. By recognizing this, you will be less inclined to overfeed. If your baby seems to want more than 24floz (700ml) of formula a day before six months, try a pacifier.

Preparing and storing formula

Make sure you use the following tips when you are preparing and storing infant formula.

PREPARING BOTTLES

To reduce the risk of infection and to make sure your baby gets the correct amount of formula, follow these tips:
• Always buy and use the formula before its expiration date.
• Use a clean, punch-type can opener to open liquid formula. After opening, use all the contents immediately.
• Follow the manufacturer's directions exactly. If you do not add enough powder, your baby will not get enough calories. Too little water will cause your baby to get too high a concentration of formula, which may lead to diarrhea, dehydration, or overfeeding.
• Because most tap water has chlorine added as a disinfectant, there is no need to first boil tap water used for formula preparation.
• Wash baby bottles in hot soapy water.

• If your water is from a well or a nonchlorinated source, use cooled water that has been boiled.
• Your baby may like formula warmed to body temperature. You can warm it in a bowl of warm (not boiling) water. Some babies will drink it unwarmed.
• Do not use a microwave oven to warm formula. There may be "hot spots" in the formula that burn your baby's mouth.
• Before giving any warmed formula to your baby, make sure you always check the temperature yourself.

STORING FORMULA

Again, it is critical to ensure that you are strictly hygienic when storing infant formula to avoid infection:
• Do not use a liquid or prepared formula that has been frozen or stored at temperatures below 32°F (0°C) or heated above 95°F (35°C).
• Place any formula prepared in advance in the refrigerator to minimize bacterial growth.

• Throw away any refrigerated formula unused within 24 hours.
• If you and your baby are going out, put the right amount of powdered formula in a few bottles, and then add warm water when your baby is ready to feed.

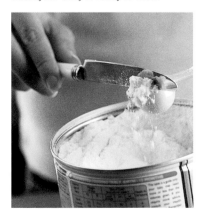

Preparing infant formula Always level off the scoop when preparing formula or you will make it too concentrated.

Introducing first foods

At about six months your baby is ready to start solid foods.

Recommendations on when to introduce solid foods to your baby's diet have changed considerably over the years. In the past, some doctors advised that children should eat a wide variety of foods as early as the first month of life. Pediatric health-care providers now advise delaying the introduction of solid foods until your child is at least four months. However, the American Academy of Pediatrics recommends breast milk as the sole nutrient source until six months of age.

When to start
The digestive system of a young baby is not developed enough to cope with solid foods until about four to six months of age and introducing solid foods any earlier can stimulate the development of

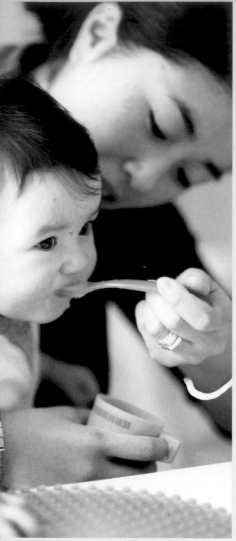

New tastes At about four to six months of age, your baby will be ready to be fed with a spoon and you will be able to add cereals, puréed fruit, and vegetables to her diet.

food allergies (*below*). Also, giving solid foods too soon could cause choking (*opposite*). Very young babies have a reflex whereby their tongue naturally pushes the food out of their mouths, but by the age of four to six months they lose this tongue-thrust reflex and so you can begin spoonfeeding. At this age, most babies can sit supported in a chair and will have developed control and coordination of their head, neck, and mouth muscles. They can eat properly, although they are likely to make a mess, so protect his or her clothes with a bib.

Spoonfeeding
The introduction of solid foods marks the beginning of a critical period during which a baby learns to eat from a spoon and accept different tastes and textures. Not coincidentally, a baby's readiness for these experiences generally corresponds to a physical need to supplement the amount of calories and nutrients available from breast milk or formula. However, milk or formula should still continue to be the major source of calories and nutrients during the remainder of the baby's first year. The common belief that solids can "fatten up" the baby or help him or her sleep better is a misconception. Most solid foods have fewer calories than breast milk or formula and should not be the sole nutrient source.

Gradual introduction
New foods should be introduced gradually—not more than every three days or longer if there is a family history of allergies—and no more than one new food at a time. Following these rules will make it easier for you to identify a food that your baby may be sensitive to or has an allergic reaction to. The table shown opposite gives general guidelines on introducing the basic five food groups.

Food allergies

These affect 4–6 percent of children in America. Even a tiny amount of an offending food can be life-threatening. Common foods that cause allergies include cow's milk, wheat, soy, eggs, honey, shellfish, fish, treenuts, such as walnuts and almonds, and peanuts. If there is a family history of allergies, delay giving dairy until one year, eggs until two, and shellfish, fish, treenuts, and peanuts, until three years.

Recognizing allergy After giving a new food to your baby, look out for signs of an allergy developing, such

as a skin rash, vomiting, or diarrhea. If your child's lips and face swell, call an ambulance as this is an emergency. Avoiding the offending food is the only prevention. (*See also pp.252–255.*)

Check labels Substances that cause allergies are often hidden in foods; for example, wheat may be in deli meats and eggs in dressings, so check food labels carefully. If you feel your child is falling short on vital nutrients because he or she has to avoid certain foods, consult your doctor or a registered dietitian.

Adding new foods to your baby's diet

Up to about the first six months of life, all the food a baby needs is breast milk or formula. After this time, you can begin to add solid foods—initially puréed—along with milk feedings, which should continue until at least 12 months. Between seven and 12 months, a baby needs 850 calories a day.

No real consensus exists among the experts regarding when and how to introduce solid foods, but you may find the chart below helpful; it shows you when you can add new foods and textures to your baby's diet. It is important not to rush your baby and take one step at a time. If he or she will not eat one particular type of food it could simply be that he or she does not like it—like adults, babies dislike some foods. Pay attention to nutrition labels if you are buying ready-prepared food for your baby, as these foods can be high in salt or sugar. When puréeing vegetables at home, do not add salt.

In terms of drinks, offer him or her occasional drinks of water. Experts feel that there is no specific need for fruit juice in a baby's diet, but if you do decide to give it to your baby, do not give more than 6floz (180ml) of diluted 100 percent fruit juice per day, and serve at mealtimes.

Foods to avoid

Children under one year are at risk of choking and at higher risk for food allergies. Do not give the following to babies under one:
- Any milk not designed for human babies, such as cow's, goat's, and soymilk
- Nuts and peanut butter
- Hard candy and marshmallows
- Whole grapes
- Egg whites
- Ice cream
- Hot dogs
- Hard raw vegetables (carrots)
- Popcorn and chips

NEW FOOD	4–6 MONTHS	7–9 MONTHS	10–12 MONTHS
Milk	• 4–6 feedings of breast milk/formula per day	• 3–5 feedings of breast milk/formula per day	• 3–4 feedings of breast milk/formula per day
Cereals and bread	• Rice, barley, or oatmeal, iron-fortified cereal mixed thinly with breast milk/formula twice daily • Teething biscuits, crackers, toast strips	• Bread and bagels • Small pieces of cooked noodles • Mashed potatoes • Unsweetened, dry cereal • Teething biscuits	• White wheat bread • Rice • Waffles • Pasta and spaghetti • Couscous
Vegetables	• Puréed, well-cooked dark yellow, orange (but not corn), or dark-green vegetables	• Cooked, mashed vegetables such as potatoes, butternut squash, and peas	• Cooked vegetables, such as boiled potatoes, carrots, and broccoli • Some raw vegetables, such as tomatoes and peeled cucumber
Fruit	• Puréed, fresh or cooked fruits • Mashed bananas • Applesauce, unsweetened	• Peeled or skinned soft fruit wedges such as bananas, peaches, pears, oranges, apples	• Any fresh fruit peeled and seeded or canned in water • Limit juice to 4–6floz (120–180ml) per day
Dairy	• No cow's milk or other dairy products at this stage	• Cottage cheese • Yogurt • Bite-size strips of cheese	• Slices of cheese, cut up • Grilled cheese
Protein sources	• Babies get all the protein they need from their milk	• Well-cooked, puréed, ground, or finely chopped chicken, fish, and lean meats (without bones, skin, or fat) • Cooked beans, such as baked beans or chickpeas • Cooked, mashed egg yolk (but not egg white)	• Small, tender pieces of chicken, fish, or lean meat • Ground lean beef or ground turkey breast • Chicken nuggets • Ravioli

Nutrition for toddlers

In the second year, a child will increase the range of foods he or she eats.

During the second year of life, children show more and more interest in food, but parents may notice that they eat less or are more choosy about what they eat. Growth rates slow at this time and

Learning to feed herself During the second year, toddlers love to sit at the table with the rest of the family and feed themselves. Offer foods that they can pick up easily, and keep a close eye while they are eating.

many toddlers seem to eat less compared to the first year of life. Those taught to eat wholesome, fresh foods will be more likely to prefer these foods for life.

Introducing cow's milk

Children at this age will usually want to eat what the people around them are eating and reach out and grab foods and drinks. It is therefore a perfect opportunity and very important to set a good example. At this time, your child will also make the transition from breast milk or infant formula to whole cow's milk and should be drinking out of a cup rather than a bottle. Their expanding palate is ready for new textures, colors, and

flavors, and it is the perfect time to offer a variety of healthy foods, not only for their three meals a day but also for their snacks.

Starting good habits now

Eating habits formed in the first two years of life are thought to persist for years, if not for life, so it is important to establish healthy habits as early as possible.

Children begin expressing personal preferences at an early age. Parents must guide a child's healthy food choices and allow the child to determine what and how much he or she wishes to eat.

At times, it may seem to you that your child is not eating enough food. But forcing children to eat something that they do not want makes them stubborn about their eating habits. By allowing some independence at this age you will be helping alleviate mealtime problems in the future.

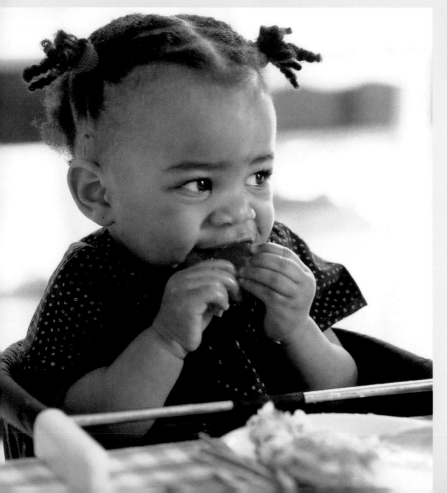

Serving sizes: 1–2 years

Children aged 1–2 years need foods from all the food groups, but with fewer and smaller servings than older children. For each food group, the daily number of servings and some examples of a serving are described below:

- 4–6 servings of grains and their products. Examples of a serving include ½ slice whole-grain bread or 1 cup cereal.
- 2–3 servings of vegetables. For example, 2 tbsp peas, 2 slices cucumber, or 2 tomato wedges.
- 2 servings of fruits. For example, ½ apple or 4floz (120ml) fruit juice.
- 2 servings of dairy products. Servings include 4floz (120ml) whole milk or 1oz (28g) cheese.
- 2 servings of protein sources. Examples include 1oz (28g) meat, chicken, or fish, ¼ cup beans, or 2floz (60ml) cottage cheese.

How much should your child be eating?

It is very important to keep in mind that your child's stomach is much smaller than an adult's and therefore, he or she does not need as much food as you or an older sibling. An example of what a 1–2-year old child can eat in a day is shown in our sample menu on the right. If your child is particularly energetic, he or she will may need another snack after dinner.

Some helpful tips to bear in mind when feeding your young child include:
• Use smaller plates for toddlers and let their appetite regulate how much food they want to eat.

• Do not force, bribe, or nag a child to finish his or her meal or "clean your plate." This negative approach will lead to arguments over food or could result in an overweight child who develops habits that are difficult to break. Your child will let you know when he or she has had enough by clamping his or her lips closed, pushing the plate away, or dropping food.
• Serve a well-balanced meal in small quantities that includes foods from all the food groups. There is no need to push second servings of anything. If your child is still hungry, he or she will

ask for more, at which time, it is best to give more vegetables or fresh fruit. He or she may eat more at the next meal.
• If your child is cutting back on the amount of milk he or she drinks, offer yogurt or cheese as a snack or dessert.

SAMPLE MENU: 1–2 YEARS

Breakfast
• 2 mini waffles with low-sugar syrup, 4floz (120ml) fruited yogurt, and 4floz (120ml) dilute apple juice (half juice, half water)

Snack
• 1 cup fruit salad and 4floz (120ml) whole milk

Lunch
• 1 cup macaroni and cheese with green peas, 4floz (120ml) milk, and ½ banana

Snack
• 2 graham crackers and 4floz (120ml) dilute apple juice

Dinner
• 2oz (55g) white-meat chicken with ½ cup cooked brown rice, ½ cup soft carrots, 2 slices of cucumber, and 4floz (120ml) water

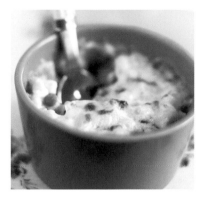

Macaroni and cheese A good source of calcium, macaroni and cheese can be mixed with peas as to make sure that your child is also getting nutrients from vegetables.

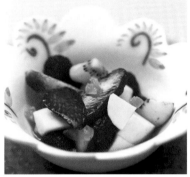

Fruit salad Full of beneficial vitamins, phytochemicals, minerals, and fiber, a small bowl of fresh fruit salad makes an ideal dessert or snack for a young child.

Introducing new foods

When most of your child's teeth have come through, he or she is ready to chew new foods. However, there is still a risk of choking, so you need to avoid certain foods (*right*).

As you can see from the sample menu above right, 1–2-year-old children need three meals and at least two snacks every day. You can start to give them table food, such as baked chicken, but it is very important to remember to cut everything up into tiny pieces so that they are not at risk of choking. Since children at this age prefer to grab everything within reach and put it in their mouth at one time, try giving a

few bites at a time so that they learn to take their time when eating. Serve water with meals in order to help them swallow these foods.

If your child rejects a new food, remove it without fuss, and reintroduce it at a later date. Your child may not be hungry, or may want something else that day. Do not emphasize that a food is new, or suggest that he or she may not like it before even trying it.

Make the effort to eat with your child often, at home, or in restaurants. This can encourage your child to try new foods. Eating with young friends can also stimulate his or her appetite.

Preventing choking

The risk of choking is particularly high for young children because they may have problems chewing. It is best to avoid giving young children small pieces of fruit, such as whole grapes, raw vegetables, or chunks of meat, such as slices of hot dog, as they could be a hazard. Instead, cut them into tiny pieces or thinly sliced sticks, and for very young children, boil well and then mash or purée foods. Wet or juicy foods may slip down a child's throat without being chewed properly, so give these foods one at a time.

Feeding preschool children

Between the ages of two and five, children need plenty of snacks.

After the rapid growth of early infancy, toddlers' growth rate slows, and they tend to eat less, although appetite fluctuations are normal and correspond to growth spurts. Therefore, your child may seem very hungry one day and not show any interest in food at all the next.

Learn to recognize when your child is hungry and offer healthy, appetizing meals, one small snack between meals, and a piece of fresh fruit before bedtime. Keep in mind that giving your child too many drinks between meals can also fill up his or her small stomach very quickly so, do not overdo it. This also applies for serving sizes; children cannot manage adult-sized portions, so try to use smaller, child-friendly plates and offer smaller amounts of food.

Giving the right food

Because appetites vary from child to child and from day to day, you may worry about your child's eating habits. For example, sometimes he or she may want to eat the same foods for every meal, and at other times that same food may get rejected outright. Inconsistency when it comes to mealtimes is very common, so offer your child a nutritious selection of food, try to remain patient and let your child choose what he or she wants to eat within reason. Over the course of a week, most children's diets will balance out. If your child is a picky eater you may need to develop some strategies for dealing with this (*see p.127*).

Monitoring your child

By monitoring your child's growth (*see p.112*) and eating habits and looking for signs or symptoms of nutritional deficiency, you can tell if he or she is getting the proper amounts of nutrients. Children who are eating enough will be growing at the appropriate rate. Growth charts (*see pp.111–113*) can be kept at home to help you track your child's height and weight for age.

It is difficult to detect deficiencies on your own, so see a dietitian or doctor for an assessment. Generally, only severe deficiencies can be physically seen, which is why regular wellness visits are vital.

What can I offer my preschool child?

Preschool children need more grains, vegetables, and protein sources as they get older. Give them low-fat milk and dairy products instead of whole milk as long as they are not underweight. The serving sizes need to be increased for the protein and vegetable groups (*opposite above*). Children at this age need three meals and at least two snacks during the day and sometimes a bedtime snack. To prevent a child from eating too much and gaining excess weight, try to serve fresh fruit for snacks. Provide water with at least one meal and one snack rather than fruit juice as it supplies additional calories and may reduce a child's appetite for the next meal. Listen to your child's appetite and use smaller plates and portions than you use for yourself.

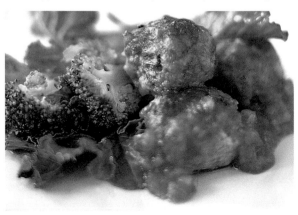

Dinner Meatballs in a fresh tomato sauce with broccoli is a popular meal for many 3-year-olds. It is rich in protein, vitamins C and K, iron, and lycopene.

SAMPLE MENU: 5 YEARS

Breakfast
- ½ cup low-sugar cereal with low-fat milk and ½ banana, sliced

Snack
- Apple with a slice of cheese and 8floz (240ml) water

Lunch
- Turkey slices on bread, carrots, and 4floz (120ml) low-fat yogurt

Snack
- 4–6 graham crackers, mandarin oranges in own juice, with 4floz (120ml) low-fat milk

Dinner
- 3 meatballs in tomato sauce, ½ cup noodles, broccoli, and tomatoes with 8floz (240 ml) water

Snack
- ½ cup oat cereal with low-fat milk

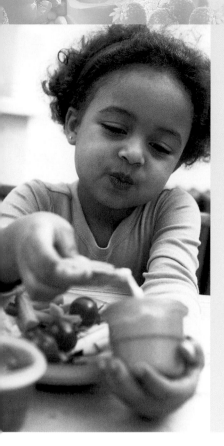

If you are concerned about your child's habits, record a "food diary" of everything he or she eats and drinks each day for a week. Record the type of food, its brand, and the amount eaten. Discuss the week's intake with a pediatric dietitian.

Computer analysis programs may be used to show you which of the food groups your child is getting enough of, the amount of calories consumed, and which, if any, nutritional deficiencies your child is at risk of developing. One of the most common nutrients lacking in a child's diet is iron, especially among picky eaters, so try to give your child plenty of iron-rich foods, such as meat, dried fruits, poultry, and legumes (see p.135).

Dipping foods Make mealtimes fun and interesting activities for children. Letting them dip food in tubs is a good way to increase the amount of vegetables they eat.

Serving sizes: 3–5 years

For 3–5-year-olds, the serving sizes of vegetables and protein sources are larger than those for 1–2-year-olds. For each food group, the daily number of servings and examples of a serving are shown below:
- 6 servings of grains and their products. Examples of a serving include 1 slice whole-grain bread and ½ cup cooked rice.
- 3 servings of vegetables. For example, 2 tbsp peas or carrots.
- 2 servings of fruits. Examples include 1 whole fruit, such as an apple or peach, or ½ banana.
- 2–3 servings of dairy products. Examples of a serving include 4floz (120ml) low-fat milk or low-fat yogurt and 1oz (28g) cheese.
- 2–3 servings of protein sources. Examples include 2oz (55g) meat, chicken, fish, or tofu, 1 vegetable burger, or 2 tbsp peanut butter.

Making food interesting to eat

An excellent way to get young children to eat nutritious food is to make meals and snacks fun and interesting and let them help you prepare them. Try some of the following tips to get your child to look forward to eating at mealtimes:
- Cut sandwiches, pizza, meats, and pancakes into small shapes. By making all the choices nutritious, your child will be eating healthy no matter which food he or she chooses.
- Let your child have fun immersing foods in a tasty dip. Some possibilities include tofu dip, cream cheese thinned with juice or milk, puréed vegetables or fruits with ranch or French dressing, yogurt, and cottage cheese. You can make cottage cheese more interesting by adding some pieces of pineapple.
- Let your child help you prepare food. Carefully teach him or her how to use a small blunt butter knife to spread cheese spread, peanut butter, and fruit concentrate onto crackers, toast, or rice cakes. You can try filling celery stalks

with peanut butter or putting some sliced cucumber or steamed spinach on a slice of toast spread with low-fat cream cheese.
- Create meals or snacks with your child. Make fresh-fruit or vegetable kabobs or smoothies. Making mini-pizzas is a great way to add variety with healthy toppings, while allowing your child to be creative in the process. Must-have ingredients for pizzas include low-fat mozzarella cheese, broccoli, tomatoes, asparagus, spinach, chicken, tuna, and pineapple chunks (see p.131).
- Most children love fruit and will eventually ask for it if you introduce it on a regular basis.
- Try to offer healthy desserts as much as possible. These include cut-up apples and oranges, canned fruit in its own juice, and fruit salad. Other healthy desserts include those made from low-fat milk, sorbet, low-fat ice cream, or angel food cake. Again, you can garnish these with fresh or frozen fruit.

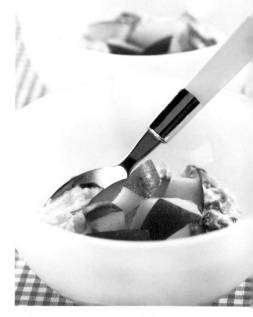

Fruit and fiber Adding chopped, fresh fruit to a dessert is a good way of getting extra nutrients and fiber into your child's diet, especially if he or she is a picky eater.

Healthy eating habits

To encourage healthy eating habits in your preschool children, follow the tips outlined below. Do not worry if you can't do everything at once; just adopting one tip at a time will make a difference to your children's eating habits.

• Serve fruits and vegetables every day, whether at mealtimes or as a snack. Canned fruits, such as pineapple, peaches, or mandarin oranges in their own juice can be kept in the cabinet, quickly opened, and any leftovers stored in the refrigerator.

• Provide water or low-fat milk with meals and snacks.

• Do not be afraid to say no to junk food, chips, soda, candy, or sweets, especially if your child has already eaten some that day.

• Serve small portions on small plates and in small cups. Giving too much and insisting that your child "cleans his or her plate" will lead to overeating and will not help your child regulate his or her own eating habits.

• Do not reward with dessert. Enticing children to eat all of their dinner to get dessert will only make dessert more important than the main course.

• When your child says that he or she has finished, ask him or her to take the plate to the sink and return to the table and sit with the family. Use arts and crafts or sticker books to keep the children entertained while the adults finish their meal. You can also adopt this strategy when you eat out together as a family.

• Keep a cabinet full of healthy snacks for when your child is hungry.

• Limit TV and video and computer games to less than two hours a day. A sedentary lifestyle will lead to excess weight gain (and overweight children).

• Encourage your child to be active, and exercise regularly as a family.

• Try to dine as a family when possible.

Being a role model

As a parent, you are responsible for setting a good example for your children when it comes to establishing healthy eating habits. Children usually want to copy what you eat and drink at a very early age and will reach out to grab whatever you are eating or drinking. If you drink soda with meals, and eat in front of the television, your child will be likely to want to do the same. However, soda is not appropriate for children—it is too high in calories and displaces the much needed calcium that they should be getting from milk—and eating in front of the TV does not promote family bonding or socialization. Think about your own food habits and make a conscious effort to eat healthy, well-balanced meals as a family at a dining table without TV.

What to give children to drink

The healthiest drinks to give young children are low-fat milk and water. Other drinks, such as fruit juices and sodas, are high in sugar and can cause tooth decay. If you do give your child fruit juice, follow these tips:

• Give your child juice from a cup as part of a meal or snack.

• Always dilute juice with water because it has a high sugar content.

• Limit juice given to 2–5-year-olds to 4–6floz (120–180ml) per day.

• Encourage your child to eat fresh fruit in place of fruit juice. This will increase your child's intake of fiber.

• Do not give your child unpasteurized fruit juices as they may contain bacteria.

• Limit any drink that does not contain 100 percent fruit juice because these drinks generally contain sweeteners, artificial flavors, or fortifiers.

Low-fat-milk drinks A healthier alternative to sugar-filled juices, low-fat milk is rich in calcium and fortified with vitamins A and D.

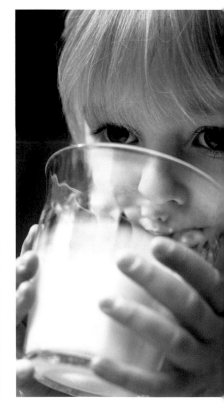

Keeping teeth healthy

Sugary and starchy foods that stick to teeth feed the bacteria that cause tooth decay. To ensure that your child's teeth develop properly and remain healthy, give a variety of foods to provide all the necessary nutrients for tooth development. Limit the amount of sugary drinks and foods, such as cookies and candies, that you provide. Good, teeth-friendly snacks include cubes of cheddar cheese, yogurt, fresh fruit, and vegetable sticks with dips. In addition, fluoride (see p.65), present in many water supplies, helps protect teeth. Make sure your child has regular dental checkups and brushes his or her teeth in the morning and before going to bed, when teeth begin to erupt.

Managing the picky eater

There are many strategies to help you overcome picky eating. If you are having problems with your child's eating habits, try following the tips below:

• First of all, be patient and sit down at the table with your child and have a conversation about his or her day.

• Offer a variety of bite-sized foods in order to allow your child to pick and choose the most appetizing and thus expand his or her diet.

• Presenting food in small shapes to make it look more appealing can often do the trick.

• Offer your child foods that pack lots of nutrition in small doses, such as avocados, broccoli, whole grains such as rice, cheese, eggs, fish, kidney beans, yogurt, pasta, peanut butter, squash, sweet potatoes, and tofu.

• Do not turn each meal into a battle if your child goes on a "food jag," in which he or she insists on eating the same foods over and over again at every meal. Offer a healthy selection of food at each meal and your child will eventually tire of the same food. The less pressure you impose, the more likely it is that your child will pass through this stage without problems.

• Do not try to force-feed your child or hover over him or her worrying about what he or she will or will not eat.

• If your child does not like different foods to be touching one another, serve them on separate plates.

• Do not become a "short-order cook" by always making your child something else if he or she refuses to eat.

• Do not give junk food if your child refuses to eat his or her meal.

• Do not punish your child for not eating a particular food; it is much better to congratulate him or her for what he or she does eat.

Finger foods Try serving dahl (mashed lentils) or hummus (ground chickpeas) in a bowl with cut-up pita bread or vegetables for dipping.

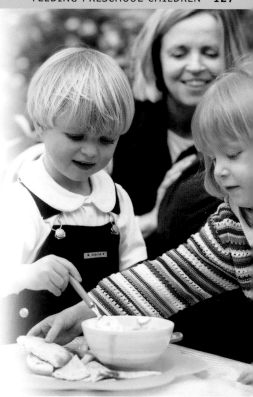

Case study Preschool child who eats only white food

Name Jodie

Age Three years

Problem Jodie will not eat anything green or red and tends to eat the same foods every day for lunch and dinner. She mostly eats white foods, such as cheese, yogurt, and macaroni.

Lifestyle This toddler's mother is concerned that her child's diet is very limited and she has become a picky eater. Jodie's mother is also concerned about whether her daughter should take a multivitamin supplement.

Although her appetite varies from day to day, Jodie's dinner usually consists of chicken nuggets, macaroni and cheese, and applesauce at least five nights a week. Sometimes, she eats pizza dipped in applesauce, but she has not been open to trying any foods that the family is eating, such as chicken, beef, rice, potatoes, or vegetables. She does like some fruits, such as canned mandarin oranges, fresh strawberries, and bananas. In addition, she often takes only a few bites of whatever foods she is offered and announces that she is done. Jodie rarely finishes what is on her plate and frequently returns to the kitchen after an hour or so asking for an ice pop or other sweets.

Advice It is normal for children at this age to have small appetites, so they may appear to be picky eaters and may need to eat every few hours. Young children often go on "food jags," preferring to eat the same food every day and then, after a week or so, move to other foods or food groups. Jodie's mother should continue to offer the foods she likes, and avoid forcing her to "clean her plate." It is best to let her regulate her own intake and avoid bribing her with dessert to get her to finish what is on her plate. If she usually leaves food, then Jodie's mother should serve smaller portions. If Jodie continues to say she is not hungry, her mother should then avoid giving juice between meals and serve water with meals. She can also try to introduce new foods at the beginning of the meal when Jodie is hungry and tell her her macaroni is still cooking.

Eventually Jodie will eat a more varied diet, but as long as she grows normally and does not lose weight she is eating enough. However, since her diet is so limited and she avoids vegetables, she may benefit from a "complete" vitamin and mineral supplement that contains iron. If fluoride is not in the water supply, her doctor can prescribe a fluoride

Nutrition for school-age children

Schoolchildren need a variety of good foods to grow and develop.

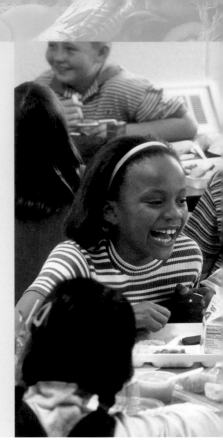

Good nutrition is essential for schoolchildren. They need enough fuel to get them through the day and for their minds to thrive and brains to develop, so give them a healthy breakfast, and if they are taking a lunchbox to school, ensure that it contains a mix of nutritious foods from the five food groups.

Limiting junk food

Junk food such as French fries, cookies, and chips are extremely tempting to children. These are high in sugar, fat, salt, and in empty calories. Sodas and fruit drinks also contain empty calories and sugar. Your child's diet can contain some foods that are high in sugar and fat as long as the total diet is well balanced and all food groups are consumed in the appropriate number of servings.

Healthy snacking

Snacking is important for children because they usually do not eat enough at mealtime to sustain their blood-sugar levels between meals. Snacks prevent children from getting so hungry that they cannot focus on school or other activities and offers an opportunity, along

What to give your school-age child

School-age children need to eat three meals and at least one snack per day. Breakfast is an important meal because it helps minds stay alert until lunchtime. School-age children can often buy lunch at school, but these meals may be high in fat and most children will end up eating dessert. Encourage your child to pack a healthy lunch a few times a week (*see p.130*). After school, children are hungry so give them a healthy snack, such as fruit or cut-up vegetables (*opposite*). Serve low-fat milk or water with the snack, which they can eat while they do their homework.

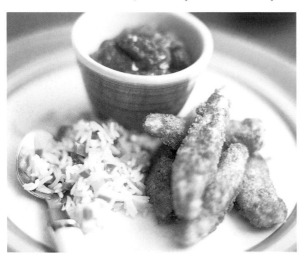

Chicken fingers Full of protein and vitamins chicken fingers, served with a tomato sauce for dipping and rice with vegetables are fun to eat. Serve with 8floz (240ml) of low-fat milk or water.

SAMPLE MENU: 10 YEARS

Breakfast
- 1 cup low-sugar cereal with 8floz (240ml) low-fat milk and banana slices, and 4floz (120ml) orange juice

Snack
- ½ bagel with peanut butter and jelly and 4floz (120ml) apple juice

Lunch
- 1 cup meat ravioli with fresh tomato sauce, 1 slice bread with margarine, 6 carrot sticks with dressing, and 1 apple

Snack
- 4 graham crackers and 8floz (240ml) low-fat milk

Dinner
- 2oz (55g) strips of breaded chicken breast with ½ cup boiled rice with vegetables, and ½ cup fresh tomato sauce, and 8floz (240ml) water

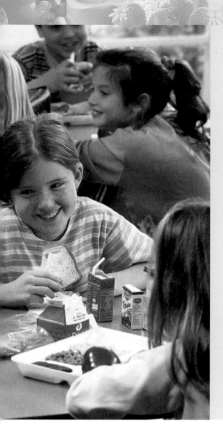

with meals, for children to get enough calories and nutrients for normal growth and development. They can contribute a significant amount of important nutrients, so snacks should be as healthy as possible. If a child does not eat fruits or vegetables at mealtimes, these foods make excellent snacks.

Empty calories

Unfortunately, many children like to snack on sweets, chips, cookies, doughnuts, and other foods low in nutritional value, but high in calories. The calories in such snacks are known as empty calories. Such snacks can cause unhealthy weight gain as your child grows

School lunches The midday meal allows children to have a break, sit down together, and enjoy one another's company while refueling for the afternoon.

Serving sizes: 6–12 years

For children aged 6–12 years, the number of daily servings from each food group and examples of a serving are shown below:
• 6–9 servings of grains and their products. Examples of a serving include 1 slice whole-grain bread or ½ cup brown rice or noodles.
• 3–5 servings of vegetables. For example, 1 serving equals 1 cup salad or ½ cup chopped raw or cooked vegetables.
• 2–4 servings of fruit. Examples of a serving include 1 apple, 4floz (120ml) fruit juice, or 1 cup berries.
• 2–3 servings of dairy products. Examples of a serving include 8floz (240ml) low-fat milk or low-fat yogurt, or 2oz (55g) cheese.
• 2–3 servings of protein sources. Servings include 2oz (55g) meat, chicken, or fish, or 2 eggs.

Healthy snacks for children

Children are often hungry, especially when they get home from school. Have healthy snacks ready for them to eat before their dinner and again in the evening. You can try some of the following ideas:
• Animal, goldfish, or graham crackers.
• Dry breakfast cereal such as oat circles or puffed grain.
• Rice cakes or pretzels.
• Cut-up vegetables, such as carrots, peppers, tomatoes, or cucumbers, with low-fat ranch or French dressing as a dip.
• Fresh fruit such as bananas, pears, plums, grapes, oranges, strawberries, peaches, and apples.

• Frozen juice cubes or ice pops.
• Fruit salad.
• Fruit smoothie with yogurt.
• Low-fat, part-skim string cheese.
• Low-fat yogurt.
• Hard-boiled egg.
• Sandwiches, such as tuna, egg salad, turkey, cheese, or peanut butter and jelly.
• Homemade trail mix (a mixture of dried fruit, such as raisins, cranberries, and apricots, unsalted peanuts, sunflower seeds, and crunchy low-sugar cereal).

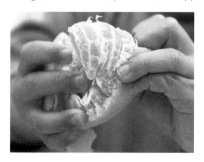

Appealing fruit Oranges and tangerines are packed with vitamin C and are a good source of fiber. They are also fun to peel.

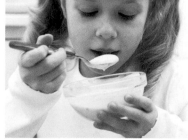

Superfood Low-fat yogurt is an ideal snack. It is rich in calcium, protein, and some of the B vitamins, and is easier to digest than milk.

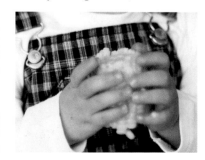

User friendly Give your child a section of boiled corn on the cob for a snack. Corn is a good source of fiber.

Preventing excess weight in childhood

Being overweight is a big problem in North American children and is also now becoming a global problem. One of the main reasons for this is that they spend more time watching television and playing video games than any other activity. Children also tend to eat more while watching television. Parents should try to limit these sedentary activities to less than two hours per day.

A recent study looking at television and video-game use and their relationship to obesity found that children who were limited to seven hours of television and video games per week had significant decreases in weight and body fat compared to a control group who were allowed to watch television or play video games for more than seven hours a week. The first group of children also ate fewer meals in front of the television.

To prevent children from becoming overweight, parents should therefore encourage children to develop skills for both indoor and outdoor activities, such as arts-and-crafts projects, creative imaginary play, jump rope, or hula hoop—basically, any activity that does not require expensive equipment or a large play area. For more information on weight management in children, see pages 206–207.

School lunch-box ideas

When preparing a school lunch box for your child, make sure to include foods from each of the food groups (*see p.71*) and vary these foods throughout the week. Variety will ensure that you are providing the maximum number of nutrients and will also prevent your child from getting bored with eating the same things.

Prepare foods that are appropriate for your child's age; for example, peeled apple or pear slices are ideal for a young child, while whole fruit is fine for an older child. You could try letting your child make his or her own sandwich, choosing healthy fillings together. If your children buy drinks at school, teach them why it is better to choose low-fat milk, bottled water, or even low-fat chocolate milk, all of which are more nutritious than sodas and juice drinks.

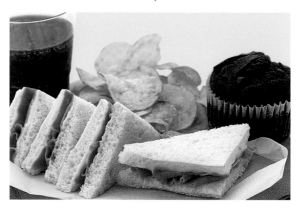

Unhealthy lunch
Ham and cheese are high in saturated fat, while white bread is low in fiber. Potato chips, chocolate-chip muffin, and cola add extra fat, sugar, and calories to this very unhealthy lunch.

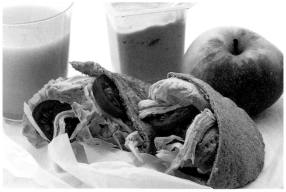

Healthy lunch
Whole-wheat pita containing sliced chicken, tomato, and lettuce is a nutritious low-fat lunch. A red apple, low-fat yogurt, and fresh orange juice are healthy choices and add vitamins, minerals, and fiber.

Lunch-box tips

Try some of these suggestions for your child's lunch box, and make sure you follow the storage tips.

Lunch menu ideas Provide a carton of long-life low-fat milk or apple juice with each lunch. Add one or more pieces of fruit, and vary the choices daily.
● Raisin bread or an English muffin spread with light cream cheese and topped with either low-sugar jelly, cucumber slices, or tomato. Serve with fruited yogurt.
● Whole-wheat pita filled with tuna, light mayonnaise, lettuce, and sweet pickle relish. Serve with cherry tomatoes and low-fat chocolate milk.
● Taco with kidney beans, topped with low-fat cheddar cheese, lettuce, and very mild salsa. Serve with baby carrots and fresh pear slices.
● Pasta salad with tuna or some shredded chicken breast, corn, cucumber slices, and chopped parsley with a low-fat dressing. Serve with a cereal bar.

Storage tips If keeping food cool at school poses a problem, freeze drinks or low-fat yogurts at home, and by lunchtime they should have become defrosted.
● Keep cold foods cold in an insulated lunch box. Include a frozen juice pack or water bottle.
● Keep hot foods warm by using an insulated portable container.

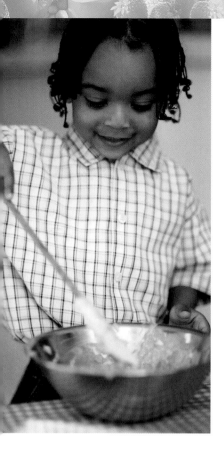

Cooking with kids

One of the most effective and fun ways to teach children about healthy eating is to involve them in the kitchen. This can begin by planning a menu and going to the supermarket together to purchase foods. Expose children to label reading, costs, and how to use coupons. This will stimulate their interest in helping you prepare, serve, and clean up the meal or snack.

SKILLS THAT STAY FOR LIFE

Children develop a sense of pride and ownership as they learn how to cook for the family. By engaging children to prepare and eat healthy meals and snacks, these skills will stay with them for life. In addition, cooking with kids and teenagers reinforces what they are learning in school, such as reading, science, biology, and mathematics.

Mixing it up Teaching children to cook lets them see which ingredients go into different foods and different meals. It also prepares them for when they eventually leave home.

Teach young children about colors, shapes, sizes, and to recognize the names of fruits and vegetables. Make a guessing game out of it when you are tossing a salad and let them help you wash the fresh vegetables. As your child grows older, he or she can participate in peeling and cutting up vegetables and be introduced to new foods, such as eggs and berries.

When you cook together, start with simple meals, such as baked chicken, brown rice, and string beans. Encourage your child to find healthy recipes he or she would like to make. Focus on lots of colors on the plate as well, such as red (tomatoes), green (peas), orange (carrots), and yellow (corn).

SAFE COOKING PRACTICES

Of course, safety is always an issue in the kitchen and children should never be left unsupervised. Teach them to ask for help and to use pot holders. This will help them to be more self-sufficient as teenagers and adults and to prepare healthy foods on their own.

Recipe Children's choice pizza

INGREDIENTS

2 cups canned tomatoes

fresh oregano

1 pizza crust

2oz (55g) sliced ham

½ bell pepper

1 cup canned artichoke hearts

½ cup black olives, optional

fresh basil

Serves 6

1 Heat a little olive oil in a skillet. Drain and chop the tomatoes, chop the oregano, and add to the pan. Bring to a boil, stirring gently, then reduce the heat and simmer until the mixture is slightly thickened.

2 Preheat oven to 425°F/220°C. Brush the crust with a little olive oil then spread the tomato sauce over the crust.

3 Cut the ham into strips, slice the pepper, quarter the artichoke hearts, and remove the olive pits. Place these on the pizza crust then drizzle a little olive oil on top.

4 Bake the pizza until the crust is just crispy. To serve, garnish with fresh basil leaves.

Suggested toppings You can use many other toppings such as corn kernels, fresh spinach, asparagus spears, broccoli florets, eggplant or zucchini slices (lightly fried), pineapple chunks, low-fat mozzarella cheese, canned tuna, shredded chicken, or anchovies.

Each serving provides

Calories 222, Total fat 7.4g (Sat. 1.3g, Poly. 0.3g, Mono. 0.8g), Cholesterol 4.8mg, Protein 8.0g, Carbohydrate 31g, Fiber 4.0g, Sodium 891mg. Good source of—Vits: A, C, K; Mins: Ca.

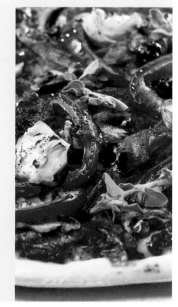

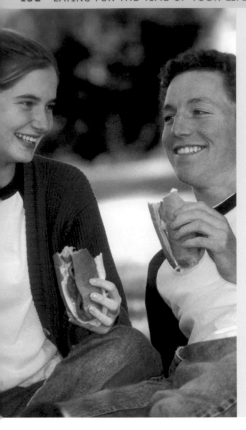

Dietary needs of adolescents

Children aged 11–18 years have increased needs for nutrients.

Girls aged 11–14 years and boys aged 12–15 years undergo major physical and psychological changes (puberty) that affect their behavior and what they need to eat. These body changes increase their energy and nutrient needs, which differ in boys and girls, although both sexes require extra calcium and iron at this stage. Wanting independence, resisting authority, and developing logical reasoning are characteristics of adolescents that you must keep in mind when you address their nutritional needs and behavior.

Becoming adults

Puberty usually starts in girls between 11 and 14 years, earlier than in boys, for whom it most often starts between 12 and 15 years. Girls usually have a rapid period of growth at the onset of puberty, whereas boys grow at their fastest after their sexual development is more advanced.

Growing adolescents have increased energy and nutritional needs to support their rapid

Growing up As they go through major body changes, adolescents often develop ravenous appetites. Make sure they fill up on nutritious foods, rather than empty-calorie junk snacks.

Encouraging teens to eat healthy

Teenagers these days are busier than ever. They leave the house at 7a.m. and may not return until dinnertime, when they grab a quick bite and are often out the door to an evening activity, then busy with homework. Finding time to properly nourish an active teenager can be quite a challenge—teenage boys are the biggest consumers of junk food, more and more teenagers are deciding to become vegetarians, and those involved in sports need more calories and fluids and often complain about being hungry all the time.

Since most teenagers are on their own when it comes to making food choices, it is helpful to plant healthy eating messages early in their lives. This is a "teachable moment" and an opportunity to provide tasty alternatives to junk food, such as those listed on the right. So try to limit how much fast food your teenager eats and pack healthy after-school snacks such as fresh fruit, peanut butter, sports bars, sandwiches, pretzels, and yogurt

POOR CHOICE	HEALTHY CHOICE
Sweetened cereals	Low-sugar cereals or oatmeal
Doughnuts	Frozen waffles with low-sugar syrup
Fried potato chips	Roasted peppers or carrot salad
Microwave popcorn	Fat-free microwave popcorn
Pizza	No-cheese tomato pie
Breaded chicken fillets or nuggets	White-meat chicken fillets
Candy bar	Sports or high-fiber breakfast bar
Cheeseburger with fries	Veggie burger with salad
Traditional TV dinner	Low-fat TV dinner (under 350cal)
Milkshake	Yogurt smoothie
Ice cream	Low-fat ice cream or frozen yogurt
Traditional muffins	English muffins or fat-free muffins
Chocolate chip cookies	Oatmeal cookies or fig bars

growth. If your child does a lot of exercise, this will further increase his or her energy requirements.

In healthy girls, menstruation usually starts about a year after their growth spurt begins. As they start menstruating, their iron (*see p.66*) and protein needs increase, as do other mineral needs associated with rapid growth (*below*).

As boys enter puberty, their muscle mass increases relative to girls, which increases adolescent boys' need for protein, calories, and overall nutrients—with the exception of iron—compared to adolescent girls.

Risk of deficiencies

If your adolescent has a poor diet, he or she may be at an increased risk of several vitamin and mineral deficiencies, most notably calcium and iron. The highest requirements for calcium are during infancy, when the first growth spurt takes

place, and during adolescence. The high calcium requirements of adolescents—1,300mg per day—are needed for bone growth and for depositing calcium within the bones. These processes are promoted by hormonal changes linked with puberty and its associated growth spurt.

Preventing overweight

Teenagers have easy access to high-calorie junk foods and may prefer sedentary activities, such as watching television and using the computer. If you are overweight, your teenager is at higher risk of becoming overweight, and overweight teens often develop high blood pressure and diabetes.

It is therefore critical that you think about your children's future health and make a commitment for your family to eat healthy, limit fast food and junk food, and be more physically active.

Serving sizes: 13–18 years

Adolescents need more servings per day from the grain and protein groups than younger children do. Their nutritional needs are now similar to those of adults. For each food group, the daily number of servings and examples of a serving are shown below.

- 6–11 servings of grains or their products. Examples include 1 slice whole-grain bread or ½ cup cooked brown rice or low-sugar cereals.
- 3–5 servings of vegetables. For example, 1 cup salad or ½ cup chopped, raw, or cooked vegetables.
- 2–4 servings of fruits. For example, 1 apple or ½ banana.
- 3–4 servings of dairy products. For example, 8floz (240ml) low-fat milk/yogurt or 2oz (55g) cheese.
- 2–3 servings of protein sources. Examples include 2oz (55g) meat, chicken, or fish, or 2 eggs.

Teens and exercise

Adolescents can improve their overall health by exercising regularly and reducing the amount of television that they watch. Participation in team sports is an excellent way for your teenager to get aerobic exercise and to meet and exercise with friends, or maybe your teen would prefer the challenge of athletics.

Encourage your teenager to join in any exercise you do as a family, such as going swimming or for a bike ride, but you may find that he or she prefers to exercise alone or with friends. At this age many young people prefer to join a gym or sports club independently. A financial contribution from you or another family member as a present would be a great incentive.

Organize activities Encourage your teenager to do plenty of exercise, either as part of a team, independently, or with friends on the weekend. Starting these behaviors now will encourage continuation into adulthood.

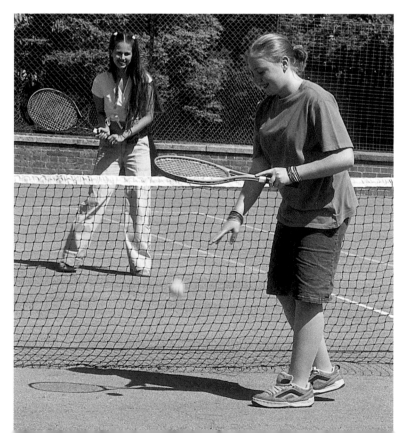

Calcium needs

Needed for the strength and structure of bones and teeth, calcium is vital in a teenager's diet. Children aged 3–8 years need 800mg of calcium per day. For 9–18-year-olds, the recommended daily amount goes up to 1,300mg for both sexes. However, most teens fail to get this amount; this has been called the "calcium crisis" because it can lead to osteoporosis (see p.242) in later life.

To make sure that your teen gets enough calcium, encourage him or her to eat or drink plenty of dairy products, which are the most efficient food sources of calcium. Use low-fat milk and low-fat cheeses in order to avoid excessive fat, saturated fat, and cholesterol. Ideally, teenagers need three to four servings a day of calcium-rich foods. The best natural sources of calcium are shown in the chart (right). Calcium fortified orange juice and breakfast cereals are good sources too. If a teenager does not eat enough calcium, he or she should take a supplement (see p.109).

CALCIUM-RICH FOOD	SERVING SIZE	CALCIUM
Milk-based liquid supplement	8floz (240ml)	500mg
Low-fat plain yogurt	8floz (240ml)	400mg
Fortified orange juice	8floz (240ml)	350mg
Low-fat fruited yogurt	8floz (240ml)	350mg
Cheese pizza	¼ of a 14in (36cm)	332mg
Fat-free and low-fat milk	8floz (240ml)	300mg
Chocolate pudding	1 cup	292mg
Low-fat cheddar cheese	1oz (28g)	204mg
Yogurt smoothie	8floz (240ml)	200mg
Low-fat ice cream	8floz (240ml)	180mg
Taco with shredded cheese	1 taco shell	174mg
American cheese	1oz (28g)	174mg
Frozen yogurt	8floz (240ml)	150mg
Tofu	4oz (110g)	145mg

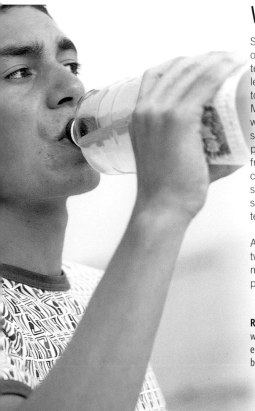

Why you should limit soft drinks

Soft drinks should generally be avoided or limited to 12floz (360ml) a day for teenagers as the high sugar levels can lead to excessive calorie consumption, tooth decay, and excess weight gain. Many studies have shown that teenagers who drink a lot of sweetened beverages such as regular sodas, lemonade, punch, sports drinks, and 100 percent fruit juice have an unnecessarily high calorie intake, which is due to the high sugar content of these drinks—most soft drinks contain between 15 and 20 teaspoons of sugar per 20floz (600ml).

According to the US Department of Agriculture, American teenagers drink twice as much carbonated soda as milk; in fact, most adolescents (65 percent of girls and 74 percent of boys)

Refreshing water The ideal thirst quencher, water does not contain any calories. Always encourage your teenager to carry a water bottle with him or her.

consume soft drinks on a daily basis. This substitution of soft drinks for milk is another factor contributing to the poor calcium intake in North America. In addition, the sugar in soft drinks can cause tooth decay and contribute to weight problems. Drinking healthier beverages, such as low-fat milk or water, can help prevent your teenager from becoming overweight. Other tips to limit the amount of soft drinks your teenager drinks include:
• Always keep a range of healthy drinks at home. In this way, even though your children will have soft drinks when he or she goes out, you are making an attempt to balance the intake of soft drinks.
• Teach your teenager to ask for diet soda when he or she is at a party or restaurant. This will address peer pressure to drink soda and limit calories when he or she does not want to drink water.
• Try serving your teenager 100 percent fruit juice mixed with sparkling mineral water as a healthy alternative.

Making sure teenage girls get enough iron

Growing adolescents have increased requirements for energy and all nutrients, but especially iron (*see p.66*) to support their rapid growth. In addition, vigorous exercise, such as running or dancing, further increases these requirements.

Since menstruation begins during adolescence, teenage girls will lose blood and therefore iron on a monthly basis and will need extra dietary iron.

IRON DEFICIENCY

The body needs iron to build red blood cells and when you do not get enough of it from the diet, you may experience fatigue and poor endurance, which can be especially difficult for those involved in sports (*see p.61*).

In addition, many teenagers skip meals, decide to become vegetarian, or follow unbalanced, fad diets in an effort to lose weight. These diets may lack sufficient iron for the body's needs. In this way, a teenage girl is at risk for iron-deficiency anemia. This condition is common in teenage girls, especially those with heavy menstrual periods and a nutrient-poor diet.

Teenagers between 12 and 18 years need 15mg of iron per day, unless they are pregnant, in which case they need 30mg per day. To achieve an iron-rich diet, encourage your teenager to eat red meat at least once a week and iron-rich vegetables and fruits, such as legumes, dried fruits, and spinach on a regular basis. She should also eat a breakfast cereal fortified with iron. The recipe (*below*) for an iron-rich bean dish will provide an iron boost.

If your teenage daughter becomes a vegetarian, she can still meet her daily iron requirements, but it will take careful planning and eating a varied diet (*see pp.100–101*). If no-one else in the family is a vegetarian, you should invest in a recipe book to get plenty of ideas for vegetarian meals. Everyone in the family will benefit from vegetarian meals a few times a week.

IRON AND VITAMIN C

In order to maximize the amount of iron absorbed from a meal, your daughter could eat foods containing vitamin C (*see p.56*) as part of the meal, as these foods aid the absorption of iron.

Citrus fruits or juices, such as orange or grapefruit, tomatoes, and broccoli are all good sources of vitamin C. Nonmeat food sources that are high in iron include broccoli, raisins, watermelon, spinach, black-eyed peas, blackstrap molasses, chickpeas, and pinto beans. Raisins make a convenient iron-rich snack, as well as being a good source of other important nutrients and fiber.

A multivitamin and mineral supplement that contains iron would also be helpful if you suspect that your daughter is not getting a sufficient amount of iron in her diet (*see p.55*). Discussing suppplements with her doctor would be important because a simple blood test can be done to test for iron-deficiency anemia prior to initiating a supplement.

Recipe **Iron-rich bean dish**

INGREDIENTS
1 onion
4 garlic cloves
1 carrot
2 zucchini
2 bell peppers
2 potatoes
4 ripe tomatoes
14oz- (400g-) can white beans
2 tbsp chopped fresh basil
black pepper

Serves 4

1 Slice the onion, crush the garlic cloves, and finely chop the carrot and zucchini. Deseed the bell peppers and chop finely.

2 Heat a little olive oil in a large pan, add the prepared vegetables, and cook over a medium heat until they are soft (approximately 5 minutes).

3 If the potatoes are old, peel first. Cut potatoes into ½in (1cm) cubes and quarter the tomatoes. Add potatoes and tomatoes to the pan along with 4floz (120ml) water. Cover and simmer for approximately 30 minutes, until all the vegetables are softened.

4 Drain and rinse the beans and add to the vegetables in the pan. Cook for a further 5 minutes, until the beans are very hot.

5 Add the basil and season with black pepper, stirring gently to combine.

6 Serve hot in warmed bowls, drizzled with a little olive oil, and garnished with chopped fresh basil. Serve with crusty wholegrain bread.

Each serving provides

Calories 260, Total fat 1.1g (Sat. 0.2g, Poly. 0.5g, Mono. 0.1g), Cholesterol 0mg, Protein 13g, Carbohydrate 54g, Fiber 11g, Sodium 37mg. Good source of—Vits: A, Fol, C; Mins: Ca, Mg, P, K, Fe.

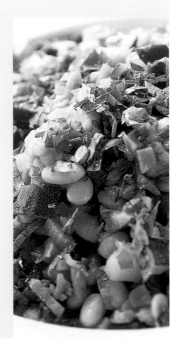

Nutrition throughout adulthood

Your food choices throughout adulthood can help ensure good health into old age.

Do you take your health for granted? If you are like most people between 20–50 years old, you have never had to worry about your health. However, you may have noticed that you cannot just eat whatever you want and stay thin like you did when you were younger. Maybe you have put on extra weight and have not been able to exercise as much as you used to due to your busy schedule at work or home. Those of us between the ages of 20 and 50 usually feel that we are healthy. We are too busy to go to the doctor and we really do not think we need to change our diets, and why should we?

What you eat and how much you exercise can significantly impact your current and future health. If you eat lots of fat and sugar and do not exercise, chances are you will feel sluggish at work and will not be motivated to exercise. But this stage of life is the most critical time to determine your future health and probably the easiest time for you to begin adopting healthy dietary habits, an active lifestyle, and to quit smoking if you smoke. By making the effort to eat a well-balanced diet and exercise on a regular basis, you will feel better today and have more energy. You will also probably live longer and the years you have will be healthier.

Eating for two

Making healthy food choices and gaining enough weight during pregnancy have been shown to improve the health of your baby. We show you which needs are increased during pregnancy (see pp.138–141) and while you are breast-feeding (see pp.142–143), as well as how to meet these needs with food and vitamin and mineral supplements. Since breast-feeding is best for your baby, we describe the benefits for you and your baby and show you how to breast-feed with success.

Nutrition for athletes

The nutritional needs of athletes vary depending on the amount and type of physical activity you are involved in. We describe the specific requirements for both

Do men have specific dietary needs?

Due to a larger muscle mass, men have a higher metabolic rate than women. This means they need more calories and also more of certain vitamins and minerals, specifically those involved in releasing energy from food.

Men's larger bodies contain more water, bone, muscle, organ tissue, and fat than women's, and their increased muscle mass requires more protein for its maintenance. Therefore, men tend to eat more food than women.

Each day, men burn up about 600 calories more than nonpregnant women do. Men's needs for carbohydrate are the same, but they need more fiber—38g per day compared to 25g per day for women. There is no recommended amount of dietary fat, but men require 60 percent more essential fatty acids than women (see p.38). While men's daily recommended intake of protein is the same as women's at 0.8g per 2.2lb (1kg) of body mass, their intake needs to be 10g per day higher on average due to their greater muscle mass. Dietary and health recommendations for men include:

• Eat lots of fruits and vegetables. Rich in nutrients, the health benefits of these foods cannot be overstated.
• Avoid saturated fats. Keep meat intake to a minimum. Use low-fat or fat-free dairy products. Limit ice cream and other fatty foods, such as french fries.
• Drink alcohol in moderation. Limiting it to 1–2 drinks per day will give you the health benefits without the risks.
• Manage stress. Stress is unavoidable and not necessarily bad for you—it is how you react to stress that determines its effects on your health. Techniques such as yoga or meditation can help.
• Do not smoke cigarettes and cigars, and try to avoid passive smoking.
• Maintain a healthy weight. Excess weight, especially around the abdomen, is a risk for heart disease and diabetes.
• Make exercise a priority. Get plenty of physical activity to stay healthy.
• Have annual medical checkups.

Nutrients for men

The nutrients below are thought to have an impact on fertility, prostate health, and the prevention of cancer and cardiovascular disease.

Lycopenes These nutrients occur in tomatoes, watermelon, and pink grapefruit and may lower the risk of prostate and lung cancer.

Vitamins B_6, B_{12}, and folate These B vitamins lower blood levels of homocysteine, thus lowering the risk of cardiovascular disease.

Selenium and vitamins C and E These antioxidants are necessary for normal fertility in men, and adequate intake or supplements may help to improve fertility.

Zinc and folate A combination of zinc and folate supplements may improve fertility in men.

endurance and nonendurance athletes, focusing on supplements and sports drinks, and provide suggestions for meals and snacks for active people (*see pp.146–149*).

Menopause and older adults

The population of older adults is rapidly expanding worldwide, and in the second half of this chapter, we address the nutritional needs for optimum health of men and women as they age—through menopause, over 50 years, and older than 70 years (*see pp.154–155*). Lifestyle changes, such as taking part in regular physical activity, can ease the symptoms and effects of aging and help you feel better as you advance in age.

Healthy choices Try to make healthy eating a priority, especially when dining out. Order an appetizer or a salad and share an entrée to prevent overeating.

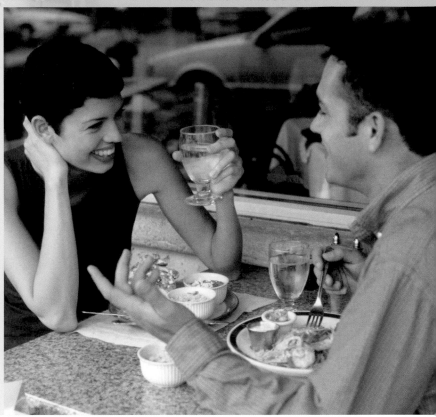

When do women's dietary needs change?

Because women are generally smaller than men and have less muscle mass they require fewer calories. However, you will need more calories during pregnancy (when you are eating for two), and if you decide to breast-feed, you will need extra calories and nutrients to produce enough breast milk. Athletic women also need more calories than those with a more sedentary lifestyle.

IRON FOR BLOOD LOSS

Throughout the reproductive years, women need more iron in their diet to replace the iron in the blood lost as a result of menstrual periods. Otherwise, you may be at risk of iron-deficiency anemia (*see p.55*), so it is important to eat plenty of iron-rich foods (*right*).

FOLATE FOR PREGNANCY

During pregnancy, women need extra calories and nutrients and more of most of the vitamins and minerals (*see pp.50–67*). The B vitamin folate is very

important. An increased intake of folate before conception and in early pregnancy prevents neural tube defects in babies (*see p.139*). Extra iron is also necessary in pregnancy, to produce new red blood cells for the mother's increased blood volume and also for her baby.

New mothers need extra calories and nutrients (*see pp.142–143*). A woman's body needs to recover after delivery. Increased amounts of iron and various vitamins and other minerals are vital for returning to normal health.

CALCIUM FOR BONE HEALTH

Breast-feeding is recommended as the best way to feed your baby for the first six months of life. Mothers need a balanced, nutritious diet not just for themselves but to produce the nutrient-rich milk for their baby. Since calcium is lost from the bones to make breast milk, mothers will need extra calcium. By restoring lost calcium, you will protect yourself from the degenerative bone disorder osteoporosis (*see p.242*) during and after menopause and into old age.

Which foods are good for women?

Folate, calcium, and iron are key nutrients for women. Try to eat foods rich in these nutrients.

Folate Good sources of folate include green vegetables, such as cabbage and spinach, and legumes, such as chickpeas and kidney beans.

Calcium This mineral is naturally abundant in milk and other dairy products, sardines, and spinach.

Iron Foods that are naturally rich in iron include spinach; dried fruit, especially prunes; and legumes, such as soybeans and kidney beans.

Eating for two

When pregnant, you need to eat for yourself and your baby.

Good nutrition is vital for both normal pregnancies and those considered high-risk, such as in a woman who is carrying twins or has gestational diabetes.

Pregnant women require more calories and nutrients than other women to provide for their growing baby (*opposite*). To achieve this, a pregnant woman should consume an extra 300 calories per day during the second and third trimesters of their pregnancy. This is about a 15–17 percent increase in calories. Otherwise healthy pregnant women need few or no additional calories during the first trimester.

Increased demands put pregnant women and their unborn babies at risk of nutritional deficiencies if these demands are not met by the diet (*opposite*) or by prenatal supplements (*see p.140*).

Key nutrients

Taking a multivitamin supplement that includes folate before and during pregnancy decreases the risk of neural tube defects, which affects about 1 in 1,000 pregnancies in North America. Since 1998, food manufacturers have been required by law to add the vitamin folate to grain products. Other key nutrients during pregnancy are iron, which is used to make red blood cells for both the growing baby and mother, whose blood volume increases by 50 percent during pregnancy, and calcium for the baby's skeleton.

Health problems

Changes in your body during pregnancy may result in temporary health problems. These include gestational diabetes, constipation, heartburn and indigestion, and nausea and vomiting. In gestational diabetes, body cells have difficulty absorbing glucose from the blood during pregnancy due to resistance to the hormone insulin (*see p.141*).

The intestinal muscles are more relaxed during pregnancy. This can cause constipation because of the slower movement of food through the body and the increased amount of water absorbed from the food by the intestine.

Heartburn and indigestion occur when the stomach contents flow up into the esophagus, causing discomfort in the chest. During pregnancy, it is usually due to the shift of organs in the abdomen to accommodate the growing baby.

Nausea and vomiting (morning sickness) are due to increased levels of the pregnancy hormone human chorionic gonadotropin, levels of which peak at about 12 weeks into a pregnancy. Tips to manage these disorders through nutrition are discussed on page 141.

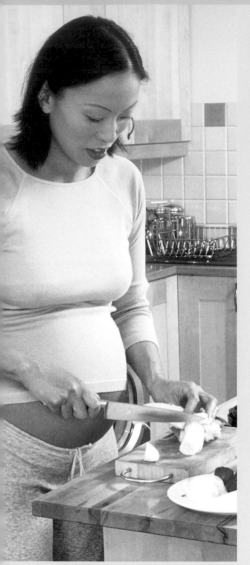

Increased needs During pregnancy you need more calories than usual—for yourself and for your growing baby. Make sure you choose nutrient-rich foods to get your extra calories.

Jargon buster

Neural tube defects Abnormalities in a fetus's brain and spinal cord and their protective coverings. Neural tube defects vary from severe (anencephaly—lack of brain) to mild (meningoceles—opening of the spinal cord that can be surgically repaired). The most well-known neural tube defect is spina bifida.

Weight gain

If you do not gain enough weight during pregnancy, you could put your baby at risk of being born prematurely or underweight, which could result in life-threatening problems. The recommendations set by the Institute of Medicine for how much weight you should gain during a normal pregnancy are based on your body mass index (BMI; *see p.26*).

- If you are underweight with a BMI less than 18.5, you should gain 28–40lb (12.7–18.2kg).
- If your weight is normal (BMI 19–24.9), you should gain 25–35lb (11.4–15.9kg).
- If you are overweight (BMI 25–29.9), you can gain 15–25lb (6.8–11.4kg).
- If you are very overweight, (BMI 30 and above), you can gain up to 15lb (6.8kg).

Increased needs during pregnancy

The most significant increases in nutrient needs during pregnancy are for protein, vitamins, and minerals; pregnant women need to almost double their intake of protein. Other key nutrients include folate (*opposite; p.56*) and iron (see *p.66*). An increased intake of calcium is not required during pregnancy but make sure you meet your normal requirements (1,000mg per day). Pregnant teenagers need 1,300mg per day.

Pregnant woman must get enough fats. Two fatty acids—docosahexanoic acid and arachidonic acid—are vital for the development of your baby's brain and vision. Water and fiber intake should also be increased. Ways of meeting your extra needs through diet are discussed below and, by taking prenatal supplements, on page 140. The table (*right*) shows the recommended daily intakes of key nutrients for pregnant and nonpregnant women aged 19–45.

NUTRIENT	NONPREGNANT	PREGNANT
Protein	46g	71g
Vitamin A	0.70mg	0.77mg
Vitamin C	75mg	85mg
Thiamine (B_1) / Riboflavin (B_2)	1.1mg	1.4mg
Niacin (B_3)	14mg	18mg
Vitamin B_6	1.3mg	1.9mg
Vitamin B_{12}	0.0024mg	0.0026mg
Calcium	1,000mg	1,000mg
Folate	0.4mg	0.6mg
Magnesium	320mg	360mg
Iron	18mg	27mg
Iodine	0.15mg	0.22mg
Selenium	0.055mg	0.06 mg
Zinc	8mg	11mg

Foods to eat during pregnancy

The best foods to eat during pregnancy are those that supply essential vitamins, minerals, lean protein, and energy.

Protein Eat about 10oz (280g) per day of healthy protein sources such as lean red meat, white-meat poultry, fish (cooked only), eggs, and legumes.

Calcium Adequate calcium intake during pregnancy is very important to prevent osteoporosis later in life. Eat or drink at least three to four servings of calcium-rich foods every day.

Folate Adequate folate is required in early pregnancy to prevent neural tube defects (*see p.56*). Folate is now added to grain products. It is also found in fresh green vegetables, legumes, liver, oranges, and poultry. So make time for breakfast, add beans to your diet, and eat five fruits and vegetables per day.

Small meals You may find it easier to eat small carbohydrate-rich meals, such as pasta with vegetables, to maintain energy levels.

Iron Necessary for the production of red blood cells in both you and your unborn baby. Iron-rich foods include: red meat, legumes, raisins, spinach, black-eyed peas, dried fruits, and green vegetables. Vitamin C helps your body absorb iron from plant sources.

Fiber Increased intake of high-fiber foods, such as vegetables and whole grains, is recommended for the prevention of constipation.

Fluids Drink at least 4 pints (2 liters) of water per day to provide fluids for blood production and to aid digestion.

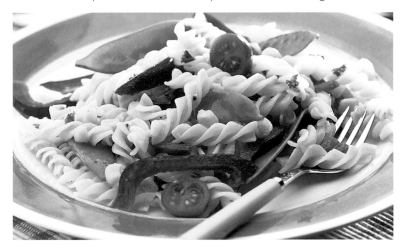

Foods to avoid during pregnancy

The chances of your unborn child becoming infected during pregnancy are small, but you should be aware of potentially risky foods to avoid eating. Foods contaminated with germs, such as bacteria, or heavy metals, such as lead and mercury, can seriously harm your growing baby.

Listeriosis The bacterium *Listeria monocytogenes*, which causes this infection, can cross the placenta and may be fatal for the baby. To prevent infection avoid eating unpasteurized dairy products, especially soft cheeses, such as camembert; cooked and then chilled prepared meals, especially those containing chicken and seafood; and liver and liver patés.

Toxoplasmosis This protozoal infection, which can cause problems in an unborn baby, is caused by *Toxoplasma gondii*. Cysts (dormant stages) of *T. gondii* are excreted in the stools of infected cats and can be passed to humans by handling cats or cat litter, by fruit or vegetables contaminated with cysts, or by eating the meat of animals that feed on food contaminated with cysts. Minimize the risk of infection during pregnancy by avoiding cats, by washing fruits and vegetables before eating, and avoiding undercooked meat, especially pork.

Salmonella This common type of food poisoning, due to *Salmonella* bacteria, does not usually harm the baby, but if severe in a pregnant woman it can lead to miscarriage or preterm labor. You should avoid undercooked eggs and poultry products to prevent infection.

Other infections You should avoid raw seafood, such as sushi, oysters, and clams, during pregnancy as they carry a risk of hepatitis and intestinal parasites.

Heavy-metal poisoning Remove heavy metals from vegetables by washing them thoroughly with water or by removing their skin. Also, seafood, especially swordfish, tile fish, king mackerel, and shark, are best avoided during pregnancy due to high levels of mercury.

Alcohol and caffeine

It is best to abstain from alcohol during pregnancy. Drinking alcohol can lead to your baby being born with fetal alcohol syndrome and learning difficulties. It is also thought that high caffeine intake can increase the risk of miscarriage in early pregnancy.

The effects of alcohol are most severe in the first two months of pregnancy, when your baby's organs are developing. Just one episode of binge drinking at this stage of pregnancy is now thought to be as harmful to your baby as excessive drinking throughout pregnancy.

Pregnant women should reduce their intake of caffeine from all sources—coffee, tea, cocoa, and cola drinks—to 200mg per day (*see p.97*). More than this amount may interfere with your baby's growth and development and increase the risk of low birth weight.

Do you need prenatal supplements?

Most healthcare providers prescribe a prenatal multivitamin and mineral supplement because many pregnant women do not eat enough to meet their increased nutritional needs, especially with regard to the B vitamin folate and the minerals calcium and iron.

NEED FOR CALCIUM

Nonpregnant women generally consume only 75 percent of their recommended calcium intake; therefore, pregnant women may need to take a supplement to achieve their recommended intake of 1,000mg per day. Even though calcium needs do not increase with pregnancy, your baby needs calcium as early as four to six weeks after conception, when teeth and bones begin to form. By 25 weeks, your baby's needs are even higher due to significant bone growth at this time. As the amount of calcium you absorb depends on your levels of vitamin D, you should spend at least 10 minutes a day in the sun when you are pregnant.

NEED FOR IRON

Iron is necessary for the production of red blood cells in both the mother and her growing baby. A mother's blood volume increases by up to 50 percent during pregnancy, requiring an extra 500mg of iron. The fetus requires an additional 300mg of iron, accumulating most of its iron stores during the third trimester; this may help to explain why iron-deficiency anemia is most common during the third trimester of pregnancy. Therefore the Dietary Reference Intake (DRI) of iron increases from 18mg per day for nonpregnant women to 27mg per day when you are pregnant.

Vitamin C also helps the body absorb iron, so taking prenatal vitamins or iron supplements with orange or grapefruit juice will aid absorption.

Special need for folate

Supplementation with the B vitamin folate decreases the risk of neural tube defects in your baby (*see p.139*). Women planning a pregnancy should start taking a multivitamin supplement before conception and switch to a prenatal vitamin during pregnancy. In fact, since about 50 percent of all pregnancies are unplanned, all young women would benefit from taking a multivitamin with folate.

The recommended daily intake of folate throughout pregnancy is 0.6mg (it is 0.4mg for nonpregnant women). Almost all prenatal vitamins are now supplemented with at least 0.8mg of folate. However, up to 4mg of folate per day may be prescribed for women who have a family history of neural tube defects. In these circumstances, a doctor will supervise the dose.

Minor ailments during pregnancy

Common ailments during pregnancy include nausea and vomiting (also known as morning sickness), which are most common in the first three months of pregnancy; heartburn and indigestion; and constipation. The suggestions below may help ease your symptoms. Tips for dealing with constipation, such as drinking plenty of water and eating lots of fiber, can be found on page 229.

MORNING SICKNESS

If you are experiencing morning sickness, try some of the following suggestions to ease your discomfort:
• Eat some dry crackers or toast first thing in the morning.
• Avoid strong food odors by eating food cold or at room temperature and using good ventilation while cooking.
• Avoid fragrances that might trigger nausea, such as perfume, household cleaners, and air fresheners.
• Drink a cup of ginger tea. Make it yourself by steeping one teaspoon of

ground or grated ginger in boiling water in a teapot for a few minutes. Strain and add honey or brown sugar to taste.

HEARTBURN AND INDIGESTION

Try some of the following tips if you are suffering from heartburn and indigestion during pregnancy:
• Eat small, low-fat meals and snacks, such as fruits, pretzels, crackers, and fat-free yogurt, slowly and frequently.
• Drink fluids between meals.
• Avoid foods that may irritate the stomach, such as caffeine, spearmint, peppermint, citrus fruits, spicy foods, high-fat foods, and tomato products.
• Take a walk after meals.
• Avoid eating or drinking for one to two hours before lying down.

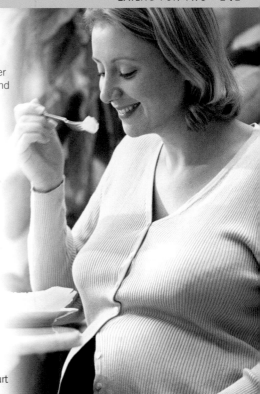

Relieving heartburn Eating a bland snack such as watery-melon or low-fat or fat-free yogurt slowly can help ease heartburn. Yogurt is also a good source of calcium.

Dealing with gestational diabetes

In gestational diabetes, there are raised levels of the blood sugar glucose during pregnancy. The disorder occurs in about 4 percent of all pregnancies. It is usually diagnosed during the second or third trimester of pregnancy when the body may become resistant to the hormone insulin, which enables body cells to take up glucose from the blood. The resistance occurs because hormones produced by the placenta have an anti-insulin effect. Symptoms can include fatigue, excessive thirst, and passing large amounts of urine, but often there are no symptoms.

In about 90 percent of cases, blood-glucose levels return to normal after delivery, but these women remain at increased risk of developing diabetes in later life (see pp.246–247).

NUTRITION GOALS

The aims of treating gestational diabetes through nutrition are to provide enough calories for the appropriate weight-gain

in pregnancy, to achieve and maintain normal levels of glucose in the blood, and to avoid the production of chemicals known as ketones.

KETONES

Because the body cannot use glucose efficiently as a source of energy in diabetes, it will then derive energy by breaking down fats, producing waste products called ketones. The buildup of ketones (ketosis) in the body causes symptoms such as fruity-smelling breath, nausea, and abdominal pain.

If you are diagnosed with gestational diabetes, you will be asked by your doctor to monitor your blood glucose levels via a finger stick test and to test your urine or blood for ketones. Most women with gestational diabetes are referred to a registered dietitian for nutritional counseling and for the design of a meal plan that will be adjusted throughout pregnancy based on levels of glucose in the blood.

MEAL PLANNING

Generally, 40–45 percent of calories in the diet should come from carbohydrates, taken throughout the day. An evening snack is recommended to prevent ketosis overnight. Carbohydrate is not as well tolerated at breakfast as at other meal times, possibly due to the levels of certain hormones, so an initial meal plan may limit carbohydrate at that time.

INSULIN INJECTIONS

If your blood sugar levels are persistently high, you will most likely have to have insulin injections. This is the best thing for your baby, and with the help of your prenatal care provider, you can have a healthy pregnancy. The main goal of this therapy is to prevent complications associated with gestational diabetes developing in both the mother and baby. If your blood sugar levels are not treated, your baby might gain too much weight and might need to be delivered by cesarean section.

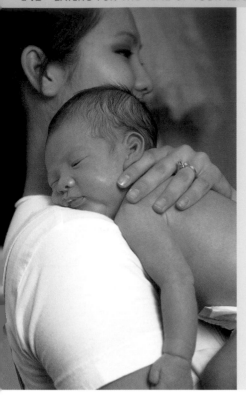

Nutritional needs of new mothers

After giving birth, women still need extra calories and nutrients.

Most women want to know how to lose the weight they gained during pregnancy as soon as possible. For some, it disappears in weeks; for others, years. Without eating well-balanced meals and exercising, you may find it difficult to lose weight.

Mother and child After giving birth, a woman must consume more calories and nutrients, not only for her body to recover but also to produce milk if she decides to breast-feed.

Calories for breast-feeding
However, taking drastic dieting measures after you deliver your baby will not help you keep up your strength or give you the important nutrients you need for healing. And if you plan to breast-feed, your body requires more calories than you needed when you were pregnant. If you decide not to breast-feed your baby, your nutritional needs will return to normal after a few weeks.

Don't skip meals
Because this is a stressful period, having a newborn and not getting enough sleep, it is important to

Requirements for breast-feeding

Mothers who are breast-feeding should be encouraged to obtain their nutrients from a well-balanced, varied diet and to drink about 4–6 pints (2–3 liters) of fluid per day to maintain their milk production. As with pregnant women, breast-feeding women have an increased requirement for calories and essentially all nutrients, especially protein, the mineral calcium, and vitamins A and C.

Calcium Mothers who are producing milk should make sure that they get their recommended 1,000mg of calcium each day. About 2–8 percent of total body calcium is used for breast-milk production. Mothers usually replace this lost calcium during the intervals between pregnancies. Women who have several children or short intervals between their pregnancies may not be getting enough calcium, putting them at risk of developing the bone disorder osteoporosis later in life (see p.242).

Iron Immediately after giving birth, the requirements for iron are high, especially if you have lost a lot of blood. However, after recovery from birth, your need for

iron when breast-feeding (9mg per day) is lower than it was during pregnancy (27mg per day). When menstruation resumes, the recommended intake of iron returns to the level of nonbreast-feeding women (18mg per day).

Vitamin supplements Prenatal vitamin supplements (see p.140) are routinely prescribed to breast-feeding women in order to ensure adequate intake of vitamin and minerals.

Foods to avoid Substances from some foods that a mother eats while breast-feeding may pass into her milk and affect the baby in adverse ways. In many cases, this will first be noted by the mother whose baby seems to be suffering from colic or having abdominal bloating and gas. Other symptoms may include diarrhea, vomiting, runny nose, bronchitis, wheezing, and skin rashes.

Foods eaten by the mother that may cause these symptoms in breast-fed babies include cow's milk and other dairy products, eggs, wheat products, citrus fruits, caffeine, chocolate, garlic, cabbage, and cucumber.

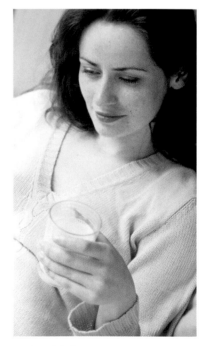

Calcium-rich diet A new mother needs to ensure she gets plenty of calcium, especially if she is breast-feeding, to keep her bones strong. Low-fat milk is an excellent source.

keep your immune system strong. To do this, it is critical to eat three meals a day and to avoid skipping meals due to lack of time or the desire to lose weight. Even if you have to grab a high-fiber breakfast bar and a piece of fruit and eat it in the car on the way to the doctor's office, it is better than nothing. You are the most important person in your baby's life. If you take proper care of yourself you will be better able to take care of him or her.

So make time for yourself by planning ahead. Bring snacks, such as fruit, rice cakes with peanut butter, and drinks such as juice or water for yourself in the diaper bag when going out. Eat on a regular schedule as much as possible, no matter how busy and on the run you are, or demanding your baby is. You will feel much better for doing this.

Weight loss after pregnancy

You should not go on a diet or take weight-loss medications immediately after pregnancy, particularly if you are breast-feeding. Weight loss after giving birth should be gradual, and this is particularly true for breast-feeding women, who burn more calories than other women in order to support breast-milk production.

A woman should not expect to return to her prepregnancy weight immediately after delivery. On average, a new mother will lose 15lb (6.8kg) within the first week after having given birth.

Many mothers are concerned about their weight gain during pregnancy and worry that they may not return to their original weight. This concern is real as some women retain 5–10lb (2.3–4.5kg) for each of

their pregnancies. Breast-feeding women who eat nutritionally balanced diets typically lose 1–2 lb (0.45–0.9kg) per month during the first 4–6 months of breast-feeding. This weight loss is more rapid than for mothers who bottle-feed their babies from the start.

A weight loss of more than 1.5lb (0.7kg) per week can decrease breast-milk production and put both mother and baby at risk nutritionally. However, there are some mothers who maintain or gain weight during breast-feeding but may lose the additional weight after they have weaned their infants.

The best way to return to your prepregnancy weight is to exercise regularly, such as walking your baby in the stroller once a day.

Case study   New mother losing too much weight

Name Suzie

Age 26

Problem Suzie is very busy with her young baby and finds it hard to sit down for a meal. Yesterday, Suzie ate cornflakes with low-fat milk for breakfast, half of a peanut-butter-and-jelly sandwich and orange juice for lunch, and some chicken breast with a baked potato and diet cola for dinner. She likes ice cream at night if she has time between feedings.

Suzie says she is now hungrier than she was during her pregnancy, but cannot find time to eat and knows she is not drinking enough because her mouth is dry. She is afraid that she is not producing enough milk because her baby always appears hungry and is not as chubby as her friend's formula-fed baby. Her mother told her not to eat vegetables and

chocolate because they would upset the baby's stomach and produce gas.

Lifestyle Suzie had a healthy 8lb, 2oz (3.7kg) baby boy, now 6 weeks old and weighing 11lb (5kg). This was her first pregnancy. She has lost 20lb (9kg) since giving birth and currently weighs 140lb (63.5kg). She is 67in (170cm) tall and weighed 130lb (59kg) before she was pregnant.

Advice Suzie is not getting enough calories to maintain her weight and produce enough breast milk for her baby. Her calorie requirements when she is breast-feeding are about 2,400 per day. She specifically needs more protein, vitamins A, B_{12}, and folate, calcium, iron, and zinc.

To increase her intake of calories, Suzie should follow the recommended servings from the five food groups (see pp.70–72) and eat a number of servings toward the higher end of the given range for each food group.

Since she lacks the time to prepare and eat balanced meals, she should buy low-fat frozen meals that can be cooked quickly in a microwave oven. Suzie can also increase her intake of whole-grains by eating a microwaved package of instant oatmeal with low-fat milk at breakfast with a cut-up banana or berries. She can add baby-carrot sticks with a glass of milk to her sandwich at lunch, and include a piece of whole-wheat bread and fresh fruit salad with her dinner. These are healthy additions that are quick and easy to prepare.

Low-fat milk or yogurt and an iron-rich food, such as dried fruit, can be added as snacks. She should continue with her prenatal vitamin supplement. To increase her fluid intake, she should drink more nutritious fluids (up to 6 pints/3liters per day), such as low-fat milk, 100 percent fruit juices, and water with meals and snacks. Suzie should keep a large bottle of water in the refrigerator, available at any time.

During and after menopause

Lifestyle changes ease the symptoms and effects of menopause.

Menopause is a natural part of aging that occurs when the ovaries dramatically reduce their output of sex hormones, especially estrogen. This change often occurs over a few years, usually between the ages of 45 and 60, but it can happen at an earlier age in some women. As sex-hormone levels drop, a woman's menstrual periods end.

What are the symptoms?
Menopausal symptoms vary greatly. Some women experience significant discomfort, while others have no symptoms. Typical symptoms are hot flashes (sudden intense waves of heat and sweating), depression, anxiety, and mood swings. There may also be urinary and vaginal problems, such as atrophy, where the vaginal tissue becomes thinner, drier, and more delicate, irregular or heavy periods until menstruation finally stops, infections, urinary incontinence, and inflammation of the vagina. Many women also notice changes to the condition of their skin and hair.

Making lifestyle changes
To prevent the consequences of low-estrogen levels and ease the transition during menopause, there are lifestyle changes that

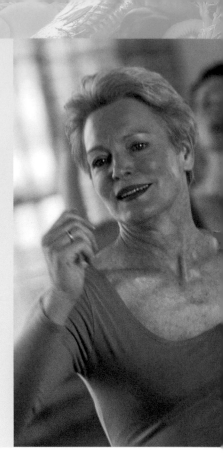

Foods that reduce symptoms

Studies show that certain dietary changes during menopause may ease symptoms. Generally, eating a healthy, balanced diet that includes moderate amounts of fat and plenty of fruits, vegetables, and whole grains will make you feel better. More specifically, soy is known to contain chemicals that ease symptoms. Calcium is also vital, not so much to ease the symptoms of menopause, but to keep bones strong and prevent or delay the onset of osteoporosis.

Soy products Foods that naturally contain soy include soymilk, soybeans, tofu, edamame, soy nuts, and tempeh. These foods are good sources of protein and phytochemicals called isoflavones. Interest has centered on two specific isoflavones—genistein and daidzen. These are similar in structure to the sex hormone estrogen. They mimic the activities of estrogen in the body and may help reduce menopausal symptoms that occur due to reduced estrogen levels, such as urinary and vaginal problems and menstrual irregularities. In addition, studies have shown that isoflavones have anticancer properties.

Calcium-rich foods The North American Menopause Society (NAMS) recommends that menopausal women get 1,200–1,500mg of calcium per day. This amount is significantly more than the average calcium consumed each day by women aged 50–65 (about 700mg). Low-fat dairy foods and dark-green leafy vegetables, such as kale and turnip greens, are good sources.

Because vitamin D is needed to help the body absorb calcium, try to get about 0.015mg of vitamin D per day (*see p.57*) from fortified dairy products or calcium supplements containing vitamin D.

Herbal supplements

Various herbal supplements, such as black cohosh, may help reduce the symptoms of menopause.

Black cohosh This woodland plant has large leaves and a thick knotted root system. It has been used for more than 100 years to help reduce the symptoms of menopause. Scientific studies have shown that this herbal supplement can reduce hot flashes, vaginal dryness, and depression.

However, do not use black cohosh for more than 6 months or if you are taking hormone replacement therapy (HRT) or any medications for high blood pressure.

Other herbal remedies Dong quai, evening primrose oil, and wild yam can also be used to ease the symptoms of menopause, but, as yet, there is not sufficient evidence to support their effectiveness.

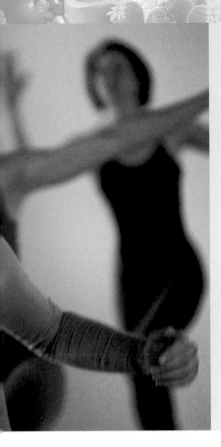

you can make. These include eating healthy nutrient-rich foods that may help ease symptoms and prevent postmenopausal problems, such as the degenerative bone disorder osteoporosis (*see p.242*). Evidence shows that soy products, some herbal supplements, and certain nutrients can be helpful (*opposite below and below*).

Physical activity

Exercise improves menopausal symptoms. Try to do at least 30 minutes a day of moderate aerobic exercise, such as walking, biking, or swimming, for the greatest effect on the health of your heart and lungs. Weight-bearing exercises, such as weightlifting, walking, or

Keeping bones strong Together with a healthy diet rich in calcium, weight-bearing exercises, such as dancing and jogging, keep bones strong and help prevent bone loss.

tennis, can also delay or prevent bone loss. Exercising is also good for preventing obesity; studies have shown that women who have successfully lost weight and kept it off tend to participate in some type of physical activity every day.

After menopause

Reduced levels of the hormone estrogen after menopause puts postmenopausal women at risk of osteoporosis. This disorder may develop because estrogen helps maintain normal bone density.

Prior to menopause, women are at a lower risk of cardiovascular disease (*see pp.214–221*) compared to men because estrogen helps lower "bad" LDL-cholesterol and raise "good" HDL-cholesterol levels in the blood. However, as estrogen declines during and after menopause, a woman's risk of cardiovascular disease becomes the same as that of a man.

Nutrients that help ease menopausal complaints

To ensure that you get plenty of the nutrients that can help ease menopausal complaints (*below*), eat a varied diet and try these tips. For breakfast, add ground flaxseeds to your whole-grain cereal. For lunch, try eggs, canned fish, or vegetable sources of protein, such as soybeans or a mixture of other legumes, grains, and corn, with whole-grain bread.

For dinner, have fish, lean meat, or poultry with a green leafy vegetable, such as spinach or collard greens. For snacks, eat at least two pieces of fruit a day and a handful of almonds at least every other day. In addition, two glasses of fat-free or low-fat milk a day will minimize an active woman's risk of troubling menopausal complaints.

COMPLAINT	NUTRIENT	TOP SOURCES
Depression, mood swings	• Omega-3 fatty acids • Folate • Vitamin D	• Flaxseed, oily fish • Whole grains, green leafy vegetables, orange juice • Oily fish, enriched dairy products
Breast soreness and lumps	• Vitamin E	• Almonds, vegetable oil, flaxseed
Heavy menstrual bleeding	• Iron	• Red meat, legumes, spinach, raisins, bran cereal
Hot flashes	• Calcium • Exercise	• Low-fat dairy products, green leafy vegetables, canned oily fish with bones (salmon, sardines) • 20 minutes per day, such as dancing, swimming, or walking
Osteoporosis	• Vitamin D • Calcium	• Oily fish, enriched dairy products • Low-fat dairy products, green leafy vegetables, canned oily fish with bones (salmon, sardines)

The extra needs of athletes

When exercising, we need extra calories and nutrients.

Proper nutrition is not only essential for the growth, maintenance, and repair of your body's tissues, but it also provides fuel for exercise. The fuel that your body uses is known as ATP (*below*).

Adjusting your diet

If you are an athlete, the best diet you can have is similar to the best diet for a nonathlete: obtaining enough calories while limiting how much saturated fat you eat.

Jargon buster

ATP This chemical, which is short for adenosine triphosphate, is a product of the breakdown of carbohydrates, proteins, and fat in the body. Whenever your body needs energy for chemical reactions and processes, it uses ATP.

To achieve an athlete's diet, you do not need to change the food you eat; you need to adjust the amount of food and fluids, the number of meals, and timing of meals (before, during, or after competition).

The need for extra calories

Calorie needs vary widely among athletes as body size, age, gender, and environment all influence the number of calories burned during exercise. The intensity, duration, and mode of exercise, your level of conditioning, and how efficiently you move also influence how many calories you burn up.

The basic energy requirement per day for a sedentary or overweight person is 20 calories per 2.2lb (1kg) of body weight. Moderately active people need 25–35 calories per 2.2lb (1kg) of body weight, with women at the lower end and men at the higher end of the scale. Very active people require more: male athletes need 37–51 calories and females 41–58 calories per 2.2lb (1kg) of body weight per day.

The fuel of choice

Carbohydrate is the fuel of choice for exercise. Compared to fat, it is more easily converted into ATP, providing energy for all working muscles and the rest of the body. At rest, when plenty of oxygen is available, the body burns mostly fat. When you begin to exercise, less oxygen becomes available, and carbohydrates become a more important energy source, especially for short, intense exercise.

Protein is stored in the body as muscle, and fat is stored as body fat. Carbohydrates are only stored in tiny amounts in the body—in the liver and muscles as a molecule called glycogen—so it is important to eat carbohydrates before you exercise. If you exercise for a long time or at a moderate pace, you exhaust glycogen stores, and the body breaks down fat for energy.

Burning up fuel Carbohydrates provide the fuel needed for the energy muscles expend during intense exercise such as sprinting.

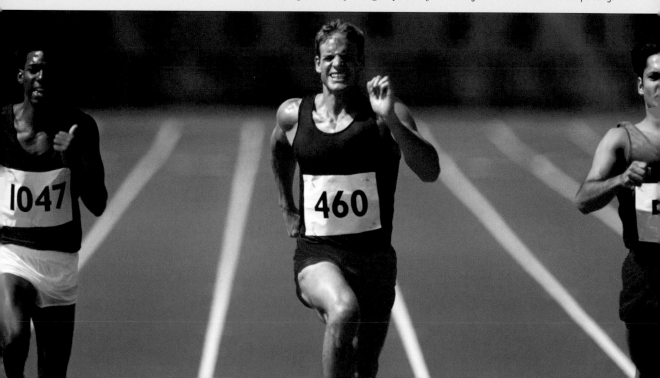

Very active people need more protein

The protein needs for athletes depend upon the type of exercise (resistance vs. endurance) and its intensity and duration. During rest, protein can supply as much as five percent of the energy the body burns up. During aerobic exercise, such as jogging, protein may then account for as much as 15 percent of the energy used. Hardly any protein is used during resistance, or strength, training.

When exercise is extremely intense or if there is no fat or carbohydrate available for the body to use as fuel, muscle will then be broken down.

People who play sports that require muscle building, such as football and wrestling, need more protein in their diet than sedentary people. If you start a program of resistance training, current recommendations are to increase protein intake during the initial weeks of your training program.

● Moderately active men and women need 0.35g of protein per lb (0.45kg) of body weight per day.
● Men who do endurance sports, such as long-distance cycling and marathons, need to increase their protein intake up to 0.65g per lb (0.45kg) per day.
● Men who do resistance training, such as weightlifting, need 0.7g of protein per lb (0.45kg) per day.
● Women athletes, participating in either endurance or resistance exercise, need 0.5g of protein per lb (0.45kg) of body weight per day.

Healthy protein sources

The best food sources of protein should also be low in fat. About 8–10oz (225–280g) a day of the following should meet the protein needs of most athletes:
● Low-fat dairy products
● Lean beef
● Poultry
● Eggs
● Fish
● Shellfish
● Tofu
● Kidney beans
● Lentils
● Nuts
● Sesame seeds
● Soybeans

Making sure you get plenty of fluids

Water accounts for 80 percent of our bodies. During exercise, our muscles generate internal heat. In order to prevent the body temperature from rising too high, we sweat—water and salts are excreted through pores in the skin to cool the body.

Dehydration If excess sweating occurs during exercise without replacing the fluid you have lost, you can become dehydrated. Symptoms of dehydration include general discomfort, headache, exhaustion, and apathy.

Keeping hydrated Because a loss of 3 percent of body weight as water can decrease athletic performance, it is vital to drink enough before, during, and after an event, especially during the meal prior to exercise.

● The day before a competition try to have at least one 8floz (240ml) drink during each meal with at least two other 16floz (500ml) drinks between meals.
● Avoid large amounts of tea, coffee, and alcohol as they have a diuretic effect, that is they increase the amount of urine produced by the body.
● During exercise, drink at regular intervals, about 8floz (240ml) every 30 minutes. Fluid intake following physical activity can also be critical in helping athletes recover quickly between bouts of training and competition.
● Take carbo drinks for carbohydrates before a competition, isotonic drinks for carbohydrates during exercise, and hypotonic drinks to avoid dehydration.

Don't drink too much water It is very important to follow the recommendations above as drinking too much water can cause problems. If you have over 7 pints (3.5 liters) while sweating profusely in competition, you are at risk of low blood-sodium levels (hyponatremia). This is a risk for athletes who participate in endurance events, such as triathlons or marathons. Symptoms include headache, nausea, fatigue, drowsiness, muscle weakness, muscle twitching or cramping, confusion, seizure, and possibly coma.

Sports drinks

There are three basic types of sports drinks, each for a different need:

Carbo drinks Rich in carbohydrate, these sports drinks should be taken before an event in order to replenish glycogen reserves in the muscles and liver.

Isotonic drinks Designed to be taken while exercising, isotonic drinks quickly deliver glucose to the muscles for extra energy.

Hypotonic drinks These drinks contain little carbohydrate. They replenish water and salts lost from the body and prevent dehydration.

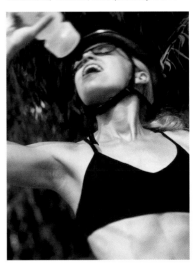

Preventing dehydration Make sure you drink plenty of fluids during prolonged exercise to prevent dehydration, especially if you are outdoors in hot weather.

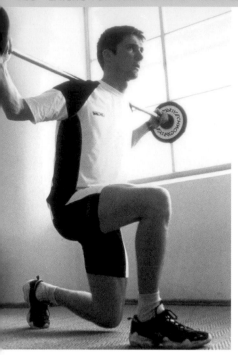

Strength training During intense short-burst exercise, such as weightlifting, muscles burn up glucose anaerobically (without oxygen).

What do nonendurance athletes need?

For nonendurance athletes, such as football, tennis, and baseball players and weightlifters, the bulk of their calorie intake (55–60 percent) should come from carbohydrates, mainly starches and a small proportion from sugars. No more than 30 percent of calories should come from fat and the remainder (10–15 percent) from protein. As with any diet, it should be well-balanced and provide all the necessary nutrients.

GLUCOSE AND GLYCOGEN

When starches or sugars are eaten, the body changes them to glucose, which is the only form of carbohydrate used directly by muscles for energy. Glucose is also stored in the liver and muscles as glycogen. During exercise, glycogen is broken down to provide energy. There is usually enough glycogen in the muscles for 90–120 minutes of exercise. Most exercise and sport games do not use up glycogen stores so eating carbohydrates during the activity is not necessary.

Here are a few tips for nonendurance athletes about what to eat and drink before, during, and after exercise:
Before Have some high-carbohydrate foods like a banana, bagel, or fruit juice. These foods are broken down quickly and provide glucose. Researchers have found that eating something between one and four hours before exercise keeps glucose available for working muscles. It is also critical to drink plenty of water beforehand to keep muscles hydrated.
During Perspiration and exertion deplete the body of the fluids necessary for optimum performance and lead to dehydration. Drink plenty of water, at least 4floz (120ml) every 20 minutes of exercise. Replace carbohydrates with a sports drink (see p.147) if the exercise lasts over 90 minutes.
After If the exercise was strenuous and lasted a long time, glycogen stores may need refueling. Foods and drinks high in carbohydrates right after exercise will replenish glycogen stores.

Do performance enhancers work?

Any substance that can improve the performance of a sport is known as an ergogenic aid. These aids include sports drinks (see p.147), caffeine, and creatine (right).
Caffeine Found naturally in tea, coffee, and chocolate, this stimulant is often added to soft drinks as a performance enhancer. Caffeine is a controlled, or restricted, drug during competition, and it should be avoided before competition and training due to its diuretic (urine-producing) effect, which can contribute to the risk of dehydration.
Supplements To prevent fatigue, some athletes use alkaline salts such as sodium bicarbonate (baking soda) to neutralize the buildup of lactic acid. This acid is a waste product of anaerobic respiration, in which muscles burn glucose without using oxygen. Creatine is used by many athletes to enhance muscle activity and increase muscle mass (right).

Professional athletes need to be careful when taking any supplement or

ergogenic aid, unless it is approved by a sports governing body. In some cases, supplements that are not banned or restricted may be chemically converted in the body into ones that are.
Vitamins and minerals Most athletes have lower blood levels of vitamins than nonathletes, regardless of whether they are taking any supplements. However, while it is true that physical activity may increase the need for some vitamins and minerals, the body's increased needs generally can be met with a balanced diet that includes a variety of foods. Despite what many athletes believe, vitamin supplements have not been shown to improve or enhance athletic performance, according to the American College of Sports Medicine.

However, some female athletes may develop an iron deficiency and therefore should eat a diet rich in iron—from foods such as red meat, spinach, and legumes—or take a supplement to prevent anemia (see p.271).

Creatine supplements

Studies have shown that creatine—an amino acid present in some proteins—may be beneficial for athletes participating in sports that involve short bursts of intense exercise, such as weightlifting, baseball, and sprinting.

Creatine works by providing quick energy for the initial phase of muscle contraction. It can also increase muscle mass and strength, necessary for these kinds of sports. It works by pulling water into muscle cells from the surrounding fluid, resulting in a larger muscle and, eventually, a stronger muscle.

Creatine occurs naturally in the body—it is manufactured by the liver—but it can also be obtained in the diet from fish and red meat. It is marketed as a supplement in the form of creatine phosphate, which is more bioavailable, or easier for the body to use.

What do endurance athletes need?

Carbohydrates are the most important nutrient for endurance sports, such as marathons and long-distance cycling, swimming, or cross-country skiing.

CARBOHYDRATE LOADING

Before an event, some athletes practice "carbohydrate loading," an approach that maximizes stores of muscle glycogen, which is the first fuel to be used during intense exercise. To achieve this, you limit your intake of carbohydrates for a few weeks before eating a lot of them in the days before the event. The initial reduction in carbohydrates makes the body extremely sensitive to them when they enter the body, allowing glycogen stores to be replenished. See below for a healthy carbohydrate-rich meal to eat the day before an event.

DAY OF THE EVENT

It is best to eat a light breakfast, such as cereal or toast and fruit juice. After breakfast, drink water in small amounts at regular intervals to ensure you start the race fully hydrated. Since the body's carbohydrate stores become depleted during the exertion of an endurance event, replace them whenever possible. Sports drinks (see p.147) help maintain diminishing stores of energy, water, and nutrients, especially salts lost in sweat, throughout the event. Up to 8–10 pints (4–5 liters) of sweat may be lost when running a marathon. Afterward, restore the body's water and energy levels as soon as possible.

WHAT TO AVOID

Endurance athletes should avoid coffee, tea, and alcohol, because they might lead to dehydration. Some athletes, however, do take caffeine just prior to a race to enhance performance.

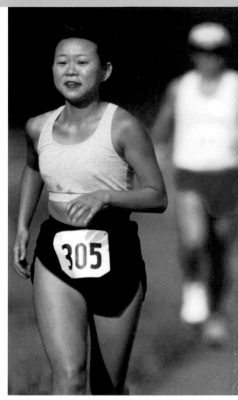

Running a marathon Always begin an endurance event fully hydrated and with replenished glycogen stores.

Recipe Carbohydrate meal for endurance athlete

INGREDIENTS
1 large onion
4 garlic cloves
2 tbsp olive oil
1 eggplant
1 tbsp reduced-salt soy sauce
13oz (400g) can tomatoes
2 plum tomatoes
fresh thyme
2½ cups fusilli pasta

Serves 6

1 Finely chop the onion and crush the garlic cloves. Heat a little olive oil in a skillet, add the onion and garlic, and fry until the onion is softened.

2 Cut the eggplant into ½in- (1cm-) cubes. Add to the skillet and cook until it is soft. If the mixture becomes too dry, add a little water.

3 Add the soy sauce to the vegetable mixture, stir gently to combine, and cook for a further 1–2 minutes.

4 Add the canned tomatoes to the skillet, stir gently to combine, cover the pan, and cook for about 20 minutes.

5 Skin, seed, and finely chop the plum tomatoes and add to the skillet, along with a little chopped thyme. Simmer for a further 2 minutes.

6 Cook the pasta in a large pan of fast-boiling water, until just firm to the bite, then drain.

7 Season the sauce with freshly ground black pepper before spooning over the pasta. If you like, garnish with chopped fresh flat-leaf parsley.

Each serving provides:
Calories 243, Total fat 5.2g
(Sat. 0.8g, Poly. 1.0g, Mono. 2.8g)
Cholesterol 0mg, Protein 9g,
Carbohydrate 50g, Fiber 6g,
Sodium 117mg. Good source of—Vits: A, Fol, C; Mins: Ca, Mg, P, K.

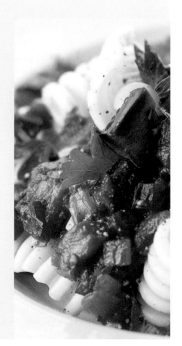

The middle-to-later years of life

Good food choices and exercise between 50 and 70 years can help you defy aging.

As people age, they tend to eat less, and therefore take in fewer calories and smaller amounts of important nutrients. In addition, it becomes more difficult for the body to digest and absorb certain vital nutrients. For example, in older people, the amounts of calcium, vitamin B_{12}, and folate in the diet often fall well below the recommended daily intakes.

For good health over 50, it is important to make sure that you eat nutrient-dense foods and remain physically active.

Changing caloric needs

Your body changes as you get older and these changes affect your nutritional needs. There is a reduction in muscle, an increase in body fat, and your total body water decreases by up to 20 percent. You need fewer calories than you did when you were younger since your basal metabolic rate (BMR; *see p.26*) decreases as muscle mass declines with age.

The good news is that moderate exercise helps preserve muscle mass and can thereby slow the rate at which this process occurs.

Gentle exercise Walking is an excellent excercise, so playing golf is an ideal activity that helps improve stamina, flexibility, and muscle and bone strength.

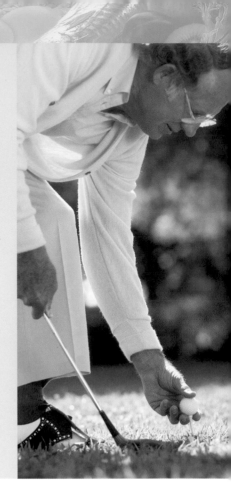

Do you need to take supplements?

If you are over 50, the key vitamins and minerals you should get enough of are vitamins B_6, B_{12}, folate, and D and calcium. It is better to meet your needs through your diet, but these are so important that you might have to take supplements. See your doctor for advice before taking supplements because high doses of certain supplements, such as vitamin B_6, can be harmful.

Vitamin B_6 Adults 50 years and older have increased vitamin B_6 needs at 1.5mg per day. Older people who suffer from depression or those taking hormone replacement therapy have lower blood levels of vitamin B_6. Post-menopausal women with osteoporosis (*see p.241*) have also been shown to have low levels of this vitamin.

Vitamin B_{12} Adults aged 50 and over are recommended to take 0.0024mg of this vitamin per day. Although most Americans who eat animal products get sufficient vitamin B_{12} from their diet, about 10–15 percent of people over 60 have lost the ability to absorb this vitamin properly due to a reduction in the secretion of acid and pepsin, which break down proteins in food, in the stomach. It is now recommended that people over age 50 meet most of their dietary requirement for vitamin B_{12} with synthetic vitamin B_{12}, which is easier for the body to absorb and is used in fortified foods or supplements.

Folate Adults aged 50 years and over need 0.4mg of folate per day. Since folate fortification of grain products is now widespread, most older people obtain enough from their diet alone.

Older adults who do need a folate supplement must also take a vitamin B_{12} supplement, as too much folate may mask a vitamin B_{12} deficiency, which can result in anemia and damage to the nervous system.

Vitamin D This vitamin aids calcium absorption and helps maintain healthy bones, but it may be difficult for older adults to get enough. For adults aged 50–70 years, the daily recommended intake is 0.01mg. Those who have limited exposure to sunlight and eat or drink very few dairy products would benefit from a supplement (*see p.269*), as they are at risk of the bone disorders osteomalacia (*see p.241*) or osteoporosis.

Calcium Osteoporosis is a major health risk for both older women and men. The daily recommended amount of calcium is 1,200mg for men and women aged 50 years and older. This amount of calcium should help retain the mineral in the bones, keeping them strong and making them less susceptible to fracture. If you have difficulty getting enough calcium through your diet, see your doctor or dietitian about taking a supplement (*see p.267*).

Regular exercise has other benefits too—it keeps your bones strong, enhances mobility and flexibility, and generally increases your well-being (*see p.153*).

The digestive system

Digestion and absorption of food appear to be well preserved as aging occurs. However, aging does affect some digestive processes. Saliva production decreases, which may affect how food is broken down in the stomach to prepare for digestion and absorption in the intestine. The stomach reduces its secretion of acid and pepsin, which may lead to decreased absorption of vitamins B_{12}, folate, and D and the mineral calcium. The smooth muscles in the intestine become less efficient, resulting in slower movement of food through the intestine and often constipation.

As you age, there is also a decline in the skin's production of vitamin D, which is necessary for the body to use calcium, making it more

difficult for the body to meet its calcium needs. Calcium is especially important for women during and after menopause (*see p.144–145*). For these reasons, older adults should eat nutrient-dense foods and may also need to take supplements.

Health problems

Chronic disorders, such as arthritis, obesity, diabetes, cardiovascular disease, and osteoporosis, are more likely to develop after age 50. The risk of other serious disorders such as cancer, heart attack, and stroke is also increased. You can reduce the risk or minimize the effects of many disorders by avoiding or eating certain foods (*see Food as Medicine, pp.210–271*).

In addition, if you have been prescribed any medications, they may affect your appetite or even prevent, or in some cases enhance, absorption of certain nutrients, vitamins, or minerals from the stomach or intestine (*see p.153*).

Drinking alcohol

Recent studies suggest that moderate drinking—about 1–2 drinks a day—may have health benefits for older adults. These include improving mood, reducing stress, maintaining mental faculties, mixing socially, enhancing bone-mineral density, and improving cardiovascular health. However, many older people, especially those living in nursing homes, drink more than this, often due to depression or loneliness.

Too much alcohol can drain the body of water-soluble vitamins and decrease the absorption of most vitamins and minerals. It can also displace important calories, resulting in poor appetite for the meals needed to prevent weight loss. The National Institute on Alcohol Abuse and Alcoholism recommend that people over 65 years should limit their alcohol consumption to one drink per day.

Easing constipation with diet

A slower intestine is one of the most common changes experienced by older people. The smooth muscles of the gut contract more slowly with age and food moves more slowly through the intestine. This can lead to constipation—difficult and infrequent passage of small, hard stools. It can usually be corrected by increasing fiber and fluid intake. High-fiber foods include vegetables, fruits, legumes, and whole grains. A bowl of raisin bran cereal or oatmeal each day is often enough to achieve bowel regularity.

Try to achieve a routine in which you go to the toilet at the same time each day. If you ignore the urge to go, stools remain in the gut longer, becoming dry and hard, and you will strain more when you do go.

DRINK PLENTY OF WATER

Try to drink at least 6–8 glasses of water daily, even if you are not thirsty. As you age, your thirst response may decrease,

so you may not always recognize when you need fluids. Keep a bottle or pitcher of water handy to remind you to drink regularly throughout the day and ensure that you get enough fluids, which will help your stools stay soft, bulky, and easy to eliminate.

TRY TAKING A NATURAL LAXATIVE

If water and fiber are not sufficient, try taking a laxative, such as psyllium fiber, which can be easily mixed with water or juice. It causes the stool to retain water as it passes through the intestine to produce soft, bulky stools.

Drink several glasses of water with the laxative and use sugar-free varieties if you are diabetic. Avoid mineral oil laxatives, as they can interfere with the absorption of fat-soluble vitamins. Persistent use of stimulant laxatives should be avoided because your colon will eventually be unable to function without them.

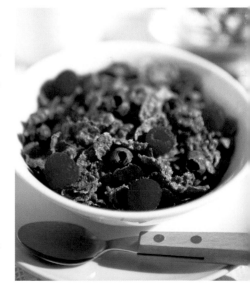

Fiber can prevent constipation A bran cereal with added fruit each day can help prevent constipation. Men over 50 need 30g of fiber per day and women over 50 need 21g per day.

Which foods can fight aging?

Certain foods are rich in antioxidants. These are substances that neutralize free radicals, chemicals that damage cells in the body and thus aggravate aging and disease.

The main antioxidants are vitamin A (*see p.52*), vitamin C (*see p.56*), vitamin E (*see p.58*), beta-carotene (a precursor of vitamin A), and the minerals selenium (*see p.67*) and zinc (*see p.67*). Some phytochemicals, such as lycopene (*see p.59*), are also antioxidants. You can try the following tips to get the maximum benefit from antioxidants:

- Make sure you eat plenty of fresh fruits and vegetables.
- Since vitamin E is one of nature's best antioxidants, do not eliminate olive and canola oils from your diet.
- Try to reduce the amount of work antioxidants have to do by preventing the buildup of free radicals. Do not smoke, spend too long in the sun, or let yourself get too stressed, and keep away from polluted areas.

ANTIOXIDANT-RICH MEALS

Ideas for modifying a snack or a meal to pack a powerful antioxidant-rich punch include the following tips:

- Fresh cantaloupe melon, cut up with low-fat or fat-free cottage cheese.
- Strawberry smoothie (*see p.81*).
- Half of a whole wheat bagel with farmer's cheese and sliced tomato.
- Grilled salmon on a bed of field greens with peppers, tomatoes, sliced mango, and sprinkled ground flaxseed.
- Heated-up leftover broccoli, green peas, and cauliflower.
- A handful of baby carrots or almonds.
- Sautéed spinach in olive oil and garlic and garnished with lemon and parmesan cheese.
- Add extra tomatoes, corn, broccoli and celery to your salad.
- Sweet potatoes instead of white potatoes in your meals.
- Sliced almonds added to string beans.
- Sliced oranges with your dessert or instead of your usual dessert.

Age spots

When free radicals—damaging chemicals in the body (*see p.58*)—build up they can produce a substance known as lipofucsin. This substance is deposited in the skin, most commonly on the face and back of the hands, in the form of brown spots or patches. These areas are commonly known as "age spots" or "liver spots." The number of age spots that you have is thought to indicate the total amount of damage that your body has suffered from free radicals.

Eating foods that are rich in antioxidants (*left*), especially those that are good sources of vitamin A, C, and E and the mineral selenium, can prevent the formation of liver spots by breaking down the lipofuscin before it is deposited. In addition, using creams that contain vitamin C may eventually make age spots disappear from the skin.

Recipe Antioxidant-rich fish with salsa

INGREDIENTS

2 lemons

4 cod steaks

1 yellow bell pepper

1 stalk celery

4 plum tomatoes

1 onion

2 chili peppers

fresh flat-leaf parsley

1 garlic clove

Serves 4

1 Grate the zest of one lemon into a shallow dish; add the juice of both lemons, and ground black pepper to taste.

2 Add the cod steaks to the lemon juice and marinate for 30 minutes, turning once, and keeping refrigerated.

3 De-seed the pepper and chop finely, along with the celery, tomatoes, onion, chilis, and some chopped parsley. Crush the garlic and add to the other ingredients, mixing together to make a salsa.

4 Preheat oven to 425°F/220°C. Lightly brush a baking dish with olive oil and arrange the

fish steaks in it. Cover each steak with a few spoonfuls of the salsa mixture. Pour the marinade juice over the salsa and add a little more olive oil.

5 Bake the cod steaks for 20 minutes in the preheated oven, until cooked through.

6 Serve with a green salad or green beans, broccoli, or spinach for an antioxidant-rich meal. Garnish with remaining chopped flat-leaf parsley.

Each serving provides:

Calories 200, Total fat 1.5g (Sat. 0.3g, Poly. 0.6g, Mono. 0.2g), Cholesterol 73mg, Protein 32g, Carbohydrate 15g, Fiber 3.0g, Sodium 113mg. Good source of—Vits: A, Fol, C, K, Mins: Ca, Mg, P.

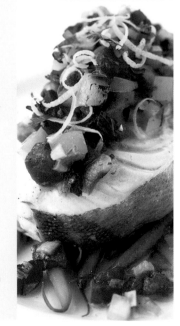

The importance of keeping fit

Regular exercise significantly slows the effects of aging. Not only does physical activity give you more energy and make you feel relaxed, but it also enables you to meet new people, boosts your self-esteem, and maintains a feeling of independence. It also reduces the risk of many age-related disorders, including diabetes, cardiovascular diseases such as stroke and heart attack, and the bone disorder osteoporosis.

Exercise for people over 50 should aim to maintain strength, bone density, balance, flexibility, mobility, and general well-being. You can increase your bone strength and density by weight-bearing exercises, such as tennis, jogging, or brisk walking. In addition, you should increase your calcium and vitamin D intake and exposure to sunlight, which allows the body to make vitamin D, to maximize bone strength.

You can increase your flexibility and mobility in the following ways:
- Be active and do plenty of walking.
- Practice yoga or simple stretches.
- Try body-weight exercises, such as squats, leg lifts, and arm raises.
- Do exercises that increase muscular strength, such as weight-training.
- Take up activities that are good for the heart and lungs, such as swimming or gardening. Remember to begin any new exercise gently to avoid injury.

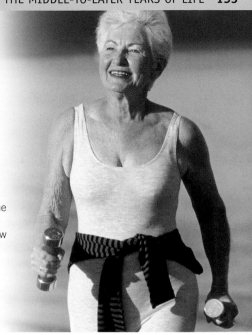

Out and around Exercising outdoors—in a park or on the beach—is beneficial for your health and well-being. Exposure to the sun also allows your body to make vitamin D.

Do your medications affect your diet?

Many people over the age of 50 years have long-term, or chronic, disorders, such as high blood pressure and arthritis, and need to take medications to control their symptoms. These medications may interact with the foods that you eat. Some block the absorption or processing of a nutrient in the body, while other medications enhance it. Conversely, some nutrients block or improve the effects of a medication. Taking medications may affect your appetite, and there is also a risk of missing out on a key nutrient due to an interaction. If you take a medication, your doctor or pharmacist should tell you which foods or nutrients may cause interactions. The most common interactions are listed below.

DRUG GROUP	REACTS WITH	EFFECT	WHAT YOU CAN DO
Analgesic drugs	• Alcohol	• Increases risk for liver damage	• Avoid alcohol
Antibiotic drugs	• Calcium and biotin • Vitamin K	• Reduces absorption of drug • Drug interferes with manufacture of vitamin K in the intestine	• Take drug on an empty stomach • Take a multivitamin supplement
Anticoagulant drugs	• Foods rich in vitamin K • Vitamin E supplements	• Decreases drug effectiveness • Increases drug effectiveness	• Limit foods high in vitamin K • Avoid vitamin E supplements
Antihypertensive and diuretic drugs	• Potassium and magnesium	• Some of these drugs increase potassium and magnesium losses	• Eat plenty of potassium- and magnesium-rich foods
Anti-inflammatory drugs	• Alcohol	• Can aggravate bleeding from the stomach	• Avoid alcohol
Cholesterol-lowering drugs	• Any food	• Enhances drug absorption	• Take with food
Steroid drugs	• Sugar • Sodium	• Drug elevates blood-sugar levels May cause fluid retention	• Reduce sweets and sodas • Limit sodium (salt) intake

Feeling good into old age

It is essential to eat healthy as you advance in age.

People aged 70 years and over are the rapidly expanding sector of the North American population. Their nutritional needs are, in general, similar to those of adults aged 50–70 (see pp.150–154), but deficiencies are more common, especially in frail or homebound older adults who rely on others for basic needs. This age group does, however, need increased amounts of some crucial nutrients, specifically calcium and the vitamins B_6, B_{12}, folate, and D.

Changes in senses

The taste buds deteriorate with age. To compensate, many older people prefer very sweet or salty foods. Adding sugar contributes empty calories (those with no nutritional value) to the diet, and adding salt to food can worsen high blood pressure. The senses of smell and sight may also deteriorate, resulting in a preference for strong-smelling foods or a loss of interest in food.

Health problems

Most older people have at least one long-term disorder, such as cardiovascular disease, arthritis, and diabetes. In addition, many are affected by dementia—which is a reduction in mental capacity due to a disorder that affects the brain.

These and other disorders affect what and how much you eat, and may require dietary restrictions, such as a low-fat or low-salt diet. The chapter Food as Medicine has more information on what to eat if you are ill (see pp.210–271).

Physical disabilities can affect nutritional health. For example, being unable to walk to the kitchen or go food shopping without help can result in poor eating habits. Emotional changes resulting from depression, grief, and loneliness can lead to loss of appetite.

Difficulty chewing

Dental problems are common in older people. Loose, decaying, or missing teeth, dentures that do not fit properly, and gum disease make it difficult to chew food and increase the risk of poor nutrition. Regular dental checkups are vital to help detect these problems before they become a nuisance.

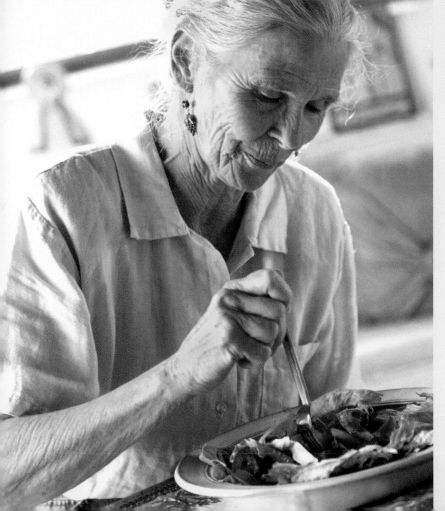

Continuing healthy eating As you age, it becomes more difficult to digest and absorb certain nutrients. Therefore, it is vital to have a varied diet of easy-to-digest, nutrient-dense foods such as the salad shown here.

Staying active

It is important to keep as active as possible later in life as this will benefit your health and well-being. Gentle activities such as walking, swimming, and neck and shoulder exercises are excellent. Even a short walk around the yard or the garden, or moving around your home during the day is beneficial. If you cannot walk easily or have difficulty moving about, think about installing or using mobility aids in your home, such as a walker.

Flavorful meals and snacks

Scientists refer to those 85 years and over as the "old-old," and for this fast-increasing group, weight maintenance is the biggest issue, with the focus on maintaining muscle mass and preventing weight loss. Therefore, making sure that you have access to meals and snacks that taste good and are easy to chew and swallow will help you feel good on a daily basis.

These meals should also be packed with nutrients and calories, such as the soup, scrambled eggs, and fruit with yogurt that are shown below. Prepared frozen meals are a good choice, too, because they can be quickly microwaved and require very little clean up, a key factor for older people who may also have difficulty preparing food in their kitchen.

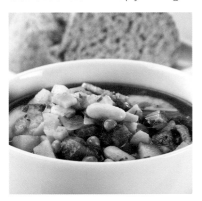

Spicy bean soup Homemade or from a can, these soups are an excellent source of protein, vitamins, minerals, and fiber.

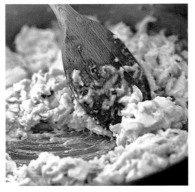

Scrambled eggs A quick and nutritious snack, scrambled eggs can be livened up by adding chopped herbs and Havarti cheese.

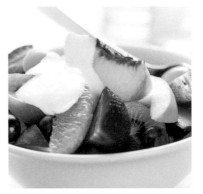

Fruit and yogurt Add low-fat yogurt—a great source of calcium—to a mixture of fresh fruits for a fiber- and calcium-rich dessert.

Case study Homebound senior with a hip fracture

Name Ben

Age 85 years

Problem Ben's diet is low in calories and he eats a poor selection of foods. His appetite has decreased since the death of his wife. His dentures are not fitting properly, so he has difficulty chewing, and he has a sore in his mouth beneath the bottom plate. He also has cracks at the corners of his mouth, which are due to poor vitamin intake. Ben slipped and broke his hip two months ago and has difficulty walking and shopping for food. He dislikes cooking just for himself. Because he is homebound, his exposure to sunlight is limited, which may result in vitamin D deficiency.

Lifestyle Ben lives alone. His wife died 3 months ago. He does not drink or smoke. He rarely sees his children,

who live out of state. Yesterday for breakfast, Ben had a jelly doughnut, one slice of white toast with jelly, and a cup of coffee. For lunch, he had a cup of chicken-and-rice soup with a few crackers and two cookies. For dinner, he had a peanut-butter-and-jelly sandwich on white bread with a few more cookies. He does not usually snack. Ben takes an iron supplement that was prescribed for anemia. He has constipation but uses laxatives and a suppository.

Advice Ben's family should be made aware of his current problems so that they can visit and arrange for a home health aid to monitor his health and diet. Ben will need to undergo physical therapy to improve his mobility. With regard to nutrition, Ben's diet needs to be higher in calories, protein, fiber, vitamins, and the mineral calcium. In addition, he should continue taking his iron supplements.

For breakfast, Ben can try instant oatmeal with low-fat milk and orange juice to give him calories, vitamin C, folate, and calcium. For lunch, he can microwave frozen meals delivered from a local agency.

He can try prepared foods, such as a tuna sandwich, or have leftovers from dinner the night before. Adding applesauce and a dessert to his dinner will also give him more calories, as would canned fruit in its own juice. He could also drink high-calorie, high-protein liquid supplements in order to increase his calories, protein, vitamins, and minerals.

Ben should make arrangements to have his dentures adjusted. His doctor can prescribe a multivitamin and mineral supplement for him. In addition, a visit to a social worker will help him get in touch with the local Council on Aging, Meals on Wheels, and other community resources that benefit elderly people.

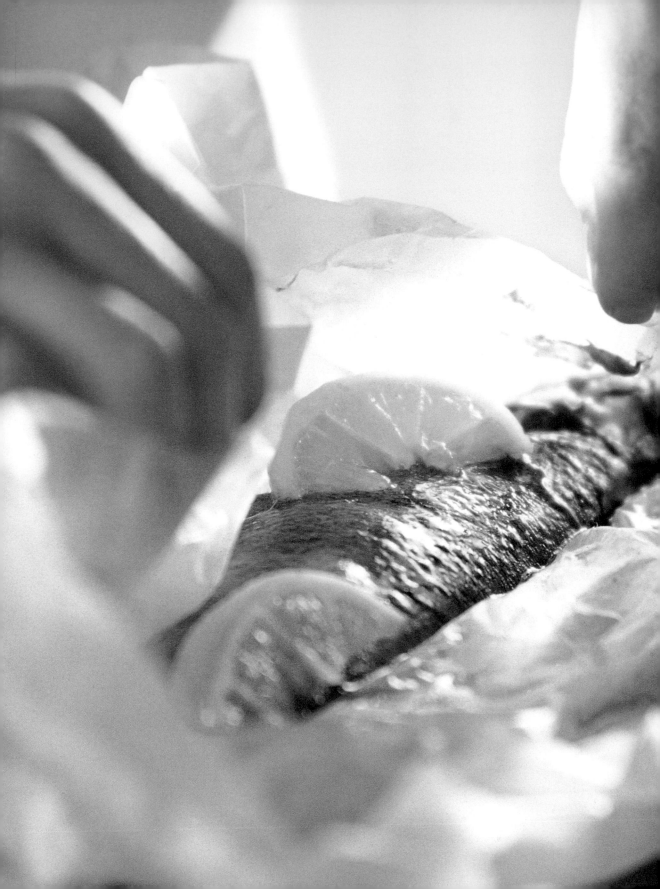

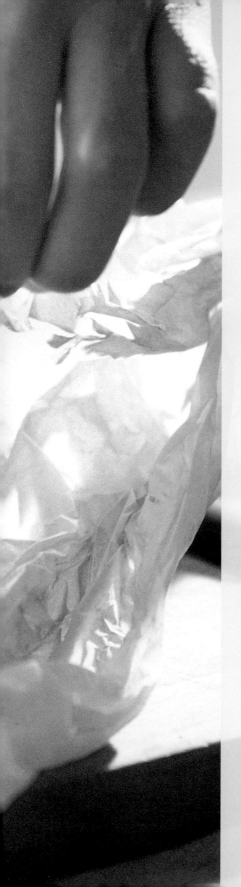

The truth about weight control

Not only does controlling your weight make you feel and look better, but there is also abundant evidence to show that keeping your weight within healthy limits decreases your risk of developing a variety of serious medical conditions, including high blood cholesterol, high blood pressure, other cardiovascular diseases, diabetes, and cancer.

Why weight control is important

Weight control means maintaining a healthy weight that is just right for your body.

If advertising for weight-loss diets and equipment is to be believed, weight control is primarily about improving your appearance. While it is true that keeping your weight in check can make you look better, it is even more important for your health and life expectancy. Being overweight increases your risk of developing a number of serious medical conditions (*right*).

Build activity into daily life Regular exercise is one of the keys to weight control for adults and children alike. Walking is a great activity for the whole of the family.

In 2000, the US Surgeon General declared that obesity had reached epidemic proportions—currently, over half of North American adults and a quarter of North American children are overweight, and these proportions have increased rapidly over the last twenty years. Such statistics highlight the importance of weight control.

Changing your "set point"

To maintain a healthy weight for your height and build, you need to adopt a strategy that will work for you in the long-term. Many of the diets on the market promise quick results, and while these may help you "kick-start" weight loss, they are not suitable for long-term weight control. The reason for this is what scientists identify as "set point"—the level at which your body defends its current weight.

If you consume extra calories (for a short period), your body will use these by generating more heat. If, on the other hand, you use more calories than you consume, your body will become more efficient at turning those calories into energy, to prevent short-term weight loss. This means that if you are trying to lose or gain weight, you have to make a serious commitment over a long period of time in order to retrain your body and readjust your set point.

Weight control for life

But where you do you start? In this chapter, we will guide you through the maze of diet plans, pointing out their strengths and weaknesses, and help you develop your own long-term weight-control strategy through good nutritional choices and regular exercise.

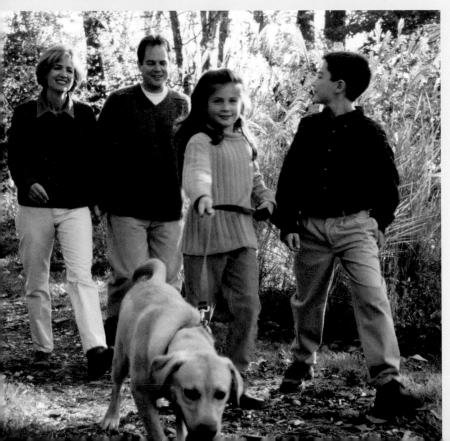

Health risks of obesity

The more overweight you are, the higher your risk of disease and premature death.

• Carrying too much weight places great strain on your heart and other organs as well as on weight-bearing joints, and puts you at greater risk of developing a range of serious medical conditions, including cardiovascular disease, such as high blood pressure, respiratory disease, osteoarthritis, gallstones, and certain cancers.

• Being obese increases your risk of complications during surgical procedures as well as creating extra difficulties for the surgeon performing the operation.

• Since being overweight makes it more difficult to engage in regular exercise, a downward spiral into increased health risk and lack of fitness is likely to ensue. A weight change of just 10 percent can reduce your risk and improve your health.

The benefits of controlling weight

Keeping your weight in check is critically important for your health. The more overweight you are, the higher your risk of developing various medical conditions (*opposite below*) and the more probable that your excess weight will shorten your life. Conversely, if you are overweight, losing weight will greatly benefit your health and well-being.

• Research shows that losing just 10 percent of excess body weight lowers blood pressure, thereby reducing the risk of cardiovascular disease, such as stroke (*see pp.214–215*).

• Losing weight lowers blood cholesterol and triglyceride levels, both of which are associated with increased risk of cardiovascular disease (*see pp.214–215*).

• Overweight people are twice as likely to develop type 2 diabetes as those who maintain a healthy weight. Losing weight reduces blood glucose levels and decreases the risk of developing diabetes (*see pp.246–247*).

• Losing weight will not only reduce your risk of developing osteoarthritis (*see p.245*), but will also reduce the stress on weight-bearing joints, such as the hips, knees, and lower spine, that are already affected by osteoarthritis.

• If you are considering surgery to replace arthritic hip or knee joints, you will almost certainly be advised to lose weight before the operation and to control your weight afterward in order to optimize the chances of a successful outcome.

• Obesity and being overweight are major risk factors for certain cancers: these include cancer of the uterus, cervix, ovary, breast, gallbladder, and colon in women; and cancer of the colon, rectum, and prostate in men. Losing weight will produce a corresponding reduction in those risks (*see pp.258–259*).

• Sleep apnea is a serious condition that is closely associated with being overweight. Weight loss usually improves this condition (*see p.225*).

• In additional, controlling your weight leads to enhanced self-esteem and a sense of well-being, as well as improving your appearance.

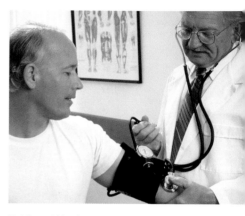

Weight and blood pressure If you are overweight, even a small reduction in weight will lower your blood pressure, which in turn reduces your risk of cardiovascular disease.

Questionnaire Are you controlling your weight?

Circle the letters that accompany your answers to these simple questions, then check your score.

1 Do you usually finish what is on your plate?
a No, I usually don't try to finish
b Yes, and then I am done
c Yes, and then I go for seconds

2 Do you ever share entreés when eating in restaurants?
a Yes, I usually share
b Sometimes, but only infrequently
c No, I don't usually share

3 Do you exercise at least 3 times per week?
a Yes, and sometimes more
b No, but I lead an active lifestyle
c No, I rarely exercise

4 Do you eat fruits and vegetables every day?
a Yes, about 5 servings a day

b Yes, a few servings a day
c No, only a few times a week

5 Do you eat low-fat dairy products?
a Yes, I always choose low-fat dairy
b Yes, a few servings a day
c No, only a few times a week or less

6 Do you try to eat low-fat meals and snacks?
a Yes, I always choose low-fat foods
b Yes, but I frequently cheat
c No, I choose high-fat foods

7 How much TV do you watch?
a I usually watch less than 1 hour a day
b I watch 2–3 hours a day
c I watch more than 4 hours a day.

8 Do you limit your intake of sweets and desserts?
a Yes, I choose fruit instead
b Yes, but I occasionally indulge
c No, I eat sweets almost every day

9 Do you drink water instead of sweetened beverages?
a Yes, I only drink water or diet soda
b Yes, but I also drink sweetened beverages and fruit juices
c No, I prefer soda and fruit drinks

Score a 1 **b** 2 **c** 3

9–13 points You are doing well and making a lot of effort to control your weight. Keep up the good work!

14–20 points Good job: you are really trying and your efforts will pay off over time. Look at the areas where you scored high and think about making some extra effort.

21–27 points Your score indicates that you are making choices that may lead to weight gain. These are just a few of the many small changes that you can make that will help you control your weight. Start slowly.

Tips for successful weight control

Maintaining a healthy weight is all about balancing your total food intake and the energy this provides, with the energy you expend in the course of your daily life. It's a simple equation, but not so simple to follow. We develop habitual ways of behaving in all areas of life, including what and how we eat and how active or sedentary our lives are. These habits build up over many years, so it is no easy matter to change them overnight. But if you find it difficult to control your weight, then you must make a serious commitment to change these habits. Here are some tips.

EAT ONLY WHAT YOU NEED
The key to controlling your weight is to balance how many calories you consume with how many you expend in the course of your daily activities (*see p.34*). Many people eat much more than they need and the excess calories are stored as fat. However, the more active you are, the more food you can consume and still maintain a healthy weight. You will benefit from both the physical activity and the weight control.

FILL UP ON FRUIT AND VEGGIES
Since there is a limit to the number of calories you can consume in a day if you want to maintain or lose weight, it is best to concentrate on those foods that supply your body with essential vitamins and minerals, such as fruits and vegetables, rather than on so-called "empty calorie foods" (*see p.99*). Eating two servings of vegetables with a meal will help fill you up and reduce your risk of snacking on less valuable foods. Similarly, eating an apple an hour before a meal will help you eat less at mealtime.

CUT OUT FATTY FOODS
Fat has more than twice the number of calories by weight as carbohydrate or protein. Therefore, if you want to cut calories and still eat enough to feel satisfied, you should eat fewer fatty foods. Even healthy oils contain 100 calories per tablespoon, so you should limit the amount of fried food you eat and replace full-fat dairy products with low-fat or fat-free varieties.

REDUCE SNACKS AND JUNK FOODS
Many people eat sensibly and healthy at mealtimes, but they consume high-calorie snacks during the day. If you are hungry and need a snack, choose healthy options, such as raw vegetables or fruits. If you snack out of boredom, try to identify the situations that trigger this impulse and devise alternative strategies for dealing with the impulse—for example, go for a walk or read a book or a magazine.

Exercise and weight control

Regular exercise is vital for long-term weight control. People who participate in physical activity at least three times a week are more likely to lose weight and keep it off than those who do not exercise. Strength training, such as lifting weights, is also helpful, since this type of activity increases muscle mass, which helps the body to burn more calories, even at rest.

To make exercise work, select an activity that you enjoy, start slowly, and stick with it. The great thing about exercise is that it makes you feel good, so it is self-reinforcing.

Exercise also combats fatigue—one of the most common reasons for which people consult their doctor. Once you start an exercise program, however, you begin to sleep better, your aches and pains vanish, your outlook on life improves, and fatigue vanishes.

Any food that has sugar listed as the first ingredient on the packaging (*see p.277*) is likely to be high in calories, and probably contains very little of nutritional value. Despite the notion that some people have a "sweet tooth," anyone can get used to less sugar in food. If you find this difficult, aim to re-train your taste by gradually eating less candy, soda, and sugary desserts.

BEAT THE FATIGUE TRAP
Feeling tired can lead people to eat foods that give a quick burst of energy, such as candy or chips. A balanced diet and a multivitamin supplement will help you maintain energy levels through the day.

JOIN A SUPPORT GROUP
Weight-loss groups offer sensible dietary advice, regular weigh-ins, and group support, which can really help with long-term motivation when trying to lose or control weight. You should choose a group that offers free weigh-ins once you have reached your target weight and, ideally, an exercise session.

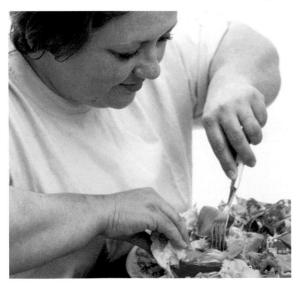

Eating healthily
The sensible approach to controlling weight is to eat vegetables, fruits, and low-fat proteins. This woman may feel she is eating healthy, but salami is high in saturated-fat, and she would also be better off eating whole-wheat bread.

Avoiding weight gain as you age

Getting older is often accompanied by steady weight gain because your body starts to digest food more slowly. For each decade between the ages of 20 and 60, the average North American gains 10lb (4.5kg) in weight. Scientists used to believe that such weight gain was normal, but we now know that it is unhealthy and brings an increased risk of developing a variety of serious medical conditions, such as diabetes and stroke.

The main reasons for weight gain in middle age are a decrease in physical activity and eating too much. In order to maintain a healthy weight, you need to recognize that your energy needs may be considerably less now than they were when you were younger, and that you must tailor your nutritional intake to your current requirements.

KEEP MOVING
Whatever your level of fitness, you should try to incorporate as much exercise into your life as possible. It may be that you

have an illness, injury, or condition such as arthritis (*see pp.240–241*) that makes it more difficult for you to continue with the level of activity or type of exercise that you enjoyed in the past. If necessary, consult your doctor for help finding an exercise program that suits your age and ability, and takes into account any medical condition from which you suffer.

It is never too late to start something new, and the benefits of embarking on a fitness program, such as improved flexibility and energy levels, and loss of excess weight, will quickly become apparent. Joining a group program can make exercise more enjoyable and help keep you motivated.

MODIFY YOUR DIET
Maintaining a healthy, balanced diet is important throughout life, but as energy requirements decrease with aging, it is even more important that you choose wisely, cutting down on sugary and fatty foods, and opting instead for a diet of

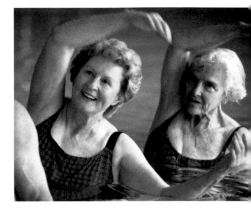

Finding suitable activities Water-based exercises are particularly beneficial for older people, allowing a good workout without putting undue strain on weight-bearing joints.

nutrient-dense fruits and vegetables, whole grains, and low-fat sources of protein and calcium. If you are trying to lose weight, make sure that you do not miss out on important nutrients. Taking a multivitamin supplement is advised.

Case study Older adult eating the same yet gaining weight

Name Marylyn

Age 65 years

Problem For most of her life, Marylyn has been able to control her weight, but recently it has become difficult. She has suffered from back pain for several years and has tried numerous treatments. Most recently Marylyn underwent surgery and her pain has lessened. However, she has not been as active and has gained 10lb (4.5kg) since last year. She finds this weight gain depressing. In addition, she has borderline high blood pressure, which did not need medication, but now her blood pressure is rising.

Lifestyle Marylyn has always led an active life. She raised three children and now spends time with her six

grandchildren. She is 62in (157cm) and weighed 110lb (50kg) for most of her life. Now she weighs 120lb (54.4kg) and complains that all her clothes are too tight. She eats small portions and snacks on fresh fruits or sometimes yogurt. She drinks soda or iced tea with meals, always has dessert with dinner, and has a snack before going to bed. She does not drink alcohol. She and her husband frequently eat out and have begun to travel quite a bit.

Advice Gaining weight as you get older is a very common problem. Marylyn cannot eat as many calories as she did when she was younger because she is not as active. Because of her surgery, her activity is limited and this is the most likely explanation for her weight gain. In addition, she has also been eating out more, and this often means larger portions.

There are a number of measures that Marylyn can take. The most important for her overall health, the strength of her back, and to prevent depression would be for her to begin a daily walking or swimming program. This will also help maintain her overall muscle mass, which declines as we age. Since Marylyn already eats small portions, the most significant change in her diet would be to switch to fresh fruit for dessert at dinner, and to substitute water or diet soda for regular soda and sweetened iced teas. She should avoid using salt when cooking and eating out because of her raised blood pressure. Marylyn does not get enough calcium so she should either drink more milk or eat more low-fat yogurt. If she can do this, then a calcium supplement of 500mg per day would be advisable. Otherwise, she may need to take a supplement of 1,000mg per day.

Looking at diet plans

There is a proliferation of weight-loss diets, not all of which are good for you.

Many of us have attempted to lose weight at one time or another, and the natural tendency is to look for a fast and easy way to shed that extra weight. As a result, weight loss is now a multi-billion-dollar industry, encompassing everything from diet books and slimming clubs to weight-loss programs selling specially formulated foods and medications.

Think long-term
Weight loss is difficult and there are no miracle solutions. To lose weight and keep it off takes time and commitment. Many popular programs appear to fulfill their promises in the short-term by restricting certain food groups for example. However, these rarely teach you how to establish and maintain healthy eating habits in the long-term and, once you return to your old eating habits, your lost weight quickly returns.

Changing your behavior
Regardless of which type of weight-loss diet you choose to follow, there are guidelines that can help you succeed in changing your eating habits.
• Avoid exposing yourself to situations where uncontrolled eating is likely to occur.
• Alter unhealthy eating habits, such as skipping meals or filling up on snacks.
• Change behavior chains: for example, if you often wind up eating ice cream late at night, don't buy it or go to bed earlier.
• Self-monitor: it has been proven that keeping a food diary helps change eating behavior.
• Think about how you will address problems and difficult situations before they arise.
• Change the way you think about your weight and your efforts to change it.
• Provide yourself with non-food rewards for accomplishing your weight-loss goals.

Seeking medical advice
Before beginning any program, especially very low-calorie or quick weight-loss types, talk to your doctor, especially if you are on any medication since the dose may have to be adjusted. Your doctor will monitor your progress and help you determine how much and what type of exercise is appropriate. He or she may also advise you to take vitamin and mineral supplements while you are on the diet program.

In general, weight-loss diets should not be undertaken by women who are pregnant or breast-feeding or by anyone under the age of 18. If you are in one of these categories and are concerned about your weight, seek advice from your doctor.

The diet directory
On the following pages, we provide you with information on many of the most popular diet programs currently available, and guidance about what to expect if you choose a particular program, including a sample day's menu from each one. We also look at the potential health benefits or hazards of each one.

There are many types of diets. Some limit certain macronutrients, such as fat or carbohydrates; others limit types of food, such as starchy carbohydrates. Some promote specific foods, such as grapefruit or cabbage soup, while others attempt to regulate your intake according to a strict formula, such as 40 percent carbohydrate: 30 percent protein: 30 percent fat.

However, other diet programs are based on theories that our bodies do not tolerate certain foods and that these must be eliminated from the diet. Most diets are aimed at helping you lose weight, but others promise a disease-free life to those who follow the program. When evaluating each of these diet plans, consider what it promises.

We firmly believe that there is no single best way for everyone to lose weight; most weight-loss diets work for some people; none works for everyone. However, with a little trial and error, everyone should be able to find a diet program that is effective for them.

Monitoring your weight When you are trying to lose weight, weighing yourself is one way of monitoring your progress—but do it just once a week, always at the same time of day.

DIET TYPE	UNDERLYING THEORY	DIET PLAN
High-carbohydrate, low-fat	Weight loss occurs on these very low-fat, high-fiber, mainly vegetarian diets because much less of such foods is required in order to feel satisfied.	• Ornish Diet (see p.164) • Pritikin Program (see p.164) • Hawaii Diet (see p.165) • Low-fat Living (see p.166) • McDougall Program (see p.167)
Carbohydrate-controlled	Based on a strict ratio of carbohydrate, protein, and fat, these diets aim to maintain stable blood-sugar levels, which helps the body break down fat, work within its "peak performance zone," and maximize weight loss.	• Atkins Diet (see p.167) • Carbohydrate-Addict's Diet (see p.169) • Protein Power Lifeplan (see p.169) • Sugar Busters (see p.170) • Zone Diet (see p.171) • Life Without Bread (see p.172) • Scarsdale Diet (see p.172) • Schwarzbein Principle (see p.173) • South Beach Diet (see p.174)
Controlling portion sizes	Based on the principle that eating large portions is a major factor in becoming overweight, these diet plans promote weight loss by controlling portion sizes.	• Picture Perfect Weight Loss (see p.175) • Volumetrics Weight-control (see p.176) • 90/10 Weight-loss Plan (see p.177) • Change One Eating Plan (see p.177)
Glycemic index	These diets are based on the theory that insulin levels and weight can be controlled by eating low-glycemic-index foods.	• Glucose Revolution (see p.178) • Montignac Method (see p.179) • Insulin-resistance Diet (see p.180)
Food-combining	Based on the belief that different food types are digested in different ways and should not be eaten together; weight loss results from correct combining of food types.	• Hay Diet (see p.180) • Somersizing (see p.181) • New Beverly Hills Diet (see p.182) • Fit for Life (see p.183)
Metabolic typing	Different blood types affect digestive processes; weight loss occurs when only correct foods for blood type are consumed.	• Eat Right 4 Your Type (see p.184) • Body Code (see p.184) • Metabolic Typing (see p.185)
Quick weight loss	Programs based on severe calorie restriction, producing specific weight loss over very short time period.	• Cabbage Soup Diet (see p.186) • 5-Day Miracle Diet (see p.187) • Grapefruit Diet (see p.188) • Rotation Diet (see p.188) • 14-day Beauty Boot Camp (see p.189)
Low-calorie, liquid meal replacement	Weight loss based on very low-calorie meal replacements supplying 100 percent of recommended daily vitamins and minerals.	• Cambridge Diet (see p.189) • Herbalife (see p.190) • SlimFast (see p.190)
Detox	Detox programs aimed at eliminating toxins from the body, since a healthy liver burns fat more efficiently and therefore aids weight loss.	• Fat-Flush Plan (see p.191) • Juice Fasts (see p.192) • Living Beauty Detox (see p.192) • Detox Diet (see p.193)
Weight-loss centers	Weight-loss programs supported by regular weigh-ins, advice, and group support; these work on the basis that dieters find it easier to maintain a diet plan in which they are accountable to others.	• Weight Watchers (see p.194) • National Slimming Centers (see p.195) • Jenny Craig (see p.196) • LA Weight Loss (see p.196) • Nutrisystem (see p.197)

Diet directory

There is a huge variety of diet plans and weight loss programs—some sensible, some bizarre, and a few that are potentially dangerous. The most widely used are reviewed here.

Ornish Diet

High-carbohydrate, low-fat

- ⊗ **Are special products required?**
- ⊘ **Is eating out possible?**
- ⊗ **Is the plan family-friendly?**
- ⊘ **Do you have to buy a book?**
- ⊗ **Is the diet easy to maintain?**

Dr. Dean Ornish is a cardiologist who has demonstrated that the buildup of fatty plaques in the arteries, which causes heart attacks (*see p.215*), is preventable and reversible by following his program. In addition to the diet, the program covers smoking cessation, anger management, exercise, and meditation and relaxation exercises.

HOW IT CLAIMS TO WORK
This diet works on the principle that by virtually eliminating fat from your diet, you get fewer calories without eating less. It is a plant-based diet that excludes all cooking oils and animal products, except fat-free milk and fat-free yogurt. It also excludes plant foods that are high in fat, such as avocados, olives, nuts, and seeds. Less than 10 percent of calories from fat is allowed, which amounts to approximately ½–1oz (15–25g) of fat per day. The diet is high in fiber and allows moderate use of salt, sugar, and alcohol.

Although this diet does not restrict total calories consumed, when you eat less fat you tend to eat fewer calories. The diet allows you to eat plenty of food and to eat frequently.

THE REGIMEN
Three meals and one or two snacks per day are allowed, of mostly fat-free foods, such as legumes, fruits, grains, and vegetables. These foods can be eaten at any time, in fairly unrestricted quantities. Fat-free products and egg whites are allowed in moderation, as are certain commercially available fat-free products such as yogurt. The diet also advocates snacking throughout the day to maintain energy levels rather than eating three large meals at long intervals, and lists ideas for healthy snacks. It recommends eating high-fiber fruits, vegetables, grains, and legumes, which help lower levels of cholesterol (*see p.40*) and the hormone insulin and contribute to weight loss.

ORNISH DIET

Breakfast
- 4floz (120ml) orange juice
- 1½ cups cold cereal with fresh berries and fat-free yogurt

Lunch
- 1 cup tofu, ½ cup broccoli, ½ cup potato, ½ cup chickpeas, mixed together
- 4oz (110g) garlic bread
- 2 cups green salad
- 1 medium apple

Dinner
- 1 bruschetta with sun-dried tomatoes and capers
- 1 cup pasta mixed with red peppers, ½ cup greens, ½ cup white beans, a little chopped garlic, and lemon zest
- ½ cup grilled asparagus with lemon, freshly ground black pepper, and caper vinaigrette
- 1 cup green salad
- 2 peaches poached in red wine

Snacks
- 1–2 snacks of fresh fruit or raw vegetables

IS IT HEALTHY?
Research shows that the low-fat, low-cholesterol Ornish diet can reverse cardiovascular disease (*see pp.214–221*) by lowering cholesterol levels and reducing blood pressure (*see p.215*). However, some critics argue that the diet is too low in fat and does not provide sufficient amounts of essential fatty acids (*see p.40*). The diet excludes fish and oil, despite evidence that fish, fish oil, and olive oil provide a protective effect against cardiovascular disease.

Dr. Ornish's patients were treated in spalike environments where the meals were prepared by chefs. For people trying to follow the diet at home, the plan may be difficult to maintain.

Pritikin Program

High-carbohydrate, low-fat

- ⊗ **Are special products required?**
- ⊘ **Is eating out possible?**
- ⊘ **Is the plan family-friendly?**
- ⊘ **Do you have to buy a book?**
- ⊗ **Is the diet easy to maintain?**

This low-fat program was developed in the 1970s by Nathan Pritikin as a means of treating cardiovascular disease. The work is continued today by his son Robert.

HOW IT CLAIMS TO WORK
This is a low-fat, primarily vegetarian diet based on whole grains, fruits, and vegetables. The author argues that you can eat a much greater volume of low-fat foods and feel satisfied, without taking in too many calories. This diet requires no calorie counting or portion control. Foods are ranked according to their caloric density, and dieters are encouraged to create a healthy balance of low- and medium-ranked foods. The diet encourages the consumption of healthy fats that are high in omega-3 fatty acids (*see p.40*).

THE REGIMEN
Processed foods, eggs, and most types of fat are eliminated in favor of whole grains, fruits, and vegetables, and low-fat carbohydrates, such as brown rice and whole-wheat pasta. The diet is

PRITIKIN PROGRAM

Breakfast
- 1 cup cinnamon-flavored oatmeal cooked with 8floz (240ml) fat-free milk with 1 banana and 1 cup blueberries

Lunch
- 4oz (110g) grilled chicken breast with 1 ear steamed corn
- 2 cups green salad with 2 tbsp fat-free dressing

Dinner
- 1 cup fat-free vegetarian chili with ½ cup brown rice
- 2 cups tomato and cucumber salad with 2 tbsp balsamic-vinegar dressing
- ½ cup pineapple slices

Snacks
- 2oz (56g) baked tortilla chips with 4floz (120ml) tomato salsa

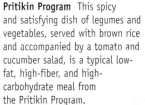

Pritikin Program This spicy and satisfying dish of legumes and vegetables, served with brown rice and accompanied by a tomato and cucumber salad, is a typical low-fat, high-fiber, and high-carbohydrate meal from the Pritikin Program.

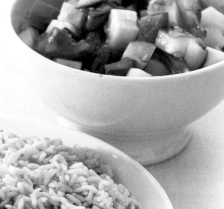

therefore high in fiber, low in cholesterol, and low in saturated and total fat. The program is based on three meals a day with snacks between meals. Less than 10 percent of total daily calories is allowed to come from fat. About 75 percent of calories should come from carbohydrates and about 15 percent of calories from protein.

IS IT HEALTHY?
Although very low-fat diets are often unsatisfying, leading some dieters to overeat or give up, the health benefits of eating less fat and more fruits, vegetables, and whole grains are well documented—especially their role in the prevention of many long-term diseases. No food groups are entirely eliminated in the Pritikin diet, and the sample menus provide a large variety of nutritional choices. The revised Pritikin diet encourages the limited use of fats that are high in omega-3 fatty acids. Overall, we feel that the Pritikin diet is safe and effective.

Hawaii Diet

High-carbohydrate, low-fat

- ⊗ Are special products required?
- ⊘ Is eating out possible?
- ⊘ Is the plan family-friendly?
- ⊘ Do you have to buy a book?
- ⊗ Is the diet easy to maintain?

This plan emphasizes the health of the whole person, including spiritual, mental, emotional, and physical aspects. This very low-fat diet is based on traditional Hawaiian foods, which the author claims can help control weight and levels of sugar and cholesterol in the blood.

HOW IT CLAIMS TO WORK
This diet teaches you to select foods based on nutrient density so you eat healthy food that makes you feel full. It includes fresh fruits, vegetables, and whole unprocessed grains, with an emphasis on plant-based foods high in complex carbohydrates (*see p.47*) and low in fat and cholesterol (*see pp.38–40*).

The selection of foods is based on the Shintani Mass Index (SMI), named after its author, Dr. Terry Shintani. The SMI value of any given food reflects its mass-to-energy ratio and represents the actual weight in pounds of that food that will provide one day's worth of calories. For example, corn has an SMI of 6.5, which means that it takes 6.5lb (3kg) of corn to provide one day's worth of calories. A cheeseburger, in contrast, has an SMI value of 2.1, meaning it takes 2.1lb (1kg) of cheeseburgers to provide one day's calories.

An apple is larger and weighs more than a doughnut, so the apple's mass-to-energy ratio will be greater than that of a doughnut because the apple is larger in mass, or bulk, though lower in calories. The higher the mass-to-energy ratio of a food, the fuller you become, because the bulk fills your stomach and signals your brain that your hunger is satisfied. At the same time you are eating fewer calories, fats, and refined carbohydrates. Foods that have a high mass-to-energy ratio are also higher in fiber and richer in beneficial nutrients such as vitamins, antioxidants, and phytochemicals.

HAWAII DIET

Breakfast
- 2 whole-grain waffles topped with 1 cup strawberries

Lunch
- 1½ cups bean stew with vegetable of your choice
- 1 cup green salad with fat-free dressing
- ½ cantaloupe

Dinner
- 1½ cups tofu and vegetable stir-fry
- 1 cup green salad with fat-free dressing
- 1 medium baked apple

Snacks
- Fresh fruit and sliced raw vegetables

THE REGIMEN

The Hawaii diet recommends that you eat three meals a day, with one or two snacks. It recommends six to 11 daily servings of whole, unrefined complex carbohydrates with most calories and protein coming from vegetable sources (three to five servings per day), and fruits (two to four servings per day). No more than 1oz (28g) of animal-based food is allowed per day. A pyramid chart helps you choose foods from each group. The diet allows very little saturated fat, but some sources of monounsaturated fat are permitted. Dairy products, refined fats, oils, sugars, and alcohol are optional in small amounts. Exercise and meditation are also recommended as part of the program to lose weight.

IS IT HEALTHY?

A major benefit of this diet is that it teaches you about the nutrient density of foods. Since it is very low in fat, the diet may help to lower blood cholesterol levels; however, it may be difficult to follow because menu-planning requires constant reference to the SMI, or memorizing the numbers. In addition, although the diet claims to be based on foods traditionally eaten in Hawaii, American fruits and vegetables are

included because they are easier to find, so it cannot really claim to be a purely Hawaiian diet. However, if you do manage to follow the diet and exercise and meditate on a daily basis, you will feel the benefits.

Low-fat Living

High carbohydrate, low-fat

- ⊗ **Are special products required?**
- ⊘ **Is eating out possible?**
- ⊘ **Is the plan family-friendly?**
- ⊘ **Do you have to buy a book?**
- ⊗ **Is the diet easy to maintain?**

This program is based on four small, low-fat meals and three low-fat, high-fiber snacks per day. The plan also advocates daily exercise.

HOW IT CLAIMS TO WORK

According to Dr. Robert Cooper, the author of this program, you start to burn fat the moment you get up in the morning. He recommends five minutes of easy physical activity every morning, followed by a low-fat breakfast rich in protein and carbohydrates. Dr. Cooper claims that eating low-fat, high-fiber snacks between meals increases your energy and metabolism and reduces the urge to overeat, especially at night. The book categorizes low-fat, high-fiber snacks, exercise, and drinking water as fat-burners, whereas high-fat, low-fiber meals or snacks and skipping meals are regarded as fat-makers.

Each meal provides fewer than 500 calories, with a maximum of 20–25 percent of those calories from fat. Snacks should be lower in calories than meals. All recommended meals need to be prepared according to recipes offered in the book. Artificially sweetened foods or beverages are not permitted, since they may stimulate an appetite for fats in some people and there is no evidence that they contribute to weight loss.

THE REGIMEN

The regimen consists of four meals and three snacks daily, which should be eaten at specific times. You should eat breakfast at 7a.m., snack 1 at 10a.m.,

lunch at noon, snack 2 at 3:15p.m., pre-dinner appetizer at 5:30p.m., dinner at 6–7p.m., and snack 3 at 8:45p.m.

Examples of foods on the Low-fat Living program include: whole-grain breads and crackers, pastas, fat-free dairy products, tomatoes, including pasta sauce, canned food packed in water, eggs (yolks and whites), fresh vegetables, herbs, spices and dry seasonings, and sweeteners, such as brown sugar, honey, maple syrup, molasses, and sugar.

Because this is a low-fat program, no fatty foods or all-fat dressings are permitted. Fat-free processed products should be consumed sparingly since they may trigger an unusually high insulin response if they are eaten in large quantities. In addition to the type of foods permitted on this program, the timing of meals and snacks is important. Also, low-intensity exercise, especially aerobics, is strongly recommended during the program.

IS IT HEALTHY?

Overall, this diet is very healthy since it is low in fat, high in fiber, and can help reduce your blood pressure and cholesterol levels, thus reducing your risk of diabetes (*see p.246–249*) and

LOW-FAT LIVING

Breakfast (7a.m.)
- 1 boiled egg with 2 slices whole-wheat bread
- 4floz (120ml) fat-free milk

Lunch (noon)
- 1½ cups (360 ml) gazpacho
- 2 low-fat whole-grain biscuits, chili-pepper-and-cheddar-cheese flavor

Dinner (5:30–7p.m.)
- 1½ cups green salad with creamy garlic dressing
- 3½oz (100g) broiled chicken cutlets with 2 cups linguine (no dressing)

Snacks (10a.m., 3:15p.m., 8:45p.m.)
- 3 low-fat, high-fiber snacks

cardiovascular disease (*see p.214–221*). You are likely to have more energy and feel good when you follow this diet, since it offers plenty of food, high-fiber snacks, and encourages daily physical activity. Since the diet is very low in fat, however, it may be difficult to follow, especially if you often eat away from home. Recipes for the suggested meals and snacks are helpful, but might require considerable preparation. You should be careful to stick to the portion sizes.

McDougall Program

High-carbohydrate, low-fat

- ⊗ **Are special products required?**
- ✓ **Is eating out possible?**
- ⊗ **Is the plan family-friendly?**
- ✓ **Do you have to buy a book?**
- ⊗ **Is the diet easy to maintain?**

This 12-day program is practiced in a live-in clinic in California, where patients experience significant weight loss, in addition to lowered levels of cholesterol and blood pressure.

HOW IT CLAIMS TO WORK
Dr. John A. McDougall, the author of the program, believes that the adoption of a vegetarian diet high in starches from fruits and vegetables aids permanent weight loss. The plan eliminates all meat, dairy products, eggs, and oils, although exceptions are made for rare occasions. The diet is low-fat, meaning that you can eat plenty without eating more calories. Daily exercise is a major element. The McDougall program does not restrict calories, instead allowing unlimited amounts of most fruits and vegetables, including frozen ones.

Dr. McDougall identifies what he terms a "rich" Western diet, high in fats and dairy products, and describes many disorders and diseases associated with such a diet. Patients on Dr. McDougall's program at the clinic experience, on average, a 2–11lb (0.9–5kg) weight loss during the 12 days, accompanied with lowered levels of blood cholesterol and reduced blood pressure.

MCDOUGALL PROGRAM

Breakfast
- 4floz (120ml) fresh fruit juice
- 1 cup hot seven-grain cereal

Lunch
- Whole-grain bread sandwich with vegetable filling
- 1 medium apple

Dinner
- 2 bean burritos, and green salad with low-sodium, fat-free Russian salad dressing
- 1 cup sunshine fruit dessert

Snacks
- Unlimited low-fat, high-carbohydrate snacks such as whole grains and rice cakes

THE REGIMEN
This program allows three meals and unlimited healthful snacks each day and encourages you to drink plenty of herbal teas and water. Animal foods, oils, refined foods, alcohol, and caffeine are eliminated but fat, sugar, and salt are permitted in limited quantities. In addition, whole-grain bread and/or additional vegetables may be added to any of the three daily meals. Within the first 12 days, no soybeans or soybean derivatives, nuts and nut butters, seeds, olives, or avocados are allowed, but these can be added later in the program.

The program incorporates medical, psychological, social, and practical preparation for the diet and exercise regime as a positive lifestyle change. Dr. McDougall's book provides a 12-day menu of meals, as well as recipes and tips on healthy eating out.

IS IT HEALTHY?
The benefits of eating more fruits and vegetables and reducing fat intake in reducing the risk of various diseases, bowel disturbances, and cancer, are proven and documented. However, while the results discussed by Dr. McDougall are encouraging, they are specific to the residential program at his clinic, located in California. The situation may have provided additional

benefits, such as social reinforcement and food preparation. In addition, the elimination of all animal products may be unwarranted given the proven health benefits of fish oils (*see p.90*) and low-fat dairy products (*see p.80*).

Atkins Diet

Carbohydrate-controlled

- ⊗ **Are special products required?**
- ✓ **Is eating out possible?**
- ⊗ **Is the plan family-friendly?**
- ✓ **Do you have to buy a book?**
- ⊗ **Is the diet easy to maintain?**

By severely limiting carbohydrate intake, this diet produces ketosis, a state in which the body uses up its stored carbohydrate and begins to burn fats for energy (*see p.168*).

HOW IT CLAIMS TO WORK
Dr. Atkins believed that weight gain is the result of fat synthesis from excess ketones (*see p.168*). He claimed that fat loss occurs when the body changes from using carbohydrates for fuel to using fats. This change requires a period on a low-carbohydrate diet.

The Atkins diet is organized into different stages. The first stage limits carbohydrates such as bread and pasta, fruits, and some vegetables and includes high-fat food to encourage your body to become ketotic and start using ketones for energy. Some carbohydrates can be reintroduced later, in the maintenance stages of the diet.

THE REGIMEN
The Atkins program begins with a 14-day induction phase to place your body into ketosis. During this period, your daily diet consists of 100g protein, which is the equivalent of eating about 14oz (400g) of meat, 75g fat, and less than 20g carbohydrates, totalling between 1,500 and 3,500 calories per day.

The induction phase is followed by an ongoing weight-loss phase, during which you continue to limit your intakes of carbohydrates to less than 30g per day—the amount of carbohydrate in 8floz (240ml) of soda or two slices of bread.

ATKINS DIET: INDUCTION PHASE

Breakfast
- 3-egg omelet with ham, cheese, bacon, and mushrooms

Lunch
- 1½ cups chef's salad of ham, chicken, cheese, and eggs, with creamy Italian dressing

Dinner
- 9oz (250g) broiled salmon and 2 cups steamed kale mixed with 1 tsp garlic, 1 tsp lemon juice, and 1 tsp sesame seeds

Snacks
- 1 cup berries with cream
- 1 or 2 cheese sticks

The program is then modified to pre-maintenance and maintenance phases, when your carbohydrate intake can be increased up to 4¼oz (120g) or eight servings per day. (For comparison, note that a typical "balanced" diet would include more than 10¾oz (300g) or 16 servings of carbohydrate per day.)

IS IT HEALTHY?

Reducing calorie intake by cutting carbohydrates is a good slimming principle, but not when taken to this extreme. You will lose weight, but the long-term health effects are not known.

Some 8–10lb (3.6–4.5kg) of weight loss during the first week or so on a low-carbohydrate diet such as this is due to water loss associated with using up stored glycogen. However, while such an immediate result provides a psychological boost to a dieter, once you start eating carbohydrates again, this weight will return.

Another criticism of the diet is that glycogen stores are needed for exercise, and exercise is a key to long-term weight maintenance. For example, scientific studies of athletes show that dietary carbohydrate is essential for optimum athletic performance.

Dr. Atkins claimed that you can eat as much as you want on his diet but, like any other diet, this works only to the extent that your caloric intake is less than your caloric expenditure. Ketosis does tend to reduce appetite but, more importantly, eliminating an entire food group is a significant dietary change that may be enough to help you begin to lose weight. For example, many combination foods are eliminated including pizza because of the crust, hamburgers and hot dogs because of the bun, and all sandwiches. These foods can be high-fat, and can come in large portion sizes. Many convenience and snack foods such as cookies, chips, and pasta are excluded, and these are replaced by structured meals and low-fat snacks, resulting in a lower total calorie intake than usual.

Jargon buster

Ketones These chemicals, also referred to as ketone bodies, are produced by your body when it does not get enough calories from carbohydrates and burns fats for energy instead.

Ketosis This is a state in which the body has used up its store of carbohydrates and is producing ketones from the breakdown of fat.

Ketogenic diet A diet that causes your body to produce ketones. This involves limiting your intake of carbohydrates. Examples include the Aktins Diet and Scarsdale Diet.

Some people find the metabolic changes that result from this diet uncomfortable. Carbohydrate cravings, for example, may or may not disappear with time. Some people develop blood-pressure problems, which can lead to dizziness on rising from a seated position, and some complain of bad breath. The lack of fiber in the Atkins diet may lead to constipation and an increase in the risk of certain illnesses, such as colon cancer, while the restricted intake of dairy products, fruits, and vegetables may lead to deficiencies in calcium, the B vitamins, vitamin C, and certain important minerals including iron.

In order to counteract these potential deficiencies, Dr. Atkins recommended the consumption of specific supplements available from his website. His claims that significant calories will be lost through excreting ketones in urine have been disproved. However, when ketones are excreted, they remove water and the minerals sodium and potassium from the body, which means that people on this program must drink plenty of water, diet soda, tea, or coffee (but not fruit juices) to avoid dehydration.

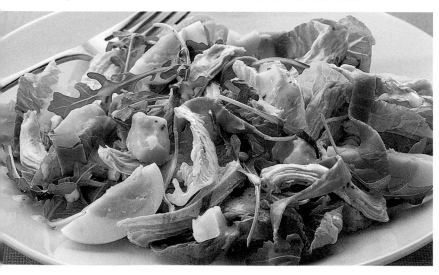

Atkins Diet High in protein and saturated fat from ham, chicken, cheese, and eggs, but low in carbohydrate and fiber, this salad is typical of meals from the induction phase of this weight-loss program.

Carbohydrate-Addict's Diet

Carbohydrate-controlled

⊗ **Are special products required?**
⊘ **Is eating out possible?**
⊘ **Is the plan family-friendly?**
⊘ **Do you have to buy a book?**
⊗ **Is the diet easy to maintain?**

This diet is based on the theory that many people have an exaggerated insulin response to carbohydrates, which creates an addiction to them.

HOW IT CLAIMS TO WORK

This diet is a modification of low-carbohydrate programs such as the Atkins diet (*see p.167*). Its authors claim that as many as 75 percent of the population are carbohydrate-sensitive. This creates an exaggerated insulin response to carbohydrate intake, leading to hunger and cravings after their consumption. Instead of limiting carbohydrates completely to create ketosis—as in the Atkins diet—this plan recommends limiting carbohydrate consumption to one hour each day, in order to balance insulin responses. The program recommends that two out of three meals each day be carbohydrate-free. These are called "complementary" meals. Unlike the other restricted carbohydrate diets, which can lead to carbohydrate craving, this diet allows one "reward" meal each day, during which any foods can be eaten, including carbohydrates, as long as they are part of a balanced meal and are consumed within a one-hour period.

THE REGIMEN

The diet is somewhat complicated because it is divided into an entry plan and four different diets. Everyone on the diet uses the entry plan, and, then once it is completed, you determine whether you will follow plan "A," "B," "C," or "D" according to how much weight you have lost and whether or not you wish to lose more. This is not as difficult as it sounds, since the different regimens are very similar. For example, plan "B"

is the same as plan "A," but you do not eat the snack.

There are also five guidelines for following the regimen:
● Eat two complementary meals daily
● Eat one reward meal daily
● Complete your reward meal within one hour
● Consume any alcoholic beverages with your reward meal
● Drink plenty of water, juice, or coffee throughout the day.

IS IT HEALTHY?

Many of us would probably lose weight if the only time we drank alcohol was with our evening meal and we cut out snacking between meals. If you are the type of person who feels tired an hour after having a piece of cake, or if you get hungry soon after having a carbohydrate-based meal, then this diet will teach you a lot about managing your appetite and avoiding cravings.

On the down side, it is difficult to confine all your carbohydrates to one hour-long period each day and it is not obvious that this provides any benefit over avoiding simple sugars altogether. The authors ran a weight-loss clinic for

CARBOHYDRATE ADDICT'S DIET

Breakfast
● 3-egg omelet with ¼ cup spinach and 1 tbsp sour cream

Lunch
● 1½ cups green beans cooked with 1 tbsp olive oil, ½ cup scallions, ½ cup basil, cloves, chilli powder, and 1 tbsp sour cream

Dinner (reward meal)
● 4oz (110g) chicken cooked with 1 tbsp olive oil, lemon juice and garlic, rosemary, salt, and pepper
● 1 cup broccoli florets
● 1 cup steamed rice
● 1½ cups cucumber salad dressed with salt, white wine vinegar, 1 tsp sour cream, sesame oil, scallions, and ginger

Snacks
● Only on some plans

years and presumably had good results with their regimen, but there is no data on its long-term health effects or its effectiveness in maintaining lost weight.

The plan is promoted as a lifelong solution to yo-yo dieting; however, there is no evidence as yet that being allowed to eat whatever you like for one hour each day will enable you to maintain the diet and lose weight.

Protein Power Lifeplan

Carbohydrate-controlled

⊗ **Are special products required?**
⊘ **Is eating out possible?**
⊗ **Is the plan family-friendly?**
⊘ **Do you have to buy a book?**
⊗ **Is the diet easy to maintain?**

This high-protein, low-carbohydrate diet program claims to help you lose weight, lower cholesterol and blood pressure levels, feel fitter, and restore your health in just a few weeks.

HOW IT CLAIMS TO WORK

The authors believe that eating more protein than is normally recommended will help balance the body's hormonal response to other foods. The plan is more detailed than the Atkins diet and somewhat more difficult to follow, since protein requirements must be calculated and daily protein intake divided between your meals and snacks. There are no food groups to avoid, so you have to make more decisions.

THE REGIMEN

Carbohydrates are restricted to between 30–55g per day, which is slightly more than allowed during the middle phases of the Atkins diet (*see p.167*). This is low enough to induce ketosis. However, this plan does not allow an unlimited intake of fat, and the authors do advise dieters to seek their doctor's advice before they begin the program. The plan focuses on high protein intake, including eggs, cottage cheese, tofu, lean meat, poultry, pork, and seafood. It recommends three meals a day with regular snacks

PROTEIN POWER LIFEPLAN

Breakfast
- 1 boiled egg with 1 slice toast with butter
- ½ cup strawberries or raspberries

Lunch
- ½ cup steamed squash
- Fresh spinach salad with vinaigrette or blue-cheese dressing
- ½ cup fresh blueberries
- ½ cup low-fat cottage cheese

Dinner
- 6oz (170g) steamed shrimps with 1 cup steamed broccoli, 1 cup sautéed red/yellow peppers, with low-fat vinaigrette
- 1 cup mixed fruit salad

Snacks
- Sliced raw vegetables including peppers, carrots, and tomatoes

in order to avoid hunger. Carbohydrates are permitted at every meal.

In addition to recommending lots of exercise, the plan also recommends taking vitamin and mineral supplements.

IS IT HEALTHY?

While this diet plan does a better job of explaining the low-carbohydrate approach than the Atkins Diet, it creates the same potential problem of calcium excretion

Jargon buster

Aerobic exercise Any repetitive exercise, such as jogging, in which the body uses oxygen to burn fat. It needs to be sustained for at least 15 minutes while you maintain 65–85 percent of your maximum heart rate to be effective.

Anaerobic exercise Any vigorous, short-burst exercise that causes your muscles to work without oxygen. Glycogen is burnt for energy. This type of excercise can cause fatigue, but if you exercise regularly your anaerobic fitness will improve.

due to excessive intake of protein. It also requires more work by the liver and the kidneys, which is not advisable for those with liver or kidney problems (*see pp.236–239*).

The authors of this plan claim that the body has no need for carbohydrate, but if that were true then muscle would store only fat and not glycogen. Glycogen is required for the generation of energy in muscles. If there is no carbohydrate in the diet, the authors claim energy will come from protein.

As yet, no studies have been carried out on the long-term effects of this diet, which may be high in saturated fat and low in many vitamins and in calcium. Recent research has demonstrated that people are more likely to lose weight when their intake of protein is higher than normal, but there is no reason to eliminate carbohydrates in order to do this. While it is true that insulin promotes fat storage, insulin production can be limited by eating complex carbohydrates (*see p.46–47*) and by eating balanced meals and snacks.

Sugar Busters

Carbohydrate-controlled

- ⊗ **Are special products required?**
- ⊘ **Is eating out possible?**
- ⊗ **Is the plan family-friendly?**
- ⊘ **Do you have to buy a book?**
- ⊗ **Is the diet easy to maintain?**

The authors of this plan believe that North Americans eat too much sugar and refined carbohydrates and this has contributed to the current high prevalence of obesity and diabetes.

HOW IT CLAIMS TO WORK

The authors of this diet recommend that by balancing the proportion of carbohydrate to protein that you eat, you will lose weight because this will increase glucagon production. Glucagon is a hormone that stimulates the release of glucose into the bloodstream.

They suggest that to achieve this, 45 percent of calories should come from high-fiber carbohydrate sources, 30–35 percent of calories from fat, and 20–25

percent from protein. This is based on the idea that eating foods high in sugar causes an overproduction of insulin and a suppression of glucagon, which then promotes fat storage in the body and inhibits weight loss.

In addition, the authors emphasize that exercise is important because it lowers insulin levels and increases insulin sensitivity.

THE REGIMEN

The authors recommend eating more unrefined foods, high-fiber vegetables, stone-ground whole grains, lean meats, fruits, and, if you choose, alcohol in moderation. Excluded vegetables (those containing less than 2.5g of fiber) include potatoes, beets, and carrots. The diet also recommends eliminating the refined sugar found in cakes, cookies, candy, and sodas, as well as high-glycemic index foods (*see p.47*) such as white flour, pasta, and potatoes.

You are allowed three meals a day, in moderate-sized portions, and the authors suggest that you limit the volume of fluids that you drink with each meal. However, they recommend that you drink at least 6–8 glasses of water a day, in addition to coffee, tea, and diet soda. Sugar Busters also permits you to snack on all types of fruits.

SUGAR BUSTERS

Breakfast
- 4floz (120ml) orange juice
- 1 package instant oatmeal made with 4floz (120ml) fat-free milk

Lunch
- 4oz (110g) turkey breast on whole-grain bread, with mustard, lettuce, and tomato

Dinner
- 6oz (170g) grilled or baked pork tenderloin with sliced onions and ½ cup brown rice, cooked in fat-free, low-sodium chicken broth
- 1 cup steamed green beans

Snacks
- 1 medium apple
- 12 nuts

IS IT HEALTHY?

While this theory has some scientific rationale, there is no evidence that the proportion of carbohydrate to protein to fat does what the authors claim. However, the focus on high-fiber carbohydrates is healthful, and there are significant potential benefits from reducing our intake of simple carbohydrates such as sugar. While there is no direct evidence that diabetes results from sugar intake, diabetes risk is related to obesity. In turn, obesity is related to calorie intake—and excess calories are often consumed in the form of simple carbohydrates, such as soft drinks, juices, candies, bakery goods, and other snacks. All of us can benefit from reducing the amount of sweet foods we eat, and a period of time following this diet might change a few of your dietary habits.

Some of the ideas presented in this plan—such as the idea that digestive juices are diluted by drinking fluids with your meals—have no scientific evidence to support them. Also, there is certainly no health risk from reducing your intake of simple carbohydrates, but most North Americans are not likely to give up their sodas and desserts completely.

More seriously, the plan's emphasis on monitoring precise proportions of carbohydrate, fat, and protein is the kind of inappropriate focus that can result in the development of eating disorders.

Zone Diet

Carbohydrate-controlled

- ✖ **Are special products required?**
- ✔ **Is eating out possible?**
- ✔ **Is the plan family-friendly?**
- ✔ **Do you have to buy a book?**
- ✖ **Is the diet easy to maintain?**

The aim of this carbohydrate-controlled diet is to make the body work within its peak performance zone for maximum energy, "fat-burning," and weight loss.

HOW IT CLAIMS TO WORK

According to the Zone Diet plan, what is important is not what you eat, but the balance between what you eat and the hormonal response it creates. In

particular, the author looks at food's impact on the body's ability to influence eiconsanoids—chemical messengers derived from dietary fats that control various metabolic processes.

The author states that people can be divided into those who produce enough insulin and those who produce too much of the hormone. He prescribes a very simple test to find out which group you fall into: have pasta for lunch at noon and see how you feel at 3p.m. If you can barely keep your eyes open, and you hungry, you are among the 75 percent who have a genetic predisposition to over-produce insulin. This diet plan is designed to limit this, and any subsequent overeating.

THE REGIMEN

Meal plans are tailored to gender, activity level, and current percentage of body fat, but all include 40 percent of calories from carbohydrate, 30 percent from protein, and 30 percent from fat. All meals and snacks follow this ratio. The North American diet generally gets as much as 50–60 percent of its energy from carbohydrates and about 35 percent from fat. The author believes that a high intake of dietary carbohydrate leads to hyperinsulinism and obesity, while a high intake of dietary protein leads to high glucagon and ketosis.

The diet calls for the consumption of a specific number of small portions of carbohydrate, fat, and protein at regular intervals throughout the day (roughly four and a half hours apart). For most people this means eating three meals a day, and two substantial snacks. The snacks should follow the same ratio of carbohydrate: protein: fat (40:30:30) as your main meals.

The plan suggests that you divide your plate into three sectors; on one third you put low-fat protein, no bigger and no thicker than the palm of your hand. The remaining two thirds of the plate should be filled to overflowing with fruits and vegetables.

IS IT HEALTHY?

There is no scientific evidence that this plan, which is based on a combination of combating insulin resistance and altering eiconsonoid levels, will produce

ZONE DIET

Breakfast
- 1 flour quesadilla filled with 2oz (56g) shredded, low-fat Monterey Jack cheese, 2oz (56g) chopped extra-lean Canadian bacon, chopped scallions, green pepper, and tomato, served with 2 tbsp guacamole
- 1 cup grapes

Lunch
- 1 slice whole-grain bread with 1oz (28g) low-fat cheese and 2oz (56g) extra-lean Canadian bacon, with lettuce, tomato slice, and dill pickle wedge
- 4floz (120ml) low-fat yogurt with ⅓ cup chopped peaches

Dinner
- 4oz (110g) pork medallions and 1 sliced apple, sautéed in 2 tsp white wine, 1 tsp Dijon mustard, and chopped rosemary, with 1¼ cups steamed broccoli
- Large green salad with 4 tsp olive oil and vinegar dressing

Snacks
- Small cooked chicken breast, 1 slice of melon, and 6 small nuts
- 1oz (28g) low-fat cheese and 1 small orange

the health effects claimed. It is more likely that your response to dietary carbohydrates is influenced by your usual diet and activity levels than by some genetic predisposition. While it is true that refined or high glycemic-index foods (see p.47) may overstimulate insulin secretion, this can be avoided by consuming low glycemic-index carbohydrates.

This is a complicated regimen that few can follow accurately. The diet may be high in saturated fat, depending on the types of proteins selected. There are also potential problems linked to high protein intake, such as bone loss.

The author sells specific "zone" food products such as snack bars that claim to retard aging. However, there is no evidence to support such claims.

Life Without Bread

Carbohydrate-controlled

⊗ **Are special products required?**
⊘ **Is eating out possible?**
⊘ **Is the plan family-friendly?**
⊘ **Do you have to buy a book?**
⊗ **Is the diet easy to maintain?**

This diet is based on the clinical experience of Dr. Lutz, an Austrian physician who claims to have helped thousands of patients to lose weight and achieve health by following low-carbohydrate diets.

HOW IT CLAIMS TO WORK

Life Without Bread is based on eating a low-carbohydrate, high-fat, high-protein diet. The authors claim that this was what humans ate during evolution, and it is what we are suited to. Today's typical high-carbohydrate, low-fat diet, they claim, is alien to our species.

The authors also describe the benefits of low-carbohydrate diets in relation to disorders such as cardiovascular disease, diabetes, gastrointestinal disorders,

LIFE WITHOUT BREAD

Breakfast
- 2 scrambled eggs with 1 slice whole-wheat bread (no spread)
- 4floz (120ml) orange juice

Lunch
- 6oz (170g) grilled chicken breast with ⅔ cup fresh green peas
- Large green salad with olive oil and vinegar dressing

Dinner
- 8oz (225g) grilled tuna steak with 1 cup string beans and 4 tbsp steamed brown rice

Snacks
- 8floz (240ml) plain, whole-milk yogurt
- 2oz (56g) cheese
- 1 medium apple

obesity and cancer. In a section on cardiovascular disease, they claim that saturated fats and cholesterol from animal foods do not contribute to cardiovascular disease, and argue that current nutritional advice on this topic is flawed.

THE REGIMEN

This diet restricts carbohydrates, of which no more than 72g (or 6 bread units, each containing 12g carbohydrates) per day should be consumed, hence the name of the diet. Examples of what one bread unit consists of include:
- ½ cup dry pasta
- 1 slice of bread
- Half grapefruit
- 8floz (240ml) milk or yogurt
- 8floz (240ml) of beer.

Foods restricted in the diet include most carbohydrate-containing foods (breads, pastries, bagels, cereals, grains, pasta, potatoes), sweet fruits, sweetened foods of any kind (yogurt, drinks, desserts, candy), and dried fruit.

You can eat all the protein, nonstarchy vegetables, cheese, and healthy fats you want from a variety of plant and animal sources, with moderate amounts of nuts, yogurt, and whole milk. Protein foods, such as meat, poultry, and fish can be fried, baked, roasted, broiled, grilled, or steamed.

The diet does not provide any specific menu plans, but it does explain how to work the low-carbohydrate eating plan into meals and snacks. A table listing grams of carbohydrate for a variety of items allows the reader to plan full menus containing a wide variety of foods.

IS IT HEALTHY?

The Life Without Bread program is a moderately low-carbohydrate, rather than an extremely low-carbohydrate diet. By limiting carbohydrates to less than 72g per day, you can follow this program without severe restrictions on healthy foods such as fruits and dairy products, both of which are permitted in limited amounts.

Although this book is entitled *Life Without Bread*, meal planning is based on "bread units," each of which contain 12g of carbohydrate. So this diet is not really about eliminating carbohydrates or bread, but limiting intake and finding

alternatives to form the basis of your meals. The diet promotes a healthy weight loss because you are reducing calories but still consuming a variety of carbohydrates.

Compared to some other plans, the book is complicated and technical, which may be difficult for the average reader to follow every day.

The authors of Life Without Bread claim that low-carbohydrate diets can help or cure diabetes, gastrointestinal disorders, cardiovascular disease, and even cancer. They do not accept that saturated fat contributes to increasing blood cholesterol or LDL levels (*see p.38–40*). On the contrary, they urge the consumption of high saturated-fat foods, such as cheese, sour cream, cream cheese, and whole milk. However, there is a huge amount of evidence that limiting saturated fat is important for the prevention of these chronic diseases, and this is a major flaw in this diet.

Scarsdale Diet

Carbohydrate-controlled

⊗ **Are special products required?**
⊘ **Is eating out possible?**
⊗ **Is the plan family-friendly?**
⊘ **Do you have to buy a book?**
⊗ **Is the diet easy to maintain?**

Similar to other high-protein, low-carbohydrate diets, this plan claims to produce weight loss by forcing the body into ketosis (*see p.168*).

HOW IT CLAIMS TO WORK

This very high-protein, low-carbohydrate, short-term, calorie-restricted diet claims to alter your metabolism and produce a 1lb (0.45kg) a day weight loss, with up to 20lb (9kg) or more in two weeks.

Because the Scarsdale Diet is very low in fat and carbohydrates, it is claimed that the body will be forced into ketosis and begin to burn stores of fat rather than carbohydrates for energy. The metabolism of fat produces ketone bodies, and the greater the amount of ketone bodies produced by the body, the more body fat is broken down, and the more weight is lost.

THE REGIMEN

The Scarsdale Diet allows 1,000 calories or fewer per day, and averages 43 percent protein, 22.5 percent fat, and 34.5 percent carbohydrates. The calories are distributed between three meals, spaced throughout the day. The only between-meal snacks permitted are carrots and celery. Oil, mayonnaise, and other salad dressings are not permitted; salads should be prepared only with vinegar and lemon. Vegetables should be eaten without butter or oil; lemon or vinegar may be used instead. Skin should be removed from chicken and turkey before eating and all meats should be lean. Alcoholic beverages are not allowed, but you are encouraged to drink plenty of water. Decaffeinated coffee, tea, diet soda, and club soda are permitted when on the diet.

Because the diet is so low in calories, it is limited to 14 days at a time. It may last five, nine, or 14 days, depending on how much weight you want to lose. After two weeks, you have to switch to the "Keep Trim Program," which offers an expanded list of foods and drinks. It includes one alcoholic drink daily, all lean meats including chicken and turkey, fish, eggs, cheeses, soups, vegetables, fruits, nuts, bread, condiments, and herbs, seasoning, and spices. Bread is

SCARSDALE DIET

Breakfast
- ½ grapefruit
- 1 slice toasted bread (no spread)

Lunch
- Assortment of lean meats (2oz/55g chicken, 2oz/55g turkey, 1oz/28g tongue, 2oz/55g lean beef) with 1 cup sliced, broiled, or stewed tomatoes

Dinner
- 6oz (170g) fish or shellfish salad
- 1 slice toasted bread (no spread)
- ½ grapefruit

Snacks
- Carrots or celery

still limited to two slices per day. Sugar, pasta, potatoes, candies or desserts, cream, whole milk, dairy products made with whole milk, and fatty meats are not permitted.

IS IT HEALTHY?

An older version of the Atkins diet (*see p.167*), this diet is dangerously low in carbohydrates and is lacking in many key vitamins and minerals found in

Scarsdale Diet This platter of lean meat and tomatoes is typical of the high-protein meals allowed during the initial phase of the diet.

carbohydrates and dairy products. If followed, it will promote weight loss, but it is a very difficult diet to maintain, as it is highly restrictive, and has very limited snacks. If you follow this diet, you are likely to be hungry between meals and need to eat a more substantial snack to satisfy your cravings. In addition, because of the Scarsdale Diet's high-protein content, it is not appropriate for people with kidney disease and may pose serious health risks if followed for more than the recommended 14 days.

Schwarzbein Principle

Carbohydrate-controlled

- ⊗ **Are special products required?**
- ⊘ **Is eating out possible?**
- ⊗ **Is the plan family-friendly?**
- ⊘ **Do you have to buy a book?**
- ⊗ **Is the diet easy to maintain?**

Created by Dr. Diana Schwarzbein, this low-carbohydrate diet claims to improve metabolism and health. Fat and protein intake are unrestricted, and starchy carbohydrates are restricted.

HOW IT CLAIMS TO WORK

The Schwarzbein Principle suggests lifestyle reform, including an end to yo-yo dieting. It also claims that a diet rich in natural fats and proteins, complemented by nonstarchy vegetables, delays the natural aging process. This is based on the belief that exposure to chemical, environmental, and physiological factors both damages body cells and results in poor metabolic function. It is impossible to escape aging, but it is possible to avoid many factors that accelerate chemical, environmental, and physiological attacks on body cells and tissues.

Alcohol, artificial sweeteners such as aspartame, caffeine, drugs and other stimulants, tobacco, stress, and a sedentary lifestyle worsen the aging process by disrupting the chemical balance that governs metabolism. For example, diets high in processed or refined carbohydrates, such as white bread, are digested rapidly, leading to a rapid increase in insulin. Although insulin is an important hormone for normal metabolic function, too much insulin contributes to a variety of health problems, including insulin resistance (*see p.47*) and type 2 diabetes (*see p.246-249*). Low-fat, high-carbohydrate diets result in chronically elevated insulin levels, which promotes cellular aging.

Fat and cholesterol, on the other hand, are essential for brain and nerve cell function, cell membrane integrity, effective immunity, and balanced levels of hormones. Not eating enough fat and cholesterol results in many conditions, including brittle nails, limp hair, infertility, constipation, mood instability, and a reduction of lean body mass.

THE REGIMEN

The Schwarzbein Principle encourages habit-purging and lifestyle reform. In addition to recommending the elimination of artificial sweeteners, hydrogenated oils, tobacco, alcohol, soda, caffeine, and low-fat and refined foods, the plan advocates stress management, exercise, hormone replacement therapy (if necessary), and the consumption of

---

SCHWARZBEIN PRINCIPLE

Breakfast
- ⅔ cup oatmeal cooked with butter and cream
- 2 scrambled eggs with 1 nitrate-free sausage and 1 sliced tomato

Lunch
- Whole-grain roll with 2oz (56g) turkey and 1 tsp mayonnaise
- 2 cups lettuce and tomato salad with olive-oil and vinegar dressing

Dinner
- 6oz (170g) broiled pork chops, ½ cup steamed lima beans, and nonstarchy vegetables with butter
- ½ cup fresh strawberries with unsweetened whipping cream

Snacks
- ½ cup sunflower seeds
- ⅓ cup hummus with carrot, bell pepper, and celery sticks

---

good oils and fats. The plan advises:
- Eat three balanced meals a day, spaced regularly throughout the day, with snacks, if necessary.
- Eat protein and fat from natural sources at every meal.
- Obtain carbohydrates from nonstarchy vegetables, such as arugula, asparagus, greens, bell peppers, green beans, broccoli, cauliflower, radishes, onions, celery, cucumber, and eggplant.
- Avoid starchy carbohydrates, such as sweet potatoes, potatoes, beets, squash, corn, and turnips.
- Restrict consumption of legumes.
- Avoid consuming bottled dressings or condiments, margarine, canned, dried, or deep-fried foods, half-and-half, cold cereal, bagels, spaghetti, noodles, breads, muffins, pizza, jams, jellies, syrups, reduced-fat dairy products, and desserts.

IS IT HEALTHY?

The Schwarzbein Principle targets refined carbohydrates as the source of the high insulin levels that underlie many health problems. These simple carbohydrates are digested quickly, contributing to a rapid increase in insulin and blood-glucose levels following a carbohydrate-rich meal.

Complex carbohydrates, such as whole grains and fiber, are digested more slowly than simple carbohydrates, resulting in a slower rise in insulin and lower blood-glucose levels following ingestion. It is important to include carbohydrates in a balanced diet, because they are essential for the normal function of body cells, along with proteins and fats.

Schwarzbein correctly advocates the inclusion of fats and proteins in the diet, and recommends monounsaturated fats (*see pp.38-43*), rather than saturated fats, which lead to elevated cholesterol and triglyceride levels in the blood, increasing your risk of cardiovascular disease (*see pp.216-221*). It would also be better if proteins were obtained from lean sources of meat.

Finally, this plan advocates exercise and stress management, which are appropriate complements to a nutritious diet and are fundamental to every health-promoting regimen.

South Beach Diet

Carbohydrate-controlled

- ⊗ **Are special products required?**
- ✓ **Is eating out possible?**
- ✓ **Is the plan family-friendly?**
- ✓ **Do you have to buy a book?**
- ✓ **Is the diet easy to maintain?**

This program is another modification of the low-carbohydrate diets and was developed by a prominent Miami cardiologist as a means of improving the health of his patients.

HOW IT CLAIMS TO WORK

The author of this diet believes that other low-carbohydrate diets, such as Atkins (*see p.167*), neglect the healthy aspects of carbohydrates by limiting intake of this food group. He also claims that other low-carbohydrate diets encourage the intake of saturated fats and proteins, which can lead to high triglycerides and cholesterol (*see pp.39-41*). This diet, in contrast, limits "bad" carbohydrates, such as white bread, processed wheat, baked goods, white rice, and potatoes, while maintaining the consumption of "good" carbohydrates, such as whole-wheat pasta and brown rice.

For the first phase of the diet, which lasts for two weeks, carbohydrates are completely eliminated, including fruits and alcohol. The author claims that this alters the way the body processes carbohydrates and reverses or prevents insulin resistance, the precursor to diabetes (*see pp.246-251*).

On completion of the first phase, carbohydrates are gradually reintroduced, along with fruit and wine. The staple of this diet becomes lean meats, vegetables, low-fat dairy products, and eggs. The diet is claimed to be easy to maintain since it allows dieters to eat until their hunger is satiated. It also encourages both midday snacking and an evening dessert in addition to a filling breakfast.

The theory of the South Beach Diet is that the structured meals and snacks prescribed in the book will maintain satiety and prevent you from snacking on bad carbohydrates, such as potato chips and baked goods.

SOUTH BEACH DIET: PHASE I

Breakfast
- 6floz (180ml) vegetable juice
- Western egg-white omelet, cooked with 2 tbsp chopped red and green bell pepper, 1 tbsp chopped scallion, 4floz (120ml) liquid egg substitute, and 3 tbsp shredded reduced-fat cheese

Lunch
- Chef's salad with 1oz (28g) ham, 1oz (28g) turkey, ½ cup low-fat cottage cheese, and 2 tbsp balsamic vinaigrette
- 1 cup sugar-free jello

Dinner
- 8oz (225g) grilled salmon, with 1 cup steamed asparagus and ½ cup mashed potatoes
- Green salad with olive oil and vinegar dressing
- 4floz (120ml) part-skim ricotta cheese, flavored with vanilla extract and sugar substitute

Snacks
- 2 sticks fat-free mozzarella
- 1 cup celery with 1in- (2.5cm-) cube light cheese

THE REGIMEN

The diet is divided into three phases. In each one you can eat three meals and a mid-morning and afternoon snack. The lists of permitted foods change in each phase. Phase I, which lasts for two weeks, excludes all carbohydrates, including fruits, candy, and alcohol.

In Phase II, the diet becomes more liberal, with the reintroduction of fruits and one forbidden food. For example, if you love chocolate, you can add chocolate to your second two weeks of the diet. Phase III of the diet serves as a maintenance phase, when more portions of forbidden foods are added, in moderation, to the diet.

Most of the weight loss occurs during the first two phases of this program, and the author claims that the diet is very flexible. If you go on vacation and gain weight, for example, you would simply revert to the initial phase for another

two weeks when you return home. Recipes are provided for each phase of the diet, including several from restaurants in the Miami area.

IS IT HEALTHY?

Certain aspects of this diet are extremely logical and probably helpful for dieters. For example, eating until you are full will help you maintain the diet for the necessary period of time. This diet is also positively healthy, because it encourages the abundant consumption of vegetables and, unlike the Atkins diet (*see p.167*), it does not allow unlimited intake of fats and proteins. Dieters are encouraged to use monounsaturated oils, such as canola and olive oil, when cooking and to stick to moderate portions of lean meats, such as fish and poultry. This is advice that should help dieters improve their cholesterol and lipid profiles as well as lose weight.

However, it is difficult to completely give up carbohydrates, even for two weeks, and those who are not used to following recipes and preparing foods every day may find it difficult to follow this diet. The absence of fruit in the first phase is also questionable.

The book is practical and dedicates a chapter to eating out and makes many suggestions of foods that could be ordered at a restaurant. The book describes glycemic index—how the carbohydrates affect blood-glucose levels (*see p.47*). For example, a baked potato is worse than mashed or boiled potato, since the body will process the former much more quickly. The author suggests that if you must eat a baked potato, heap some cheese on top, which will make it healthier by slowing the body's absorption of carbohydrate.

This diet claims to be scientifically proven, but no real data is presented, apart from the results witnessed by the author. The idea that snacking will be prevented simply by maintaining satiety is also unproven. Finally, although the author addresses the use of medication in weight control, he neglects to cover the benefits of exercise, implying that the South Beach Diet itself is enough to maintain health. This is a serious omission, since exercise is an essential component of weight control.

Picture Perfect Weight Loss

Controlling portion sizes

- ⊗ Are special products required?
- ⊘ Is eating out possible?
- ⊘ Is the plan family-friendly?
- ⊘ Do you have to buy a book?
- ⊗ Is the diet easy to maintain?

This program, which was devised by Dr. Shapiro, gets its name from the pictorial comparisons of foods that it employs to show the calculated calorie content of different food choices.

HOW IT CLAIMS TO WORK

Drawing on his years in clinical practice counseling those who wish to lose weight and keep it off, Dr. Shapiro has developed a program that he calls "Food Awareness Training," which teaches his clients how to make mindful choices about food. His principle is that people must change their relationship with food and learn to select low-calorie foods that may be eaten in filling, satisfying portions, rather than choosing high-calorie alternatives that result in weight gain.

Successful weight loss following this plan comes from applying Dr. Shapiro's principles to adhere to a reduced-calorie diet and also by increasing your levels of physical activity.

THE REGIMEN

Dr. Shapiro has developed a flexible, nonrestrictive program in which no food is taboo, and no prescription is offered for when to eat or for "correct" portions. When beginning this program, you are asked to keep a food diary faithfully for at least a week, detailing when and what foods you ate along with the degree of hunger and the situation in which eating occurred. Keeping the diary serves as an awareness tool to increase forethought and responsibility for food choices and to highlight pitfalls in your eating habits. Once conscious of your current eating habits, you will make healthier choices and modify your eating behavior. To assist you in making better choices, Dr. Shapiro provides pictures that graphically demonstrate the number of calories in various portions of foods. Dr. Shapiro also includes a list of foods that you should stock to eat any time, a supermarket shopping guide, an exercise guide, and a selection of menus from restaurants and nationwide chains, with options highlighted.

IS IT HEALTHY?

The strength of Dr. Shapiro's plan is its emphasis on a healthy, reduced-calorie diet and regular exercise. He offers good advice on how to rethink your relationship with food, and diets in particular. The food diary is an important tool for success, especially if you have someone you can share it with in order to establish support and accountability.

If you use it correctly, this program will accomplish calorie reduction without feelings of deprivation. Calorie counting is not necessary, but some people may find it difficult to visualize the calorie and portion comparisons. In this respect, the lone dieter may have a more difficult time than those dieters who are able to visit Dr. Shapiro's clinic on a weekly basis in order to meet with his nutritional counselors and dietitians.

PICTURE PERFECT WEIGHT LOSS

Breakfast
- 1 cup chopped banana and melon
- 3 slices smoked salmon
- 1 pumpernickel roll

Lunch
- 2 cups tossed salad with shrimp and light dressing
- 1 sourdough roll

Dinner
- 4floz (240ml) Manhattan clam chowder
- 1 cup pasta primavera
- 1 cup mixed berries and raspberry sorbet

Snacks
- 8floz (240ml) low-fat yogurt
- 1 piece of fruit
- 2 rice cakes
- 3 tbsp almonds

Volumetrics Weight-control

Controlling portion sizes

- ⊗ **Are special products required?**
- ⊘ **Is eating out possible?**
- ⊘ **Is the plan family-friendly?**
- ⊘ **Do you have to buy a book?**
- ⊘ **Is the diet easy to maintain?**

The concept of satiety, or feeling of fullness after a meal, forms the basis of this weight-loss and maintenance program. The authors believe that the fuller you feel at the end of a meal, the less you are likely to eat between meals or at the next meal.

HOW IT CLAIMS TO WORK

The aim of this program is to create satiety by choosing low-calorie foods in quantities that make you feel full, rather than eating the same volume of high-calorie foods. Successful weight loss on the plan occurs by reducing caloric intake through food choices that satisfy your appetite and meet daily nutritional requirements, as well as by increasing how much exercise you do. They claim that dieters can expect to lose 1–2lb (0.45–0.9kg) per week. Subsequent weight maintenance is achieved by making the same food choices, but matching calorie consumption with calorie expenditure.

THE REGIMEN

During the weight-loss phase, which should not exceed six months at a time, the authors suggest reducing caloric intake by 500–1,000 calories per day. Three meals each day plus snacks are recommended, and the proportions should follow those of the United States Department of Agriculture's Food Guide Pyramid (*see p.72*), which suggests that 20–30 percent of total calories should come from fat; 55 percent from carbohydrates, in the form of whole grains, vegetables, and fruits, (aiming for 20–30g of fiber daily); and 15 percent of total calories from proteins, including low-fat fish, poultry without the skin, and lean meats. Moderate

VOLUMETRICS WEIGHT-CONTROL

Breakfast
- 1 cup citrus fruit salad
- 1 English muffin with 2 tsp low-calorie margarine and 4 tsp low-sugar jam
- 8floz (240ml) low-fat milk

Lunch
- Bean and cheese burrito with 8 baked tortilla chips and 4floz (120ml) salsa
- 2 peaches

Dinner
- 3oz (85g) steak and ½ cup vegetable kabobs with asparagus
- 2 cups romaine salad with low-calorie dressing
- ½ cup watermelon with 4floz (120ml) cup fat-free frozen yogurt

Snacks
- 20 mini pretzels

amounts of sugar and alcohol are allowed, as are tea and coffee. Water (72floz/2.2 liters a day for women and 96floz/2.9 liters a day for men) may come from food or drinks. No foods are eliminated from Volumetric Weight-control, but foods with a high-energy density should be limited.

IS IT HEALTHY?

The Volumetrics Weight-control Plan is based on sound, sensible principles for weight loss and maintenance and is backed by short-term studies that confirm its potential for success. Long-term studies are underway. The book provides a clear explanation of the diet's underlying principles as well as comprehensive guides for choosing low-calorie, low-energy dense foods. Sample menu plans and recipes are also included. Followed correctly, weight loss is safely accomplished by making wise food choices, reducing calories while meeting nutritional needs, and increasing physical activity. Because no food is eliminated, the feeling of deprivation is avoided, which makes this program sustainable.

This is a safe and effective weight-control program for everyone from the moderately overweight to the obese. If you follow it, try to keep your calorie intake to at least 1,000 calories per day and eat a variety of foods.

90/10 Weight-loss Plan

Controlling portion sizes

⊗ **Are special products required?**
⊗ **Is eating out possible?**
⊘ **Is the plan family-friendly?**
⊘ **Do you have to buy a book?**
⊗ **Is the diet easy to maintain?**

This is a low-calorie plan, high in fiber, phytochemicals, and antioxidants and low in saturated fat. The title refers to the concept of eating healthily 90 percent of the time, while for the other 10 percent you can enjoy "fun foods."

HOW IT CLAIMS TO WORK
On this 14-day plan, which may be repeated until you achieve your goal weight, you lose weight by limiting your calorie intake to between 1,200 and 1,600 calories daily, depending on your current weight and activity level. Ninety percent of each day's calories should come from the menus provided, and the remaining 10 percent from a list of "fun foods." The program relies on portion control and, by allowing foods we often crave, encourages you to eat those foods in moderate amounts. Physical activity is emphasized as an important component in both losing weight and keeping it off.

The author, Joy Bauer, claims that you may lose up to 10lb (4.5kg) in the first two weeks but admits that much of that is usually water loss; in subsequent weeks, ½–2lb (0.2–0.9kg) is average. The author discourages quicker weight loss, which is unsafe and runs the risk of losing lean muscle mass.

THE REGIMEN
In the 90/10 Weight-loss Plan, you follow a daily menu, which includes breakfast, lunch, dinner, and snacks.

Each day, you choose one item from the list of fun foods or snacks that may be eaten at any time during the day. Calorie counting is not necessary if you follow the menus, but the calorie range for each meal is given in case you are not able to follow the menu provided. The plan offers menus for 14 days, while additional main course menus are available to lend diversity to the program. Multivitamin and calcium supplements are suggested, and the plan encourages drinking plenty of water, coffee, tea, and seltzer.

Before you begin the diet, the author suggests taking a "before" photograph, writing down your clothing size and body measurements, and, if possible, having your body fat measured. She then recommends repeating this two weeks later, so that you can track your progress in other ways besides weight.

IS IT HEALTHY?
The 90/10 Weight-loss Plan is based on the interesting concept of eating healthy for 90 percent of the time, while being allowed to "cheat" for the remaining 10 percent. The menus are designed to be low in saturated fat and high in fiber, phytochemicals, and antioxidants.

Even if you substitute some of the other dinner plans provided, this program may become monotonous, since you are asked to repeat the menu repertoire every two weeks for as long as it takes to achieve your target weight loss. The

---

90/10 WEIGHT-LOSS PLAN

Breakfast
● 1 whole-grain waffle with ½ cup berries

Lunch
● 8floz (240ml) cottage cheese with ½ cup fresh fruit salad

Dinner
● 4oz (115g) spinach lasagna
● 1 cup green salad with olive oil and vinegar dressing

Snacks
● Granola bar or cereal bar
● ½ cup potato chips (fun food)

1,200-calories-per-day program included in the book is very restrictive, and few will be able to follow it successfully for extended periods of time. The book includes tips for subsequent weight maintenance, but it could be more instructive in teaching you how to determine sensible portion sizes and how to make healthy meal choices, especially when you are dining out.

Change One Eating Plan

Controlling portion sizes

⊗ **Are special products required?**
⊘ **Is eating out possible?**
⊘ **Is the plan family-friendly?**
⊘ **Do you have to buy a book?**
⊘ **Is the diet easy to maintain?**

Based on the idea that it takes time to adjust to new habits, this 12-week plan advises making just one change to your eating habits each week. Online support and information are available.

HOW IT CLAIMS TO WORK
The program starts by overhauling your breakfast routine and then, over the first month, works through lunch, snacks, and dinner. Each chapter provides a guide to staying within a 1,300 calorie-per-day allowance (or up to 1,600 calories per day for the active or significantly overweight) by focusing on portion control. Change One is based on the principle that it is not what we eat, but how much we eat, that is at the root of our weight problems. The menus provide reduced calories without compromising nutritional value or fiber intake. Since exercise is included as part of the program, you can expect to lose weight in safe amounts—1–3lb (0.45–1.35kg) per week—and maintain weight loss. A limited trial showed that volunteers who followed the program over the 12-week period lost an average of 17lb (7.7kg).

THE REGIMEN
In the first week of the diet, the focus is on breakfast. Lower-calorie, nutritionally balanced meals begin the day, but you

CHANGE ONE EATING PLAN

Breakfast
- 8floz (240ml) yogurt layered with granola, fruit, and coconut

Lunch
- Chef's salad with 1oz (28g) turkey breast, 1oz (28g) ham, and 1oz (28g) grated cheese, with 2 tbsp low-fat dressing
- 1 medium whole-grain roll
- ½ cantaloupe, cubed

Dinner
- 4oz (110g) grilled halibut steak with ½ cup grilled onions and ⅛ cup scallions, ½ cup ziti, and ½ cup zucchini
- Frozen fudge bar

Snacks
- 10 baked tortilla chips with salsa

are encouraged to eat as usual for the rest of the day. In the following three weeks, changes are gradually made to lunch, snacks, and dinner, until you have totally overhauled your entire daily eating habits.

In the last eight weeks, you focus on how to make good choices when dining out and during weekends and holidays, how to stock a healthy kitchen, and how to incorporate other good habits, such as regular exercise, to help you keep on track toward your goal. All foods are allowed in appropriate amounts, and moderate amounts of good fats are also included in the plan.

Change One offers meal suggestions and recipes. It also covers potential pitfalls, and dieters are encouraged to keep a food diary. Each chapter has a guide suggesting optimum strategies for speeding up weight loss.

IS IT HEALTHY?
The Change One Eating Plan offers a sensible, sound regimen that will lead safely to weight loss and weight control without compromising good nutrition. The recipes, meal plans, and shopping guides provide helpful tools and structure throughout the 12-week plan. The online support and additional information may also prove valuable, since those who have the backing of a support group tend to be more successful in their weight-loss efforts than those people who try to go it alone.

Glucose Revolution

Glycemic index

- ⊗ Are special products required?
- ✓ Is eating out possible?
- ✓ Is the plan family-friendly?
- ✓ Do you have to buy a book?
- ✓ Is the diet easy to maintain?

Based on the glycemic index (GI; *see p.47*), diets such as this were developed originally to help people with diabetes, but the emphasis on unrefined grains and other useful carbohydrates, low-fat foods, and plentiful fresh fruit and vegetables will aid healthy weight loss for a wide range of people.

HOW IT CLAIMS TO WORK
The Glucose Revolution is based on extensive research of the glycemic index, which is a numerical way of describing how the carbohydrate in individual foods immediately affects blood-sugar levels. High-GI foods increase blood-sugar levels, causing a rapid rise and subsequent fall in blood sugar, stimulating a counter-regulator response and possibly an increased appetite. This diet claims to ensure that you eat enough and eat the right kind of carbohydrates. It is directed at helping people with diabetes and those with excess fat in the abdominal area.

THE REGIMEN
The diet is based on a selection of low-GI foods. These have the advantage for weight loss of containing more fiber, so they fill you up and satisfy your hunger. In addition, such foods tend to be less processed and contain less sugar than high-GI foods. Suggestions include eating five servings of vegetables and legumes every day, two servings of fruits, four servings of bread and cereals, eating regularly, and decreasing your intake of total fat and saturated fat.

IS IT HEALTHY?
The concept of a glycemic index has been controversial in North America for a number of years because of variations in the technology used to measure the

Glucose Revolution Roast chicken breast, baked sweet potato, and broiled peppers provide a typical low-fat, low-GI, high-fiber meal on this program.

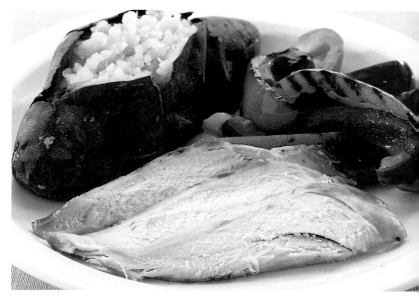

response. However, with modern methods and standardization of measurements, GI is one way to evaluate how carbohydrates can affect blood-sugar levels, either when eaten alone or with meals. This concept is particularly important for people with diabetes and abdominal obesity, since the insulin resistance that accompanies these conditions makes it difficult for their bodies to metabolize large amounts of carbohydrates. The glycemic index has also been distorted to form the basis of other well-known diets, and this has created some misunderstanding of the concept. This book recommends a more balanced long-term approach that can be maintained.

The plan advocates eating plenty of fiber-rich vegetables and legumes every day. Maximizing fresh fruits, whole-grain breads, and cereals that have a low-GI value, and minimizing saturated fat intake, this program will promote a sensible, well-balanced, healthy weight loss. The Glucose Revolution diet may be especially helpful for people with type 2 diabetes (see pp.246–251).

Specific advice on quantities, for both small and average eaters, is supplied in the book's weight-loss section.

GLUCOSE REVOLUTION

Breakfast
- 1½ cups bran cereal with low-fat or fat-free milk
- 1 slice whole-grain bread with low-sugar jam

Lunch
- 2 slices whole-grain bread
- 4oz (110g) grilled chicken, turkey, or ham
- 2 cups green salad

Dinner
- 6oz (170g) roasted chicken with baked sweet potato and ½ cup broiled green and red bell peppers
- 1 cup low-fat ice cream with ½ cup green pears

Snacks
- 2 medium fresh fruits

Montignac Method

Glycemic index

- ⊗ **Are special products required?**
- ⊘ **Is eating out possible?**
- ⊘ **Is the plan family-friendly?**
- ⊘ **Do you have to buy a book?**
- ⊘ **Is the diet easy to maintain?**

Developed by Michel Montignac, this diet plan combines a reduction in high glycemic-index (GI) foods (see p.47) with recommendations for specific combinations of foods.

HOW IT CLAIMS TO WORK
The diet is based on reducing high-GI foods and increasing low-fat, high-fiber, low-GI foods, along with some specific food combinations. The diet does not require calorie-counting and you can eat as much as you wish, as long as it is the right kind of food.

Foods are categorized in the diet as carbohydrates (good and bad), lipids (meat, dairy, and oils), carbohydrate-lipids (nuts, avocados, organ meats), and fiber (vegetables and whole grains). Combinations of carbohydrates and lipids in the same meal are not allowed.

THE REGIMEN
The diet is divided into phases:
- Phase I of the diet consists of three meals per day, following the food-combining principles (fruits—which are classified as good carbohydrates—must be eaten alone, not with or close to any other meal).
- Phase II allows you to gradually reintroduce some "bad" carbohydrates. You can begin to drink some wine and eat a little unsweetened dark chocolate.

You should minimize drinking with a meal, but can drink plenty of water at other times. Aim to avoid coffee and tea altogether.

IS IT HEALTHY?
Weight loss on this diet is promoted by the reduced calorie intake that occurs when you give up foods such as pastry, doughnuts, and french fries. The fact

MONTIGNAC METHOD

Early morning
- 20 grapes

Breakfast
- 1 cup cooked oatmeal with 8floz (240ml) fat-free milk

Lunch
- 6oz (170g) roasted chicken with 1 cup whole-grain rice, ½ cup tomatoes, ½ cup zucchini, 1oz (28g) fat-free cheese, and 8floz (240ml) applesauce

Dinner
- 3 cups endive salad with 1 cup sliced tomato, 2 hard-boiled eggs, 2oz (55g) grated hard cheese, and sugar-free dressing

Snacks
- Not allowed in Phase 1. Dark chocolate in Phase 2.

that you can eat some chocolate and drink a little wine in Phase 2 may explain the diet's popularity. However, the author is not a health-care professional and makes claims that are unscientific and even wrong. For example, he claims that North Americans have reduced their caloric intake by 30 percent in the last hundred years while becoming more obese. In fact, over the past 20 years, Americans have increased their calorie intake by about 200 calories per day.

Montignac fails to consider levels of physical activity, which are also markedly lower now than a century ago, but it is our sedentary lifestyle, combined with increased calorie intake, that is leading to the increase in excess weight and obesity in both adults and children.

Montignac also believes that bad carbohydrates—those with a high GI—interfere with the absorption of fats when they are consumed together, resulting in fats being stored. But if absorption is blocked, then fats cannot be stored. The best way to prevent fats from being stored is to avoid eating them in the first place. If you follow this diet, make sure you also take a vitamin and mineral supplement every day.

Insulin-resistance Diet

Glycemic index

- ✖ **Are special products required?**
- ✔ **Is eating out possible?**
- ✔ **Is the plan family-friendly?**
- ✔ **Do you have to buy a book?**
- ✔ **Is the diet easy to maintain?**

This diet is based on a combination of limiting high glycemic-index foods and controlling insulin by balancing the intake of protein and carbohydrate.

HOW IT CLAIMS TO WORK

Insulin resistance—a condition in which the body does not respond appropriately to an increase in insulin levels following a meal (*see p.47*)—is often associated with diabetic status and, according to Dr. Cheryle Hart, the author of this diet, is present in 75 percent of overweight people. Dr. Hart believes that this is what makes them overweight.

The Insulin-resistance Diet is based on the concept of the glycemic index (GI; *see p.47*)—a numeric description of how quickly insulin is released following the ingestion of specific carbohydrate-containing foods. High-GI foods are those that more rapidly increase blood-sugar levels, with subsequent increases in levels of insulin. In addition to limiting high-GI foods, the diet follows recent evidence suggesting that foods with a high protein to carbohydrate ratio consistently have a lower glycemic index. This diet is directed particularly toward people who suffer from type 2 diabetes (*see p.246–251*) and/or metabolic syndrome (*see p.214*).

THE REGIMEN

Dr. Hart acknowledges the controversy surrounding the glycemic index and therefore chooses to focus additionally on the protein to carbohydrate ratio. An integral part of her program is the "Link-and-Balance Eating Method," which suggests eating (linking) a protein every time you eat a meal, and, at the same time, balancing one serving of high carbohydrate with one serving of

high protein. To satisfy hunger, you may have a greater amount of protein, but not of carbohydrates.

In addition to the balanced protein–carbohydrate ratio, this diet encourages the consumption of low-GI foods and limits those with high-GI values. Alcohol is permitted, in moderation, and the plan also includes suggestions for healthy choices at restaurants and fast-food chains and restaurants. Three "balanced" meals a day are suggested, with limited consumption of liquids.

IS IT HEALTHY?

The concept of insulin resistance is very important because people who have this condition are at greater risk of becoming diabetic. Individuals with metabolic syndrome (*see p.214*) may also be more insulin resistant.

We know that eating low-GI foods is beneficial for some people with pre-diabetes or diabetes because it helps lower their blood-sugar levels. However, whether or not a low-GI diet is effective for weight reduction is questionable. The author claims that most people are overweight because they are insulin-resistant, which may or may not be

---

INSULIN-RESISTANCE DIET

Breakfast
- 2 frozen waffles with ½ cup low-fat cottage cheese and 1 cup raspberries

Lunch
- 1 cup pasta primavera, with ½ cup steamed vegetables and 3oz (85g) Italian sausage
- 1 cup green salad with reduced-fat or fat-free dressing
- 1 slice low-fat garlic-herb bread

Dinner
- 6oz (170g) marinated London broil, with ½ cup vegetable kabobs and 8floz (240ml) mushroom gravy
- 2oz (55g) fat-free sour-cream chocolate cake

Snacks
- ½ cup sugar-free ice cream

---

true. In addition, although the primary treatment for metabolic syndrome is weight loss and increasing exercise, eating a low-GI diet may only improve metabolic syndrome if the individual has insulin resistance.

If you are planning to follow this diet, bear in mind that the key to weight reduction is reducing portion sizes and increasing your physical activity level.

Hay Diet

Food combining

- ✖ **Are special products required?**
- ✔ **Is eating out possible?**
- ✔ **Is the plan family-friendly?**
- ✔ **Do you have to buy a book?**
- ✖ **Is the diet easy to maintain?**

The Hay Diet was introduced in the 1930s by Dr. William Hay, who believed that eliminating refined foods from the diet and avoiding eating protein and starch at the same meal allows the body to heal itself. Loss of excess weight is an additional benefit.

HOW IT CLAIMS TO WORK

This diet is based on the belief that weight gain stems from a metabolic imbalance resulting from poor digestion. According to this theory—which was based on experiments conducted in the 1920s, using techniques that are now outdated—the imbalance occurs because we eat a mixed diet, and the enzymes required for the digestion of carbohydrate and protein operate optimally in different chemical environments. Eating foods in the wrong combinations, therefore, causes the body to be in an acidic rather than an alkaline state. Dr. Hay states that protein and starch foods need different conditions in the digestive tract for digestion and should never be combined at the same meal, with four hours between each meal. In the diet, food is classified according to its chemical requirements for efficient digestion:
- Fruits and vegetables are alkali-forming foods and are good for us.
- Most protein foods (meats, fish, eggs, poultry, and cheese) are acid-forming foods and should be limited.

HAY DIET

Breakfast
● 8floz (240ml) yogurt with sliced apple and sliced almonds

Lunch
● 1 toasted banana sandwich
● ½ cup grapes, hazelnuts, and raisins combined
● 1 medium yellow pear

Dinner
● 6oz (170g) grilled cod with ½ cup carrots, peas, and cauliflower
● 1 cup fruit salad of pineapple and fresh orange

Snacks
● 1 medium fresh fruit
● 1 cup chopped vegetables

● Starchy foods are also considered to be acid-forming and, as with protein foods, should be limited.

THE REGIMEN
This diet prescribes completely natural whole foods, with at least 50 percent from fresh fruit, vegetables, and salad. No processed foods, such as white flour and sugar, are permitted. The "food combining" element of the diet means that concentrated proteins, such as meat and cheese, should be eaten at separate meals from carbohydrates.

The diet's rules for a healthy diet include eliminating processed and refined foods, eating only whole grains, minimizing milk intake, and avoiding combinations that clash. Neutral foods include vegetables, nuts, seeds, and oils and form the foundation of your diet. These can be eaten with either proteins or starches.

IS IT HEALTHY?
While there is no scientific basis for the claim that an acidic condition counteracts the body's healthy alkaline state, this diet promotes weight loss by decreasing your intake of calories. Eating more fruits and vegetables, whole grains rather than refined and processed foods, and limiting protein intake is a healthy idea.

Somersizing

Food combining

⊗ **Are special products required?**
✓ **Is eating out possible?**
✓ **Is the plan family-friendly?**
✓ **Do you have to buy a book?**
⊗ **Is the diet easy to maintain?**

Suzanne Somers, the author of this diet plan, incorporates ways to splurge and enjoy foods into her own version of a food-combining program.

HOW IT CLAIMS TO WORK
Somersizing claims to reprogram your metabolism to burn fat by providing a constant source of energy, with frequent small meals and plenty of fresh fruit and vegetables throughout the day. No portion monitoring or calorie counting is required, but you do need to think about which types of food to eat at any one time. The plan advocates eating proteins and fats with vegetables and no other carbohydrates, and eating carbohydrates with vegetables and no fat. It also eliminates sugar, white flour, alcohol, and caffeine and suggests that fruit should be eaten on its own or on an empty stomach.

SOMERSIZING

Breakfast
● 1 slice whole-grain toast with 2 tbsp fat-free cottage cheese

Lunch
● 4oz (110g) grilled fish with 1 tbsp lemon-butter sauce, ½ cup snow peas tossed in butter
● 1 cup green salad, with 2 tbsp sugar-free dressing

Dinner
● 4½oz (130g) pot roast with ¼ cup onions, ½ cup tomatoes, and ½ cup steamed asparagus
● 2 cups green salad with vinaigrette dressing

Snacks
● 2 peaches

THE REGIMEN
Somersizing prohibits all alcoholic and caffeine-containing drinks (decaffeinated coffee is allowed). So-called "funky" foods, such as sugar, corn syrup, honey, beets, carrots, white flour, pasta, white rice, corn, bananas, potatoes, sweet potatoes, pumpkin, and winter squashes, are discouraged. Nuts, olives, avocado, liver, coconuts, milk (other than fat-free), tofu, and soymilk are also restricted because they are "combination foods" that contain both carbohydrates and proteins, which the diet claims should not be eaten together.

The main points of the Somersizing diet to remember are:
● Fruits should be eaten alone or on an empty stomach.
● Carbohydrates should be eaten only with other carbohydrate-rich foods.
● Proteins and fats can be eaten together.

IS IT HEALTHY?
By following the rules of this diet, you are likely to be successful in losing weight because you are cutting out food groups and reducing your daily calorie intake. With exercise, this combination does promote weight loss.

Reducing some processed foods that are low in fiber and high in sugar and eating plenty of fresh vegetables is a healthful approach, but restricting foods that contain both carbohydrate and protein (such as avocados) makes no sense, since that is the way they are available in nature. We also know that nuts, olives, and avocados are excellent sources of monounsaturated fats, which are helpful in preventing cardiovascular disease (*see pp.214–221*).

However, it does not make any sense to suggest that fat and protein can be eaten together while carbohydrates and protein cannot. The author claims that when carbohydrates and protein are eaten together, their enzymes cancel each other out, halting the digestive process and causing weight gain. The fact is that most foods naturally contain all of the three macronutrients (proteins, fats, and carbohydrates) in various combinations, so there is no reason to believe that they cannot be digested together in the body successfully.

New Beverly Hills Diet

Food combining

- ⊗ **Are special products required?**
- ⊘ **Is eating out possible?**
- ⊗ **Is the plan family-friendly?**
- ⊘ **Do you have to buy a book?**
- ⊗ **Is the diet easy to maintain?**

According to the author of this program, which claims to be a 35-day lifestyle eating plan rather than a diet, the key to losing weight and feeling healthy is to improve digestion by combining fats, proteins, and carbohydrates correctly.

HOW IT CLAIMS TO WORK
The author, Judy Mazel, believes that when carbohydrates are eaten with proteins, they become trapped and are not digested properly. She goes on to claim that when carbohydrates are not digested, they are stored as fat. The premise is that proteins are the most difficult foods to digest, carbohydrates are easier, and fruits are the easiest. Fats do not interfere with the digestion of either protein or carbohydrates, but must not be eaten with fruit. Since fruits are digested very quickly, they have to be eaten alone, or they will become trapped in your stomach by other foods. Ideally, proteins should be eaten with other proteins, carbohydrates with carbohydrates, and fruit eaten alone.

THE REGIMEN
Unlike the first edition of the book, this New Beverly Hills Diet includes foods from all food groups, including animal protein, for the first ten days. The plan recommends beginning each day with fruit: you may eat as much fruit as you want, but should avoid mixing fruits. After eating proteins or carbohydrates, you should not eat fruit.

If you eat a carbohydrate food (such as starches, vegetables, salads, cereals, or grains) after eating fruits, you may eat carbohydrates without restriction until you eat a protein.

Once you eat protein (such as meat, fish, milk, yogurt, cheese, nuts, seeds or ice cream), then 80 percent of what you eat for the rest of the day should be protein only.

If you want to eat what the author calls your "open meal" (in which you combine carbohydrates and proteins, such as a hamburger and french fries), you have to eat only carbohydrates for lunch and snacks that day.

Fats (such as butter, mayonnaise, oil, sour cream, and heavy cream) can be combined with carbohydrates or proteins. Diet sodas and artificial

NEW BEVERLY HILLS DIET

Breakfast
- ½ cup dried apricots

Lunch
- 1½ cups salad of spinach, leeks, mushrooms, and Mazel dressing (rice vinegar, sesame oil, cloves, garlic, ginger, and pepper)

Dinner
- 1½ cups cooked pasta with marinara sauce and 1 cup broccoli

Snacks
- All carbohydrates, protein, or fruit, depending on the day.

sweeteners are not permitted in the diet. Most alcoholic drinks are considered carbohydrates and should be consumed only with other carbohydrates. However, wine is considered a fruit and must be combined only with other fruits.

The plan also includes antidotes and precedotes to offset the negative side effects of eating foods that are difficult to digest. Antidotes are foods eaten for breakfast the day after you eat food that is difficult to digest. Precedotes are foods eaten for breakfast the day you know you are going to eat a difficult-to-digest food. For example, before you eat greasy, creamy, or cheesy foods, you have to eat plenty of pineapple or strawberries as a precedote. Alternatively, you can eat one of these fruits as an antidote for breakfast the day after you have consumed a difficult-to-digest food.

Supplements are not essential for the diet, but nutritional yeast flakes mixed with water can be taken in order to supply B vitamins, sesame seeds as a calcium source, and blue-green algae as a source of natural nutrients. Also, a supplement of 1,000mg of vitamin C with bioflavonoids is recommended.

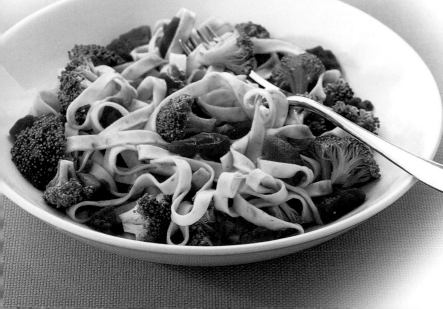

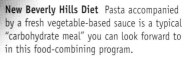

New Beverly Hills Diet Pasta accompanied by a fresh vegetable-based sauce is a typical "carbohydrate meal" you can look forward to in this food-combining program.

IS IT HEALTHY?

This program is based on the concept of food combining—a theory that has no scientific evidence to support it. The idea that carbohydrate is stored as fat because it is improperly digested makes no sense from a medical perspective.

There is no scientific evidence that food composition affects the way in which enzymes digest food. In any case, most foods found in nature contain some proteins, fats, and carbohydrates, making it very unlikely that our bodies are not adapted to dealing with combinations of nutrients. It is true that the absorption of carbohydrates will be delayed if they are combined with other foods, but no matter what we eat with carbohydrates, they will always be absorbed. If you select high fiber, complex carbohydrate sources, such as whole-wheat bread, they will take longer to be absorbed by the body than simple carbohydrates such as candy or soda.

You may lose weight with the New Beverly Hills Diet due to a significant reduction in the calories you consume, but trying to remember which foods to eat when, and in what combination, can be confusing, time-consuming, and often very frustrating, especially when you are eating out or preparing meals for a family.

The New Beverly Hills Diet is an improvement on the old version, but in our opinion it is still nutritionally unbalanced and restrictive.

Fit For Life

Food combining

⊗ **Are special products required?**
⊘ **Is eating out possible?**
⊘ **Is the plan family-friendly?**
⊘ **Do you have to buy a book?**
⊗ **Is the diet easy to maintain?**

Fit For Life is another diet claiming that combining food in certain ways improves digestive processes and thereby leads to successful weight loss.

HOW IT CLAIMS TO WORK

This is essentially a no-processed-food regimen. The diet is high in fruits and vegetables and limited in dairy products and meats. It also recommends that foods be eaten in specific combinations at certain times of the day. The goal is rapid weight loss based on when and how you eat. It draws on various theories, including natural body cycles, water content of food, food combining, "proper" fruit eating, and detoxification.

The theory behind this food-combining program is that the body is not designed to digest more than one "concentrated" food in the stomach at the same time. (Any food that is not a vegetable or a fruit is considered concentrated.) The authors cite research carried out in the 1940s suggesting that carbohydrate and protein cannot be digested when consumed together. In addition, they suggest that eating two concentrated foods together will cause the food to rot because it cannot be digested properly.

The idea behind high water-content foods such as fruit is to maintain and replenish the body's water content to prevent waste accumulation.

The book also espouses "natural hygiene"—a theory that the body is constantly seeking to clear itself of waste, and that helping this process along will improve health.

According to the authors, the body operates in cycles:

FIT FOR LIFE

Breakfast
● Fruit salad of ½ banana, ½ grapefruit, and 1 medium apple

Lunch
● 1½ cups salad of chopped lettuce, cucumber, tomato, olives, Brussels sprouts, and sunflower or sesame seeds
● 1 slice whole-grain bread

Dinner
● 16floz (480ml) creamy cauliflower soup
● 6oz (170g) roasted chicken breast with 1 cup string beans and 1 cup green salad
● 8floz (240ml) vegetable juice

Snacks
● ¼ cup almonds

● Noon to 8p.m. is for appropriation (eating and digestion).
● 8p.m. to 4a.m. is for assimilation (absorption and use).
● 4a.m. to noon is for elimination (of body waste and food debris).

THE REGIMEN

This diet advises that in the mornings you eat only fruits; for lunch, you eat raw vegetables with some whole-grain bread or vegetable soup; and for dinner you have salad with grain and meat. The authors are against cooking where possible, as they claim it removes water from food and destroys its natural enzymes. If your diet does not include enough high water-content foods, they recommend drinking distilled water, since the minerals in natural water are presumed to bind with cholesterol and form plaques. Eating fruit is highly recommended, but it should be eaten separately and never immediately following any other foods.

IS IT HEALTHY?

By restricting certain foods at each meal, you will take in fewer calories overall and you will lose weight. The scientific basis for food combining is unfounded, and there is no reason for most people to avoid combining foods. However, if you often have difficulty digesting certain foods, or experience abdominal discomfort after eating, it may be worth following this regimen for a few weeks to see if you feel better.

Most foods promoted on this diet are healthy, but the rules do not promote flexible, long-term habits that are easy to maintain. The concept of daily cycles is based on normal hormonal changes in the body, but there is no scientific evidence to support the claim that these fluctuations influence nutritional requirements and how and when you should eat specific types of food.

In addition, the authors argue that calories are the enemy only if they are consumed in foods that are highly processed or ill-combined, rather than encouraging sensible portion control. Overall, this program has serious flaws and if followed for more than several weeks, could lead to deficiencies of vitamin D, calcium, and iron.

Eat Right 4 Your Type

Metabolic typing

⊗ **Are special products required?**
⊘ **Is eating out possible?**
⊗ **Is the plan family-friendly?**
⊘ **Do you have to buy a book?**
⊗ **Is the diet easy to maintain?**

This diet is based on the idea that your blood type reflects your anthropological background and that this influences your body's reaction to food.

HOW IT CLAIMS TO WORK

The author of this diet plan claims that people's metabolic profiles differ and that these can be matched to specific dietary constituents. In order to avoid the complexity that renders some metabolic-profiling systems useless, this plan categorizes all people by their blood type. The author proposes that your anthropological background—whether your ancestors were hunters, cultivators, enigmas, or nomads—is reflected in your blood type; that the antibodies on the outside of blood cells vary with blood type; and that these react in varying ways to food antigens, causing intolerance and illness. If you eat the right foods for your type, you will lose weight and have more energy.

EAT RIGHT 4 YOUR TYPE: TYPE O

Breakfast
● 1 slice cinnamon and raisin toast with 1 tbsp cream cheese

Lunch
● 4oz (110g) grilled chicken with green salad and low-fat dressing

Dinner
● 6oz (170g) broiled lamb chops with ½ cup asparagus and ½ cup string beans and carrots

Snacks
● Slices of tofu or tofu-based low-fat dessert

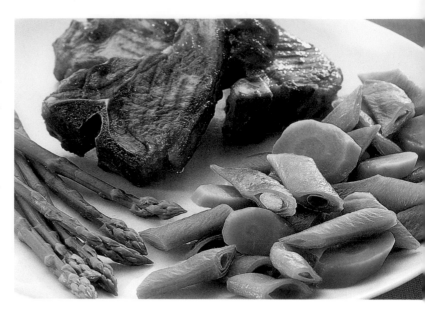

Eat Right 4 Your Type Lamb with vegetables is a high-protein meal recommended by this program for people with blood group O.

THE REGIMEN

Lists of permitted and nonpermitted foods are available for each blood group. The recommended diets range in caloric value from about 1,500–1,800 per day.
● Persons with Type O blood are believed to be the oldest in evolutionary terms and are therefore more adapted to a red-meat-based, low-carbohydrate diet, with few grains and no wheat.
● Type As are younger evolutionarily, as humans moved from being hunter-gatherers to a more agrarian lifestyle. This group tolerates vegetables better and are advised to follow a vegetarian, high-carbohydrate, low-fat diet.
● Type Bs emerged when the races were merging from Africa, Europe, Asia, and America. According to this plan, Type Bs tolerate a more balanced diet that includes a variety of vegetables, fruits, dairy products, grains, and meats.
● Type ABs represent the newest group from interbreeding. They have fewer restrictions and tolerate more foods.

IS IT HEALTHY?

The idea of basing your dietary needs on your blood type has no scientific foundation. Neither has the premise that your risk of certain diseases is based on your blood type. If it were, people's blood types would be tested as routine when they are admitted to the hospital or for laboratory visits.
   A serious drawback of the diet plan for Type A and O blood types is that dairy products are limited, and, consequently, the diets are low in calcium.

Body Code

Metabolic typing

⊗ **Are special products required?**
⊘ **Is eating out possible?**
⊘ **Is the plan family-friendly?**
⊘ **Do you have to buy a book?**
⊗ **Is the diet easy to maintain?**

This plan is based on the theory that humans can be classified into different genetic types, with different dietary requirements. For every type, however, the focus is on a nutritious diet and regular exercise.

HOW IT CLAIMS TO WORK

According to the authors of this program, not every diet, lifestyle, or exercise plan is suitable for all people. They classify the human body into two basic genetic types—strong and sleek. Strong types are generally more solid and muscular than sleek types and require a low-protein, plant-based diet and plenty of physical activity. Sleek types, on the other hand, are generally leaner and more delicate than strong types. They need less physical activity and more protein in their diets.

Each of these two body types is subdivided into two further categories. Strong body types may be "warriors" or "nurturers," while sleek types may be "communicators" or "visionaries."

According to the authors of this plan, the four body types are influenced by a specific gland that governs food intake and energy balance. Your diet and exercise plan depend upon what body type you are:

• Warrior-type people are healthiest on a plant-based diet that includes whole grains, fruits, and vegetables.
• Nurturers need to eat plenty of soy and flaxseeds and minimize their intake of meat and fish.
• Communicators need a diet high in leafy vegetables, monounsaturated fats, and lean protein, including all white meats, fat-free dairy products, eggs, some nuts, and soy protein.
• Visionaries need an Asian-style diet that includes lots of cooked vegetables, whole grains, and protein, especially those derived from soy.

THE REGIMEN
The Body Code embraces a holistic philosophy, founded on a balance of body and spirit. Unlocking the "Body Code" enables people to define their types, which are characterized by prototypical physical features and personal attributes:

• Warriors need a diet based on plant foods. This is because animal foods over-stimulate their dominant adrenal glands, leaving them out of balance. Their everyday diet should include plenty of vegetables, fruits, roots, and grains to stimulate the nondominant glands and to create energy balance. Higher-calorie plant foods, such as nuts and seeds, should be restricted if weight loss is desired. Warriors should avoid consuming saturated and hydrogenated fats including red meats in favor of white meats, alcohol, salts, and refined grains and flour and include herbs, teas, and

---

BODY CODE: WARRIOR TYPE

Breakfast
• ½ cup whole-grain cereal, cherry sauce, and 8floz (240ml) fat-free milk

Lunch
• 2 cups DeLayne's tomatoes and rice (recipe in book)

Dinner
• 4oz (110g) chicken Parmesan with 1 cup whole-grain pasta and red sauce
• 2 cups green salad

Snacks
• 4floz (120ml) fat-free yogurt
• ½ cup vegetable sticks
• Unlimited fruits, vegetables, whole grains, white and pink fish, white poultry, egg whites and substitutes, fat-free dairy, ginger tea, flaxseeds, and alfalfa

---

condiments that will help control their appetite and balance the biochemical reactions in the body.
• Nurturers are curvy and pear-shaped; charismatic, compassionate, and selfless. They need a diet based on plants and high water-content foods. Their everyday diet should include plenty of plant foods, especially fruits and vegetables. Since the nurturer's appetite is stronger in the evening, they should eat a substantial meal at this time of day.
• Communicators are lanky, long-limbed, lively, creative, and unpredictable. They need a diet based on monounsaturated fats, vegetables, protein, and small amounts of carbohydrate. They can eat as much protein as they like, including red meat, as long as they are careful to limit saturated fat.
• Visionaries are thin and youthful, calm, intellectual, and reserved. Their basic nutrition is based on proteins, whole grains, and cooked vegetables. The best foods for this diet are soy proteins and vegetables.

IS IT HEALTHY?
The positive aspects of the Body Code diet are that it teaches a way of life, rather than a quick fix. The program

---

states that weight loss and health maintenance require a nutritious diet complemented by regular exercise, which we support. They also stress that healthy eating requires a commitment and perseverance for success and that physical and emotional fitness need to be part of your lifestyle.

However, there is little evidence to support the idea of a dominant gland leading to physiological imbalance as a principle factor in weight management. There are many glands at work in the body, and, in good health, these glands work in synchrony and harmony. In a few cases, glandular disease is a relevant consideration, but it is not a basic tenet of weight management, and it is not appropriate for most people. Omitting or favoring entire food groups can lead to deficiency in essential vitamins and minerals, including iron.

Metabolic Typing

Metabolic typing

⊗ **Are special products required?**
✓ **Is eating out possible?**
⊗ **Is the plan family-friendly?**
✓ **Do you have to buy a book?**
⊗ **Is the diet easy to maintain?**

This diet is based on the belief that people vary in their nutritional needs according to their body types, which reflect their unique ancestral histories.

HOW IT CLAIMS TO WORK
The Metabolic Typing diet proposes that our unique body types derive from variations in our ancestors' diets, which were determined by diverse geographic and environmental circumstances. It is suggested, for example, that people with tropical ancestral origins have different nutritional needs from those originating from temperate zones.

The authors of Metabolic Typing assert that universal diets are ineffective for the varied physiologies and nutritional needs of different populations. Instead, they identify individual biochemical profiles and nutritional needs in order to produce customized diets designed to promote vigor and well-being in each individual.

METABOLIC TYPING: PROTEIN TYPE

Breakfast
- 2 scrambled eggs with 1 slice bacon and ½ cup potatoes fried in butter

Lunch
- 4oz (110g) dark meat chicken with ½ cup carrots, ½ cup cauliflower, and 2 tbsp olive spread

Dinner
- 4oz (110g) broiled steak with ½ cup peas, ½ cup corn, and ¼ cup avocado marinated in olive oil and vinegar

Snacks
- 8floz (240ml) full-fat yogurt with 1 tsp sunflower seeds and 1 tsp cashews

THE REGIMEN

The first step in this program is to establish your type by completing a 65-point questionnaire that evaluates physical appearance, anatomical and structural characteristics, psychological characteristics, behavioral habits, as well as food preferences and reactions. Specific combinations of fat, protein, and carbohydrate for optimum nutrition are then recommended, according to your classification as a "Protein Type," "Carbohydrate Type," or "Mixed Type."
- Protein Types are advised to include meat, seafood, and dairy at every meal. Organ meats (beef or chicken liver), sardines, anchovies, or caviar, and whole-fat dairy products are particularly recommended. Sprouted-grain breads are the only breads allowed; unripe apples and pears are acceptable but in moderation. All nuts and oils are allowed, but alcohol, caffeine, and fruit juices should be avoided by people who are Protein Types.
- Carbohydrate Types are advised to base their meals on high-starch vegetables, such as potatoes, sweet potatoes, and rutabaga, as well as on any type of whole grain. Nuts and oils should be eaten sparingly and only light meats and fish, such as chicken breast or catfish, should be included.

Dairy products must be fat-free or low-fat, and legumes should be avoided. Alcohol and caffeine are restricted.
- Mixed Types must include ample foods from both the Protein- and Carbohydrate-types regimens.

IS IT HEALTHY?

Few people can claim to have a single ancestral lineage. Most of us are a mix of races, ethnicities, and genes, and this complicates any historical correlations between geography and optimum nutrition. However, it is important to remember that the foods our ancestors ate were natural, and natural foods contain all three macronutrients in variable proportions. Fats, proteins, and carbohydrates are essential for life, and we are all equipped with the genetic tools to digest and benefit from these macronutrients. On the positive side, this diet may encourage you to eat more natural, unprocessed foods.

In addition, human nutrition must adapt to and accommodate changes in our lifestyle due to new developments in technology, wider availability of foods from around the world, prosperity, illness, and level of physical activity. These factors affect our nutritional status and demand a diet designed to suit individual needs.

Cabbage Soup Diet Unlimited quantities of homemade vegetable soup form the basis of this short-term, quick-weight-loss program.

Cabbage Soup Diet

Quick weight loss

- ⊗ Are special products required?
- ⊗ Is eating out possible?
- ⊗ Is the plan family-friendly?
- ⊘ Do you have to buy a book?
- ⊗ Is the diet easy to maintain?

This extremely low-calorie diet should be followed for only seven days at a time. It is not nutritionally sound or a safe way to lose weight.

HOW IT CLAIMS TO WORK

The diet claims that you can lose 10–15lb (4.5–6.8kg) by eating as much cabbage soup as you want to for seven days. The cabbage soup includes a variety of low-calorie vegetables with canned tomatoes, flavored onion-soup mix, and bouillon or vegetable juice.

THE REGIMEN

In addition to eating unlimited amounts of homemade cabbage soup, this plan allows combinations of foods each day, such as fruit and milk one day, vegetables and milk the next, and beef the next day. No bread, alcohol, or carbonated beverages are allowed.

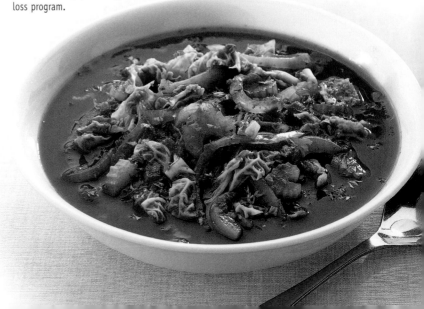

CABBAGE SOUP DIET

Unlimited cabbage soup plus:

Day 1
• Any fruit except bananas

Day 2
• Unlimited vegetables
• Baked potato with butter

Day 3
• Any fruit except bananas
• Unlimited vegetables

Day 4
• Up to 8 bananas, plus unlimited fat-free milk

Day 5
• 10–20oz (280–560g) beef with 20oz- (560g-) can tomatoes
• 6–8 glasses water

Day 6
• Unlimited beef and vegetables

Day 7
• Brown rice
• Unsweetened fruit juices

Snacks
• Cabbage soup

Recipe: Cabbage Soup This recipe makes about six servings of soup. You can make and eat as much the soup as you like throughout the day.
• 6 large onions, chopped
• 2 green bell peppers, seeded and chopped
• 1–2 20oz (560g) cans tomatoes
• 1 bunch celery, chopped
• Half head cabbage, chopped
• 1 package onion soup mix
• 1–2 cubes bouillon (optional)
• 6-pint (3-liter) carton vegetable juice with 2 pints (1 liter) of water, or just use 6 pints (3 liters) of water.

Sauté onions and bell peppers, and then add other vegetables. Add bouillon and water or juice. Bring to a boil and then simmer for up to 2 hours. Season to taste with salt and freshly ground black pepper and your choice of fresh chopped parsley or curry powder.

IS IT HEALTHY?

The diet offers quick weight loss, most of which is water weight. It is neither nutritionally balanced nor a safe method for achieving long-term weight reduction and is likely to promote cravings as soon as you come off the diet. If you do try it, be sure to eat sensible, well-balanced meals once you have completed the seven days.

5-Day Miracle Diet

Quick weight loss

⊗ **Are special products required?**
⊘ **Is eating out possible?**
⊘ **Is the plan family-friendly?**
⊘ **Do you have to buy a book?**
⊘ **Is the diet easy to maintain?**

This program aims to control the food cravings that often cause people to abandon their attempts to lose weight by maintaining stable blood-sugar levels throughout the day.

HOW IT CLAIMS TO WORK

The author claims that a drop in blood-sugar levels results in uncontrollable cravings, often for foods such as sweets and alcohol. After you eat, insulin levels rise to reduce blood-sugar levels, and this leads to a drop in blood sugar, which prompts the urge to eat more. This diet recommends eating at specific, regular times during the day, and advocates consuming certain types of foods in specific combinations.

THE REGIMEN

According to this program, breakfast should be eaten within 30 minutes of waking up, snacking within two hours of breakfast, lunch by 1p.m., followed by an afternoon snack three hours later, and dinner several hours after having the snack.

In addition to specifying the times of the meals, specific types of foods to be eaten at each meal are listed.
• Breakfast: protein and bread.
• Lunch: protein, fresh vegetables, with optional fruit.
• Dinner: a variety of vegetables, protein, and bread.

Men can eat three starchy foods per day, while women can eat these foods only on alternate days.

Recommended snacks include fresh fruits and vegetables. Plenty of water is advised, and coffee is allowed. Pasta is limited to twice a week and and can only be eaten at dinner, but you are can eat one or two foods a week that you "absolutely adore."

IS IT HEALTHY?

This is a sensible diet that does not advocate any bizarre eating habits. It is essentially a calorie-controlled plan that will help you lose weight by reducing portion sizes and limiting your intake of carbohydrates. Starches are permitted only twice a day, mostly at breakfast and at lunch or dinner, but not both. If your eating habits are very different from this, such that you skip meals and eat a lot of sweets, you may feel better and be able to regulate your blood-sugar levels by eating at specific times each day. However, there are no miracles when it comes to dieting and losing weight, and you will certainly need to follow this program for longer than five days in order to see long-term results.

5-DAY MIRACLE DIET

Breakfast (½ hour after waking)
• 1 egg
• 1 slice toast with spread

Lunch (by 1p.m.)
• 2–4oz (56–110g) tuna with 1 cup spinach and tomato salad with balsamic-vinegar dressing
• 1 orange

Dinner
• 2–4oz (56–110g) grilled chicken with ½ cup spinach, ½ cup chopped tomato, ¼ cup chopped bell pepper, ½ cup chopped lettuce, and 1 tsp balsamic-vinegar dressing
• 1 slice of bread

Snacks (2 hours after breakfast; 3 hours after lunch)
• 1 nectarine, ½ cup grapefruit, carrots, or raw cauliflower

Grapefruit Diet

Quick weight loss

- ⊗ **Are special products required?**
- ⊘ **Is eating out possible?**
- ⊗ **Is the plan family-friendly?**
- ⊘ **Do you have to buy a book?**
- ⊗ **Is the diet easy to maintain?**

This diet is based on the idea that eating grapefruit with every meal helps you to lose weight by burning fat.

HOW IT CLAIMS TO WORK
The theory behind the program is that grapefruit contains enzymes that make the body burn fat for energy. Calories are limited to fewer than 800 per day, which promotes quick weight loss—primarily due to loss of body water.

THE REGIMEN
The Grapefruit Diet advocates eating half a grapefruit before every meal and before any caffeinated drinks. The diet restricts dairy products, other fruits, and most vegetables. You can drink black tea or coffee with meals.

IS IT HEALTHY?
There is no evidence to support the idea that eating grapefruit helps burn fat. Any weight loss that occurs is due to the extremely low calorie intake. If

you like grapefruit, you may be able to stay on this diet for about a week, but with fewer than 800 calories daily, any weight loss that occurs will be mostly due to loss of water weight.

This diet is not nutritionally balanced. It is low in fiber and essential vitamins, and minerals such as iron and calcium. Because the caloric intake is so low, causing you to be in a ketotic state (*see p.168*), you are likely to lack energy, and any attempt to exercise may make you dizzy or light-headed.

GRAPEFRUIT DIET

Breakfast
- ½ grapefruit

Lunch
- ½ grapefruit
- 1 egg and 1 cup garden salad with tomatoes and carrots
- 1 slice whole-wheat toast

Dinner
- ½ grapefruit
- 2 eggs, half lettuce, ½ cup chopped tomato, and dressing
- Black tea or coffee

Snacks
- Not allowed with this diet plan

Rotation Diet

Quick weight loss

- ⊗ **Are special products required?**
- ⊘ **Is eating out possible?**
- ⊗ **Is the plan family-friendly?**
- ⊘ **Do you have to buy a book?**
- ⊗ **Is the diet easy to maintain?**

This diet is designed to reduce overall caloric intake without causing the body to go into "starvation mode," which leads to additional weight gain when normal eating is resumed.

HOW IT CLAIMS TO WORK
This plan recommends a rotation of diets of varying calorie levels that will create a caloric deficit great enough to produce significant weight loss, without causing the body to lower its metabolic rate as it does in fasting. The author recommends two cycles of rotation diet, each followed by no dietary restriction for one to four weeks. The author's rationale is that low-calorie diets cause a reduction in the body's metabolic rate, which sets the dieter up for rebound weight gain when he or she stops dieting and reverts to a normal calorie intake.

The author describes the "starvation response," which is the body's response to caloric restriction. To preserve essential functions, the body lowers its metabolic rate—the rate at which calories are burned at rest (*see p.34*).

THE REGIMEN
The diet advocates different calorie levels for men and women, and recommends an extremely low calorie regimen for

---

ROTATION DIET: 1,200 CALORIES

Breakfast
- ½ grapefruit
- 1 slice whole-wheat bread with 1 slice cheese
- Noncalorie beverage

Lunch
- 3oz (85g) salmon with unlimited "free" vegetables
- 5 whole-wheat crackers
- Noncalorie beverage

Dinner
- 3oz (85g) baked chicken with 1 cup cauliflower and beets
- 1 apple
- Noncalorie beverage

Snacks
- Any from the list of "safe" fruits, such as apples, oranges, and berries

---

three days, followed by a more modest calorie restriction for four days, and then a week of mild calorie restriction.
- Women are allowed:
600 calories per day for 3 days
900 calories per day for 4 days
1,200 calories per day for 7 days.
- Men are allowed:
1,200 calories per day for 3 days
1,500 calories per day for 4 days
1,800 calories per day for 7 days.

This level of caloric restriction is likely to cause more hunger than most of us are willing to tolerate. To compensate, the diet recommends filling up on "free vegetables," such as asparagus, celery, chicory, Chinese cabbage, cucumber, endive, escarole, lettuce, radish, spinach, watercress, and zucchini.

The diet recommends "safe" fruits for snacking on when you are hungry; these include apples, berries, grapefruit, melon, oranges, peaches, and pineapple. It also recommends standard serving sizes, based on the Food Guide Pyramid (*see p.72*), and there is no specific restriction on caffeine and alcohol.

IS IT HEALTHY?
This extremely low-calorie program should be attempted only under medical supervision. The claim that

it prevents rebound weight gain is unproven. Because the diet produces a caloric deficit of 7,200 calories in the first week and 6,300 calories in the second week, it is designed for men or women to lose 6–7lb (2.7–3.2kg) in two weeks. However, the diet actually claims to produce weight losses of 14lb (6.4kg) in three weeks, which does not seem possible. The diet will result in significant weight loss if it is followed, but will also result in severe hunger and dehydration, which is likely to cause people to stop following the program.

The rotational aspect of this diet seems like a gimmick, but people who are able to tolerate this level of caloric restriction will lose a significant amount of weight in a short period. However, whether or not they maintain the weight loss in the long-term is more likely to be due to what they eat after reverting to normal eating than to the diet they followed while losing the weight.

A psychologist and obesity expert has devised this program, and its strength lies not in the actual diet recommended but in the many suggestions given for behavioral management in relation to eating and appetite. This section of the book is the most helpful.

14-day Beauty Boot Camp

Quick weight loss

- ⊗ **Are special products required?**
- ⊘ **Is eating out possible?**
- ⊘ **Is the plan family-friendly?**
- ⊘ **Do you have to buy a book?**
- ⊘ **Is the diet easy to maintain?**

HOW IT CLAIMS TO WORK
This diet is low in sugar, and high in protein, complex carbohydrates, fiber, and vegetables. Drinking water is an important element in the program.

According to the author, water helps convert food to energy and drinking plenty of cold water can burn up to 250 extra calories each day and can give a feeling of fullness.

THE REGIMEN
In addition to eating three times a day, plus a snack, which will provide about 1,000–1,200 calories, you are advised to drink 8–10 glasses of ice water daily, flavored with lemon or lime juice. Drinking three cups of green tea daily is also recommended for its antioxidant effect (*see p.20*) and some coffee is allowed. You should not eat dinner after 8p.m. or in the three hours before going to bed, to prevent overeating and to help you feel more alert in the morning. Eating high-fiber foods is also recommended to satisfy hunger and suppress appetite.

IS IT HEALTHY?
Of all the quick weight-loss diets, this offers the most healthful suggestions. Eating high-fiber foods and plenty of

---

14-DAY BEAUTY BOOT CAMP

Breakfast
- 1 cup bran flakes with ⅔ cup blueberries
- 8floz (240ml) fat-free milk or soymilk

Lunch
- Pizza: half pita pocket topped with 1oz (28g) shredded mozzarella cheese, 1 chopped tomato, oregano, garlic powder, Italian seasoning, and black pepper
- 1½ cups salad of mixed greens, carrots, tomatoes, and celery, with 2 tbsp fat-free dressing or balsamic vinaigrette

Dinner
- 14oz (390g) broiled chicken or fish, with 2 cups cooked vegetables, drizzled with lemon, and 1 small baked potato topped with 1 tsp plain yogurt

Snacks
- 1 medium apple
- 2 tbsp reduced-fat peanut butter

---

vegetables, including low-fat and fat-free regular milk and soymilk, and drinking 8–10 glasses of water every day will all definitely help you feel good and probably look better.

This diet allows only 1,000–1,200 calories per day. Since this is likely to be less than your usual intake, the diet will promote weight loss, assuming you follow the plan and limit portion sizes. Drinking lots of water and eating plenty of high-fiber foods may help curb your hunger, although it is unlikely that water actually burns calories.

You should keep in mind that any weight loss you experience during the first two weeks of any diet is usually water weight, so you would need to continue to follow this program for more than two weeks to see any more permanent changes in your weight.

You should also take a multivitamin and mineral supplement, as well as calcium, while following this program.

Cambridge Diet

Low-calorie, liquid meal replacement

- ⊘ **Are special products required?**
- ⊗ **Is eating out possible?**
- ⊗ **Is the plan family-friendly?**
- ⊗ **Do you have to buy a book?**
- ⊗ **Is the diet easy to maintain?**

This program is based on eating only specially manufactured, low-calorie foods that are designed to provide 100 percent of the recommended daily allowance (DRI) of all vitamins, minerals, and trace elements.

HOW IT CLAIMS TO WORK
This very low-calorie diet—in which the dieter consumes about 400 calories a day—involves drinking shakes for at least the first two weeks. This "sole source" period is marked by rapid weight loss because of the ketosis that results from the low-carbohydrate content and severely restricted calories (*see p.168*).

THE REGIMEN
For the first two weeks, you are allowed to drink three or four shakes every day (the shakes are available in eight flavors).

<table>
<tr><td colspan="1">CAMBRIDGE DIET: SOLE SOURCE</td></tr>
</table>

CAMBRIDGE DIET: SOLE SOURCE

Breakfast
• High-protein shake

Lunch
• High-protein shake

Dinner
• High-protein shake

Snacks
• Not allowed

You are also encouraged to drink 48floz (2 liters) of calorie-free fluids daily. After two weeks, you may introduce the specially formulated bars and soup.

The diet recommends remaining on the 400-calorie regimen for a maximum of eight weeks. After achieving your target weight, you follow a maintenance plan, which can include varying calorie levels (from 800–1,500 calories daily) and incorporates regular foods.

IS IT HEALTHY?

Very low-calorie diets with liquid meal replacements are effective for weight loss because of the dramatic reduction in calories, but these diets are particularly ineffective in promoting long-term weight maintenance. In fact, once they return to eating regular food, most people regain all the weight they have lost—and in many cases more.

Very low-calorie diets, such as this one, have been shown to create mineral imbalances that can result in sudden death and they should therefore be undertaken only under the supervision of a medical professional. Currently, the products associated with this diet are available via independent counselors who provide screening, advice, and monitoring. However, it is unlikely that these counselors are medically qualified, since most health professionals do not advocate such programs for weight loss.

If you decide to follow this program, make sure that you have a complete physical and discuss your plans with your doctor. It may be better to drink two shakes a day and to eat a well-balanced meal and healthy snacks to decrease hunger cravings.

Herbalife

Low calorie, liquid meal replacement

- ✅ **Are special products required?**
- ✅ **Is eating out possible?**
- ❌ **Is the plan family-friendly?**
- ❌ **Do you have to buy a book?**
- ❌ **Is the diet easy to maintain?**

This is another weight-loss program based on replacing meals with specially manufactured, low-calorie replacements and supplements, including shakes, soups, and bars.

HOW IT CLAIMS TO WORK

The Herbalife diet promotes weight loss by limiting your intake of calories to about 1,000 calories per day, with meal replacement drinks and bars. It also claims to lower fat absorption through the use of "fat-burning" pills and to produce feelings of satiety by taking Herbalife fiber supplements. The authors of this program claim to have helped many people lose significant amounts of weight.

THE REGIMEN

Herbalife sells products designed for people following their "Green" and "Gold" weight-loss plans. Both plans require replacements of two meals a day with liquid supplements, soups,

HERBALIFE (GOLD PLAN)

Breakfast
• Herbalife protein bar
• Piece of fruit

Lunch
• Herbalife shake
• Large green salad

Dinner
• Herbalife shake
• Large green salad
• Steamed vegetables

Snacks
• Herbalife soup mix
• Herbalife roasted soy nuts
• Piece of fruit

or bars. Both also prescribe specific vitamin, mineral, herbal, and fiber supplements. The Gold plan offers a high-protein, low-carbohydrate shake for people who are carbohydrate-sensitive. In addition to the shakes and soups, dieters are encouraged to eat steamed vegetables and/or green salad at mealtimes, and to snack on fruit once or twice a day.

IS IT HEALTHY?

This program is an expensive way to lose weight, and it does not teach you how to eat sensibly in the long-term. You are required to buy not only drinks or shakes, but also bars, soups, and an array of vitamins, minerals, and fiber supplements. A few of the supplements contain ephedrine, an ingredient that has caused some deaths and is likely to be banned by the US Food and Drug Administration (FDA).

SlimFast

Low-calorie, liquid meal replacement

- ✅ **Are special products required?**
- ✅ **Is eating out possible?**
- ❌ **Is the plan family-friendly?**
- ❌ **Do you have to buy a book?**
- ❌ **Is the diet easy to maintain?**

This plan is based on reducing total calorie intake by replacing two meals and snacks each day with specially manufactured, low-calorie products including SlimFast shakes in various flavors, soups, and bars.

HOW IT CLAIMS TO WORK

The program is based on a daily intake of 1,200–1,500 calories which should promote weight loss in most people. The program suggests eating slimfast meal replacements with one sensible meal each day, and it emphasizes portion control when planning your main meal and follows standard nutritional guidelines (*see pp.70–73*). SlimFast also advocates 30–60 minutes of exercise per day. Their website gives information on lifestyle changes, exercise plans, healthy meal and snack ideas, and achieving long-term weight maintenance.

SLIM-FAST

Breakfast
- SlimFast shake or bar
- 4floz (120ml) orange juice

Lunch
- SlimFast shake or bar
- 1 medium fresh fruit

Dinner
- 4–6oz (110–170g) lean meat with medium baked potato, 1 cup steamed vegetables, and 1 cup salad
- 1 medium fresh fruit

Snacks
- 2 cups air-popped popcorn
- 1 medium fresh fruit
- 1 cup fresh vegetables
- SlimFast bar

THE REGIMEN

The SlimFast plan does not advocate using their products as the sole source of nutrition, but recommends eating at least 1,200 calories per day, since fewer may cause unhealthy, rapid weight loss. They recommend losing no more than 2lb (0.9kg) per week after the first week. The diet plan suggests limiting alcohol consumption and how often you eat out, and controlling portion sizes.

IS IT HEALTHY?

This plan will promote weight loss and may be helpful for people who eat on the run and need quick meals, but want to avoid fast-food restaurants. The shakes and soups are quick and easy to prepare. However, your diet will be low in calcium and most other minerals, and drinking shakes and bars every day will become monotonous after a while, making the diet difficult to maintain.

Essentially, the SlimFast diet promotes weight loss by cutting down on calories. The key to long-term success with this diet is the sensible evening meal, which limits portion sizes and does teach you how to eat healthy, at least at dinner. SlimFast has data showing successful weight loss and effective management from people who have followed this diet for several years.

Fat-Flush Plan

Detox

- ✅ Are special products required?
- ❌ Is eating out possible?
- ❌ Is the plan family-friendly?
- ✅ Do you have to buy a book?
- ❌ Is the diet easy to maintain?

This is a detox diet aimed at cleansing your liver of toxicity, which contributes to weight gain and other conditions, including cellulitis, high blood pressure, and mood swings.

HOW IT CLAIMS TO WORK

Claiming to melt fat from the hips, waist, and thighs in just two weeks, this diet's underlying theory is that "hidden weight gain" is caused by five factors:
- Liver toxicity
- Waterlogged tissues
- Fear of eating fat
- Excess insulin
- Stress fat.

The author claims that liver toxicity (caused by caffeine, sugar, trans fatty acids, medications, certain herbs, and lack of dietary fiber) is responsible for weight gain, cellulitis, bloating, elevated blood pressure and blood cholesterol levels, mood swings, and skin rashes.

The author also claims that fear of eating fat results from consuming the wrong types of fat (saturated), while excess insulin results from excessive intake of refined carbohydrates.

The book also states that some medical researchers have suggested high levels of cortisol (a hormone that is produced in stressful situations) in the blood is linked to abdominal obesity, which they refer to as stress fat.

THE REGIMEN

The plan recommends special fat-flush supplements and a drink claimed to cleanse the system, enable natural weight loss, and help melt away accumulated fat. The drink is made from unsweetened cranberry juice with purified water and psyllium or ground flaxseed, hot water, and lemon juice. You have the drink when you rise, mid-afternoon, and 20 minutes before you eat lunch and dinner.

Other foods are included for claimed detox properties, such as red meat for l-carnitine; eggs for taurine, cysteine, and methionine; and cruciferous vegetables, garlic, onions, and some specific herbs (dandelion root, milk thistle, turmeric, and Oregon grape root).

Flour, sugar, margarine, shortening (and all products containing these), artificial sweeteners, and caffeinated beverages are not allowed.

The diet is divided into three phases:
- Phase 1—the weight-loss phase—during which the liver detoxification is primary and about 1,200 calories a day are consumed.
- Phase 2, during which 1,200–1,500 calories are allowed, is a transition to a more long-term diet.
- Phase 3, when 1,500 calories are allowed, is a long-term lifestyle diet.

IS IT HEALTHY?

If you decide to go on the Fat-Flush Plan because you are looking to "flush" or "melt" fat from your body, you are likely to be disappointed. Aerobic exercise, such as running, biking, swimming, and aerobic dancing, is the only proven way to burn body fat.

FAT-FLUSH PLAN

Breakfast
- 2 scrambled eggs with ½ cup spinach, green peppers, scallions, and parsley

Lunch
- 4oz (110g) broiled salmon with lemon and 1 cup asparagus
- ½ cup mixed green salad with ½ cup broccoli florets, ½ cup cucumber, and 1 tbsp flaxseed oil for dressing

Dinner
- 4oz (110g) broiled pork chop, with a pinch of mustard powder, and 1 cup steamed kale
- Baked summer squash with 1 tbsp flaxseed oil

Snacks
- ½ large grapefruit
- 1 apple

The concept of liver toxicity is often used by alternative practitioners to explain a variety of common problems, but there is little evidence to support the idea that the liver is responsible for "hidden weight gain." The regimen proposed to improve liver toxicity is an extreme diet and may be beneficial to only a very small number of people, although the drink may provide some vitamins and minerals.

Eliminating dairy, wheat, sugar, and yeast-containing foods may be helpful for people who are affected by food sensitivities or food allergies, but how this relates to weight loss is questionable. It is difficult to eliminate these foods entirely from your diet, so if this is necessary because of allergies, you may lose weight simply because you have cut your calorie intake.

The most beneficial advice that this diet offers is to increase water and add flaxseed oil because of its high content of omega-3 fatty acids.

Juice Fasts

Detail

Detox

⊗ **Are special products required?**
⊗ **Is eating out possible?**
⊗ **Is the plan family-friendly?**
✔ **Do you have to buy a book?**
⊗ **Is the diet easy to maintain?**

This diet claims that fruit- and vegetable-juice fasts cleanse the body of harmful toxins. Juice Fasts recommends freshly squeezed juice from organic produce, rather than pasteurized varieties, which should be avoided.

HOW IT CLAIMS TO WORK
This plan claims to offer a safe and easy way to detoxify the body and lose weight. It claims that fruit and vegetable juices are concentrated nutritional elixirs easily assimilated and that the nutrients present in juices bind with harmful toxins and carry them out of your body.

THE REGIMEN
You are allowed to drink as much fruit and vegetable juice as you like, made from a range of produce, at any time of

day. The recommended amounts vary from 8–16floz (240–500ml), but not more than 20floz (600ml) in one serving.

Fruits such as apples, pears, grapes, and watermelon contain high amounts of water and this, it is claimed, will flush your digestive tract and kidneys and purify your bloodstream.

Advocates of juice fasting also claim that fruits have a purging effect on the liver and gallbladder. Pineapple, for example, contains the enzyme bromelian, which encourages the secretion of hydrochloric acid from the body and helps digest protein. Many other claims are made for the detoxifying effect of fruit and vegetable juices. For example, grapes and apples are potent cleansing agents; watermelon juice is a diuretic (increases urine production); prune and apricot juice are natural laxatives that help promote bowel movement; and cabbage juice is soothing for intestinal gas and ulcers.

Some fruits, such as papaya, coconut, banana, strawberry, peach, cantaloupe, honeydew, plum, and avocado, do not release water when they are blended so they are better eaten whole. Dried fruits can be added to improve the nutritional content of juice.

Vegetable and fruit juices can be combined. For example, carrot can be combined with apple, alfalfa, ginger, watermelon, and lemon rind.

You can also prepare green juices, which are claimed to heal, stabilize, and calm the body and give energy by relaxing and centering. Examples of green juice combinations include celery and spinach; celery, spinach,

JUICE FASTS

Ingredients for one day's juice:
- 4floz(120ml) grape juice
- ½ cup beets
- 2 bunches carrots
- 1 red bell pepper
- 4–5 stalks celery
- Handful spinach
- 1 garlic clove
- ⅕ habanero pepper

Snacks
- Fruit or vegetable juice

and tomato; cabbage, celery, and tomato; and celery, spinach, cabbage, dill, tomato, lemon, garlic, ginger, cayenne, and tamari. Only one green juice should be consumed per day.

IS IT HEALTHY?
Fasting has been recorded throughout history as part of many different religious practices. However, fasting to detoxify your body or to get you started on a quick weight-loss program has become very popular in recent years. Juice fasting should not be continued for more than three days, because you will not take in adequate protein and may become lightheaded and dizzy as a result of the low-calorie level and inadequate sodium intake. Because of the high carbohydrate content, juice fasting is not an appropriate diet for people with diabetes.

A number of weight-loss programs advocate a juice fast combined with high-protein foods to help achieve immediate weight loss. However, such diets should not be followed by people with high blood pressure, diabetes, cardiovascular disease, kidney stones, gout, or high uric-acid levels in the blood, because of the high protein and carbohydrate intake.

Living Beauty Detox

Detox

✔ **Are special products required?**
⊗ **Is eating out possible?**
⊗ **Is the plan family-friendly?**
✔ **Do you have to buy a book?**
⊗ **Is the diet easy to maintain?**

This detox program, aimed specifically at women, proposes internal cleansing as a means of achieving exterior beauty. It claims that the body's appearance is a reflection of inner well-being.

HOW IT CLAIMS TO WORK
According to Living Beauty Detox, a woman's physiology fluctuates daily, weekly, monthly, and annually, and the program provides seasonal guides for

LIVING BEAUTY DETOX: TYPE I

On rising
- Living Beauty Elixir
- 2 high-fiber supplements
- 16floz (480ml) water

Before breakfast
- 8floz (240ml) dandelion-root tea

Breakfast
- ½ grapefruit
- 2 boiled eggs
- ½ cup steamed kale and ½ cup red bell peppers with 1 tbsp chopped fresh thyme

Lunch
- 4oz (110g) broiled spring-lamb patty and 1½ cups watercress and mung-beansprout salad, with dressing of flaxseed oil, lemon juice, and chives

Mid-afternoon
- 16floz (480 ml) water

4 p.m.
- 1½ cups strawberries

Dinner
- 4oz (110g) poached salmon with ½ cup Brussels sprouts and 1½ cups salad (parsley, tomatoes, and scallions) with dressing of flaxseed oil, fresh lime juice, and mint

Mid-evening
- Living Beauty Elixir
- 2 high-fiber supplements
- 16floz (480 ml) water

Snacks
- As specified

hormonal, nutritional, emotional, and spiritual balance throughout her life. Seven elements are proposed as the foundation of the program:
- A cleansed, detoxed system to maintain liver function.
- Purified water to dilute toxins and flush the body.
- Powerful proteins to maintain healthy skin, hair, and nails.

- Beautifying oils, such as omega-3 in order to stabilize blood sugar and suppress appetite.
- Energizing, immune-boosting organic fruits and vegetables to limit bloating.
- Revitalizing vitamins, minerals, and protective antioxidants.
- Balanced hormones.

Living Beauty Detox claims that by including the seven elements in their diets and eliminating manufactured and/or hydrogenated oils (see p.38), sugar, caffeine, alcohol, and refined white-flour products, women will rejuvenate their inner wellness and reveal their outer beauty.

THE REGIMEN
Lasting from three days to two weeks, this diet of balanced fruits, vegetables, and lean protein with supplements of vitamins, minerals, antioxidants, herbs, and spices is complemented by a specially made elixir that is designed to cleanse the body of harmful pollutants. You are encouraged to drink plenty of water and dandelion tea.

Each season, women should analyze their appearance to identify their type and discover sources of underlying internal imbalance. The appropriate detox diet should be maintained during each season of the year.
- Type 1 manifests symptoms of toxin-overload in the spring.
- Type 2 will be susceptible in the summer months.
- Type 3 is vulnerable in autumn.
- Type 4 exhibits imbalance in the winter months.

IS IT HEALTHY?
This plan is time-intensive and may be costly to follow. It is also low in carbohydrates, which makes it quite difficult to maintain.

The human body is designed to maintain a balance between internal and external environments. The skin, lungs, and immune system provide an external barrier, while the liver, kidneys, and gastrointestinal tract cleanse the body of metabolic wastes or toxins. A diet rich in fruits, vegetables, whole grains, and lean protein and dairy products, complemented by regular exercise, should be adequate to

maintain normal, healthy physiological function. If your body's innate detox systems are compromised by illness or disease, an extreme or alternative dietary regimen may do more harm than good by placing your organ systems under further stress. In such circumstances, you should consult your doctor or a registered dietitian, who will formulate an appropriate diet for your needs.

Detox Diet

Detox

- ✖ Are special products required?
- ✔ Is eating out possible?
- ✖ Is the plan family-friendly?
- ✔ Do you have to buy a book?
- ✖ Is the diet easy to maintain?

According to Dr. Elson M. Haas, the author of this plan, detoxification is the missing link in the North American diet and she recommends this diet as a way of losing weight and improving health.

HOW IT CLAIMS TO WORK
This detoxification plan claims to renew health, increase energy and vitality, as well as promote weight loss. Dr. Haas is a practicing physician of integrated medicine and the founder and medical director of the Preventive Medical Center in California. She believes that health problems often arise from nutritional deficiencies, or from congestion resulting either from a reduced ability to eliminate toxins from the body or from the over-consumption of substances such as caffeine, alcohol, nicotine, refined sugar, and food chemicals.

Dr. Haas claims that people who are deficient in a variety of nutrients may experience problems such as fatigue, coldness, hair loss, or dry skin. Such people need to be nourished with wholesome foods and to follow a detox diet to aid healing.

Congestive problems include acute and chronic diseases that result from clogging of tissues and tubes and the suffocating of cells and vital energy. Colds and flu, cancer, cardiovascular diseases, arthritis, and allergies are all examples of congestive disorders.

Dr. Haas claims that such problems may be prevented or treated, at least in part, and often dramatically improved by cleansing and detoxification.

Dietary changes, including more fruits, vegetables, and water, fewer animal fats and proteins, and the elimination of damaging substances from the body, mark the beginning of a rejuvenation process for the human body.

THE REGIMEN

The plan includes three meals a day with drinks including vegetable water and water with lemon juice in place of snacks. Special guidelines include:
• Chewing your food thoroughly and taking time when you are eating.
• Relaxing a few minutes before and after a meal.
• Eating in a comfortable sitting position.
• Consuming plenty of steamed fresh vegetables and some fresh greens.
• Drinking only herbal teas after dinner.

Dr. Haas recommends following this diet for 5–7 days and explains that

DETOX DIET

Breakfast
• 1 medium fresh fruit

15–30 minutes later
• 1½ cups cooked whole grain, sweetened with 2 tbsp fruit juice

11 a.m.
• 8–16floz (240–480ml) vegetable water with a little sea salt

Lunch
• 1½ cups steamed vegetables, including carrots, green beans, and broccoli

3 p.m.
• 8–16floz (240–480ml) vegetable water with a little sea salt

Dinner
• 1½ cups steamed asparagus, zucchini, and onions

Snacks
• Not allowed

although you may feel a little weak or have a few symptoms for the first couple of days, this stage will pass. Symptoms may include irritability, fatigue, flulike feelings, headaches, and mild sinus congestion. Clarity and feeling good should appear by the third or fourth day, if not before.

If you start to feel weak or hungry while you are following this diet, assess your intake and elimination of fluids. If necessary, you can eat a small portion of protein food (3–4oz/85–110g) in the mid-afternoon. This could be fish, free-range, organic chicken, chickpeas, lentils, mung beans, or black beans.

IS IT HEALTHY?

The claim that medical problems may be prevented or improved by cleansing and detoxification is not based on any sound scientific evidence. The Detox diet is very low in calories, protein, fat, and carbohydrates. It is therefore rather difficult to maintain and may promote nutrient deficiencies if followed for more than a few days. It is true that making the suggested dietary changes—such as eating more fresh vegetables and fruits, drinking more water, limiting animal fats and animal-based protein sources, and eliminating caffeine, alcohol, nicotine, and refined sugars— will help you feel better and lose weight, but it is questionable whether following the Detox Diet menu several times a year is necessary for optimum health.

Weight Watchers

Weight-loss centers

⊗ **Are special products required?**
✓ **Is eating out possible?**
✓ **Is the plan family-friendly?**
✓ **Do you have to buy a book?**
✓ **Is the diet easy to maintain?**

This popular and comprehensive weight management program is based on a points system for choosing food that promotes healthy weight loss and long-term weight maintenance. In additon, Weight Watchers provides group support and professional counseling, and also encourages regular physical activity.

WEIGHT WATCHERS

Breakfast
• 1 small bagel with 2 tbsp light cream cheese
• 1 cup cantaloupe chunks with honey

Lunch
• 8floz (240ml) Weight Watchers tomato soup
• 7 fat-free saltines
• ½ cup chicken salad with 1 cup mixed greens and baby carrots, with 2 tbsp fat-free ranch dressing
• 1 medium apple

Dinner
• 8oz (225g) grilled salmon fillet with ½ cup mashed potato and 1 cup steamed green beans
• 1 cup reduced-calorie butterscotch pudding prepared with fat-free milk

Snacks
• 3 graham crackers
• 8floz (240ml) fat-free milk
• 8floz (240ml) fat-free, sugar-free fruited yogurt

HOW IT CLAIMS TO WORK

Weight Watchers' aim is to teach people how to modify their lifestyles, with the help of trained counselors and group support. A "Winning Points Plan" assigns every food a number of points based on its fat, fiber, and calorie content. There are no forbidden foods, which allows for flexibility and encourages healthy menu selections. This program facilitates immediate weight loss and enables life-long maintenance of a healthy diet. Weight Watchers At Home and Weight Watchers Online are available for those who are unable or choose not to take part in the weekly group sessions.

THE REGIMEN

There is no weighing or measuring of foods on this program. Instead, each weight-watcher is assigned a daily point quota, to which every food and drink that is consumed contributes. To help the dieter, Weight Watchers also sell

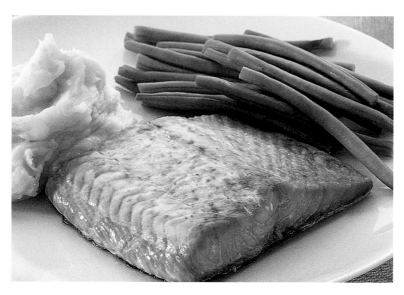

Weight Watchers Eating well-balanced, nutritious meals, such as grilled salmon with mashed potato and green beans, is encouraged by this points-based diet program.

special products, ranging from soups and yogurts to ready meals, but they are not an essential part of the program. Individual quotas are based on BMI (*see pp.26–27*) and the amount of weight to be lost. Dieters may satisfy their daily point quotas by consuming any combination of foods and drinks, but high-calorie foods have higher point values, while healthful foods have lower values. For example:
- 1 slice pizza = 9 points
- 1 scoop ice cream = 4 points
- 12floz (360ml) beer = 3 points
- 1 cup grapes = 1 point.

The plan encourages drinking plenty of water, and allows tea and coffee (with fat-free milk) and low-calorie drinks.

Encouragement to exercise regularly, routine weight plotting, and counselor support are all offered by this program, which teaches life-long habits for healthy eating and exercise.

IS IT HEALTHY?

Weight Watchers allows people to be flexible in their choices of food while teaching healthy habits for weight loss and long-term weight maintenance. The program offers professional advice on

the behavioral aspects of weight control and encourages personal accountability for the lifestyle choices that you make. The regimen thus promotes permanent changes in behavior, which contribute to its resounding success. Menus and recipes incorporate foods from all food groups in balanced proportions, and the meals are easy to prepare, which promotes long-term maintenance of the goal body weight.

Weight Watchers is ideal for people who wish to lose weight steadily and derive benefit from long-term lifestyle reforms. The group sessions are helpful for support and offer an opportunity to meet new people. This program is sensible and highly recommended.

National Slimming Centers

Weight-loss centers

⊗ **Are special products required?**
⊘ **Is eating out possible?**
⊘ **Is the plan family-friendly?**
⊗ **Do you have to buy a book?**
⊘ **Is the diet easy to maintain?**

This program, which promotes weight loss and maintenance in the context of a healthy lifestyle, is well supported in the United Kingdom by a network of

centers with counselors and physicians, but, at present, it is less well known in North America.

HOW IT CLAIMS TO WORK

The plan is based on lowering daily caloric intake and encourages regular exercise to achieve weight loss. It endorses adopting modified eating habits for long-term weight and health maintenance, and promotes a reduced-fat and low-sugar intake along with the avoidance of alcohol. Lessons in food preparation and checking food labels make the adoption of healthy nutritional habits easier, leading to permanent, health-promoting lifestyle changes and long-term weight management.

THE REGIMEN

Anyone who contacts a center is offered a free consultation with a counselor or physician in order to determine whether the program is the best choice for that individual. If you choose to participate in the program, a low-calorie diet with reduced fat and sugar is formulated. Suggestions include using low-fat spread (rather than butter or margarine), lean meats, low-fat dairy products, and fewer processed foods and condiments. Dieters consume three meals per day that contain equal shares of lean proteins (meat, fish, chicken, and

NATIONAL SLIMMING CENTERS

Breakfast
- 1 scrambled egg
- 2 slices toast with low-fat spread
- 8floz (240ml) grapefruit juice

Light meal
- 2 slices ham with lettuce
- 2 slices whole-grain bread
- 8floz (240ml) low-calorie yogurt
- 1 piece of fruit

Main meal
- 1½ cups cooked spaghetti with ½ cup bolognese sauce
- Large green salad with oil and vinegar

Snacks
- Dried apricots

eggs), starchy carbohydrates (bread, potatoes, rice, and pasta), and fruits and vegetables. Dieters can drink tea, coffee, and low-calorie drinks.

National Slimming Centers offer vitamin supplements and supervised swimming and cycling classes to provide a comprehensive healthy living program. Adherence to diet and exercise plans is facilitated by complimentary diet sheets, diaries, and guides.

IS IT HEALTHY?

This program emphasizes changes in behavior as the cornerstone of long-term success. Lifestyle modifications in diet and exercise are the most reliable means of achieving immediate weight loss and long-term weight-management. National Slimming Centers endorse this philosophy and offer excellent options for people committed to changing habits and embracing healthy living. There is ample and accessible support to participants throughout the United Kingdom, but the program is not well-marketed in North America, which limits widespread usage.

Jenny Craig

Weight-loss centers

- ✅ **Are special products required?**
- ✖ **Is eating out possible?**
- ✖ **Is the plan family-friendly?**
- ✖ **Do you have to buy a book?**
- ✖ **Is the diet easy to maintain?**

This program includes ready-made, reduced-calorie meals that are delivered to clients' homes, personal or telephone counseling, and exercise videos.

HOW IT CLAIMS TO WORK

The Jenny Craig plan provides all meals to control calorie intake and promote a new relationship with food. It includes one-on-one counseling and phone consultations to provide support. The plan encourages regular exercise.

THE REGIMEN

Age, height, current and desired weight, and gender determine the optimum daily calorie allowance. Ready-made

meals are available for delivery to your home in 2–4-weekly batches. You are also given a multivitamin and mineral supplement, which you are encouraged to take twice daily. Clients are allowed to personalize their menus to include their favorite foods and to allow for dining out. Planned menus are also available for busy clients who need all their meals provided for them.

Additional fruits, vegetables, dairy products, and whole grains may be consumed with meals or as snacks to satisfy the recommended calorie intake.

Personal counselors are available to help design menus for individuals who prefer more structured diets, while continued contact with a counselor via telephone aids the ultimate goal—the transition from Jenny Craig meals to personal menus designed for weight maintenance. Finally, because regular

JENNY CRAIG

Breakfast
- Six 2½in (6cm) silver-dollar pancakes with reduced-calorie syrup
- 1 vegetarian breakfast patty
- 8floz (240ml) fat-free milk
- 1 medium orange, small grapefruit, medium pear, or ½ cup berries.

Lunch
- 3oz (85g) grilled chicken breast, with 2 tbsp mustard sauce, in whole-wheat bun
- 2 cups green salad with tomatoes and 2 tbsp fat-free dressing
- 1 cup baby carrots

Dinner
- 6oz (170g) steamed flounder
- 1 cup linguine marinara
- 1 cup steamed green beans with lemon juice

Snacks
- 1 cup low-fat macaroni and cheese with 1 cup steamed green beans and carrots
- ½ cup mixed fresh fruit
- 8floz (240ml) fat-free milk

exercise complements a calorie-restricted diet for effective weight-loss, Jenny Craig exercise videos are also available for purchase.

IS IT HEALTHY?

The Jenny Craig regimens are developed and approved by medical professionals, including registered dietitians. These regimens are based on current nutrition research, weight management, and disease prevention.

Jenny Craig clients purchase ready-prepared entrées, thus eliminating daily meal planning and providing examples of healthy portion sizes. While this program is costly if you buy all your meals from Jenny Craig, it can be very convenient for busy people who do not have enough time to shop for and cook healthy foods.

The program is helpful for weight loss because it cuts calories, but long-term weight maintenance is questionable since you may not learn how to shop, cook, and eat healthy foods and control portion sizes. If you have a family, you will also need to consider how to prepare food for the family while you are eating your special meals. Individualized counseling may help with long-term weight management, but you should be aware that most counselors have no formal training in nutrition.

LA Weight Loss

Weight-loss centers

- ✅ **Are special products required?**
- ✅ **Is eating out possible?**
- ✖ **Is the plan family-friendly?**
- ✖ **Do you have to buy a book?**
- ✖ **Is the diet easy to maintain?**

This is essentially a calorie-restricted weight-loss and maintenance program, tailored to individual activity levels, and offering personal counseling during the weight-loss phase.

HOW IT CLAIMS TO WORK

This program, which is individualized according to weight, weight-loss goals, level of exercise, lifestyle, and medical issues, promises that you can eat the

LA WEIGHT LOSS: RED PLAN

Breakfast
- ½ cup egg white substitutes
- 2 slices low-calorie bread
- 1 small orange

Lunch
- 8oz (225g) grilled chicken breast with 1 cup lettuce, celery, and tomato, with 1 tsp oil for dressing
- 1 rice cake

Dinner
- 7oz (200g) broiled halibut with 1 cup broccoli, ½ cup cucumber, and ½ cup brown rice

Snacks
- LA Lite bar
- LA Lite shake made with 4floz (120ml) fat-free milk
- 1 small apple

---

foods you like and still lose weight. An extensive medical history questionnaire is completed at the onset of the program, which offers a three-step guide to weight management. This program consists of weight loss (without loss of lifestyle), weight stabilization, and weight maintenance. Specially formulated bars, shakes, and supplements are available to facilitate the program's sequential process.

THE REGIMEN
The program begins with a three-day high-protein food plan, followed by a calorie-restricted program aimed at a weight loss of 1½–2lb (0.7–0.9kg) per week. All the foods listed are available in regular grocery stores so it is quite easy for you to prepare your own meals. In addition, the program offers ideas for dining out.

Depending on your level of physical activity, you will be prescribed one of three levels of calories; the red, gold, and yellow plans. LA Weight Loss does not advocate exercise, but it does suggest that vitamin and mineral supplements are mandatory for weight loss and long-term maintenance. The plan also offers counseling throughout the weight-loss phase of the program.

IS IT HEALTHY?
LA Weight Loss provides a reduced-calorie meal plan to help control weight. This plan consists of high-protein, low-carbohydrate foods along with food supplements. Personalized counseling is available several times a week, but most of the counselors have no medical or nutritional training and are really just selling supplements, bars, and shakes.

This program is a good option for individuals who may be sensitive to a high-carbohydrate, low-fat diet, but its maintenance requires continued supplementation with costly products and nutrient bars. Weekly weigh-ins are helpful for accountability during all phases of the program.

Nutrisystem

Weight-loss centers

- ✅ Are special products required?
- ❌ Is eating out possible?
- ❌ Is the plan family-friendly?
- ❌ Do you have to buy a book?
- ❌ Is the diet easy to maintain?

This weight-loss plan provides nutritionally balanced, portion-controlled, prepacked meals for dieters. In addition, the plan offers online and telephone counseling as and when required.

HOW IT CLAIMS TO WORK
The plan revolves around prepackaged meals that are in line with traditional guidelines for balanced nutrition, being made up of 60 percent carbohydrate, 20 percent fat, and 20 percent protein, in addition to controlling portion sizes. This leads to weight loss as calories are controlled, while providing a range of food groups. Currently an online weight-management program, Nutrisystem offers dieters telephone, email, and chat-room consultations with agents or diet counselors.

THE REGIMEN
Ready-made Nutrisystem meals offer choices for three meals a day, including breakfast, lunch, and dinner. The plan also suggests snacks. This eliminates personal choice in menu-planning and

standardizes the quantity of food consumed, which reduces deviation from a balanced diet and limits the daily calorie intake. Exercise is highly encouraged, and regular contact with personal counselors is recommended for successful, steady weight loss. Both online and telephone support are available as required.

IS IT HEALTHY?
This program encourages the purchase of most meals online, which may not be possible or appropriate for every dieter. Prepackaged meals may contain high amounts of additives, such as sodium, that are restricted for some individuals. The reliance on prepackaged foods makes this a high-cost program, which is not conducive to long-term dieting. Nor does it teach people how to eat a healthy diet and control portion sizes for themselves.

The long-term effectiveness of the system may also be compromised by the elimination of individual choice in food planning during the weight-loss period. This may cause difficulties for dieters in developing and maintaining balanced diets once they start preparing meals themselves.

NUTRISYSTEM

Breakfast
- Nutrisystem blueberry muffin with banana
- 8floz (240ml) fat-free milk

Lunch
- Nutrisystem Chicken Cacciatore and salad with fat-free dressing
- 15 grapes

Dinner
- Nutrisystem Fettuccini Alfredo and salad with fat-free dressing
- 1 cup broccoli with 1 tsp margarine
- Nutrisystem Chocolate Decadence
- 8floz (240ml) fat-free milk

Snacks
- 4floz (120ml) fat-free yogurt
- 1 apple

Extra help with weight loss

Some people may need extra help to regain control of their weight.

Research shows that weight-loss programs that include behavior-change counseling are the most effective at helping people lose weight. The success of these is probably due to the accountability involved—you know you are going to be weighed at each visit and you will most likely be keeping a food diary, recording everything you have consumed.

Weight-loss centers

Group programs, such as Weight Watchers and individual counseling centers, such as Nutrisystem and LA Weight Loss, provide you with the opportunity for support and monitoring (see pp.194–197). The best program for you depends on when you would like to attend the sessions and your level of comfort at sharing your experiences with a group. For example, if you like meeting people and do not mind opening up about your progress and pitfalls, Weight Watchers would be a good choice.

The important considerations for sticking to a program include finding the right counselor who will listen and get to know you, rather than just try to sell you products; convenience of location; and selecting a program that includes a maintenance plan for at least a year after you have achieved your goal weight. Remember, with any weight-loss center, even if you do

not lose weight every week, at least you are focusing on healthy eating and feeling better.

Seeing a nutritionist

If you seek professional help for weight loss, seeing a nutritionist or dietitian is a good option, especially if you have a medical condition such as diabetes or cardiovascular disease. Ask your doctor for a referral or contact the American Dietetic Association for a registered dietitian in your local area (see p.326). Your insurance may cover these visits if medically necessary.

Other options you can try for help with weight loss include medically supervised residential programs and weight-loss camps for children (opposite). Both of these options are expensive but are effective in helping you lose weight.

Seeking medical advice When excess weight or obesity is seriously undermining health, a nutritionist can help formulate the most appropriate therapeutic approach.

Is there a fat gene?

We have all heard that obesity runs in families: children with two obese parents are almost twice as likely to become obese as children with one obese parent.

The genetics of obesity, however, are very complex. What your genes determine is your metabolism—the rate at which your body burns calories. We all know someone who can eat whatever they want and never gain weight, while for others just looking at sweets seems to add weight. Only some of this difference is determined by genes.

Despite recent news heralding the discovery of the "fat gene," genetics accounts for no more than one third of variations in body weight. Since there has been no change in the human gene pool over the past decade, the dramatic increase in the prevalence of obesity both in children and adults in North America is likely to be a reflection of environmental rather than genetic influences.

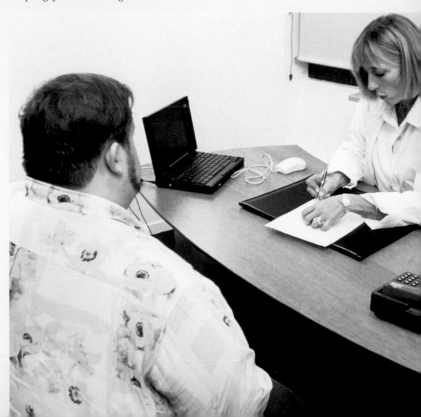

Where can I go for help?

If you know that your weight has become out of control, but you cannot find the motivation and commitment to change your eating and activity patterns in the long-term way that is essential for real weight control, you may look for outside sources of help. For those who can afford it, a personal trainer will create a tailor-made exercise program and coach you while you achieve your goals.

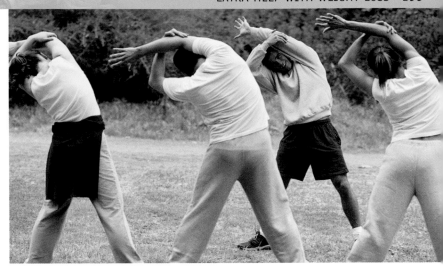

MEDICALLY SUPERVISED CENTERS

Staying in a medical clinic for a week to a month may be helpful if you have severe health problems and need to get motivated. What and how much you eat is strictly controlled, and your time is taken up with a choice of activities, including exercise, relaxation therapy, and nutrition classes. You will lose weight and your health will improve, but unless you continue the regime once you are back home, it is likely to rebound quickly. Serious weight loss requires long-term commitment to a change of lifestyle, involving eating healthily and exercising regularly.

CHILDREN'S WEIGHT-LOSS CAMPS

Eating healthy food for six to eight weeks, having limited access to junk food, and being physically active all day has been shown to produce 2–4lb (0.9–1.8kg) weight losses per week for children who

Intensive program A stay in a residential establishment may help get you started on a weight-loss program, but the lessons learned must be continued in normal life.

attend weight-loss camps. Parents must also show commitment to their children's eating and lifestyle habits in order for them to carry forward into normal life the lessons they learned in the camps.

Surgical and pharmacological treatment of obesity

In particularly severe cases of obesity, when conventional diet and exercise approaches have failed, surgery or treatment with medications may be considered. These are undertaken under the strict supervision of doctors working closely with your dietitian.

Surgical treatment There are surgical options to treat obesity. To qualify, you must have a BMI of more than 35 (see pp.26–27), a history of failed weight loss, and no history of substance abuse or psychiatric disorders.

The most common surgical method, known as a gastric bypass, involves "stapling" the stomach, thus limiting and controling intake of food. This procedure typically results in a weight loss of between 25 and 50 percent of body weight, which is generally well maintained. Patients must be able to follow a strict post-surgical diet that includes eating very small amounts of food, mostly protein, for the first 6 weeks, and taking vitamins and minerals daily.

Side effects include malabsorption of nutrients, undernutrition, and dumping syndrome—a condition in which food passes too rapidly from the stomach to the intestine, causing sweating, fainting, and palpitations.

Medication Recently, the Food and Drug Administration have approved two different medications. They are: sibutramine (Meridia) and orlistat (Xenical). Sibutramine is a serotonin and norepinephrine reuptake inhibitor (SNRI) that works by decreasing food intake. It should not be taken by people who are also taking selective serotonin reuptake inhibitors (SSRI), such as Prozac. Nor should it be taken by those with a history of cardiovascular disease or those taking monoamine oxidase inhibitors (MAOI).

Orlistat blocks the breakdown of triglycerides in the stomach and intestine. This results in about 30 percent of ingested fat remaining unabsorbed, to be excreted in the stool. People taking orlistat have to follow a low-fat diet to minimize side effects. The drug is not suitable for pregnant or breast-feeding women, or for those with problems absorbing nutrients or with liver problems such as cholestasis.

Over-the-counter products Many weight-loss products are available over the counter, but their safety and effectiveness have not been confirmed by clinical trials.

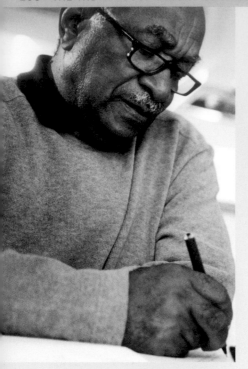

Planning ahead If you are trying to lose weight, make a list of your goals before you start. In addition, keep a food diary to help you identify your habits.

Your personal diet plan

Set realistic goals that you can achieve and maintain over time.

Many people lose weight by going on a very low-calorie diet for a short period; but once they start eating normally, the weight piles back on. This is because they have not changed their eating habits or tastes, their activity level, or reset their "set point" (see p.204).

Setting realistic goals

Once you have decided to make a change (see pp.30–31) and start a new diet or exercise program, try to set realistic targets. The key to losing weight and keeping it off is to set goals that you can achieve and maintain. Once you have achieved these goals one step at a time and they have become established, then you can raise your sights higher. When you are trying to lose weight, one percent of your body weight per week is a safe, steady amount to lose. If you lose more than this, you may be losing muscle or fluid and may become weak or dehydrated.

Focus on how you feel

If you are eating less and exercising more, and yet not losing weight, do not give up. There are numerous benefits to eating healthy and being more active. You will feel better, have more energy, and have lower levels of cholesterol in your blood. In addition, you will also have a reduced risk of cardiovascular disease, diabetes, and cancer.

Keys to safe weight reduction

The secret of lifetime weight control is to eat sensibly and maintain an active lifestyle. Here are some tips to help you.

Lead an active lifestyle Aim to be more active in your daily life. Participate in exercises that you enjoy, and aim for variety so you do not get bored.

Follow a balanced diet Do not skip meals: eat three balanced meals a day, including foods from each food group (see pp.72–73). Many diets advocate eliminating one or two food groups, but they do not teach you how to control your eating habits in the long-term.

Eat a healthy breakfast Have a low-fat, high-fiber breakfast, such as whole-grain cereal with fat-free or low-fat milk and some orange juice. Studies show that people who skip breakfast are more likely to eat fatty foods all day long.

Cut back on calories High-protein, high-fat, and high-carbohydrate diets work only because they force people to eat fewer calories. If you want to lose weight you have to eat fewer total calories than you do normally.

Eat healthy fats Most North Americans eat far too much red meat, which is high in saturated fat and calories. Instead, opt for white-meat poultry, fish, shellfish, legumes, eggs, low-fat cheese, and tofu, all of which are excellent sources of protein, nutrients, and healthy fats.

Eat smaller portions North Americans eat larger portions than the citizens of other countries, and we have the highest rates of obesity. Learn to eat until you are satisfied, and then stop.

Snack only when you are hungry If you are hungry between meals, eating a small snack will keep you from making poor food choices at your next meal. Choose healthy snacks like fruits or nuts.

Drink plenty of water Sometimes thirst is misinterpreted as hunger, so you may end up eating when all you really need is a drink. Drinking a large glass of water half an hour before eating will help you eat smaller meals.

Compensate for overindulgence If you eat too much one day, make a conscious effort to eat less for the next few days and try to increase your activity level.

Stop late-night snacking This bad habit can add hundreds of extra calories at a time when you are least likely to burn them off:

● Clean the kitchen right after dinner and try to avoid going back in there.

● If you find yourself drawn to the kitchen during TV commercials, look at a book or magazine instead.

● Exercise often reduces your hunger and will help you sleep better; take a short walk after dinner, ride an exercise bike, or walk on a treadmill.

● If you are so hungry that you cannot sleep, eat a piece of fruit, followed by a glass of low-fat or fat-free milk.

Everyday changes for weight loss

To lose weight, you have to consume fewer calories and exercise more, but it is important that you still obtain the nutrients you need. This means thinking very carefully about what you eat, filling up on nutritious but low-calorie foods and avoiding high-calorie low-nutrient foods such as candy, chips, cookies, and sugary drinks.

Here are some guidelines to help you achieve a balanced diet that will allow you to lose weight while maintaining your health. Every day you need:

At least three servings of vegetables
Vegetables are filling, low in calories, and a valuable source of phytochemicals, which have many health benefits (*see pp.76–77*). Eat vegetables raw or cook using healthy methods such as steaming or microwaving, and skip added fat such as butter, margarine, or cheese. Alternatively, you can stir-fry or sauté, using a small amount of olive or canola oil or a vegetable spray.

At least two servings of fruits Fruits make great between-meal snacks when you are hungry, and are ideal as desserts (*see pp.78–79*). If you like fruit juice, be sure to choose 100 percent real juice and limit it to 4floz (120ml) servings diluted with water.

Six servings of breads and cereals
Select whole-grain varieties, which have more fiber and fill you up more than refined grains (*see pp.74–75*). Include some grains at breakfast, lunch, and dinner and mix with vegetables or legumes to create a protein-rich meal.

Three servings of dairy products High calcium intake has been shown to aid weight loss and prevent weight gain (*see p.63*), but choose low-fat or fat-free sources of dairy products. If you have trouble tolerating milk, look for products with lactase enzyme added (*see p.232*).

Two to three servings of protein There is no need to eat meat every day— particularly red meat. Fish, eggs, dairy products, soy products, and legumes are all good sources of protein and most are low in unhealthy saturated fat. To help you lose weight, choose fish, white-meat poultry with no skin, and lean cuts of meat (*see pp.86–91*).

Tips for eating out

There is no reason to avoid eating out if you are trying to lose weight, but you will need to think carefully about what you order, and about how to avoid consuming more calories in the course of one meal than you really need.

● Have a small snack before setting out for the restaurant so you will not feel hungry when you arrive. You will then be less likely to want an appetizer or bread.

● Listen to your stomach and stop eating when you are full. Ask the waiter to remove your plate once you have finished.

● Order wine by the glass instead of the bottle and learn to make one glass last for the entire meal. If you are thirsty, drink water.

● Ask your server not to bring you any bread, tortillas, and chips, or to remove them if they are already on the table. Most people do not eat bread with their meal at home, so should not when eating out.

Lunch makeover

Going out for lunch often means a visit to a deli restaurant, with a mouth-watering array of meats and other fillings to choose from. However, many of these fillings are very high in saturated fat and calories, and need to be limited if you are trying to lose weight.

It is still possible to enjoy the deli experience by making some judicious changes in what you order.

● Choose a whole-grain bread or roll for your sandwich, rather than a refined-flour variety. In this way, you are adding essential fiber and other nutrients to your lunch.

● Opt for lean meats such as white-meat turkey or chicken rather than corned beef, pastrami, or salami, which are high in saturated fat.

● Add healthy fillings such as lettuce, avocado, tomato, and mustard rather than high-fat ingredients such as processed cheese and mayonnaise.

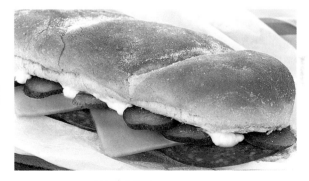

High-fat option
This white-flour roll with salami, processed cheese, gherkins, and mayonnaise has over 1,500 calories, with over 100g of fat, 38g of which is saturated. It also contains 240mg of cholesterol.

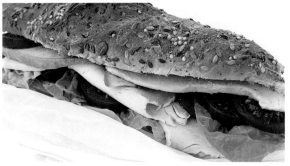

Healthier choice
With 730 calories, this rustic whole-grain roll with turkey breast meat, lettuce, avocado, and tomato has 44g of fat, 8.7g of which is saturated. The cholesterol level (61mg) is low, too.

Regular exercise and weight loss

Exercise is a vital component of any weight-loss program.

According to the US Centers for Disease Control and Prevention, 70 percent of North Americans do not get enough exercise and 40 percent say they never engage in any leisure-time physical activities. Such inactivity carries with it a list of life-threatening ramifications; it is also a major contributing factor in the current epidemic levels of overweight and obesity.

If you are trying to lose weight, increasing your level of physical activity is as important as how much you eat. Physical activity refers to all the bodily movements that result in energy expenditure and includes routine activities such as gardening and walking as well as structured exercise and sports.

Begin gradually

If you have been sedentary for a while, it is advisable to start by gradually increasing the amount of activity in your daily life. For example, walking around your

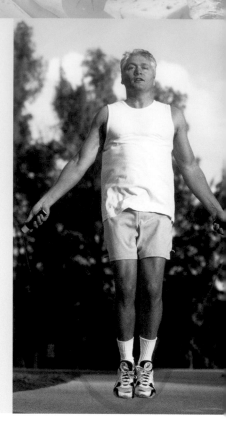

Aerobic exercise Jumping rope is a great workout for the cardiovascular system, as well as helping burn calories. It is even more enjoyable and beneficial if done outdoors.

How to get started

Once you have been cleared by your doctor to begin your exercise program (*opposite above*) and have planned a balanced routine that includes a mixture of aerobic exercise, strength training, and stretching, there are a few points to bear in mind to help you get the most out of your new routine.

SET REALISTIC TARGETS

Remember to start any new exercise program slowly and to increase your efforts gradually. The same holds true when using new exercise equipment. If you start a program that pushes you too hard, you increase your risk of injury and will be less likely to stick with it.

Set short- and long-term goals that are based on your current activity level. If you have not exercised for some time, aim to introduce a little exercise two or three times a week, such as a walk or swim during your lunch break. You can then gradually increase the intensity, duration, or frequency of your exercise sessions as you become more active.

PLAN YOUR PROGRAM

Select an activity you enjoy, get started slowly, and stick with it. The great thing about exercise is that it makes you feel good, so once it becomes a habit, you will not want to miss the opportunity to do it. Aim for a variety of exercises, so you stay motivated.

Choose exercises that will work all your major muscle groups, burn calories, and improve your flexibility. Swimming, cycling, or skipping, and other aerobic exercises will raise your heart rate, improve your cardiovascular fitness, and burn calories.

When you lose weight, the body tends to lose fat and muscle, so it is important for you to preserve muscle mass as you burn calories. Strength training with free weights or resistance machines will help increase your muscle mass and raise your metabolic rate. It also will improve the appearance of your body by toning the underlying muscles.

You should always allow at least five minutes before and after each exercise session for stretches. This activity will help prevent injury and complete your balanced work-out.

DON'T EXPECT INSTANT CHANGE

Do not give up exercising before the benefits start to kick in. People tend to lose motivation at about the two-month mark: they think they should see an improvement in the way they look and feel and, when they do not, they give up, thinking all that sweat and hard work did not make a difference.

In reality, most people will not see a significant improvement until they have been exercising regularly for at least three months. So do not give up. Be patient and hang in there; it is worth the wait and the effort.

And remember, as you build muscle and lose fat, your weight may not change initially but you will know that you are shaping up when your clothes start to fit better. You will also feel better after about three months, even if the scale does not change.

neighborhood or in a local park is a great way to work your body and enjoy the outdoors at the same time. When you do start on an exercise regimen, do so slowly and increase your effort gradually. If you push yourself too hard you risk injury and are more likely to give up. While exercise should be challenging, it is more important that you design for yourself an enjoyable program that you will continue to follow and develop.

Exercises for weight loss

There are many forms of exercise, but if you are trying to lose weight, the perfect prescription includes both anaerobic (strength training) and aerobic exercise. Anaerobic exercise refers to activities that use resistance, such as lifting weights. This type of exercise strengthens, tones, and conditions your muscles, and improves your endurance. It

also increases your lean muscle mass and, as a result of this, raises your metabolic rate, which affects the rate at which your body uses up calories. Because your body tends to lose fat and muscle when you lose weight, it is essential to include anaerobic exercise in your exercise program.

Aerobic exercise, such as dancing and swimming, raises your heart rate and burns calories, especially from fat. Therefore it should form an important component of your weight-loss program.

Maintaining flexibility

While stretching exercises do not directly affect weight, they are an important part of physical fitness. Be sure to include a 5–10-minute warm-up and cool-down before and after your exercise program. This will help you avoid injury and improve flexibility.

Seeking medical advice

It is important for your doctor to give you a physical examination before starting an exercise program, especially if you have any medical problems, are overweight, are over the age of 40, or have not done any exercise for some time.

Your doctor may recommend a stress test to check the blood flow to your heart. During this test, you ride a stationary bike or walk on a treadmill, gradually increasing the effort, while your heart rhythm and blood pressure are monitored. This test is a good indication of any potential problem in the blood supply to your heart, such as a blockage in the arteries. If your stress test is abnormal, you will be advised not to exercise until further tests are performed, in order to avoid any risk of heart attack.

Tips on incorporating activity into your daily routine

In addition to starting on an exercise program at the gym or fitness center, it is important to start incorporating more physical activity into your daily routine. As with all behavioral changes, the aim is to make changes gradually (*see pp.30–31*). Choose just one new activity that you think you can succeed in building into your regular schedule. Only when that has been established should you try to include another one.

• Schedule a 30-minute walk at the same time each day. It may help if you can arrange to exercise with a friend or a family member, or make a special time to take the dog for a walk.
• Take the stairs instead of the elevator at work or when shopping.
• Walk whenever you can instead of driving, including when going to work.
• Get off the bus at the stop before your office and walk the rest of the way.
• Park in the space farthest away from the stores so you have to walk there.

• Do more chores yourself, such as cleaning the house, washing the car, raking leaves, or gardening.
• Invest in some exercise equipment to use at home, such as a stationary bicycle.
• Make time to exercise and schedule it as you would an appointment; many people find that exercising in the morning before the day gets too busy helps them accomplish this goal.
• Buy a fitness video or DVD and get the whole family to join in the routine as a change from watching TV or playing computer games.
• Accustom children to the idea of walking to school or to the bus stop; use the time to talk about what you see and where you are going.

Start them young Get children used to walking places. You can make it fun by playing games such as "I Spy" or "Hop, Skip, and Jump" as you go along.

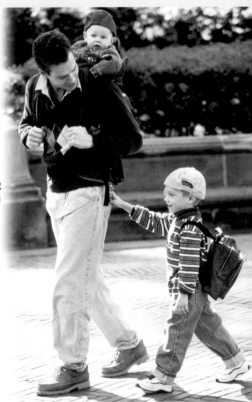

Calories expended in different activities

There are tremendous benefits, both mental and physical, to getting even a small amount of physical activity each day. All activity is good for you (and will burn calories), but it is worth noting that you do not have to be an athlete to be active. Regular activities such as mowing the lawn and playing soccer with the children all count toward keeping fit.

   The amount of calories expended during exercise varies according to your gender and weight. Because of their greater muscle mass, men burn more calories than women while doing the same activity; and the heavier you are, the more calories you will burn. Conversely, when you lose weight, your calorie requirements decrease, even if you continue with the same level of physical activity.

ACTIVITY 30 MINUTES	CALORIES MAN (175LB/80KG)	CALORIES WOMAN (135LB/60KG)
Baseball	334	258
Basketball	280	225
Cycling	334	258
Dancing	188	145
Football	334	258
Gardening	209	161
Hiking	251	193
Horseback riding	167	129
Housework	188	145
Jogging	292	225
Lawn mowing	251	193
Playing with kids	167	129
Skating	292	225
Soccer	292	225
Softball	209	161
Step aerobics	180	140
Stretching/yoga	167	129
Swimming	334	258
Tennis	292	225
Walking	167	129
Weight training	162	127

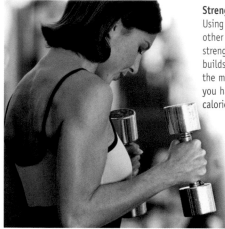

Strength training
Using weights and other forms of strength training builds muscles; and the more muscle you have, the more calories you burn.

How to increase metabolic rate

Metabolic rate is the rate at which your body uses energy to keep it functioning, and it varies among people, depending on age, weight, and fat to muscle ratio.
• The more you weigh, the higher your metabolic rate will be.
• Metabolic rate increases during rapid growth periods, such as adolescence.
• People with a high proportion of body muscle to fat have a higher metabolic rate than those with a lower proportion.

FALSE CLAIMS
Many diets claim to increase metabolic rate through special fat-burning foods and exercises. In fact your metabolic rate falls if you start losing weight.

INCREASING EXERCISE
Exercise is the only effective way to increase your metabolic rate. Not only do we use up calories during exercise, but the increased metabolic rate that occurs while we exercise continues for several hours afterward. The amount that the metabolic increases varies from person to person but even a modest increase will help to counteract the body's natural tendency to decrease metabolic rate.

   It is not known why exercise has this effect, but some researchers believe that exercise preserves more of our lean body tissue as fat tissue is lost during weight loss.

What is "set point"?

Short-term diets are doomed to fail. You may lose some weight but when you return to your usual diet your weight will return to its usual level. This is due to what scientists call "set point"—the level at which the body defends its current weight. If you burn more calories than you eat, your body will become more efficient at converting those calories into energy, so that you will not lose weight. If you are trying to slim, you have to make a serious commitment over a long period in order to retrain your body and readjust your set point.

Benefits of different types of exercises

Whereas physical activity refers to all the body movements that result in energy expenditure, exercise refers to planned and structured repetitive movements designed specifically to improve fitness and health. These include activities you can do at home, in the gym, or outdoors. Whether you do exercise indoors or out, however, it is also categorized according to whether it is aerobic or anaerobic.

AEROBIC EXERCISE

This is defined as any activity that uses large muscle groups, can be maintained continuously, and is rhythmic in nature. It is a type of exercise that overloads the heart and lungs and causes them to work harder than when at rest. Examples of aerobic exercise include running, swimming, dancing, jumping rope, and cycling. This type of exercise has many health benefits, which include:
• Improved cardiovascular function
• Lowered blood pressure
• Increased HDL and decreased LDL
• Reduced body fat and improved weight control
• Improved glucose tolerance and reduced insulin resistance.

ANAEROBIC EXERCISE

In contrast to aerobic exercise, anaerobic exercise involves short bursts of exertion followed by periods of rest, as a result of which you develop muscle strength. Although anaerobic exercise does not burn fat, it contributes to weight loss since bigger muscles burn more calories. Examples of anaerobic exercise include push-ups, stomach crunches, pull-ups, and lifting weights.

FOLLOW A TAILORED PROGRAM

Before starting on an exercise program, it is essential to discuss your aims with a professional who will assess your level of fitness and plan an appropriate program. As you progress, this should be reviewed and adjusted as necessary.

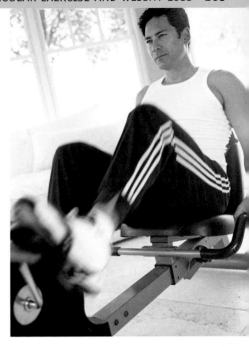

Indoor rowing An ideal aerobic exercise, rowing strengthens the muscles of both the upper and lower body, as well as improving your cardiovascular function.

Case study Overweight middle-aged man needing exercise

Name Danny

Age 45 years

Problem Danny is 50lb (23kg) overweight and his doctor has recently told him that he needs to exercise in order to improve his overall health. He has a family history of cardiovascular disease and diabetes—his mother is obese and has type 2 diabetes and his father has cardiovascular disease.

Lifestyle Danny is a regional manager for a pharmaceutical company, and he travels a lot. He says he does not have time to exercise and believes that he is active enough with his job. Danny is 70in (180cm) tall and weighs 230lb (104kg). His weight has been steadily increasing by about 5lb (2.3kg) each year since he was in college. Because Danny is on the road, driving to visit his sales representatives, he spends most of his day sitting. At night he spends time with his children then returns to his computer in order to check emails and his schedule for the next day. Danny does not own any exercise equipment and he does not belong to a gym.

Advice In order for Danny to begin a regular exercise program, he needs to understand the benefits and decide that he is going to make the effort to change his behavior. First his doctor recommended that he takes a stress test to clear him for exercise. The next step is for Danny to figure out when, where, and how he could be more physically active. For example, since he is traveling and staying in hotels at least once a week, he could bring his exercise clothes and shoes and schedule time to work out while he is away from home. If joining a gym near his house is feasible, this would be a relatively effective method to get more active if he could go at least once a week to start with, before or after work. When he is at the gym, he could walk on the treadmill for about 20–30 minutes and lift weights for about 10–15 minutes. This will help him feel better and give him more energy as well.

If Danny does not think that he has time to go to the gym, before, during, or after work, it might be better for him to purchase a treadmill or exercise bicycle for him to use at home. He could then use it at his convenience, either before or after work, and also on the weekends. As Danny's parents are sick, he should be motivated to listen to his doctor's advice or he is likely to develop health problems. So this is a good time for him to begin an exercise program.

Children and weight management

Overweight in children and adolescents is a serious problem in North America.

According to official figures, the percentage of overweight children in North America aged six to 11 increased from four percent in 1965 to 13 percent in 1999; the figures for those aged 12–19 also show an increase from five percent in 1970 to 14 percent in 1999.

These increases are thought to be due to a variety of cultural factors, including easy access to high-calorie foods, decreased opportunities for exercise, and increased interest in sedentary activities, such as watching TV or sitting in front of a computer. Overweight children are likely to remain overweight as adults and are at risk of the same health problems as adults.

What causes obesity?

Studies suggest that genetics plays a major role in the incidence of obesity. According to current estimates, a child with two obese parents has an 80 percent chance of becoming obese, while a child with just one obese parent has a 40 percent risk.

Children who lead an inactive life are at risk of obesity, especially those who watch more than two hours of TV each day. The large number of food commercials aimed at children during TV programs may be a factor, along with the increase in portion sizes, fast food, and soft drink consumption.

Is my child overweight?

In order to check whether your child's weight is within normal limits, plot his or her BMI score (*see p.113*). A score in the 85–95th percentile indicates that he or she is considered at risk of being overweight; a score above the 95th

Health risks of obesity

Numerous tracking studies have demonstrated that an obese child runs an increased risk of becoming an obese adult. Obese children may be even more obese as adults than they would have been if they had first become overweight in adulthood. Thus, preventing or treating childhood obesity should significantly decrease the likelihood of adult obesity and its associated medical problems.

Overweight and obese children and adolescents are at risk from the same health problems as adults who are overweight (*see p.158*). These problems include diabetes, high blood pressure, high blood cholesterol levels, sleep apnea, asthma, gallbladder disease, bone and joint disorders, and liver problems (*see pp.214–251*).

percentile indicates overweight. A child's progress should be tracked over time, since it is common for overweight prepubertal children to be taller than their normal weight counterparts. Overweight children enter puberty earlier and have their growth spurt earlier.

Weight management rather than dieting is usually the way forward, and there are a number of changes that can be made to cut down on calories and to increase physical activity. However, the greatest influence on a child's habits is his or her parents, so the best thing you can do is lead by example.

Underweight children

Adolescents in particular are also susceptible to eating disorders. These may develop into serious medical problems that require professional help (*opposite*).

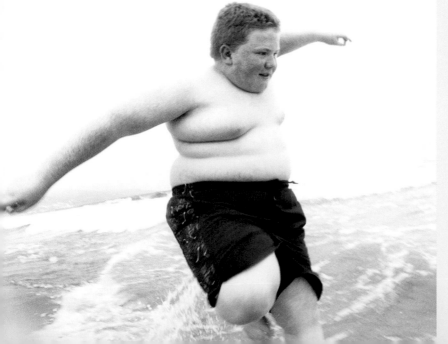

Enjoying physical activity If your child is overweight, help him find physical activities that he enjoys and it will help him if the whole family can participate too.

Focus on eating healthy and being active

The best way you can help your child maintain a healthy weight is to make healthy eating and exercise a normal part of your daily lives.

• Focus on healthy eating, not "dieting." Provide interesting, varied food that all the family will enjoy and be sure to serve fruits and vegetables every day.

• Provide an environment that includes only healthy food choices. Cut down or stop buying unhealthy food, such as chips and soda. It is unfair to expect your child not to eat a food that you or other family members are eating.

• Make eating a sociable and enjoyable occasion; try to eat together, without the television on in the background.

• Drink water or fat-free milk with meals and snacks, rather than soda.

• Serve smaller portions using small plates and cups, and provide more vegetables or a fruit dessert for people to fill up on if they are still hungry.

• Don't force your children to clean their plates: let them be guided by

their appetite and stop eating when they are fully satisfied.

• Limit fast food to less than once a week, and choose carefully. Children who eat a lot of fast food will be eating too much saturated fat, and they may be missing out on important nutrients such as fiber, vitamins, and minerals, especially calcium.

• If your child suffers from allergies or food intolerances, you should consider working with a dietitian for ideas and nutritional advice.

• Encourage your children to find physical activities that they enjoy and take an interest in their progress.

• Look for activities that you can do together as a family.

• Try to build exercise and physical activity into your daily routine.

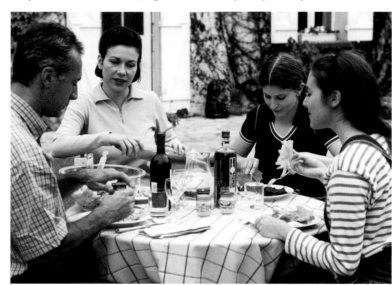

Eating together To encourage healthy eating habits in children, eat together as a family. Offer nutritious food and treat mealtimes as a chance to enjoy one another's company.

Warning signs of eating disorders

Eating disorders most commonly affect adolescents and college-aged women and occur across all the social groups. Figures suggest that about 20 percent of teenagers engage in abnormal eating behavior, while about five percent have a diagnosed disorder.

Those with anorexia nervosa typically have an altered perception of their own body image (*right*) that leads to severe restriction of calories and a resulting loss of weight. Parents should look out for changes in eating behaviors, such as skipping meals and exercising for at least three hours every day. Because anorexia nervosa often leads to the cessation of menstrual periods, it is important for parents to be aware of changes in their daughter's cycle.

Another type of eating disorder, bulimia nervosa, is characterized by episodes of binge eating, followed by purging (*right*). Those affected tend not to lose weight so the problem may be less obvious. You should look for changes in your daughter's teeth. She may complain of heartburn from vomiting and spend a lot of time in the bathroom after meals.

WHERE TO GET HELP

Eating disorders are considered to be psychiatric conditions. Treatment for such disorders is complex and requires a team approach combining medical management, psychological intervention, and nutritional counseling. It is crucial to get a diagnosis first from a psychiatrist familiar with eating disorders.

Jargon buster

Anorexia nervosa This condition, which occurs mainly, though not exclusively, in adolescent girls, involves an intense fear of gaining weight or becoming fat, a disturbed perception of body weight or shape, and doing intensive exercise. The condition leads to changes in hormone levels that affect growth and menstruation.

Bulimia Like anorexia sufferers in terms of concern with weight and body shape, people with bulimia alternate periods of binge eating with strategies to avoid weight gain, such as forcing themselves to vomit and using laxatives.

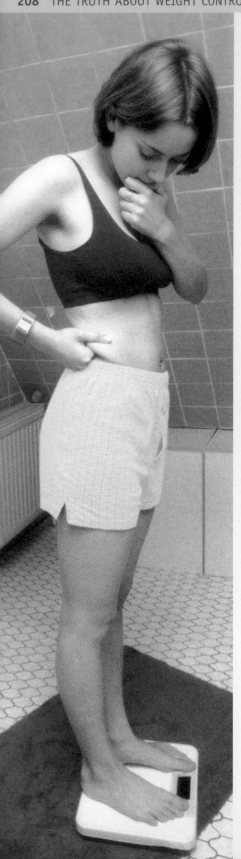

Weight check Being underweight, especially due to unplanned weight loss, may be a cause for concern. Check your weight and seek advice if you are concerned.

When you need to gain weight

Being underweight has as many health implications as being overweight or obese.

Obesity may be major problem in North America, but there are many people who exhibit varying degrees of underweight. For example, adults and teenagers with a BMI below 18.5 (see pp.26–27 and p.113) are considered underweight, as are children with a BMI for their age below the 5th percentile (see p.113).

As with overweight and obesity, being underweight has many health consequences, including impaired wound healing, higher incidences of infection, and possibly pressure sores. If you lose too much weight, you may develop heart problems since heart function declines with severe malnutrition.

Causes of underweight

Unplanned weight loss is often a problem in older people; it is also frequently a sign of serious illness. Some of the most common causes of weight loss include:
• Cancers of the colon, lung, and pancreas, and leukemia.
• Gastrointestinal disorders such as peptic ulcer, inflammatory bowel disease, celiac disease, and chronic pancreatitis.
• Endocrine diseases, such as diabetes and thyroid conditions.
• Infections, such as tuberculosis, fungal disease, parasites, and HIV.
• Psychiatric conditions such as depression, schizophrenia, and Alzheimer's disease often cause weight loss because of poor appetite or forgetting to eat.
• Some medications because they cause loss of appetite, nausea, and diarrhea (see p.153).

Treating underweight

The aim of nutritional therapy is to increase energy intake and to provide essential vitamins and minerals, without increasing the overall volume of food eaten.

Nutritional reasons for failure to thrive in infants

Children whose weight or rate of weight gain is significantly below that of other children of similar age and gender are considered to be failing to thrive. It could be due to medical reasons and you should talk to the doctor, but 80 percent of cases are due to diet and errors in preparing formula. If not caught early, failure to thrive may lead to loss of muscle mass, impaired respiratory and heart function, and a weakened immune system. If caught early, however, delayed growth can be resolved with diet. The main reasons are:

• Being fed over-diluted or improperly prepared formula.
• Being given fat-free or reduced-fat milk instead of full-fat milk between 12 and 24 months of age.
• Inappropriate feeding practice for children, such as the consumption of 12floz (360ml) or more fruit juice every day.
• Being fed foods low in nutrients and high in calories instead of age-appropriate nutrient-dense foods between 12 and 24 months of age.
• Being fed puréed or liquid food at a stage when ready to eat solid food.

How to gain weight

The first step in treating people who are underweight is to identify and address the underlying specific causes of unplanned weight loss. This may involve taking nutritional supplements or medication or undergoing psychosocial therapy.

DEALING WITH WEIGHT LOSS

Weight gain can be much harder to achieve than weight loss, particularly if your appetite is poor or you are feeling nauseous. The target is to increase energy intake and to provide essential vitamins and minerals, without increasing the overall volume of food consumed. Eating frequent, smaller high-calorie nutritious meals and snacks throughout the day allows a greater intake and should prevent further weight loss and promote weight gain if needed.

Nutritional therapy, including dietary education and/or the use of liquid supplements supervised by a dietitian, is usually beneficial. The severity of weight loss should be determined by a nutritional evaluation, which includes laboratory tests combined with a dietary history and evaluation of a person's psychosocial situation.

The goal of nutrient intake in people with low body weight and pronounced weight loss is 30–35cal per 2.2lb (1kg) of body weight per day. At least 20 percent of the calories consumed should come from protein. Malnourished older people and those with mild to moderate illness need to consume 40cal per 2.2lb (1kg) of body weight per day in order to treat underweight.

HELP WITH WEIGHT GAIN

Here are some tips on dietary changes that may help you gain weight:
• Serve butter or margarine with vegetables and use oil-based dressings.
• Add cheese to egg dishes such as omelets and scrambled eggs.
• Add cream, evaporated milk, or whole milk to soups, desserts, and puddings.
• Add fish, or ground meat, chicken, or turkey to tomato-based pasta sauces.
• Use butter or full-fat margarine, or mayonnaise in sandwiches.
• Choose full-fat dairy products rather than low-fat or fat-free varieties.
• Eat at least three times a day, and use a clock to remind you when to eat.
• Snack between meals on slices of cheese, protein bars, peanut-butter sandwiches, avocado or cream-cheese dips, whole-milk puddings, and yogurts.
• Drink whole milk or juices with meals.
• Don't drink too much before eating since this can reduce your appetite.

Liquid supplements

Nutritional supplement drinks can be beneficial for people who are trying to gain weight because each can contains a minimum of 200 calories. They are available with different calorie and protein quantities to suit different needs and may be bought without a prescription in pharmacies and supermarkets.

All of these supplements provide 100 percent of the daily value for vitamins and minerals, most are lactose-free, and a few have added fiber. They are available in a variety of flavors, such as vanilla, chocolate, and strawberry. To enhance their taste, it is usually best to serve the supplements chilled.

Liquid supplements should be used only as part of a balanced diet—they are not intended to provide all your nutritional needs. Most types contain little or no fiber, so they will not improve bowel function or prevent constipation. In addition, they do not contain the phytochemicals that occur in fruits and vegetables, which can help in reducing the risk of cancer and cardiovascular disease.

Tips to boost your appetite

Loss of appetite is a common problem following illness or while taking certain medications or undergoing various therapies. However, these are also the times when your body has most need of good nutrition, to help you regain your strength and boost your immune system. Here are some suggestions for ways of boosting your appetite and helping you look forward to mealtimes.
• Choose different foods each week at the supermarket to add interest and variety to your diet.
• Arrange to go out for lunch or dinner once a week and try new dishes.
• Get together to eat with your family and friends.
• Even if you do not feel very hungry, try to eat something at every mealtime.
• In the summertime, eat outside in the garden, have a picnic, or eat by an open window.
• Make your food look appetizing with different colors and textures on the plate, attractively presented.
• Take time to arrange the table with your best flatware, china, and placemats. Add flowers, too.
• Take a short walk in the fresh air before sitting down to a meal.

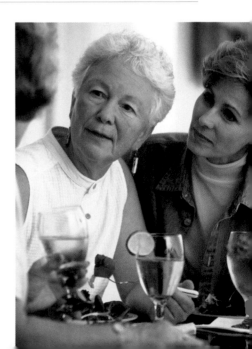

Regaining your appetite Eating with friends and family may help you regain your appetite after a debilitating illness. Sharing a meal remains a pleasant social experience.

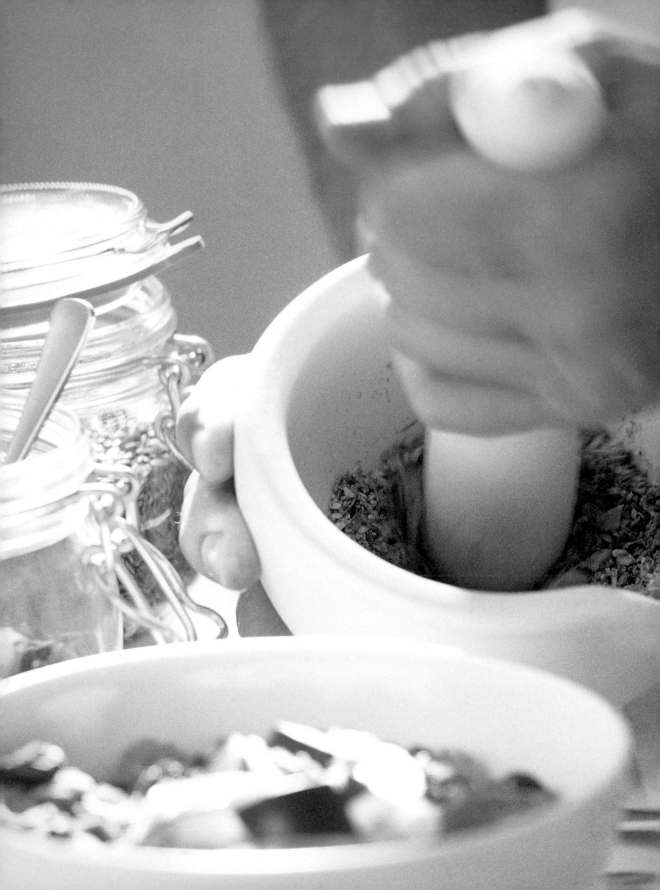

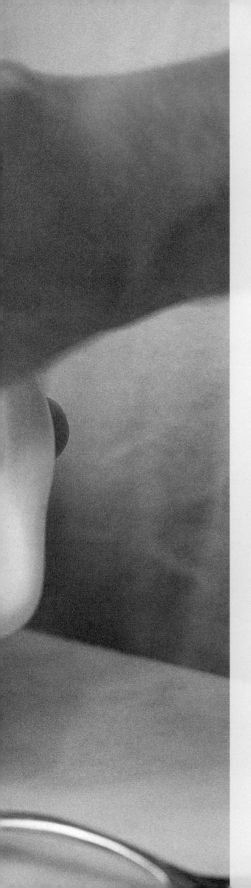

Food as medicine

There is no doubt that healthy eating can make you feel better, improve your quality of life, and even help you to live longer. This chapter looks at the key role that food can play in the prevention and treatment of a variety of diseases and medical conditions.

Improving health through diet

The foods you eat are critical in determining both your current and future health.

This chapter presents an overview for anyone who is interested in preventing health problems. But more important, it is a starting point for improving health if you already have one of the disorders discussed in this chapter.

Protection against disease

Each week, more proof emerges showing that a healthy diet and regular exercise help ward off cardiovascular disease, diabetes, cancer, and osteoporosis. Those who eat healthy throughout their lives are more likely to remain disease-free than those who follow the typical North American diet, which is high in artery-clogging fat and low in nutrients.

Healthy eating can help treat health-related problems. The risk of cardiovascular disease has decreased dramatically in North America as we have reduced our reliance on fatty foods. However, people are still eating more than they should and exercising less, resulting in a rise in obesity rates. As we gain weight the risk of cardiovascular disease rises, and we need to increase our exercise levels and control portion sizes to continue to reduce this risk.

Maintain a healthy weight

Research shows that if you are overweight and lose weight, your life expectancy increases. It also shows that by improving your diet and exercise habits to lose weight, your health will also improve.

Regular exercise, combined with a balanced, nutritious diet, is the key to managing many of the diseases discussed in this chapter.

Aging and diet

As we age, our bodies and our dietary needs change. Ongoing research looking at the impact of calorie restriction on health and longevity indicates that adults can improve their health by eating less. If you are overweight, the reasons for losing weight are clear. But even if you are a "healthy" weight, it may be possible to live longer and live better by eating less. This does not mean starvation, it means making smart choices and eating foods that give maximum nutritional benefit for the calories.

Talk to your doctor

Your doctor is your single best source of advice. The information here should not, therefore, be used to prescribe or provide treatment for yourself. This chapter should serve as a starting point to help you determine the most important dietary changes you can make to improve your health. Seeing a qualified nutritionist can also help you make the required dietary and lifestyle changes that your doctor may have recommended.

Healthy choices At any stage of life, a nutritious, balanced diet can help prevent and, in many cases, treat existing disorders.

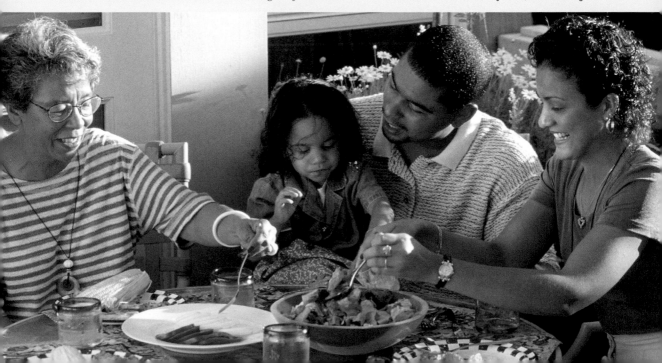

The top 15 super foods

These foods are highly valued for the health-giving, disease-preventing properties of the nutrients they supply.

Blueberries These contain valuable amounts of fiber, vitamin C, and B vitamins. They also contain flavonoids that improve the circulation and aid the body's defenses against infection.

Broccoli This is a star ingredient, rich in vitamins and minerals, particularly vitamin C and beta-carotene, as well as folate, all of which can protect against cardiovascular disease and cancer.

Flaxseed Rich in omega-3 fatty acids, which is beneficial in treating high blood cholesterol and high blood pressure.

Legumes A significant source of soluble fiber, which can help lower cholesterol levels if eaten regularly. They are also high in iron, folate, and potassium.

Low-fat yogurt Rich in calcium, which is vital for bone health, and protein.

Nuts Packed with selenium and vitamin E, nuts can help lower cholesterol levels. Recommended as part of the DASH diet to reduce high blood pressure (*see p.220*).

Oatmeal Oats are a great source of soluble fiber, and can help lower blood-cholesterol levels. They are also a useful source of magnesium and zinc.

Oily fish Tuna, salmon, mackerel, and trout are examples of oily fish and are rich in omega-3 fatty acids, which may help control cholesterol levels.

Olive oil An excellent source of healthy monounsaturated fat, which is good for maintaining levels of "good" cholesterol in the body (*see p.40*).

Oranges This fruit is one of the best-known sources of vitamin C, which may help prevent free-radical damage to the cells and tissues.

Peppers Bell peppers are a great source of beta-carotene and vitamin C, both of which are antioxidants and can help ward off cancer.

Quinoa Originating in South America, this "super" grain is part of the traditional Andean diet. It is gluten-free, and high in fiber and protein.

Red grapes These contain antioxidants that can protect against cancer.

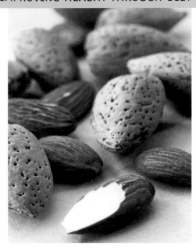

Almonds Considered by many to be the most nutritionally balanced nut, almonds are a good source of protein, vitamin E, and selenium.

Spinach This folate-rich vegetable is also rich in lutein and vitamin E and has antioxidant properties.

Tomatoes Rich in the antioxidant lycopene, tomatoes can help in the fight against cancer. Absorption of lycopene is improved by cooking tomatoes in oil.

Healthy habits to adopt now

Eating a varied diet, based on a wide range of nutritious ingredients, can help control your weight, reduce cholesterol levels, treat infections, and ensure that you get an adequate intake of vital vitamins and minerals.

What you eat and drink Planning your meals is one of the best ways of ensuring that you eat a healthy, well-balanced diet:

• Aim to eat at least five servings of fruits and vegetables every day.

• Cut back on the amount of fat you eat, especially your intake of saturated fat; use monounsaturated or polyunsaturated fats instead.

• Base meals and snacks around whole-grains, including whole-grain bread, brown rice, whole-wheat pasta and cereals—these are low in fat, high in fiber, and will fill you up.

• Choose foods that are a rich source of soluble fiber, such as oats, lentils, peas, corn, and legumes.

• Eat fish regularly—aim for at least three servings a week; one or more of these should be an oily fish (*above*).

• When buying meat, choose lean cuts of meat and poultry.

• Drink or eat at least three low-fat dairy foods a day, such as fat-free milk, low-fat yogurt, and low-fat cheese.

• Reduce your sodium intake and use fresh herbs or milled spices instead to add flavor to your food.

• Drink six to eight 8floz (240ml) glasses of water every day.

How you eat Thinking carefully about your eating habits and behaviors, will help you pinpoint areas where changes could be beneficial to your present and future health:

• Instead of eating on the run, sit down and eat your meal at a table; eating with your family at mealtimes will enhance your enjoyment of food and prevent digestive problems.

• Get into the habit of eating smaller portions and stop eating when you are full; you don't have to clean the plate each time (nor do your kids).

• Snack on healthy foods, such as fruits, or a handful of nuts or seeds; eat less junk food, candy, and sweets, which provide only "empty" calories with no useful nutrients.

• Eat less fast food (no more than once or twice a week), and when you do have it, modify your choices to include healthier options.

• If you love cakes or other sweet treats and find it difficult to eliminate these from your diet, look for low-fat versions and buy small portions.

Cardiovascular disease

The heart and blood vessels can be affected by several disorders.

Cardiovascular disease, which affects the heart and blood vessels, describes any of several disorders, including high levels of cholesterol in the blood (hyperlipidemia), high blood pressure (hypertension), heart attack, and stroke.

What can go wrong
In cardiovascular disease, there is a disruption of the heart's pumping action or the flow of blood through the blood vessels. Arteries can be damaged by high blood pressure and be narrowed by fatty deposits, especially cholesterol, restricting blood flow. A heart attack occurs if the coronary arteries, which supply the heart muscle with blood, become narrowed (coronary artery disease) and blocked. If the flow of blood in the brain is disrupted, it will cause a stroke.

Common disorders
Two very common cardiovascular disorders that can lead to other more serious problems are high blood pressure and high blood cholesterol. If you are at risk of developing, or suffer from, persistent high blood pressure—greater than 140mmHg (systolic) over 90mmHg (diastolic)—then you are putting strain on your heart and arteries.

Elevated levels of total cholesterol (greater than 200mg per dL), LDL-cholesterol, or triglycerides in the bloodstream (see p.23) is known as hyperlipidemia. This condition can lead to a buildup of plaque (deposits of lipids) in the arteries, increasing the risk of inadequate blood supply to parts of the body.

Major cause of death
Cardiovascular disease still ranks as the number one killer in North America despite improvements in diet, advances in medical treatment over the last 20 years, and more

screening, which have all helped reduce the number of deaths. However, you can still significantly reduce your risk of cardiovascular disease by making lifestyle changes such as exercising more, losing weight if you are overweight, and quitting smoking.

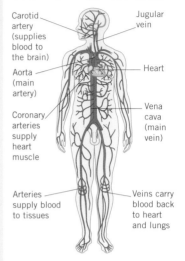

The circulatory system
This includes the heart and blood vessels: arteries, shown in red, carry oxygenated blood; veins, shown in blue, carry deoxygenated blood.

Carotid artery (supplies blood to the brain)

Jugular vein

Aorta (main artery)

Heart

Coronary arteries supply heart muscle

Vena cava (main vein)

Arteries supply blood to tissues

Veins carry blood back to heart and lungs

Who is most at risk for cardiovascular disease?

Most at risk of cardiovascular disease (and diabetes) is anyone diagnosed with metabolic syndrome, which is a precursor of cardiovascular disease.

METABOLIC SYNDROME
A condition that affects up to 25 percent of North Americans, metabolic syndrome may be diagnosed if you have at least three of the following five factors:
- Elevated fasting blood sugar levels of 110–125mg/dL, or diabetes.
- Blood pressure above 130/85mmHg, indicating prehypertension.
- Low HDL blood levels, defined as less than 40mg/dL for a man and less than 50mg/dL for a woman.

- Abdominal obesity, which is a waist circumference above 40in (101cm) for a man and 35in (89cm) for a woman.
- Elevated triglyceride levels in the blood greater than 150mg/dL.

CORONARY ARTERY DISEASE
This form of cardiovascular disease can result from metabolic syndrome or any of the following nine factors. If you are at risk, changing your diet and lifestyle can help (opposite).
- Elevated LDL blood levels (greater than 130mg/dl).
- Elevated homocysteine or C-reactive protein levels.
- Diabetes.

- Cigarette smoking and/or exposure to tobacco smoke.
- High blood pressure, defined as greater than 140/90mmHg, or taking antihypertensive medication.
- Low HDL cholesterol, defined as less than 35mg/dL for men or 45mg/dl for women. (HDL greater than 60mg/dL counts as a "negative" risk factor; its presence removes one risk factor from the total count).
- A family history of early cardiovascular disease (a heart attack before age 55 for men and 65 for women).
- Age (men older than 45 years; women older than 55 years).
- Obesity: BMI over 30 (see pp.26–27).

What is cardiovascular disease?

Cardiovascular disease covers a range of disorders in which strain is put on your arteries, other blood vessels, or the heart, leading to narrowed or blocked arteries and preventing the heart from pumping blood efficiently.

Lifestyle and diet have a large part to play both in the prevention and treatment of cardiovascular disease. Changing the way you eat, from cutting out saturated fat, and increasing omega-3 fatty acids and monounsaturated fats, to eating more fruits and vegetables, can make a big difference to your health and well-being. The table below defines each cardiovascular disorder and outlines the main dietary and lifestyle changes you can make to treat the condition.

In addition to the advice given below, it is very important to give up smoking if you are a smoker, avoid exposure to cigarette smoke, limit your intake of alcohol (or avoid it completely if your triglyceride levels are high), lose weight if you are overweight, and increase your level of physical activity.

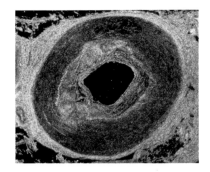

Atherosclerosis This cross-section of an artery shows its thickened walls, caused by a diet high in saturated fats.

DISORDER	WHAT IS IT?	HOW YOU CAN HELP
Hyperlipidemia	A combination of high levels of cholesterol, LDL, and/or triglycerides in the blood (see p.23), which can lead to narrowing of the blood vessels and clogged arteries. If untreated, you could develop angina and eventually suffer a heart attack.	• Reduce dietary saturated fat, trans fats, and cholesterol • Increase monounsaturated fats and omega-3 fatty acids • Avoid alcohol if triglycerides are high
High blood pressure (hypertension)	Persistent blood pressure above 140mmHg (systolic) and 90mmHg (diastolic), which may increase the risk of most other cardiovascular diseases.	• Reduce sodium and alcohol intake • Increase dietary intake of fruits, vegetables, and low-fat dairy products
Coronary artery disease	This occurs when the arteries surrounding the heart become clogged and narrowed by plaque (deposits of lipids such as cholesterol). This buildup is known as atherosclerosis, and can restrict blood flow to the heart, potentially causing angina or a heart attack.	• If you have hyperlipidemia, see above • Eat whole grains for magnesium and fruits and vegetables for potassium • Get regular exercise; limit alcohol • Take one aspirin daily
Angina	Chest pain that occurs when the heart muscle does not receive enough oxygenated blood due to the narrowing of the coronary arteries. It is triggered by exercise or stress.	• Consult your doctor before starting an exercise regime if you are over 50 • Reduce stress and saturated fat
Heart attack	A heart attack (myocardial infarction or MI) occurs when one or more of the coronary arteries become blocked by a combination of plaque (deposits of lipids such as cholesterol) and/or a blood clot (coronary thrombosis).	• Eat a low-fat diet and reduce dietary saturated fat, trans fats and cholesterol • Increase monounsaturated fats and omega-3 fatty acids
Stroke	A stroke can be caused by a blood clot blocking a blood vessel in the brain; by a blood vessel breaking (interrupting the flow of blood to an area of the brain and destroying brain cells); or by bleeding into the brain from a broken blood vessel. Stroke can lead to a loss of abilities, such as speech, movement, and memory.	• If you have hyperlipidemia, see the above entry for advice • If you have high blood pressure, see the above entry for advice • Anticoagulation medication may be prescribed for high-risk patients
Heart failure	Heart failure occurs when there is a reduced efficiency of the heart, which is defined as the amount of blood pumped by the heart in one minute. The disorder is characterized by the pooling of fluid in the extremities, especially in the legs and ankles, sodium retention, organ failure, and undernourishment caused by loss of appetite.	• Reduce your sodium intake • Increase protein-rich foods if you are underweight • Avoid stress • A medically supervised exercise program can be beneficial

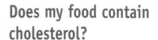

Cardiovascular disease and nutrition

There is a strong link between diet, exercise, and the development of cardiovascular disease.

Nutrition plays an essential role in the treatment of cardiovascular disease, especially in high blood pressure and coronary artery disease, which are very common problems in North America.

Cholesterol levels

Because an excessive amount of cholesterol in the blood is a major risk factor for other cardiovascular diseases—causing narrowing of the arteries—your first priority is to lower cholesterol levels.

You should reduce your intake of saturated fats and increase your intake of polyunsaturated and monounsaturated fats, which can actually help lower your blood cholesterol levels (see pp.40–41). A diet high in monounsaturated fats lowers LDL-cholesterol and triglyceride levels in the blood without lowering beneficial HDL-cholesterol levels. See the table opposite for more information.

High blood pressure

Another contributor to other types of cardiovascular diseases is high blood pressure (see pp.214–215). As the pressure exerted on blood vessels increases, they narrow, making it more difficult for the blood to get through, thereby increasing the strain on the cardiovascular system.

Diet and exercise are critical in the effective treatment of high blood pressure; in some cases, changing your diet and increasing your activity level can eliminate the need for medication or reduce the dosage required.

Changing your diet

There is a clear link between the consumption of saturated fats, which will raise LDL levels in the blood, and cardiovascular disease.

Does my food contain cholesterol?

The National Cholesterol Education Program recommends limiting your daily dietary intake of cholesterol to 200mg for a heart-healthy diet. Dietary cholesterol is present only in foods of animal origin, such as eggs, meat, poultry, fish, seafood, whole milk, and other dairy products. Cholesterol is not found in foods of plant origin, such as vegetables, fruits, grains, nuts, and seeds.

The highest amounts of dietary cholesterol come from egg yolks, caviar, liver, and other organ meats; you should limit these foods in your diet. For example, the yolk of one medium-sized egg contains about 200mg of cholesterol.

The American Heart Association recommends limiting dietary saturated fat intake to less than seven percent of total calories.

You should also reduce sodium in your diet, particularly if you have high blood pressure or suffer from heart failure, and increase your intake of potassium- and calcium-rich foods (see p.220).

Changing your lifestyle

Lifestyle changes, such as giving up smoking, losing weight, and increasing your exercise level, will help ease the burden on your cardiovascular system and reduce the effects of high blood pressure and high cholesterol. If you have angina, however, check with your doctor before embarking on an exercise program.

If you suffer from heart failure, make sure you eat enough to achieve and maintain optimum weight, limit sodium intake, and maintain a tolerable activity level.

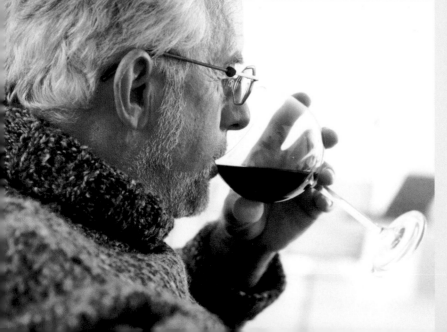

Red wine can be beneficial Red wine has been shown to increase HDL, or "good" cholesterol levels, but drink in moderation.

Reducing total cholesterol, LDL, and triglyceride levels

The first step in treating cardiovascular disease is to lower LDL-cholesterol and triglyceride levels in the blood. LDL-cholesterol is usually the primary target and lowering its levels in your blood entails making changes to what you eat, specifically by reducing the amount of saturated fat in your diet. Other lifestyle behaviors, such as weight loss, taking regular exercise, and stopping smoking can also significantly reduce your risk of cardiovascular disease. In addition to lowering LDL and triglyceride levels through nutrition, raising beneficial HDL levels through diet can also reduce the risk.

GOAL	HOW TO ACHIEVE GOAL	NUTRITIONAL AND LIFESTYLE ADVICE
Decrease LDL-cholesterol levels	• Decrease intake of saturated fat • Use mono- and polyunsaturated fats • Limit dietary cholesterol • Increase soluble fiber • Limit trans-fatty-acid intake	• Chose lean meats and low-fat or fat-free dairy products • Use only canola or olive oil for cooking and baking • Limit egg yolks, butterfat, and fatty meats. • Add oatmeal, legumes, and apples to your diet • Use soft, trans-fat free margarine; limit baked goods, such as pie crust, made with partially hydrogenated oils
Decrease triglyceride levels	• Use mono- and polyunsaturated fats • Include omega-3 fatty acids • Avoid high-carbohydrate diets • Eliminate alcohol • Lose weight if overweight	• Use only canola or olive oil in cooking and baking • Eat more cold-water fish, flaxseeds, and flaxseed oil • Cut down on high-carbohydrate foods • Reduce alcohol intake as much as possible • Exercise, limit saturated fat, and reduce portion sizes
Raise HDL-cholesterol levels	• Use mono- and polyunsaturated fats • Limit trans-fatty-acid intake • Lose weight if overweight	• Use only canola or olive oil in cooking and baking • Use soft, trans-fat free margarine; limit baked goods, such as pie crust, made with partially hydrogenated oil • Cut out saturated fat, reduce portion sizes, and exercise to help weight loss

Case study Busy accountant with metabolic syndrome

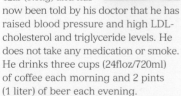

Name Harry

Age 52 years

Problem In the past three years, Harry has gained 12lb (5.5kg) and has now been told by his doctor that he has raised blood pressure and high LDL-cholesterol and triglyceride levels. He does not take any medication or smoke. He drinks three cups (24floz/720ml) of coffee each morning and 2 pints (1 liter) of beer each evening.

Lifestyle Harry is an accountant and has a high level of stress at work and at home. Work commitments mean he often orders a pizza for lunch and eats at his desk. After work and his commute home, Harry is too tired to

exercise. He often eats a steak for supper and snacks on ice cream and chips at night. He rarely eats fruit.

Advice Harry has metabolic syndrome (see p.214), which places him at risk for cardiovascular disease. He needs to lose weight and take some exercise. Based on blood tests (see p.23), his goal is to lower total cholesterol, LDL-cholesterol, and triglycerides, and to raise his level of HDL-cholesterol. He can achieve this by following the Therapeutic Lifestyle Change Diet (see p.218) and reducing his total intake of calories.

Harry's diet is high in saturated fat and cholesterol. He should substitute monounsaturated fat and omega-3 fatty acids for saturated fat (see p.39) and cut back on portion sizes and increase his activity level. Eating

more fruits and vegetables, whole grains, beans and legumes, low-fat or fat-free dairy products, white-meat chicken without skin, fish, or lean meats will help. If he likes eggs, he can include two in his diet per week.

For breakfast, Harry could have oatmeal with fat-free milk and an orange. For lunch, he could order a tuna or turkey-salad sandwich or have two slices of vegetable pizza. For dinner, he could order fish and chicken more often and limit red meat to less than once a week.

Harry could increase his daily intake of soluble fiber to 1oz (28g) from oats, psyllium, legumes, and fruits. Margarines containing plant stanol/sterols could replace other spreads to further lower his LDL-cholesterol. He may also benefit from reducing his salt intake (see p.221).

Therapeutic lifestyle changes (TLC) diet

If you have cardiovascular disease you need to think carefully about what you eat as it could have a major impact on your condition. Changes such as substituting low-fat products for full-fat ones, cutting the amount of saturated fat in your diet,

substituting low-fat dairy foods for high-fat varieties, using monounsaturated oils and increasing your intake of omega-3 fatty acids can all be beneficial. The Therapeutic Lifestyle Changes (TLC) diet, as outlined below, is a great starting point.

FOOD GROUP	GOOD CHOICES	POOR CHOICES
Breads and cereals (6 servings daily)	Low-fat crackers and cookies, whole-grain bread, cakes, and cereal bars; brown rice and pasta; lentil burgers; low-fat hummus; low-fat popcorn	Products high in saturated and trans fats, such as doughnuts, croissants, pastries, pies, and cookies; refined rice and pasta; chips and snack mix; full-fat crackers; buttered popcorn
Vegetables (3–5 servings daily)	Steamed vegetables and baked root vegetables (no butter); roasted vegetables drizzled with olive oil; raw vegetables with low-fat dips	Vegetables fried or prepared with butter, cheese, or cream sauce; baked potatoes with butter; raw vegetables with full-fat dips
Fruits (2–4 servings daily)	Fresh fruits; canned fruit in own juice; baked fruit served with low-fat sour cream or yogurt; and low-fat fruit tarts and pies	Fruits served with butter or cream; canned fruit in sugary syrup; and fruit pies with pastry made with shortening or butter
Dairy products (2–3 servings daily)	Low-fat (1 percent) milk; low-fat yogurt; fat-free frozen yogurt; low-fat or part-skim cheeses	Whole or 2 percent milk; cream; whole-milk yogurt; ice cream; full-fat hard and soft cheeses; sour cream; cream cheese
Eggs (2 yolks a week)	Egg whites; egg substitutes; omelets made from egg whites or egg substitutes	Egg yolks; whole eggs; omelets made from whole eggs
Fish, poultry, and meat (5oz/142g daily)	Grilled or barbecued fish; baked or broiled skinless meat and poultry; lean cuts of meat, such as loin or leg; cold cuts and sausages made with lean meat or soy protein, fat-free hot dogs	Fried fish; fried poultry with skin; fatty cuts of meat such as ribs or T-bone steak; sausages; cold cuts such as salami or bologna; organ meats; pastrami; corned beef, hot dogs
Fats and oils (1–2 tbsp daily)	Canola and olive oil; stanol-supplemented margarines; trans-free tub margarine	Butter; shortening; lard; stick margarine; full-fat salad dressings; coconut cream

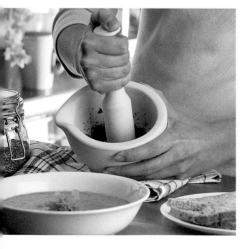

Flaxseeds are rich in omega-3

This seed has been valued for its therapeutic properties since ancient times. This nutty-tasting seed is one of the best sources of omega-3 essential fatty acid, and is excellent for regulating blood pressure (see pp.39–40). Flaxseeds contain both soluble and insoluble fiber. Soluble fiber helps reduce cholesterol, while insoluble fiber helps eliminate toxins from the bowel.

Grinding flaxseeds Boost your omega-3 intake by crushing flaxseeds with a pestle and mortar and sprinkling over soups and salads.

It is easy to incorporate flaxseeds into your diet. Ground flaxseeds provide the greatest nutritional benefit since the body cannot digest whole seeds. Crushed or milled seeds can be added to breakfast cereals, yogurt, salads, soup, or smoothies. You can also add flaxseeds to muffins, meat loaf, and sauces before baking or cooking.

Flaxseed oil is also an excellent source of omega-6, but does not contain the fiber. It can be used as a salad dressing, but is unsuitable for cooking and must be refrigerated at all times because it is sensitive to light, oxygen, and heat.

Nutrients that help cardiovascular disease

In addition to limiting your intake of saturated fats, increasing omega-3 fats, and including more fiber in your diet, there are specific changes that you can make in order to help prevent and treat cardiovascular disease.

CHOOSE SOY PRODUCTS
Studies have shown that 1oz (28g) of soy protein per day will lower LDL-cholesterol levels by about five percent. The Food and Drug Administration has approved a health claim for soy foods that encourages eating at least 1oz (28g) of soy protein daily, as part of a diet low in saturated fat and cholesterol, to reduce the risk of cardiovascular disease.

REDUCE HOMOCYSTEINE LEVELS
An emerging risk factor for developing cardiovascular disease is a high level of an amino acid called homocysteine in the blood. This can be caused by a genetic defect in the enzymes that break down homocysteine, as well as by a diet low in folate. Vitamins B_6 and B_{12} are also needed to break it down in the body, so most doctors prescribe a supplement that contains these three vitamins for anyone with elevated homocysteine levels. If you are at risk of cardiovascular disease, ask your doctor about taking a multivitamin supplement.

EAT PLANT OILS
Plant sterols and stanols, derived from natural plant oils, have been shown to significantly lower LDL-cholesterol levels in the blood by up to 14 percent. These have been incorporated into some brands of spreads.

The National Cholesterol Education Program recommends including 2g of plant stanol/sterol (esters) daily as part of a diet low in saturated fat and cholesterol for those with elevated LDL levels. In the gastrointestinal tract, sterol/stanols compete with cholesterol for absorption, so less dietary and biliary cholesterol is absorbed by the body.

Since spreads with added sterol/stanol are the main source of these compounds, it is important to substitute these for other added fats, such as butter, margarine, oil, or cream cheese, so that your total calories will not be inccreased by adding these to your diet.

What about alcohol?

The antioxidant properties of red wine may protect your heart by increasing HDL-cholesterol levels and reducing LDL-cholesterol from being oxidized and deposited in arteries. However, if you regularly have more than two drinks a day (for men) or one drink a day (for women), you may increase your risk of developing high blood pressure, elevated triglyceride levels, enlarged heart, and stroke. So you should make sure that you drink alcohol in moderation.

Boosting your fiber intake

Since a high-fiber diet has been proven to reduce the risk of heart attack and other cardiovascular diseases, it is vital that you eat lots of fiber-rich foods.

HIGH-FIBER FOODS
Eating at least 10g of soluble fiber daily has been shown to reduce LDL-cholesterol by about five percent.

Foods that are high in soluble fiber include oatmeal, whole oats, and legumes, as well as fruits, which are rich in the soluble fiber pectin. They will help decrease harmful LDL-cholesterol levels and reduce your risk of cardiovascular disease.

One meal that is easy to transform into a fiber-rich one is breakfast (*right*). By making simple changes, such as substituting whole-grain cereals and breads for refined varieties and adding fruit, you can increase the amount of soluble fiber that you eat every day.

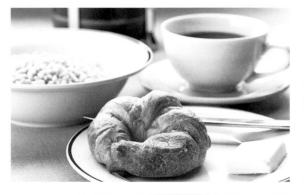

Low-fiber breakfast
This breakfast of sweetened, puffed-wheat cereal, coffee, and a croissant provides just 2.3g of fiber, as well as 27g fat and 105mg cholesterol.

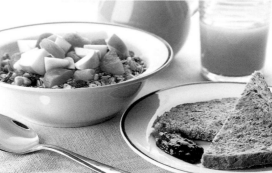

High-fiber breakfast
With whole-grain muesli and fruit, whole-grain toast, and orange juice, this version provides 12.5g fiber, 7g fat, and only 4.9mg cholesterol.

Dietary advice for high blood pressure

By making some simple changes to your diet you can can help reduce high blood pressure. In addition to the changes outlined here it is also important that you reduce the amount of salt in your diet (*opposite*). Always talk to your doctor before implementing changes.

POTASSIUM AND CALCIUM

The DASH diet recommends increasing your dietary intake of potassium and calcium (*below*). Potassium can be found in all the food groups—fruit and vegetable sources include oranges,

Potassium-rich acorn squash Make a tasty vegetarian meal by baking acorn squash halves, scooping out the seeds, and filling with a mixture of spicy chickpeas, warm baby-leaf spinach, and tomato paste.

pears, acorn squash, spinach, and artichokes. Dairy products are excellent sources, too, as are protein foods, such as red meat, poultry, and lima beans. Dairy products are of course rich in calcium (be sure to opt for low-fat versions), as are green leafy vegetables, such as kale and broccoli (*see p.62*).

ALCOHOL

People who drink large amounts of alcohol are more likely to develop high blood pressure, whereas small amounts of alcohol raise HDL-cholesterol levels and are beneficial for cardiovascular health. Larger amounts of alcohol cause blood vessels to constrict or narrow, forcing the heart to pump harder. Alcohol can thus raise your blood pressure and make your high blood pressure more difficult to manage.

DASH diet for high blood pressure

The Dietary Approaches to Stop Hypertension (DASH) diet for people with high blood pressure promotes increasing the intake of potassium and calcium in your diet (*above*) by eating plenty of fruits and vegetables and low-fat dairy products. Meat portions are limited, and nuts provide magnesium and additional fiber. Saturated-fat intake is limited to less than seven percent of total calories, and cholesterol to less than 200mg per day. Sugar and sweets can be eaten only sparingly.

BENEFITS OF THIS DIET

Research shows that people on the DASH diet were able to reduce their diastolic blood pressure (the lower measurement of blood pressure, taken between heartbeats when the heart is relaxed) by up to 5mmHg, regardless of their age, gender, ethnicity, or initial blood pressure levels. For those with high blood pressure that ranged from 140/90 to 159/99mmHg, the DASH diet's effectiveness was similar to that of medication for high blood pressure.

FOOD GROUP	INTAKE	SERVING SIZES AND SUGGESTIONS
Breads, pasta, cereals, and whole grains	7–8 daily servings	• 1 slice whole-wheat bread • 1 cup dry cereal • ½ cup cooked rice or pasta
Vegetables	4–5 daily servings	• 1 cup (56g) raw leafy vegetables • ½ cup (75g) cooked vegetables • 6floz (180ml) vegetable juice
Fruits	4–5 daily servings	• 4floz (120ml) fruit juice • 1 medium fruit • ½ cup fresh, dried, frozen, or canned fruit
Low-fat or fat-free dairy foods	2–3 daily servings	• 8floz (240ml) milk • 8floz (240ml) yogurt • 1½ oz (40g) cheese
Meats, poultry, and fish	2 or fewer daily servings	• 3½oz (100g) cooked meat, poultry, or fish
Fats and oils	2–3 daily servings	• 1 tsp soft margarine • 1 tbsp low-fat mayonnaise • 2 tbsp light salad dressing • 1 tsp vegetable oil
Nuts, seeds, and dry beans	4–5 servings per week	• 3 tbsp nuts • 3 tbsp seeds • ½ cup cooked beans

Dietary advice for heart failure

Many people with heart failure tend to lose weight and become undernourished because they follow restrictive diets and may not get enough calories. They need to work with their doctor to find a way of reducing their sodium intake and limiting their fluid intake. They should also try to maintain or increase body weight with high-calorie, nutrient-dense foods and food supplements.

MAINTAIN A HEALTHY WEIGHT
It is important to maintain an adequate calorie intake to prevent weight loss. If you have already lost weight due to loss of appetite, you may need to take in more calories. Having small, frequent nutrient-dense and high-calorie meals may help you meet your caloric needs. See page 224 for suggestions for nutrient-dense snacks and meals.

REDUCE SODIUM INTAKE
People with heart failure retain sodium and fluid, so restricting sodium (salt) in the diet is usually necessary. The level of sodium restriction varies depending on the severity of the condition. Those with long-term heart failure with symptoms

such as shortness of breath should reduce their dietary intake of sodium to less than 2000mg per day.

If you suffer from heart failure you must do more than just "stay away from salt." You must check food labels for sodium content, select only foods with less than 400mg per serving, and use herbs and other nonsalt seasonings when cooking. These dietary changes will help you feel better and maintain your health longer (right).

LIMIT FLUID INTAKE
People with heart failure may be advised by their doctor to limit fluid intake to six to eight glasses per day, which is about 3–4 pints (1.5–2 liters). Fluids may be restricted slightly more than this for patients in hospital.

TAKE FOOD SUPPLEMENTS
High-protein, high-calorie supplements can help increase calorie intake in a relatively small volume, and are especially useful for those with a poor appetite. These supplements are available in both liquid and dessert forms and in a variety of flavors.

Reducing salt intake
People who suffer from heart failure and those with high blood pressure should follow a low-salt diet. Reducing sodium is proven to be one of the best ways of lowering high blood pressure.

Tips for cutting down sodium
Convenience foods, canned foods, and eating out frequently all contribute to the higher sodium intake among North Americans today, so if you are following a low-sodium diet read labels carefully.
- Use fresh herbs, seasonings, and spices, such as basil, cinnamon, or cumin, to flavor vegetables.
- Avoid using a salt shaker.
- Use soy sauce sparingly: 1 tsp contains about 1,200mg of sodium.
- Buy either fresh, plain frozen, or canned "no salt added" vegetables.
- Rinse canned foods, such as tuna, to remove sodium.
- Choose ready-to eat breakfast cereals that are lower in sodium.
- Buy low- or reduced-sodium or no-salt-added versions of foods.

Recipe Low-sodium spicy chicken kabobs

INGREDIENTS

4 skinless chicken breasts

black pepper

3 lemons

1 tbsp grated fresh ginger

3 garlic cloves, crushed

½ tsp ground cumin

1 green chili

Serves 4

1 Cut each chicken breast into 1-in (2.5-cm) cubes. Season with black pepper and the juice of one lemon. Cover and refrigerate for 30 minutes.

2 In a small bowl, combine the grated ginger, crushed garlic, ground cumin, and chopped chili. Rub mixture into the chicken, cover, and

3 Cut remaining two lemons into wedges. Thread the chicken cubes and lemon wedges onto skewers.

4 Grill over medium-hot coals until chicken is opaque. Or cook under preheated broiler for 5 minutes each side.

If you like, serve the kabobs with cucumber–yogurt sauce.

Each serving provides
Cal. 205, Total fat 2.2g (Sat. 0.6g, Poly. 0.5g, Mono. 0.5g) Cholesterol 99mg, Protein 40g, Carbohydrate 5.1g, Fiber 1.0g, Sodium 124mg. Good source of—Mins: Ca, Mg, P, K, Se.

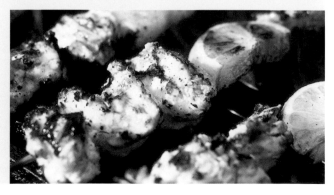

Respiratory disorders

If you suffer from a respiratory disease, changing your diet and lifestyle can help.

The respiratory system—the lungs and airways—together with the cardiovascular system (*see p.214*), is responsible for delivering oxygen from the lungs to every cell in the body and for removing carbon dioxide and returning it to the lungs to be exhaled.

How we breathe

With each breath, a fresh supply of oxygen enters the bloodstream. Red blood cells transport oxygen from the lungs to the tissues. The work of emptying and filling the lungs is done by the respiratory muscles.

The main respiratory muscle is the diaphragm, a layer of muscle situated between the chest and the abdomen. As this contracts and relaxes, air is drawn in and forced out at regular intervals. Other muscles that contribute to respiration are located between the ribs, in the neck, and in the abdomen. Any disease affecting these muscles, the bones of the chest wall, or the passage from the nose to the lungs will interfere with normal respiratory function.

Respiratory disorders

Chronic obstructive pulmonary disease (COPD) is a result of progressive damage to the lungs, and is due mainly to smoking.

Sleep apnea is a condition in which breathing is interrupted, usually by the soft tissues of the throat relaxing and blocking the flow of air. It most commonly occurs in overweight people. When the airway is obstructed, breathing becomes labored and can stop for at least 10 seconds, leading to dangerously low levels of oxygen in the blood.

In asthma, there is an intermittent narrowing of the airways, causing shortness of breath and wheezing. If asthma is severe, just trying to breathe can cause exhaustion.

Dietary and lifestyle changes

Some dietary changes can help relieve these disorders. Since COPD often leads to weight loss, making sure you have a nutrient-dense

The respiratory system

This includes the upper airway (the nasal passages to the trachea), the lower airways, and lungs.

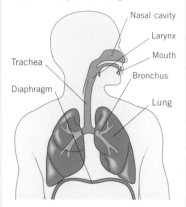

Nasal cavity
Larynx
Mouth
Trachea
Bronchus
Diaphragm
Lung

diet will help. Conversely, if you have sleep apnea you may be overweight, and losing a little weight may successfully treat the disorder. If you have asthma and know of a particular food that triggers an attack, make sure you avoid that food.

Lifestyle changes are also very important. Giving up smoking and increasing your level of exercise will benefit all respiratory disease. You should consult your doctor, however, before embarking on an exercise program.

Who is most at risk for respiratory disorders?

There are a number of risk factors for the respiratory diseases discussed in this section. The most common of these are outlined below.

Diet and lifestyle Excess body fat, especially around the neck, can cause sleep apnea, which is also more common in people who are overweight, smoke, and drink too much alcohol. Chronic obstructive pulmonary disease (COPD) is almost always due to smoking. In addition, smoking can trigger asthma in some people.

Age Asthma is more common in children, while COPD is more common in people over the the age of 40.
Gender COPD is twice as common in men, whereas adult-onset asthma is more common in women.
Family history Asthma has been found to run in families.
Other risk factors Children with eczema or other allergies are at greater risk of developing asthma. Dust, noxious gases, and other lung irritants can cause COPD and trigger asthma.

Warning signs

A morning cough and shortness of breath are two early signs of chronic bronchitis and emphysema, which together are known as chronic obstructive pulmonary disease (COPD).

Since smoking cigarettes greatly increases your risk of emphysema, it is important to take the symptoms seriously—you should avoid people who smoke and kick the habit if you do smoke. Quitting smoking will produce dramatic effects in improving your lung function.

What are respiratory disorders?

Chronic obstructive pulmonary disease (commonly known as COPD), asthma, and sleep apnea are three common respiratory disorders that you can either avoid or help treat by making sensible changes to your diet and lifestyle—as summarized in the chart below.

COPD and asthma are disorders of the lungs and the lower airways (bronchioles), whereas sleep apnea results from obstruction of the upper airway (usually the nasopharynx—the passage leading from the back of the nasal cavity to the throat).

In general, the changes that you need to make are sensible and include maintaining a healthy nutrient-dense diet, cutting out or limiting the amount of alcohol that you drink, and giving up smoking or avoiding passive smoking.

Chronic bronchitis Damage to lung tissue is shown in this X-ray of chronic bronchitis, which is usually caused by smoking.

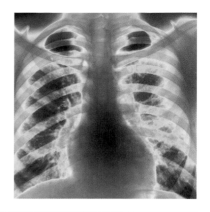

DISORDER	WHAT IS IT?	HOW YOU CAN HELP
Chronic obstructive pulmonary disease (COPD)	People with COPD usually have two lung conditions— chronic bronchitis and emphysema. In COPD, the airways (bronchi and bronchioles) and tissues of the lungs become damaged over time, causing a shortness of breath. Damage to the lungs caused by COPD is usually irreversible.	• Eat nutrient-dense foods in order to prevent or reverse weight loss and undernutrition, which are both common with this condition • Quit smoking
Sleep apnea	Obstructive sleep apnea is defined as recurrent episodes of apnea, which is the cessation of breathing during sleep, caused by blockage of the upper airway.	• Lose weight • Avoid alcohol • Quit smoking
Asthma	Asthma is a form of chronic lung disease caused by inflammation and swelling of the lining of the airways in the lungs. It is associated with exposure to allergens (substances that trigger an allergic reaction).	• Maintain a healthy diet • Avoid foods that trigger attacks • Exercise to improve your stamina • Quit smoking

Nutritional advice if you have COPD

Many people with chronic obstructive pulmonary disease (COPD) do not eat enough. Weight loss is very common and can increase breathing difficulties. It is therefore very important that people with COPD eat a balanced diet and take in enough calories to avoid undernutrition.

Recent studies suggest that foods high in antioxidants, such as fruits and vegetables, and omega-3 fatty acids (see p.90), such as oily fish, may be helpful in protecting against COPD. Taking a multivitamin supplement will also help you get the right nutrients.

MAINTAIN ADEQUATE CALORIES
If you are underweight and trying to regain your strength, gradually increase the amount you eat with small, frequent, nutrient-dense meals that are easy to

consume (see p.224). Other ideas that can help include:
• Eat three small meals and between-meal snacks to get the calories you need. Smaller meals may help you breathe more easily and may be less tiring to eat than large meals.
• Time your main meal for when you have the most energy and feel your best (often in the morning), and rest before and after mealtimes.
• Avoid foods that cause uncomfortable gas or bloating.
• Increase your intake of fiber-rich foods to avoid constipation.

Fruit salad is a healthy dessert Fruit is high in antioxidants, which have been found to help protect against COPD.

• Select soft foods that are easy to chew.
• Choose meals that can be cooked in the microwave, such as healthy frozen dinners (check labels for salt and saturated fat levels).
• Make sure you drink enough fluids—at least eight glasses of water or caffeine-free drinks per day to keep your body hydrated.

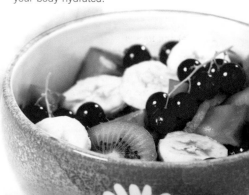

High-calorie meals to counteract weight loss in COPD

If your condition has led to weight loss and you are trying to gain weight, it does not mean that you should simply eat fatty foods, such as cheese, mayonnaise, and butter, although you can eat them in moderation. High-calorie snacks should be as healthy as possible and packed with nutrients, especially vitamins, minerals, and proteins. Bearing in mind the benefits of whole grains and the need to moderate saturated fat, try:
● Guacamole with raw vegetables or baked tortilla chips.
● Tuna, chicken, or salmon salad on whole-wheat bread.

● Full-fat cheese, cream cheese, ham salad, or peanut butter stuffed in pita bread.
● Two-egg omelet with cheese, and ham or tomato.
● Falafel in pita bread with salad, red peppers, and hummus.
● Whole-grain cereals with whole milk.
● Fruits with full-fat yogurt.
● Nuts, such as almonds or brazils, or homemade trail mix.
● An 8floz (240ml) glass of whole milk, or a mug of hot chocolate made with whole milk.

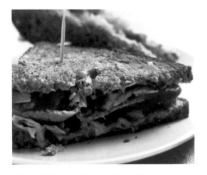

Ham salad sandwich Packed with protein and fiber, this whole-wheat-bread ham sandwich is quick to prepare and easy to eat.

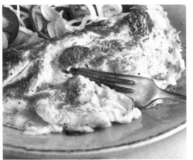

Omelet Easy to prepare, an omelet made with two eggs and grated cheese is high in protein and calcium. Serve with a bagel.

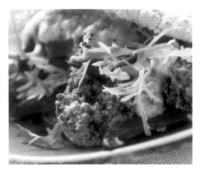

Falafels in pita bread Spicy chickpea croquettes, served in pita bread with salad, peppers, and hummus is a nutritious snack.

Case study Woman with severe COPD who is losing weight

Name Patty

Age 53 years

Problem Patty was diagnosed with COPD eight years ago. Her symptoms include shortness of breath, which seems to worsen when she is sick, stressed, cold, or in high humidity, or after a large meal. She is often too tired to prepare food and gets short of breath when she chews and swallows because these affect her breathing. Patty complains of being tired all the time and feeling weak, especially at mealtimes. Within the last year, she has lost 10lb (4.5kg).

Lifestyle Patty lives with her husband and has four children and fourteen grandchildren. She retired last year because of her illness. Lately, she has

been too tired to go out. Her husband has recently taken over shopping for food. Patty usually follows a low-salt, low-fat diet at home. She smoked for 30 years but quit five years ago.

In the morning, Patty eats cereal and a slice of toast. She has a low-fat yogurt and apple juice for lunch and a chicken breast, baked potato, and a vegetable for dinner. She often has a piece of fruit after dinner. Her caloric intake is about 1,000 calories per day. She is 62in (157cm) and weighs 147lb (67kg). Her usual weight is 165lb (76kg).

Advice Patty is eating only about 1,000 calories per day, which is two-thirds of her needs. Because of reduced lung function, she requires more energy to breathe; the normal daily intake of calories required to maintain body weight is not enough to meet the excessive demands of breathing for people with COPD.

Providing enough calories and protein to restore and maintain her weight and keep her respiratory muscles strong is the major goal of nutritional treatment for people with COPD.

Patty's dietitian advised her to rest before mealtimes and to eat foods that are easy to chew, such as soft meats and casseroles. She can get additional calories from high-protein, high-calorie shakes, drinking at least one can per day. Eating small, frequent meals consisting of nutrient-dense foods, such as peanut butter and jelly sandwiches, will help meet her nutritional needs. Using extra tub or liquid margarine on her bread, potatoes, and vegetables will also supplement her intake of calories.

Patty should have her main meal at a time of the day when her energy level is highest. She should also limit her intake of fluids during meals, and drink fluids between meals.

Tips for treating sleep apnea

Obesity contributes to the development of sleep apnea (*see p.223*) and weight loss of as little as 10lb (4.5kg) can dramatically improve symptoms.

WEIGHT-REDUCTION TIPS

If you need to lose weight because of sleep apnea, you should to consult a dietitian for nutritional counseling. However, you may find the following suggestions useful as well.

● Stay out of the kitchen after dinner. Eating late at night adds extra calories.

● If you are hungry and have to snack, have fresh fruit or cut-up vegetables ready in the refrigerator. Use low-calorie dressings for dipping.

● If you are tempted by snacks and junk food around the house, don't buy or bring those foods into your home. If you have lots of snack foods for the children, consider them "off limits."

● Be aware of your portion sizes both at home and when eating out: order an appetizer or a salad, not both, share one entrée with your partner, and skip the butter on the bread. If you want a dessert, share it and skip the wine.

● Regular exercise, such as walking, swimming, or bicycling, will give you more energy and help you sleep better.

● Alcohol may promote throat closure during sleep and should be avoided.

OTHER TIPS FOR SLEEP APNEA

In addition to losing weight, there are important lifestyle factors that can help improve your condition.

● Avoid smoking.

● Do not go to sleep immediately after eating, take a walk instead.

● Treat allergies, colds, or sinus problems. Avoid using antihistamines or tranquilizers.

● Try sleeping exclusively on your side or with the head of the bed elevated.

Asthma and nutrition

People with asthma generally have the same nutritional needs and food considerations as anyone else, but if you have asthma it is important to make a healthy diet a regular part of your life. Asthma can place additional stress on your body—especially if you take oral corticosteroids, which can deplete your body of vitamins and minerals.

EAT A HEALTHY DIET

Eat plenty of fruits and vegetables, whole-grain breads, cereals, legumes, moderate amounts of low-fat dairy products, lean meats, fish, chicken, and small amounts of fats, oils, and sugar. A healthy diet and regular exercise go a long way toward helping improve your well-being. Certain foods and additives, however, have been found to trigger or exacerbate asthma in some people.

FOODS THAT TRIGGER ASTHMA

Asthmatics are usually affected by at most two or three foods; it is a common misconception that people are sensitive to a wide variety of foods.

The factors that set off and exacerbate asthma symptoms are called "triggers." Identifying and avoiding asthma triggers are essential in preventing flare-ups. The most common trigger foods are milk, yogurt, and other dairy products, eggs, shrimp, fish, citrus fruits, soy, and wheat. These foods are more likely to trigger asthma in children than in adults, and fortunately most children outgrow such allergies. Check food labels since additives found in many canned, processed, or convenience foods, such as sulfur, monosodium glutamate, tartrazine, and benzoic acid can trigger asthma. If you can identify the specific food or additive that triggers your asthma, you should simply avoid it.

Avoiding additives By feeding your toddler homemade meals, you can be sure that she is getting the best ingredients, without the addition of potentially harmful chemicals.

Asthma in babies

This illness is sometimes related to allergies, which may be prevented by close attention to your baby's diet. Early exposure to infant cereals has been linked to an increase in asthma triggered by grass pollen. Just breast-feeding for three months may prevent this.

Probiotic foods, such as yogurt with live cultures, promote the development of bacteria in the gut (*see p.48*). The bacteria may play a role in assisting the digestion of proteins that cause food allergy.

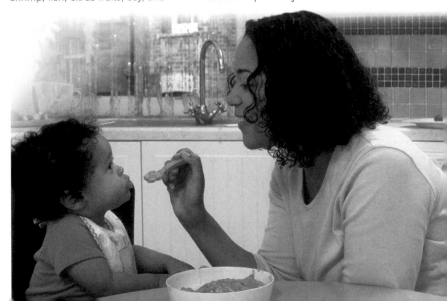

Digestive disorders

The digestive tract and associated organs can be affected by many disorders.

The digestive system is made up of the digestive tract, the salivary glands, liver, gallbladder, and pancreas. The digestive tract is essentially a long tube. In total, it is about 24ft (7.3m) long and composed of a series of joined sections made up of the mouth, esophagus, stomach, small and large intestines, rectum, and anus.

How it works
The role of the digestive tract is to break down food and transport nutrients throughout the body for energy, growth, and repair. It is also responsible for eliminating waste from the body.

The rhythmic contraction of the muscles lining the esophagus is called peristalsis. This action moves food into the stomach and prevents any stomach contents from going backward into the esophagus

(reflux). To aid in this function there is a ring of muscles at the bottom of the esophagus called the lower esophageal sphincter.

Medical problems occur when there is a structural or functional change along the digestive tract or in the associated organs.

What can go wrong?
Disorders of the digestive system that can in some way be relieved, treated, or prevented by dietary or lifestyle measures are outlined in the chart on the opposite page.

The most common digestive disorders are usually short-term problems and include indigestion, diarrhea, and constipation. A common cause of indigestion is gastroesophageal reflux disease (GERD), in which acidic stomach juices are regurgitated. Peptic ulcers, which affect either the stomach or the duodenum (the first part of the small intestine) may persist or recur.

Some disorders, for example, Crohn's disease and ulcerative colitis, cause inflammation of the intestine and affect the absorption

of nutrients. Other disorders, such as lactose intolerance and celiac disease, are a result of a reaction to a substance that is present in food. The dietary and lifestyle changes you can make to combat these disorders, and treat any side effects, are discussed in detail on the following pages.

The digestive system

The digestive system includes the digestive tract (from mouth to anus) and associated organs, such as the liver and gallbladder.

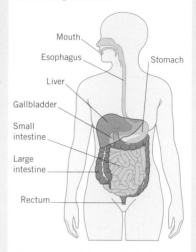

Mouth
Esophagus
Stomach
Liver
Gallbladder
Small intestine
Large intestine
Rectum

What are the risk factors for digestive disorders?

Some of the known risks for digestive disorders are outlined below. These include diet and lifestyle, age, gender, and family history.

Diet and lifestyle A diet that does not include a sufficient amount of fiber may lead to some digestive diseases. For example, diverticular disease is more common in the West, where intake of fiber tends to be low because of the popularity of refined grain products.

Anyone who is overweight or has a high-fat diet is at risk of developing gallstones. Drinking alcohol, smoking cigarettes, and emotional stress may all trigger or aggravate existing stomach ulcers or interfere with their healing.

Age As people grow older, the motility of their intestinal tract decreases, and therefore food and waste move through the intestine at a slower rate, which increases the risk of constipation.

Similarly, diverticular disease is more common in people over the age of 50, and over half of 60- to 80-year-olds and nearly everyone over 80 in North America has this disorder.

About 11 percent of people in the US suffer from irritable bowel syndrome (IBS), a condition that is most common in those aged 20–30 years. Similarly, Crohn's disease and ulcerative colitis most commonly first develop in young people aged 15–30.

Gender Some gastrointestinal diseases, such as peptic ulcers, do occur more commonly in men than in women. But gallstones and IBS are more common in women than in men.

Family history Some digestive disorders, such as celiac disease, are genetic and can run in families. Family members of people who have been diagnosed with a genetic digestive disorder may be offered tests to see if they are at risk of developing the disorder.

Between 15 and 30 percent of people with Crohn's disease and ulcerative colitis have a family history of these conditions, suggesting that genetics are involved in their development, too.

What are digestive disorders?

Diarrhea, constipation, and indigestion are common, and there are measures you can take to prevent and treat them. However, diarrhea may be a symptom of an infection or a long-term problem, such as irritable bowel syndrome (IBS) or an inflammatory bowel disorder such as ulcerative colitis or Crohn's disease. If diarrhea persists, see your doctor.

Gastroesophageal reflux (GERD) is a common disorder of the esophagus and a cause of indigestion. Attacks can be mild, but may leave your esophagus scarred. Peptic ulcer is commonly due to a bacterium called *Helicobacter pylori.*

Many digestive disorders can be managed by following your doctor's advice and making lifestyle changes. See the table below for tips.

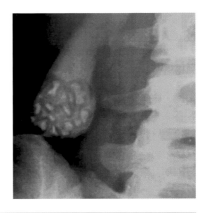

Gallstones A gallbladder full of gallstones is visible in this color-enhanced X-ray. The stones are in the green area on the left of the image.

DISORDER	WHAT IS IT?	HOW YOU CAN HELP
Indigestion	Pain or discomfort in the upper abdomen that usually develops after eating	• Avoid foods that irritate the stomach such as spicy foods and citrus fruits • Eat small, low-fat meals and snacks
Constipation	Infrequent and difficult passage of stools	• Eat plenty of soluble and insoluble fiber • Drink plenty of fluids
Diarrhea	Frequent passage of loose, watery stools, often caused by an infection	• Avoid high-fiber foods if short-term • Increase soluble fiber if long-term • Avoid sorbitol, and drink plenty of fluids
Irritable bowel syndrome (IBS)	A combination of abdominal pain, bloating, excessive gas, and changes in bowel habits	• Follow a low-fat, high-fiber diet • Avoid caffeinated drinks
Gastroesophageal reflux disease (GERD)	Regurgitation of acidic stomach juices into the esophagus, causing pain in the chest	• Follow a low-fat, high-fiber diet • Control weight; quit smoking
Peptic ulcer	Damage to the stomach lining and part of the small intestine (duodenum)	• Eat three meals daily; quit smoking • Limit alcohol, caffeine, and spicy foods
Cholecystitis and gallstones	Inflammation of the gallbladder often with stones formed in the gallbladder	• Follow a low-fat, high-fiber diet • Lose weight; exercise regularly
Lactose intolerance	The inability to digest lactose, the natural sugar present in milk	• Avoid milk and milk products • Opt for low-lactose or lactose-free drinks • Take calcium with vitamin D supplements
Celiac disease	Damage to the small intestine caused by a reaction to gluten, resulting in malabsorption	• Exclude gluten from your diet • Read labels and choose gluten-free food
Crohn's disease	An inflammatory disorder that affects mainly the ileum and the colon of the intestine	• Follow a diet low in fat, fiber, and lactose • Take a vitamin and mineral supplement
Ulcerative colitis	Inflammation and ulcers affecting the rectum and the colon (large intestine)	• Eat plenty of insoluble fiber • Take a vitamin and mineral supplement
Diverticular disease	Small pouches in the colon (diverticulosis) that may become inflamed and painful (diverticulitis)	• Eat plenty of insoluble fiber • Drink plenty of water • If you have abdominal pain, see a doctor

Nutrition for digestive disorders

What you eat and how you eat can have a major impact on digestive problems.

Nutrition plays a big role in many digestive disorders because what you eat has an important effect on your gastrointestinal (GI) tract.

The role of nutrition
If your GI tract is abnormal in any way, your doctor will suggest specific dietary changes to help alleviate some of your symptoms.

Some of these dietary changes may help correct and prevent the problem. For example, increasing the amount of fiber in your diet and drinking more water will help prevent constipation, and excluding gluten, a specific type of protein, may be required for the rest of your life if you have celiac disease. Although this may sound difficult, it could save your life and you will

be grateful to be able to enjoy your meals again without suffering from painful symptoms afterward.

Your doctor may advise you to change your lifestyle. For example, if you have reflux disease, you should avoid lying down after eating; and, if you have a peptic ulcer, you may need to limit foods and drinks containing caffeine.

Changing your diet
Making the appropriate changes to manage your digestive disorder requires patience and a trial-and-error period. You may find it helps to write down the offending foods that give you gas or cause you to feel bloated. If this continues to happen over and over again, then eliminating these foods may be beneficial to you. But remember, if you eliminate food groups from your diet you may need to take supplements. For example, those who avoid dairy products will need a calcium supplement to prevent osteoporosis from developing.

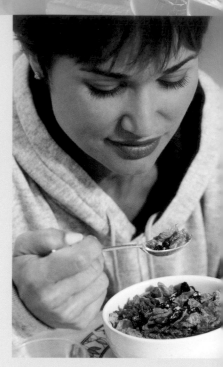

High-fiber breakfast To increase your fiber intake and keep your digestive tract active, start your day with a bran or whole-wheat cereal, topped with dried or fresh fruit.

A lot has changed over the years with regards to nutrition for digestive disorders and we have provided the most up-to-date advice in this chapter.

Tips to treat indigestion

The following suggestions can help relieve mild attacks of indigestion—pain or discomfort in the stomach or upper abdomen that usually comes on after eating a meal. The complaint may be accompanied by nausea, belching, and bloating. It is caused by eating or drinking too much, or stress, or may be a symptom of an underlying disorder such as a peptic ulcer (see p.227).
• Avoid foods that may irritate the stomach, such as caffeine, spearmint, peppermint, citrus fruits, spicy foods, high-fat foods, and tomato products.
• Some people find that an herbal tea, such as peppermint, fennel, or chamomile, provides relief.
• Eat small, low-fat meals and snacks, such as fruits, pretzels, crackers, and fat-free yogurt frequently, and at regular times during the day.
• Always eat slowly and chew your food thoroughly.
• Have drinks between meals, rather than with meals.

• Take a walk after meals, but do not do any strenuous exercise for at least one hour after eating.
• Avoid lying down for at least two hours after eating a meal.
• Try having a warm milk drink before bed, and use extra pillows to raise your head.
• If stress might be a cause of your indigestion, try to include relaxation techniques in your life, such as yoga or meditation.
• If you smoke, you should try to quit, since smoking may worsen the symptoms.
• Try an antacid medication, which can relieve the symptoms of indigestion by neutralizing stomach acid.
• Do not take aspirin or ibuprofen for pain relief since these medications can irritate the stomach.
• If you are overweight, which may worsen symptoms, try to lose weight.
• See your doctor if your symptoms become worse or do not improve after two weeks or if your indigestion recurs.

Treating constipation

A diet that is high in animal fats, such as meat, cheese, and eggs, and refined sugar but low in fiber from vegetables, fruits, and whole grains is a common cause of constipation.

The infrequent and difficult passage of stools is particularly common in older people. This is because gut motility decreases with age, resulting in food and waste taking longer to pass through the intestine. Stimulant laxatives can make the intestine sensitive to their effects, so you should avoid taking them regularly. It is far more effective to treat constipation through changes to your diet.

In addition, regular exercise will help stimulate intestinal activity and improve the motility of the intestinal tract.

INCREASE YOUR FIBER INTAKE
Dietary fiber in food (*see pp.48–49*) traps water and adds bulk to the stool, making it move through the gut more quickly.
● Gradually increase your fiber intake to 28g per day by eating more whole grains, vegetables, fruits, and legumes. Aim to eat six servings of grains and grain products daily.
● Make sure that you eat lots of fresh fruits and vegetables. Include foods with a natural laxative effect, such as prunes or prune juice, apricots, and apples.
● Eat a high-fiber breakfast cereal. Bran

cereals are particularly high in fiber and can be livened up with toppings, such as sliced banana, raisins, or strawberries.
● Switch from white bread, pasta, and rice to whole-wheat varieties.
● Avoid eating processed or highly refined foods, which are high in sugar and carbohydrates and low in fiber.

INCREASE YOUR FLUID INTAKE
If you suffer from constipation, increase your fluid intake. Aim to drink about 4 pints (2 liters) of water a day. Dry stools are more difficult and painful to pass, but drinks add bulk and fluid to the stool, making it easier to expel. Limit alcohol and caffeine because they can lead to dehydration, creating stools that are hard and more difficult to pass.

MAGNESIUM AND EXERCISE
Magnesium can help loosen stools, so increase your intake of magnesium-rich foods, such as spinach, almonds, Brazil nuts, raisins, and artichokes (*see p.68*). Alternatively, you can take a magnesium supplement (*see p.271*).

Eat dried fruit Soak dried fruits in juice or water for a nutritious fruit salad. Apricots, figs, and raisins are high in soluble fiber, and raisins are also high in magnesium.

When should I see my doctor?

If you have recently become constipated and the problem has lasted for more than two weeks—even after increasing your intake of fiber and fluids and your level of activity—you should make an appointment to see your doctor.

In addition, if you notice blood in your stool, consult your doctor, because bleeding from the intestine can be a symptom of a serious disorder such as colorectal cancer.

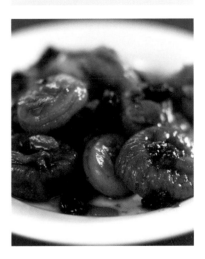

Tips to prevent diarrhea

Good hygiene and awareness of the sources of food contamination will help you to avoid diarrhea:
● Wash your hands after using the toilet and changing diapers.
● Frequently wash bathroom and food preparation surfaces.
● When traveling overseas, drink only bottled water, carbonated soft drinks, and drinks made with boiled water, such as tea and coffee. Do not drink tap water or ice that has been made from tap water.
● Avoid meat or fish that is raw or rare, or that is not served hot.
● Peel fruits and vegetables.

Treating diarrhea

Diarrhea is the frequent passage of loose, watery stools, and is often caused by infections from contaminated food or water. The following suggestions will help ease your symptoms:
● Replace lost fluid and electrolytes (minerals dissolved in fluids) with water, fruit juices diluted with water, rehydration drinks, or sports drinks. Try to drink at least 16floz (500ml) of fluid every one to two hours to prevent dehydration.
● Avoid very hot or very cold liquids, coffee, alcohol, or caffeinated soft drinks, all of which can irritate the intestine.
● Read product labels and check with your pharmacist about sorbitol- or lactulose-containing medications or diet

products, which can cause diarrhea; discontinue taking them if possible.
● If you can tolerate food, eat yogurt with live cultures (to replace gut flora) and avoid insoluble fiber (whole grains) until the diarrhea has resolved.
● Eat bland, nonfatty foods that are easily digested, and avoid milk, red meats, and highly seasoned food.
● If the diarrhea is a short-term problem, avoid high-fiber foods, such as whole grains and fresh fruits and vegetables, which can be difficult for the irritated intestine to digest. If the diarrhea lasts for more than two weeks, increasing soluble fiber intake may help, but you should see your doctor.

Treating irritable bowel syndrome

Doctors believe that in people with irritable bowel syndrome (IBS) the colon (the major section of the large intestine) is abnormally sensitive to stimuli such as excess gas, stress, high-fat or fiber-rich foods, caffeine, and alcohol. These stimuli can irritate the colon and cause pain, cramps, and diarrhea. Women with IBS may have more symptoms during their menstrual periods, suggesting that reproductive hormones can aggravate the condition. Many people state that the symptoms occur after they eat or when they are under stress.

IDENTIFY PROBLEM FOODS

A balanced diet can help alleviate IBS symptoms. You may find it helpful to keep a food diary to identify which foods cause the most discomfort and try to eliminate these from your diet. These foods may be different for each person; for example, some people may find onions and mushrooms cause gas, bloating, and discomfort; while others may find relief from omitting wheat.

CHOOSE DAIRY PRODUCTS

Even if you find that most dairy products are difficult to tolerate (see p.232), do not rule out yogurt. Yogurt may be better tolerated because it contains organisms that supply lactase, the enzyme needed to digest lactose (the sugar in milk). Lactose-free milk is also an option. Since dairy products are an important source of calcium, consider drinks enriched with calcium or take a calcium supplement if your body cannot tolerate dairy products.

OTHER DIETARY FACTORS

High-fiber foods, such as whole-grain breads and cereals, legumes, fruits, and vegetables help avoid intestinal cramps and spasms, and constipation —although, if you suffer from diarrhea, a low-fiber diet is better. It is also best to avoid caffeinated drinks such as tea, coffee, and cola, which stimulate the colon. Many find herbal teas, especially peppermint and fennel, soothing. Fruit juice contains a lot of fructose, which

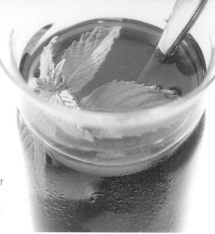

Peppermint tea A great alternative to normal tea or coffee, peppermint has anti-spasmodic properties, and can ease IBS symptoms by calming the intestinal tract.

can aggravate symptoms of IBS and contribute to diarrhea. It is best to stick to drinking mineral water to help flush out your system. In addition, smoking can exacerbate the symptoms of IBS, so it is important to quit if you smoke.

Case study Young woman with irritable bowel syndrome (IBS)

Name Megan

Age 25 years

Problem Five years ago, Megan was diagnosed with irritable bowel syndrome (IBS). She complains of crampy abdominal pain, which is relieved by a bowel movement. She often has loose stools or diarrhea followed by no bowel movements for several days. Her movements are irregular and her symptoms worsen when she is stressed. Her weight is stable and she does not have a fever or bleeding when going to the toilet.

Lifestyle Megan is a lawyer and is always busy and often stressed out. Her symptoms occur several times a week and affect her work. She has

two meals a day (pizza or a sandwich for lunch and pasta or take-out for dinner), often on the run. Because of the diarrhea, she is not sure what to eat, but she drinks apple juice to prevent dehydration. She does not take a multivitamin supplement and does not exercise.

Advice Several factors contribute to Megan's IBS. She is stressed at work and would benefit from yoga and exercise. She should eat breakfast— such as whole-grain toast or wheat cereal—to encourage more regular bowel movements and to help increase the fiber in her diet.

Megan also experiences cramping and gas from certain foods, the most common being legumes, onions, prunes, and cruciferous vegetables, such as cabbage and broccoli. Megan could try to eliminate these foods one

by one to determine any associations. She could also temporarily eliminate dairy products, since an intolerance to lactose (milk sugar) can cause symptoms similar to IBS. She may find, however, that she can tolerate yogurt, which is also high in calcium.

Increasing dietary fiber will help relieve Megan's symptoms, and she should have regular, firmer bowel movements. However, it can be hard to get enough dietary fiber, particularly if she eliminates fiber-rich foods that cause gas. She would benefit from taking a psyllium or methylcellulose fiber supplement.

Megan should make sure she drinks plenty of water with the supplements to reduce the symptoms of excessive gas, which may occur initially. The fructose in the apple juice can also contribute to diarrhea, so drinking water instead could help.

Treating gastroesophageal reflux disease (GERD)

GERD is a common cause of indigestion that occurs when acidic stomach juices are regurgitated into the esophagus (the tube from the throat to the stomach). The stomach juices irritate the esophagus, causing inflammation and pain (heartburn), and can cause permanent scarring if the condition persists. The main causes of GERD are poor tone in the ring of muscle at the end of the esophagus (lower esophageal sphincter) and increased pressure in the abdomen due to obesity or pregnancy. It is important to follow a low-fat diet since high-fat meals tend to decrease sphincter pressure, slowing the movement of food to the stomach and exposing the esophagus to irritants. Other key ways to treat GERD include losing weight if you are overweight and avoiding fatty foods, alcohol, chocolate, and coffee as much as possible.

AIM	TREATMENT
Decreasing the frequency and amount of regurgitated stomach juices	• Eat small, frequent meals • Drink fluids between meals rather than with meals • Eat plenty of fiber to avoid constipation, as straining increases abdominal pressure
Decreasing irritation in the esophagus	• Avoid or limit foods that may give you symptoms of GERD or aggravate the condition. These vary with different people but may include fatty foods, citrus fruits, tomato products, spicy foods, and carbonated drinks
Improving clearance of food from the esophagus	• Do not recline after eating—sit upright or, even better, take a walk • Avoid eating for two to three hours before bedtime or prior to lying down • Raise the head of your bed
Avoiding scarring the esophagus	• Choose soft foods that are easy to swallow, such as low-fat cottage cheese
Losing weight	• Eat smaller portions, follow a low-fat diet, and exercise regularly

Treating and preventing peptic ulcers

The goals of nutritional treatment for peptic ulcers—damage to the stomach lining (stomach ulcer) or the first part of the small intestine (duodenal ulcer)— are to reduce and neutralize stomach acid and to maintain the stomach lining's resistance to the acid. Reducing stomach acid helps alleviate symptoms and allows sores to heal.

There is no specific diet for ulcers— each person must discover which foods cause discomfort and avoid them. You may find the following tips helpful:

• Eat three meals daily, avoid skipping meals, and limit your intake of spicy, fatty, or other foods that cause discomfort.
• Avoid bedtime snacks, since symptoms often occur in the night.
• Limit caffeine intake by reducing your intake of coffee, tea, cola, and chocolate.
• Limit alcohol intake and avoid drinking on an empty stomach.
• Avoid smoking and passive smoking as smoke may increase the secretion of stomach acid, increase the frequency of duodenal ulcers, and delay healing.

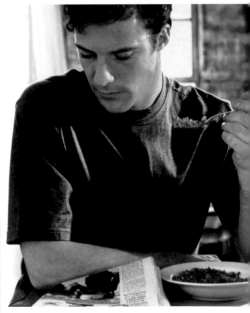

Helicobacter pylori infection and peptic ulcers

Peptic ulcers are commonly associated with *Helicobacter pylori* infection. The infection is thought to be spread by unsanitary living conditions. It infects the stomach and releases substances that reduce the effectiveness of the layer of mucus that protects the stomach lining from its own acidic juices. The acidic juices then erode the lining of the stomach or the duodenum, allowing a peptic ulcer to develop. A combination of antibiotics and ulcer-healing drugs will usually clear up the ulcer.

Make time for regular meals It is very important not to skip meals, including breakfast, if you suffer from a peptic ulcer.

Preventing and treating gallstones

Gallstones are formed from bile, a cholesterol-rich liquid made by the liver and stored in the gallbladder, that aids the digestive process. Gallstones are more common in women, in people over the age of 40, and those who are overweight and eat a high-fat diet. A family history of gallstones is a risk factor.

LOW-FAT, HIGH-FIBER DIET

Avoiding fatty foods and increasing your consumption of fiber (*see p.49*) by eating more high-fiber foods, such as bran, soy, guar gum, and pectin, which is found in many fruits and vegetables, can help prevent gallstones and relieve the discomfort caused by existing stones. Regular exercise may also decrease the risk of developing gallstones.

If you are obese, you are at increased risk of developing gallstones. Therefore, following a low-fat diet and increasing your exercise level will not only help you lose weight but also reduce your risk of developing gallstones. However, rapid weight loss can cause the formation of gallstones in some people, so you should lose weight gradually.

GALLBLADDER SURGERY

Surgical removal of the gallbladder is the most effective means of curing gallbladder disease—the effects are immediate. Once the gallbladder has been removed, however, there is no reservoir of bile, and fat absorption may be affected. In this case, following a low-fat diet may be helpful.

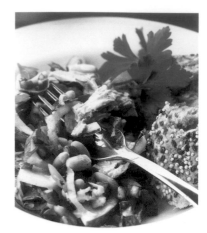

Healthy high-fiber dish Tuna and bean salad and a hunk of whole-grain bread make a low-fat, high-fiber meal that can help prevent the formation of gallstones.

Dealing with lactose intolerance

Normally, the enzyme lactase breaks down lactose (a natural sugar found in milk and other dairy products) in the intestine to form the sugars glucose and galactose. These are then easily absorbed through the intestinal wall into the bloodstream.

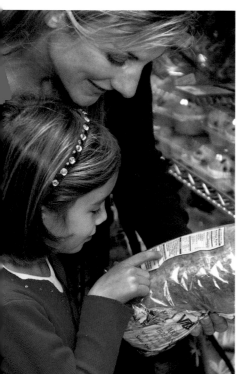

Checking ingredients If you or your child has a lactose intolerance, it is important that you check food labels carefully and learn to spot ingredients that contain lactose.

If this enzyme is absent or its levels are low, the unabsorbed lactose ferments, producing painful symptoms, such as abdominal bloating and cramping, diarrhea, and vomiting. The condition usually develops in adolescence or adulthood and is uncommon in babies and young children. No treatment can improve the body's ability to produce lactase, but symptoms can be easily controlled through diet.

LIMIT OR AVOID LACTOSE

Some people can benefit from just reducing the amount of foods they eat containing lactose, such as milk, yogurt, cheese, cream, and butter, and most are able to tolerate a small amount of lactose without symptoms. However, some people will develop symptoms from just a tiny amount of lactose. For those who cannot tolerate even small amounts of lactose, lactase enzymes are available, which will help them digest foods that contain lactose.

READ FOOD LABELS

If you are lactose-intolerant, check food labels for hidden dairy products. Small amounts of lactose may be hidden in breads, cereals, soups, margarine, lunch meats, dressings, candies, pancake mixes, cookies, and many other foods.

LACTOSE-FREE FOODS

There are lactose-free forms of milk, cheese, and yogurt available, but if you find that you cannot tolerate these, try soymilk products, which are naturally lactose-free yet supply many of the same nutrients that are in cow's milk. Different brands of soymilk have different tastes, so try a few until you find one that you like.

WATCH YOUR CALCIUM INTAKE

Dairy products are our prime source of dietary calcium, which is important for maintaining bone health. You should therefore try to include some lactose-free dairy or soy products in your diet every day. Other calcium-rich foods include salmon, spinach, and collard greens (*see p.63*). If you fall short on calcium, a supplement of 800–1,200mg per day is advisable to maintain recommended daily calcium levels.

Coping with Crohn's disease and ulcerative colitis

People with an inflammatory bowel disorder, such as Crohn's disease or ulcerative colitis, cannot absorb nutrients properly and are at risk of nutrient deficiencies and becoming underweight.

GETTING ENOUGH NUTRIENTS
If you have an inflammatory bowel disorder, make sure you get enough nutrients. A dietitian can help you in dealing with deficiencies, which can develop because the damaged intestine is not absorbing nutrients effectively. This is very important for children, who are growing and developing.

Symptoms such as nausea, diarrhea, and recurrent abdominal pain can occur at mealtimes, which often leads to decreased appetite and food intake. In Crohn's disease, inflammation of the intestine can result in overgrowth of bacteria. This, combined with the effects of any previous surgery to remove diseased sections of the bowel, can decrease the absorptive surface area of the intestine and reduce the absorption of essential nutrients. People who have undergone surgery may have

problems absorbing fats and this, coupled with frequent bouts of diarrhea, may also cause deficiencies to develop.

It is crucial to increase the amount of protein you eat since inflammatory bowel disorders can cause excessive intestinal secretion of protein-rich fluids through the inflamed wall of the intestine. Good sources include lean meat, poultry, oily fish, and legumes (*see pp.84–85*).

PROTECTIVE FOODS
Various foods can help relieve as well as prevent the troublesome symptoms of an inflammatory bowel disorder.
- Complex carbohydrates (*see p.46–47*) from whole grains, vegetables, and fruits are a good source of fiber, which helps the intestine function properly. If the extra fiber causes gas, take an over-the-counter product to reduce gas.
- Drink lots of fluids, mainly water, but avoid caffeinated drinks. Green tea is thought to be beneficial.
- Eat plenty of foods containing omega-3 fatty acids, such as canola oil, flaxseed, soybeans, and oily fish.
- The herb sage may be helpful too.

FOODS TO AVOID
Certain foods may cause symptoms. Common things to avoid are alcohol, sugary foods, including sweet fruit such as grapes and pineapple, and caffeine, as they can all cause inflammation; foods containing gluten, which is found in wheat, oats, and barley; milk and dairy products; foods that are common causes of allergic reactions, such as soy, eggs, and peanuts; and vegetables of the brassica family, such as Brussels sprouts, cabbages, and broccoli.

TAKING SUPPLEMENTS
People who have Crohn's disease or ulcerative colitis are advised to take a multivitamin supplement. Deficiencies of the fat-soluble vitamins (A, D, E, K), vitamin B_{12}, and folate are common. A folate supplement is vital for anyone taking sulfasalazine (a drug prescribed for chronic inflammation), which can interfere with folate's absorption. Some patients may need injections of vitamin B_{12}. Persistent, watery diarrhea may require supplementation with the minerals zinc and magnesium.

Recipe Omega-3-rich trout stuffed with sage

INGREDIENTS

2 fresh trout, boned and cleaned

bunch of fresh sage

2 lemons

freshly ground black pepper

3 tbsp olive oil

Serves 2

1 Preheat the oven to 350°F/180°C. Line a baking dish with a large sheet of foil and place the trout on it.

2 Stuff several sprigs of sage into each fish and season with the juice of one lemon and freshly ground black pepper.

3 Cut the remaining lemon into wedges and place around the trout. Drizzle with olive oil.

4 Bring the foil up and over the trout and seal to form a parcel. Bake for 35 minutes or until the fish is cooked.

5 Carefully remove the trout from the foil onto serving plates. Garnish with sprigs of fresh sage. If you like, serve with baby new potatoes and lightly steamed green beans.

Each serving provides
Cal. 306, Total fat 25g (Sat. 4g, Poly. 3g, Mono. 16g), Cholesterol 47mg, Protein 17g, Carbohydrate 6g, Fiber 1.3g, Sodium 33mg. Good source of— Vits: A; Mins: Ca, Mg, P, K.

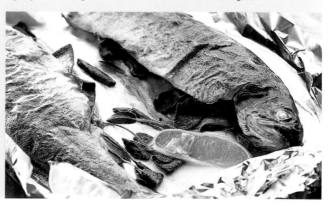

Diverticular disorders

Diverticulosis is the presence of small pouches (known as diverticuli) in the wall of the colon, which occur when parts of the intestine bulge outward through weak areas. The increase in pressure in the colon is commonly caused by constipation due to lack of fiber in the diet.

From time to time, one or more of these "pouches" may become inflamed. This condition is known as diverticulitis, and it is possible to treat it with a low-fiber, "soft" diet.

HIGH FIBER FOR DIVERTICULOSIS

Diverticulosis is very common among older people and, although it often does not produce specific symptoms, some people may develop cramps, bloating, and irregular bowel movements, with no sign of fever or infection.

Treating and preventing diverticulosis through nutrition often involves just increasing insoluble fiber in the diet; this helps keep stools soft and easy to pass and prevents constipation, and therefore prevents the development of diverticulosis.

The recommended daily amount of fiber is 25g for a woman and 38g for a man. Fruits, vegetables, and grains are

good sources of dietary fiber, and can easily be incorporated into your daily diet (see pp.48–49).

If you suffer from diverticulosis, it is important that you follow a high-fiber diet, and make sure that you also drink plenty of fluids (preferably water)—about 4 pints (2 liters) a day. It is important that you avoid becoming constipated, since hard stools or straining when you go to the toilet will cause more diverticuli (pouches) to form and make your symptoms worse.

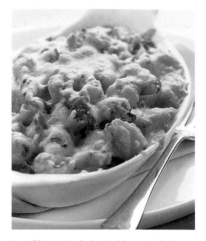

Low-fiber pasta bake A white-pasta bake with tuna, topped with low-fat hard cheese, is a great low-fiber option for people suffering from diverticulitis.

LOW FIBER FOR DIVERTICULITIS

Diverticulitis is an acute infection or inflammation of the diverticuli that may flare up if a stool gets caught in one of the "pouches." Symptoms can include abdominal pain, fever, and nausea. An infection usually lasts for about a week.

When someone with diverticulosis develops diverticulitis, the nutritional advice changes. Rather than following a high-fiber diet, you should instead follow a low-fiber one, which allows the passage of stools through the inflamed, typically narrowed segment of the colon.

In addition, you should eat a soft diet, which means that you should eat things that do not require much chewing, such as soup, mashed potatoes, well-cooked pasta, and bananas. Once the infection has cleared up, patients should go back to their high-fiber diet.

EATING SEEDS AND NUTS

In the past, doctors recommended that people with diverticulosis should avoid eating nuts and seeds because they could lodge in the diverticula and lead to diverticulitis. There are no known cases of such a blockage, however, and so there is no proven benefit in avoiding seeds and nuts. If you have suffered rectal bleeding, your doctor may still advise you to avoid seeds and nuts, but otherwise you can safely enjoy these items as part of a high-fiber diet.

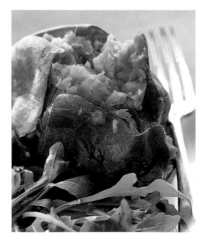

High-fiber sweet potato A baked sweet potato served with arugula is a high-fiber dish that is nutritious, easy to prepare, and will help in the treatment of diverticulosis.

Gluten-free diet for celiac disease

In celiac disease, the intestine cannot absorb food properly due to a reaction to gluten, a protein found in wheat, rye, barley, and oats. The only treatment, therefore, is a gluten-free diet, which must be followed for life. A gluten-free diet will improve symptoms within days of starting it, allow existing damage to heal, and prevent further intestinal damage. The table below is a great starting point for anyone embarking on a gluten-free diet. Remember to always check food labels for hidden gluten, as it can appear in different forms in places you wouldn't expect to find it, for example in hydrolyzed vegetable protein (HVP).

FOOD TYPE	FOODS ALLOWED	FOODS NOT ALLOWED
Breads, pasta, cereals, flour, and grains	Bread, pasta, or noodles made from corn, rice, soy, corn-starch, potato starch, potato flour, whole-bean flour, tapioca, sago, rice bran, sorghum, quinoa; cereal containing rice or corn; corn tacos and tortillas	Breads containing wheat, rye, barley, oats, bran, semolina, kamut; pasta made from wheat, wheat starch, couscous; cereals made from wheat, rye, triticale, barley, oats
Fruits and vegetables	Fresh, frozen, and canned fruits and vegetables (avoid emulsifiers and stabilizers from unknown sources)	Fruit pie filling, creamed or breaded vegetables (read labels)
Dairy	Milk, cream, buttermilk, yogurt, cheese, cream cheese, processed cheese, cottage cheese	Malted milk; thickened milkshake (check labels on processed cheeses products)
Protein sources	Fresh meat, fish, and poultry; lentils, chickpeas, peas, legumes, nuts, seeds, tofu	Luncheon meats, sausages, and canned ham or tuna may contain HVP (check labels)
Fats and oils	Butter, margarine, vegetables oils (except canola)	Canola oil; sprays with grain alcohol
Alcohol	Wine, potato vodka, rum and tequila, sake	Beers and ales, grain alcohol, most liqueurs
Miscellaneous	Homemade soup; wheat-free soy sauce; non-grain vinegars, such as wine or fruit vinegar	Canned soup and soup mixes; most soy sauces; white vinegar made from grains

Recipe Gluten-free quinoa-stuffed peppers

INGREDIENTS

½ cup quinoa

1 onion

text ves garlic

1 zucchini

½ cup canned chick peas, drained

1 lemon

4 bell peppers

Serves 4

1 Cook the quinoa according to the instructions on the package. When done, leave, covered, in a warm place for 15 minutes.

2 Preheat the oven to 400°F/200°C. Peel and chop the onion, crush the garlic, and dice the zucchini. Heat a little oil in a skillet, add vegetables, and fry for a few minutes until softened but not browned. Stir in the quinoa, the drained chick peas, and 1 tsp of lemon juice. Season with freshly ground black pepper.

3 Cut tops off peppers and remove seeds. Divide quinoa mixture between peppers and replace tops. Place in oven-proof dish, and brush with oil.

4 Bake in a preheated oven for about 45 minutes, until the peppers are tender and lightly browned. Serve with lettuce and tomatoes.

Each serving provides:
Calories 219, Total fat 2.5g (Sat. 0.3g, Poly. 1.1g, Mono. 0.6g), Cholesterol 0mg, Protein 8.4g, Carbohydrate 46g, Fiber 7.1g, Sodium 103mg. Good source of—Vits: A, Fol, C; Mins: Ca, Mg, P, K.

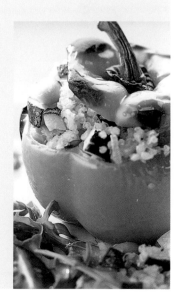

Disorders of the urinary system

The urinary system rids your body of waste, so it is crucial that it functions well.

The urinary system, also known as the urinary tract, consists of a pair of kidneys; the bladder; the ureters, which connect each kidney to the bladder; and the urethra, through which urine leaves the body.

Role of the kidneys

The main job of the kidneys is to remove waste and excess water from the body in the form of urine, keep a stable balance of salts and other substances in the blood, and produce hormones that stimulate red blood cell production and regulate blood pressure.

Every day, the kidneys filter about 50 gallons (190 liters) of blood and produce about 4 pints (2 liters) of waste products and water—the amount varies depending on how much food and drink you have consumed. The waste and water become urine, which is held in the bladder until you go to the bathroom. The waste products in your blood come from the normal breakdown of body tissues and the foods you eat. If your kidneys are not able to remove these wastes properly, they build up in the blood and can cause significant medical problems.

Potential problems

Most kidney diseases affect the filtration capacity of the kidneys, causing them to lose function.

Kidney disorders are broadly classified as acute—the sudden failure of a kidney, which may be fatal—or there may be a gradual reduction in function over months or years, in which case it is chronic.

Although the urinary system is structured in a way that helps ward off infection, infections can occur. They are caused by germs that get into the urethra, which can spread to the kidneys.

The urinary system

This is different in men and women. The urethra from the male bladder passes through the prostate gland.

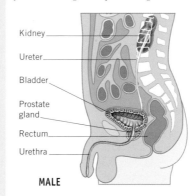

Kidney
Ureter
Bladder
Prostate gland
Rectum
Urethra

MALE

The female bladder sits under the uterus. Urination is controlled by the muscles in the neck of the bladder.

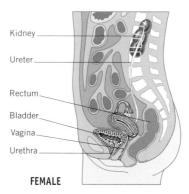

Kidney
Ureter
Rectum
Bladder
Vagina
Urethra

FEMALE

Who is most at risk of developing urinary disorders?

The following are some of the risk factors for disorders of the urinary system discussed in this section:

Diet and lifestyle People who live in hot climates and who are susceptible to kidney stones are at increased risk if they do not drink enough fluid to replace that lost through perspiration.

Gender and age About 20 percent of women will have a urinary tract infection (UTI) at some point in their life. The reasons for this are not fully understood, although it may be because a woman's urethra is short, allowing bacteria quick access to the bladder. Kidney stones are more common in Caucasians, in men, and in those between the ages of 20 and 40.

Family history You are more likely to develop a stone if someone in your family has had a kidney stone. Similarly, anyone who has a kidney stone is at increased risk of having another.

Other factors Any abnormality of the urinary tract that obstructs the flow of urine (a kidney stone, for example) sets the stage for a urinary tract infection. An enlarged prostate gland can also slow urine flow, thus increasing the risk of infection. Sexually active women or those who use a diaphragm for birth control may be more likely to have a UTI. People with diabetes have a higher risk of a UTI because of changes in their immune systems.

People with ulcerative colitis or Crohn's disease, or who have had intestinal bypass surgery for weight loss, are at risk of developing oxalate kidney stones, and these people may be prescribed preventive treatment.

People with diabetes or high blood pressure, or who have suffered repeated kidney infections are at greatest risk of developing kidney failure.

Disorders of the urinary system

The table below deals with the major disorders affecting the urinary system, which comprises the kidneys, bladder, and urethra. It keeps the body's chemistry in balance by removing waste products and excess water.

One of the most common disorders of the urinary system, kidney stones are formed from deposits of calcium, oxalate, uric acid, or citrate. The risk of developing kidney stones is increased by inadequate fluid intake. Kidney failure may be acute (short-term) or chronic (long-term). Chronic failure develops slowly over the years, with symptoms so mild that people may not recognize that they have a kidney disease.

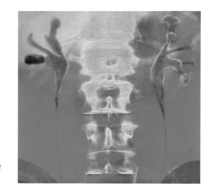

Kidney stone A reddish brown kidney stone can be clearly seen in the right kidney on the left of this X-ray image.

DISORDER	WHAT IS IT?	HOW YOU CAN HELP
Urinary tract infection (UTI)	An infection can occur in any part of the urinary tract when a bacterium, fungus, or virus invades. If the infection reaches the kidneys, it can cause a fever or lower back pain.	• Drink plenty of water and cranberry juice to flush out the system • Do not resist the urge to urinate
Kidney stones	Stones are one of the most common kidney disorders. A kidney stone is a hard mass that develops from crystals that separate from urine and build up in the kidney. Most stones pass on their own and require no treatment other than pain management. Dietary measures may be effective at reducing the risk of another occurrence. Stones can also form in the bladder from substances in urine.	• Maintaining hydration with plenty of fluids is essential • Maintain your calcium intake and reduce intake of high-oxalate foods • Eat a low-protein, low-sodium diet • Choose complex carbohydrates • Eat more fresh fruit and vegetables
Kidney failure	Damage to the kidney compromises its ability to filter out and eliminate waste products and water, which build up in the blood, disrupting its chemical balance.	• Control your blood pressure and blood sugar • Eat a low-protein, low-sodium diet

Urinary tract infections

Infections can occur if bacteria get into the body via the bloodstream or the urethra. Urinary tract infections (UTIs) are more common in women.

THE SPREAD OF BACTERIA

Despite containing fluids, salts, and waste products, urine is sterile (free from germs, such as bacteria). An infection occurs only when bacteria begin to grow. A woman's urethral opening lies near sources of bacteria from the anus and vagina. Infections often start in the urethra (urethritis). From there, the bacteria can move up into the bladder, causing an infection (cystitis), and if the infection is not treated, it can spread to the kidneys, causing pyelonephritis, which is serious and can damage the kidneys.

TREATING A UTI

There are steps you can take to ease painful symptoms, such as a frequent urge to urinate, a burning feeling when you urinate, and general discomfort.
• Drink plenty of water.
• Drink cranberry juice—it reduces the ability of bacteria to "stick" to the bladder lining and fights off infection.
• Urinate when you feel the need.
• Wipe from front to back.
• Avoid using feminine hygiene sprays.
• Take showers instead of baths.
If symptoms persist, see your doctor, who may prescribe antibiotics.

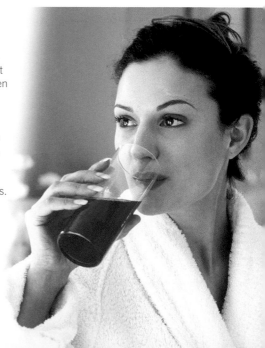

Cranberry juice Drinking pure cranberry juice can not only treat but can also prevent urinary tract infections.

Dietary treatment for kidney stones

Kidney stones occur when the urine is saturated with waste products that can crystallize into stones or when the chemicals that normally inhibit this crystallization process are absent. The most common type of stone contains calcium with either phosphate or oxalate. Some stones contain uric acid, and these are more common in people with gout (*see p.245*).

The goal of nutritional treatment is to eliminate the diet-related risk factors for stone formation and to prevent the further growth of existing stones.

THE IMPORTANCE OF FLUIDS

First, and most importantly, a regular intake of plenty of fluids is essential for people with kidney stones. This will dilute the urine, thus reducing the concentration of stone-forming substances in the urine.

Water is the fluid of choice. Some drinks, including grapefruit and apple juice, may increase the risk of kidney stone formation.

On the other hand, a moderate intake of alcohol, coffee, and tea may help reduce the risk of stone formation—

due, presumably, to the diuretic effect of the caffeine in these beverages.
• A daily intake of about 5–6 pints (2.5–3 liters) of fluid is recommended.

MAINTAIN CALCIUM INTAKE

Most calcium stones are not, in fact, attributable to a diet high in calcium-rich foods. As explained in the box (*right*), it is important to maintain a moderate calcium intake if you suffer from kidney stones. This is because a low intake may promote the formation of calcium oxalate stones.
• A calcium intake of approximately 600–800mg per day is recommended for people with kidney stones.

CUT OUT HIGH-OXALATE FOODS

A reduction in dietary intake of foods containing high levels of oxalate (*right*) is important for susceptible people, since this is an important factor in the formation of calcium oxalate stones.

Vitamin C supplements should also be avoided by people at risk of kidney stones since this vitamin can break down to oxalate, which is excreted in the kidney (*see p.269*).

RESTRICT ANIMAL PROTEIN

A high intake of animal protein is acidic and increases the excretion of urinary calcium. In addition, the binding effect of sulfate in dietary protein decreases kidney calcium reabsorption. Therefore, it is recommended that people with kidney stones should limit their intake of animal proteins from meat, fish, poultry, and egg to 60–70g per day.

REDUCE SODIUM INTAKE

A high intake of sodium (*see p.221*) increases calcium excretion, which can result in an increase in calcium-containing crystals in the urine. A reduction of high-sodium foods is therefore recommended, with an intake of no more than 2–4g per day.

High-sodium foods include most canned, processed, and packaged foods. Any labeled food that has a sodium content greater than 400mg sodium per serving is considered to be high in sodium.

COMPLEX CARBOHYDRATES

It is also advisable for people with kidney stones to reduce their intake of simple sugars and products made from refined flour (such as white bread, cakes, and cookies), in favor of whole-grain foods, such as whole-wheat bread, barley, oats, and brown rice, that are high in complex carbohydrates (*see pp.46–47*), as well as more fresh fruits and vegetables.

Avoid high-oxalate foods

Although high calcium excretion in the urine is commonly seen in people with calcium stones, kidney stones do not result from a high dietary intake of calcium. On the contrary, a diet that is very low in calcium increases the absorption and subsequent excretion of the chemical oxalate, which promotes the formation of calcium oxalate stones in susceptible people.

The amount of oxalate in the diet, however, is an important factor in the formation of calcium oxalate stones, and people who are prone to this type of kidney stone are advised to cut back on high-oxalate foods in order to help prevent the formation of stones. Foods that are rich in oxalate include:
• Dark leafy greens, such as spinach, Swiss chard, beet greens, endive, escarole, and parsley
• Other vegetables and legumes including: beets, celery, eggplant, leeks, okra, summer squash, sweet potatoes, and beans
• Fruits, including blackberries, gooseberries, raspberries, rhubarb, strawberries, and red currants
• Beverages such as draft beer, tea, and instant coffee
• Cocoa, chocolate, chocolate drinks, and carob powder
• Nuts and nut butters.

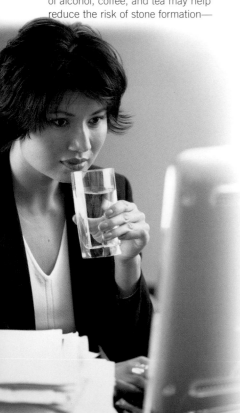

Drink plenty of water If you have kidney stones, maintain your fluid intake throughout the day to dilute your urine and reduce the concentration of stone-forming substances.

Nutrition in kidney failure

Kidney (or renal) failure occurs when the kidneys cease to function normally. People who have kidney disease will be prescribed special diets by their doctor and nutritionist, specifically to reduce their dietary protein, sodium, phosphorus, and potassium intake, depending on the results of weekly blood tests.

Dialysis can be done by filtering the blood through a machine (hemodialysis) or by infusing and removing a saline solution through the abdomen (peritoneal dialysis). People receiving dialysis must also watch their diets with extreme care and may need extra calories to prevent weight loss. The following general dietary points can be made.

CONTROL PROTEIN INTAKE

Because people with kidney failure have a decreased ability to excrete urea (the product of protein metabolism), it is advisable to control the intake of protein in the diet to help minimize the buildup of these nitrogen-containing wastes in the blood. Recent research suggests that restricting the intake of protein early in the course of kidney failure may slow the progression of the disease and delay the need to initiate dialysis therapy. The generally accepted level of

protein for people with kidney failure is to eat less than 0.6g per 2.2lb (1kg) of body weight per day.

OBTAIN CALORIES FROM FAT

Since people with kidney failure are at risk of undernutrition, additional dietary fat intake, in the form of mono- and polyunsaturated fats, may be advised as a way of providing adequate calories. However, elevated levels of "bad" LDL-cholesterol and total cholesterol are found in 20–70 percent of people with kidney failure, so regular monitoring of blood-lipid levels is important.

MAINTAIN SODIUM BALANCE

As kidney failure progresses, the ability of the kidneys to excrete sodium declines and dietary intake may have to be limited (*see p.221*). Sodium balance can usually be maintained by limiting sodium intake to 2,000–3,000mg per day.

RESTRICT POTASSIUM

A restriction on dietary potassium may be necessary during the later stages of kidney failure, or if certain medications lead to high levels of potassium in the blood. A limit of 2,000–3,000mg per day may be initiated.

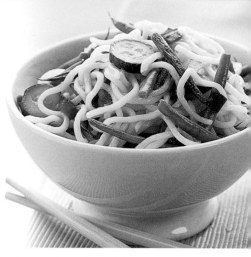

Low-protein meal Restricting protein intake may help slow the progression of kidney failure, so low-protein meals, such as noodles with fresh vegetables, are recommended.

MAINTAIN FLUID BALANCE

Fluid intake in people with kidney failure is determined by the ability of the kidneys to eliminate fluid. As long as the daily urine output essentially equals the daily fluid intake, balance will be maintained. In the later stages of kidney failure, however, fluid intake may need to be restricted in order to prevent fluid retention.

Maintaining dietary balance

It is usually advisable for people with kidney failure to follow a very specific diet to slow the progression of the condition, alleviate symptoms, and prevent nutrient deficiencies. This will usually be implemented under the supervision of a registered dietitian.

Since many people with chronic kidney failure also have other medical conditions such as high blood pressure, diabetes, and, possibly, high levels of blood cholesterol, the right balance of food is very important; otherwise, the dietary restrictions will cause them to lose weight and become malnourished. The challenge is to make sure that you get enough calories, the right kind of fat (monounsaturated) to maintain a healthy weight, and enough vitamins

and minerals. Since protein is usually reduced, calories can be added from olive and canola oil and margarine, and from small frequent meals and snacks.

NUTRITIONAL SUPPLEMENTS

Due to dietary restrictions, people with kidney failure need supplements of the vitamins thiamine (B_1), riboflavin (B_2), niacin (B_3), vitamin B_6, folate, vitamin C, and vitamin D. Vitamin A, however, may build up as kidney failure progresses and should not be supplemented.

Kidney failure usually leads to anemia due to decreased production by the kidneys of the hormone erythropoietin, which is needed to make red blood cells. Anemia can treated with erythropoietin therapy and iron supplementation.

KIDNEY FAILURE MENU PLANNER

Breakfast
- 1 scrambled egg, on a slice of whole-wheat toast with margarine
- 1 slice of cantaloupe melon

Lunch
- 2oz (55g) low-salt turkey breast, with salad on whole-wheat bread
- 8floz (240 ml) of lemonade

Dinner
- 1½ cups cooked spaghetti with low-salt marinara sauce
- 1 cup string beans
- Baked apple with low-fat yogurt

Snacks
- Raw vegetables with low-fat dip

Bone and joint disorders

Nutrition plays a vital role in the health of bones and joints.

Bones and joints make up the body's framework, protecting our internal organs and working in conjunction with our muscles to keep us mobile. Good nutrition throughout life is essential for the formation and maintenance of strong bones, while regular exercise is an important factor in maintaining the healthy function of bones and joints.

Osteoporosis

One of the most common bone diseases, osteoporosis involves a gradual loss of bone tissue, leaving the bones less dense and more prone to fracture. Osteoporosis is a major public-health problem in North America, affecting over 45

million people. The number of affected people is likely to increase as the population ages.

Adequate calcium intake is crucial for the formation and maintenance of bones (*see p.62*). This mineral must be replaced by dietary means because it is not manufactured by the body. If your dietary intake is inadequate, calcium is lost from the bones, making them weaker.

Vitamin D is also essential for bone health (*see p.57*) because it is needed for calcium absorption, with deficiency contributing to low bone density and disease (*below*). Researchers also believe that isoflavones from soy and other phytoestrogens (*see p.144*) may help increase calcium absorption.

Osteomalacia and rickets

A disease of adults, osteomalacia is characterized by soft bones due to a failure of bone to absorb calcium. The disorder is caused by various factors including too little vitamin D in the diet, insufficient exposure to sunlight, and malabsorption of vitamin D in the intestine due to conditions such as celiac disease (*see p.235*) or after gastrointestinal surgery. Osteomalacia can lead to pain in the legs, ribs, hips, and muscles, and to easily broken bones and impaired mobility.

In children, the same condition is known as rickets and is usually caused by a vitamin D deficiency. Babies who are breast-fed for more than a year (with no vitamin D supplements) and children deprived of sufficient sunlight are most at risk of developing rickets.

However, the incidence of rickets has been significantly reduced in North America, where most milk and other dairy foods are now fortified with vitamin D.

Key anatomy

Joints occur where bones meet, and enable our bodies to be flexible. The ends of bones are lined with cartilage.

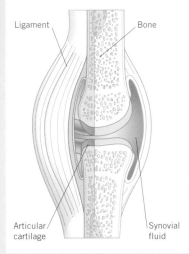

Ligament

Bone

Articular cartilage

Synovial fluid

Arthritic conditions

There are many different types of arthritis, but in general the term refers to inflammation of one or more joints, accompanied by pain, swelling, and stiffness. Rheumatoid arthritis is the most common form of inflammatory joint disease and is found in up to one percent of North Americans. Many tissues in the body may be involved, but the joints are most severely affected.

Osteoarthritis is another common form of arthritis that affects about one in seven North Americans. The condition is characterized by a gradual loss of cartilage from the joints and, in some people, joint inflammation. It most commonly affects the joints of the hands, knees, spine, and hips.

Gout is another form of arthritis that usually affects the joint at the base of the big toe. The condition is caused by high levels of uric acid in the bloodstream—which is known as hyperuricemia—leading to the deposition of uric-acid crystals in the joint. The joint becomes red, swollen, and tender, and the attack may be accompanied by fever.

Fibromyalgia and nutrition

Fibromyalgia is a complex chronic muscle disorder that affects over 10 million North Americans. The symptoms including widespread body pain, fatigue, headache, difficulty concentrating, disturbed sleep, depression, and anxiety.

While there is little scientific support for dietary treatment, many people turn to nutritional and herbal supplements, including vitamins, magnesium, and amino acids. Studies show that the pain and tenderness of fibromyalgia may be relieved by supplements of magnesium hydroxide and malic acid (a naturally occurring substance in our bodies).

Who is most at risk of bone and joint disorders?

Adult bone mass is determined by the amount of bone formed during childhood, with accumulation (known as peak bone mass) complete by age 35. Bone mass is influenced by a number of factors: up to 80 percent of bone mass is influenced by genetic factors, while about 20–40 percent is environmental. **Diet and lifestyle** A life-long diet low in calcium and vitamin D is one of the major risk factors for many bone disorders. Smoking and heavy alcohol consumption, which are often accompanied by poor nutrition and lack of physical activity, are also associated with low bone density. Gout is often associated with a rich diet and heavy alcohol consumption. **Age** Bone and joint disorders are more common among middle-aged and older adults. The onset of rheumatoid arthritis most commonly occurs between ages 40 and 60, and osteoarthritis between ages 60 and 80. Gout most commonly develops between the ages of 40 and 50 in men

and over 60 in women. Asian and Caucasian women over age 65 have a particularly high risk of developing osteoporosis. On the other hand, African–American women tend to have a higher bone mass than Caucasians and a lower risk of osteoporosis. **Gender** Osteoporosis is more common in women since they have less bone mass than men to begin with. Women who have short intervals between pregnancies or several children are at increased risk of this disease. In addition, because the levels of estrogen—necessary to retain calcium in the bones—decrease in women after menopause, their risk increases at this stage. Women have twice the risk of developing rheumatoid arthritis as men. However, gout is twenty times more common in men. **Family history** Both osteoporosis and gout are conditions in which a family history increases the risk of developing the disease. A history of a maternal hip fracture after age 50 is also considered a risk factor for osteoporosis.

What are bone and joint disorders?

Disorders that affect the musculoskeletal system are common and range from mild problems, such as gout, to more severe problems such as rheumatoid arthritis and osteoarthritis. The most common symptoms are pain and physical disability, which can have a major impact on people's lives. Some 30 percent of North Americans have symptoms related to their bones and

joints, but people rarely die from these conditions. Treatments for bone and joint disorders include medications, physical therapy, surgery, and nutritional therapy.

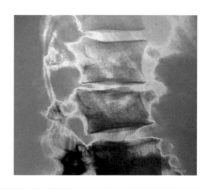

Osteoporosis This colored X-ray shows how the lower spine is compacted in a person with osteoporosis. The vertebrae (dark blocks) are touching, causing back pain and immobility.

DISORDER	WHAT IS IT?	HOW YOU CAN HELP
Osteoporosis	Loss of bone density, leaving bones brittle, and prone to fracture. Since it occurs without symptoms, it is often diagnosed only after a bone is fractured in a fall or a vertebra collapses, causing back pain.	• Ensure adequate intake of calcium and vitamin D; quit smoking; exercise regularly
Osteomalacia	Softening and weakening of bones in adults, due to a failure of bone to absorb the mineral calcium.	• Increase vitamin D intake • 15 minutes sunshine daily
Rickets	Childhood condition causing retarded growth, joint malformation, and swelling and tenderness at bone ends. May lead to bowed legs, spinal curvature, and chest-bone malformations.	• Increase vitamin D and calcium intake • 15 minutes sunshine daily
Rheumatoid arthritis (RA)	Inflammation of synovial membrane, which encloses joints, causing joint stiffness, pain, and swelling, and may lead to a loss of movement and deformity of joints.	• Eat a varied diet rich in essential vitamins and minerals • Exercise regularly
Osteoarthritis	Degeneration of cartilage covering bone ends, within joints, causing pain, swelling, and stiffness, usually in knees and hips.	• Exercise regularly • Lose weight if overweight
Gout	Deposits of uric acid crystals within joints, causing sudden pain and inflammation. Joint at base of big toe most commonly affected.	• Avoid high purine foods • Restrict alcohol intake

Treating osteoporosis

One of the most common bone diseases, osteoporosis involves a gradual loss of bone tissue, leaving the bones less dense and more prone to fracture. Osteoporosis is very common in North America, affecting over 45 million people. It is possible to slow the progress of the condition by making changes to your diet and lifestyle:

Take adequate calcium The body does not manufacture calcium, and it is lost from the body every day. It is therefore important to maintain adequate daily intake (*below*).

Take adequate vitamin D This vitamin is needed for normal calcium absorption by the body, as well as playing a role in the uptake of calcium into bone (*see p.57*). It is important that you get sufficient vitamin D from your diet as well as from exposure to the sun.

Quit smoking Studies have shown that smokers have poorer bone density than nonsmokers. Quitting smoking, even later in life, may help limit bone loss. Research shows that while hormone replacement therapy protects women from bone fractures, this may not be the case in female smokers, as tobacco may have an antiestrogenic effect. In addition, smokers tend to drink more alcohol and exercise less.

Limit alcohol intake Those who drink alcohol heavily are more prone to bone loss and fractures, mainly because of poor nutrition but also due to their increased risk of falling.

Exercise regularly Regular physical activity helps increase bone mass and reduce bone loss. Weight-bearing exercises such as walking, dancing, and weightlifting are best.

Checking bone density

A DEXA scan is currently the most widely used method of measuring bone-mineral density of the spine and extremities. Scanning takes a few minutes and is a sensitive and accurate test of bone density. The report compares your values with those of a young person and with a person of your age with normal bone density (age-related bone loss is normal). You are at risk of osteoporosis if you take medication, such as steroids, that affects your bones; if you have a history of menstrual cycle cessation; if you have inflammatory bowel disease; or if you had early menopause. In such circumstances, ask your doctor about having a baseline bone scan which can be repeated over time.

Boosting your dietary calcium intake

Calcium is vital for bone formation and keeping bones strong. It is important to boost your calcium intake if you are at risk of developing, or if you already suffer from, osteoporosis.

The recommended calcium intake is 800mg per day for children aged 3–8 years; 1,300mg per day for those aged 9–18 years; and 1,000mg for adults. Anyone over 50 years old should be increasing their intake to 1200mg per day. Adequate calcium intake is critical for women going through menopause as bone mass can decrease at this time.

CALCIUM-RICH FOODS

The mineral calcium is absorbed by the body better in food than as a supplement, so increase your intake of calcium-rich foods. Obvious sources of calcium are dairy products, such as milk, yogurt, and cheese, but calcium is also found in spinach, watercress, green beans, broccoli, canned sardines and salmon with bones, tofu, dried apricots, and figs.

Once you know how, it is relatively easy to transform meals into calcium-rich ones—see right for an easy lunch transformation to boost calcium intake.

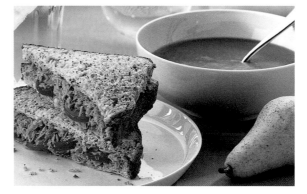

Low-calcium lunch
Although healthy in many respects, this lunch of tomato soup, tuna–tomato sandwich in whole-wheat bread, fresh pear, and a glass of water provides just 94mg of calcium.

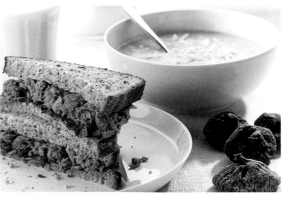

High-calcium lunch
This lunch of cream of broccoli soup topped with grated low-fat cheese, a salmon–watercress sandwich, dried figs, and a glass of low-fat milk provides 821mg of calcium.

Preventing and treating osteomalacia and rickets

Osteomalacia and rickets (the name given to osteomalacia when it occurs in babies and children) are caused by a deficiency of vitamin D in the body (see p.57).

INCREASING VITAMIN D
Deficiency is due to inadequate dietary intake of foods containing vitamin D, or to insufficient sunlight, which is necessary for the conversion of vitamin D in our skin to its active form (a form that the body can use). There are few dietary sources of vitamin D, but many common foods, such as margarine, dairy products, and orange juice, are fortified with the vitamin. Good natural sources of vitamin D include cod liver oil, egg yolks, butter, canned salmon and sardines (with bones), herring, green leafy vegetables, and tofu.

If you do not regularly consume dairy products and live in an area where you are not exposed to the sun for certain seasons of the year, you should consider a supplement that supplies at least the DRI for vitamin D (0.005mg per day).

Treating rheumatoid arthritis

Depending on the stage of the disease, treatment of rheumatoid arthritis varies but initial treatment is usually aimed at reducing inflammation while minimizing the side effects of such treatment. The presence of other disorders, particularly liver or kidney complaints, also affects the type of treatment. In some cases, treatment may involve surgery.

INCREASED NUTRIENT INTAKE
People with active rheumatoid arthritis may have a poor dietary intake due to loss of appetite. At the same time, some of the medications that treat rheumatoid arthritis, such as anti-inflammatory drugs, may increase the requirement for certain nutrients and reduce their absorption.

Like osteoarthritis (see p.245), weight loss is recommended for overweight and obese people to reduce the stress on inflamed joints. Nutritional guidelines, therefore, focus on eating a varied diet that provides essential nutrients while helping control weight.
• Sufficient intake of vitamin E (see p.58) is important for the health of your joints; vitamin E-rich foods include oils, fish, nuts, and seeds.
• You should also choose foods that provide an adequate intake of B vitamins (see pp.53–56), vitamin D (see p.57), calcium (see p.62), iron (see p.66), and omega-3 fatty acids (see p.90).
• Include adequate amounts of antioxidants (see p.20) in your diet.

MAINTAINING BONE DENSITY
Rheumatoid arthritis causes bone loss, which can also lead to osteoporosis (see p.241). Bone loss is more likely with an increasing level of disability, resulting from rheumatoid arthritis and the decreasing level of weight-bearing activity. The use of steroid drugs further accelerates bone loss, particularly in postmenopausal women.

Bone loss can be countered by making sure you consume adequate amounts of calcium (1,000–1,500mg per day) and vitamin D (0.01–0.02mg per day), either in the diet or by taking supplements.

EXERCISE AND MOBILITY
Pain and stiffness often cause people with rheumatoid arthritis to stop using their inflamed joints. However, such decrease of activity can lead to loss of joint motion and loss of muscle strength, which leads to decreased joint stability and increased fatigue. Exercise can help prevent and reverse these effects, but exercise programs should be designed by a physical therapist and tailored to the severity of your condition, the former activity level, and your body build.

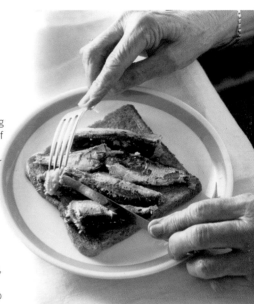

Sardines are good for rheumatoid arthritis
Containing high levels of calcium, iron, B vitamins, and omega-3 fatty acids, sardines on toast makes an easy and nutritious snack.

Omega-3 fatty acids and rheumatoid arthritis

Studies have shown that people with rheumatoid arthritis who were treated with fish-oil supplements for between 3 and 4 months had a reduction in the number of affected joints.

It is thought that omega-3 fatty acids, which are found in oily fish and in some plant oils (see p.90), might reduce inflammation and help alleviate the troublesome symptoms of rheumatoid arthritis by reducing the number of inflammatory "messenger molecules" made by the body's immune system.

High doses of omega-3 fatty acids should be taken under the supervision of a doctor to prevent side effects or interactions with medications that you may be using to treat rheumatoid arthritis. Eating oily fish, such as tuna, salmon, and mackerel, at least twice a week should be an integral part of your diet if you suffer from rheumatoid arthritis.

Can diet cure arthritis?

Theories abound that eliminating certain foods, such as tomatoes, potatoes, and peppers, taking specific supplements, or adding honey, vinegar, or herbs to the diet will alleviate arthritis. However, with the exception of gout, which may benefit from a change of diet, there is no scientific evidence that diet can cure joint disorders.

Tests have shown that diets low in saturated fats, or that include certain omega-3 fatty acids, seem to have a mild anti-inflammatory effect, but there is insufficient evidence that these are

useful in the treatment of arthritis. (You should note that cod liver oil is not a source of these oils and should not be taken in large quantities.)

Neither is there any evidence that fasting and "cleansing" diets, which are sometimes promoted as methods of treating arthritis, have any long-term benefits. On the contrary, these may lead to malnutrition and health problems.

GLUCOSAMINE SUPPLEMENTS

There is a certain amount of evidence that glucosamine, in a dose of 1,500mg per day, may help relieve the pain of osteoarthritis, and studies are now underway to try to determine whether this supplement helps preserve or regenerate damaged cartilage. Since glucosamine may affect the action of insulin in the body and may cause digestive upsets and allergic reactions,

it should be taken only under medical supervision and avoided entirely if you are pregnant or breast-feeding. The usefulness of other supplements, such as S-adenosylmethionine, chondroitin sulfate, copper, and zinc is uncertain.

TIPS FOR ARTHRITIS

If you suspect that a certain food is aggravating your arthritis, try keeping a food diary for a month, writing down everything that you eat and drink, and then see your doctor for advice. If you eliminate a food, be sure to find an alternative source for the nutrients that this food supplies. The best advice is to maintain a healthy lifestyle and eat a balanced diet, choosing foods low in sugar and fat and including a variety of food from the five major food groups every day. Other general dietary tips for people with arthritis include:

- Avoid crash dieting or fasting.
- Increase dietary calcium intake.
- Drink plenty of nonalcoholic fluids.
- Keep within a normal weight range.
- If you do drink alcohol, make sure you do so in moderation.

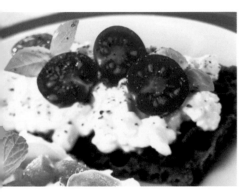

Cottage cheese on crispbread Maintaining calcium levels is critical for arthritis sufferers, but it is important to choose low-fat dairy products to help control weight.

Case study Short-order cook with severe foot pain

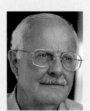

Name Michael

Age 62 years

Problem Michael woke up in the night with uncomfortable tingling at the base of his right big toe. Over the next two hours the pain became more severe and he noticed swelling and redness on the toe. He could not sleep all night and called his doctor in the morning for an emergency appointment.

Lifestyle Michael is a short-order cook at a neighborhood diner. He stands on his feet for 10–12 hours a day and is very upset because this pain in his foot will prevent him from going to work. He has a history of

mild high blood pressure, for which his doctor has prescribed diuretic medication. Michael is moderately overweight and he gets some exercise playing golf on weekends.

Michael's doctor diagnosed an acute attack of gout and placed him on anti-inflammatory medication. He is advised to stay off of his foot for 5–7 days and then to make a follow-up appointment to discuss how to prevent future attacks of gout. His doctor also advised him to reduce his intake of purines (*opposite*).

At his follow-up visit, Michael's doctor explained that gout has been linked to "rich" diets high in meat and wine. Michael's doctor changed his blood-pressure medications because diuretics may make gout worse, and explained that he wanted to check

his blood levels of uric acid and LDL-cholesterol. He explained that gout can be a sign of a serious condition, known as metabolic syndrome, which he may have because he is overweight and has high blood pressure (*see p.214*).

Advice By losing weight and limiting his intake of alcohol and foods high in purine, Michael can reduce his risk of another attack. Gout is more common in those who overeat or are overweight. Rapid weight loss can precipitate a gout attack, so a reduced-calorie diet for gradual weight loss is important. Too much alcohol can cause an attack and so should be avoided or limited. Some beers even contain purines. Plenty of water is recommended to ensure dilute urine and prevent the formation of uric-acid kidney stones.

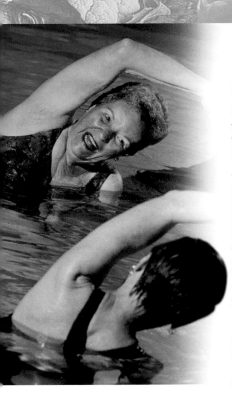

Benefits of increasing physical activity for osteoarthritis

People who exercise regularly to control their weight and manage their arthritis typically are in less pain and function better than those who are inactive.

THE BENEFITS OF EXERCISE

Being overweight not only increases the likelihood of developing osteoarthritis, but also worsens the stress on weight-bearing joints, such as the hips, knees, and lower spine, that may already be affected by the condition. Therefore, it is important for you to increase your exercise level to control your weight if you have osteoarthritis.

Joint-friendly exercise Exercising in water minimizes stress on any joints affected by arthritis, while helping to maintain flexibility, strengthen muscles, and control weight.

Regular stretching routines and exercises will help increase flexibility and reduce stiffness by keeping your joints moving, whereas strengthening exercises, which should also be performed regularly, will help maintain or increase muscle strength, and increase bone mineral density. Having strong muscles will help keep your joints stable. Cardiovascular exercise can also help with weight loss.

DIFFERENT TYPES OF EXERCISE

When starting to exercise, build up gradually, as your joints may be stiff. Water exercises such as swimming or aquaerobics, are particularly good for arthritis sufferers, as your body weight is supported by the water. In addition, low-impact exercises such as walking or Tai Chi are gentle on the joints, and easy to incorporate into a daily routine.

Nutritional therapy for gout

A common form of arthritis, gout is a very painful condition, usually affecting the base of the big toe. The condition is due to high levels of uric acid in the blood, leading to the deposition of uric-acid crystals in joint tissue. Treatment is therefore aimed at controlling uric acid in the blood and involves weight loss, where appropriate, reduction or elimination of alcohol intake, and possibly the discontinuation of diuretic drugs or other medication.

PROTEIN AND PURINE FOODS

Because foods with high protein and purine content contribute to high uric-acid levels, eliminating such foods may be beneficial for people who suffer from gout. Beer, in particular, contains high levels of purines in addition to alcohol. Milk, eggs, and cheese are good sources of protein and do not contain high levels of purine, but if you are trying to lose weight, you should choose low-fat or fat-free varieties of dairy products.
- Restrict or avoid alcohol; in particular, you should stop drinking beer.

- Avoid high purine meats, such as liver, kidneys, and brains.
- Cut down or avoid meat extracts, such as gravy made from meat drippings.
- Eat no more than 3–4oz (85–115g) of meat at any meal.
- Avoid foods that are high in fat.
- Cut down or, better still, avoid shellfish and anchovies.
- Do not overeat, especially on a regular basis. Control your portion sizes, and share entrées when eating out.
- Take your time when eating.
- Lose weight if necessary, but do it gradually and avoid going on a very low-calorie diet.
- Drink plenty of nonalcoholic fluids.
- Do not take vitamin C supplements.
- Exercise regularly.
- Take your medications if you have high blood pressure or high cholesterol.

Low-purine protein Since they are low in purine, eggs are an excellent source of protein for gout sufferers. Here, eggs, potato and leeks are wrapped in filo pastry.

Jargon buster

Purine This is a product of protein breakdown that causes a high level of uric acid in the blood. Fish and meat that are naturally high in purine include herring, anchovies, mackerel, sardines, scallops, game meats, all organ meats, and meat extracts such as gravy. High purine vegetables include asparagus, spinach and cauliflower.

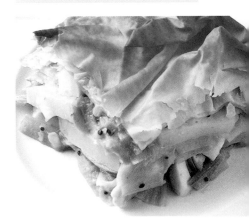

Diabetes

Nutrition plays a vital role in the treatment of this chronic illness.

Diabetes is a condition that affects how the body uses carbohydrates for energy (*see p.46*). It is diagnosed when the concentration of glucose in the blood is abnormally high (more than 126mg/dL).

Role of insulin

The body's main source of energy comes from carbohydrates, which are turned into glucose in the body. For glucose in the bloodstream to be able to enter into body cells, the hormone insulin, produced by the pancreas, is required.

Sometimes, the body cannot make enough insulin or use the insulin it does make effectively—this is known as insulin resistance—which causes blood glucose levels to rise. The reasons why insulin

resistance develops are becoming more defined. It is now known that genetics, diet, and level of physical activity are all involved.

Insufficient insulin action and the resulting high blood-glucose levels can lead to diabetes. Most of the treatments for diabetes are aimed at restoring and maintaining normal blood-glucose levels.

How common is diabetes?

One of the most common chronic diseases in North America, diabetes affects about 17 million adults in the US, and is on the rise, most likely as a result of increased rates of obesity. In addition, more than 20 million adults in the US have reduced glucose tolerance and/or

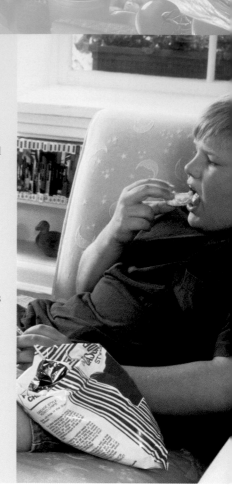

Control your child's eating Children who snack on fatty foods, such as chips, and have a low level of activity are at risk of becoming overweight and developing diabetes.

Who is most at risk of diabetes?

By identifying the risk factors for diabetes you can detect it early, and prevent or delay the complications of the disease.

General risk factors Whatever your age, if you have any of the risk factors below, ask your doctor to measure the levels of glucose in your blood.

• A family history of diabetes. If anyone in your family has type 2 diabetes, you should exercise regularly and maintain a healthy weight in order to minimize your risk of developing the condition.

• A body mass index (BMI) above 25 (*see pp.26–27*). Overweight people often suffer from insulin resistance, which is associated with type 2 diabetes because the accumulated fat cells interfere with the action of insulin.

• If you are a member of a high-risk ethnic group (*right*).

• You have been diagnosed with gestational diabetes during pregnancy.

• You have high blood pressure.

• You have HDL cholesterol levels of less than 40mg/dL (men), 50mg/dL (women), and/or a triglyceride level greater than 150mg/dL (same for men and women). This could indicate metabolic syndrome and the risk of your developing type 2 diabetes and cardiovascular disease is high (*see p.214*).

• You had borderline elevated glucose levels on previous testing (prediabetes).

• You are a woman with polycystic ovarian syndrome.

Age The risk of diabetes increases with age, and those over the age of 65 have the highest rates. At age 45, you should talk to your doctor about having your blood tested for glucose levels—even if the results are normal, you should repeat this test every three years. Children should be screened if:

• They are overweight with BMI above

the 85th percentile for age and gender (*see p.113*).

• They have two or more of these risk factors: family history of type 2 diabetes, from a high-risk ethnic group (*below*), signs of insulin resistance (such as gray-brown skin pigmentation around the neck).

Gender Women with polycystic ovarian syndrome are at increased risk. The risk of gestational diabetes (*see p.141*) is more likely in overweight women and those with a family history of diabetes. Women with a history of delivering a baby weighing more than 9lb (4kg) at birth, or a history of miscarriages or stillbirths, are also at risk. If you are at risk, your doctor will measure your blood-glucose levels during pregnancy.

Ethnicity African–Americans, Native Americans, Hispanic people, and Asian–Americans are at higher risk of diabetes than Caucasians.

insulin resistance, and may have mildly elevated blood sugar levels, which is known as prediabetes.

Type 1 diabetes

This accounts for 5–10 percent of all diagnosed cases of diabetes, and is the form that is more likely to affect children and people under 30 years of age. Type 1 diabetes, also known as insulin-dependent diabetes, is due to the destruction of the insulin-producing cells of the pancreas, thus causing insulin deficiency. It can be treated with injections of synthetic insulin.

Without sufficient insulin, people with type 1 diabetes may develop weight loss, excessive thirst and hunger, frequent need to urinate, lack of energy, nausea, vomiting, and dehydration. If it is untreated or poorly controlled type 1 diabetes can also lead to ketoacidosis (*right*).

Type 2 diabetes

The development of type 2 diabetes, or noninsulin-dependent diabetes, is strongly related to lifestyle factors.

Increasing the amount of exercise you do, losing weight if necessary and maintaining a healthy weight, increasing your fiber intake, and cutting down on your fat intake (particularly saturated fats), have been shown to delay or prevent the development of type 2 diabetes in susceptible people.

Type 2 diabetes accounts for 90–95 percent of all diagnosed cases of diabetes, and is the type that usually occurs in adults over age 40 who are often overweight. It is now increasingly common in overweight adolescents, too.

People with type 2 diabetes do not need insulin injections because the pancreas continues to secrete insulin. Symptoms develop slowly and are not usually obvious. Some people may simply feel tired, but when blood-glucose levels are very high symptoms similar to type 1 diabetes can develop. Eventually about 40 percent of people who have type 2 diabetes will require insulin to maintain adequate control of their blood-glucose levels.

Gestational diabetes

This type of diabetes occurs in some women during pregnancy due to an increase in hormones, some of which may have anti-insulin properties. Women who are diagnosed with elevated blood-sugar levels in pregnancy can usually control the problem with diet and exercise, although some may have to take insulin (*see p.141*).

Jargon buster

Ketoacidosis When the body's tissues cannot take up glucose from the blood, fat is broken down for energy instead. The breakdown of fat produces chemicals called ketone bodies, or ketones. When these build up to high levels, a ketoacidosis occurs. The symptoms of ketoacidosis include abdominal pain, rapid deep respiration, fruity breath odor, weakness, fatigue, confusion, stupor, and shock. It can lead to severe dehydration, coma, or even death.

Managing diabetes

Diabetes is a chronic disease requiring important changes to your lifestyle. These include diet, physical activity, managing the condition on a daily basis, and, for many people, medications.

DEALING WITH YOUR CONDITION

Taking responsibility for your diabetes will improve your quality of life both in the short- and long-term. Achieving the best possible control of your blood sugar, cholesterol, and triglyceride levels and blood pressure can prevent or delay any complications while minimizing low-blood-sugar episodes and weight gain.

Many doctors encourage people with diabetes to self-manage their condition, with the support of their family. Some doctors, in addition to giving medical care, provide their own nutrition and physical-activity programs, and you may even find that your doctor or clinic

can put you in contact with dietitians, nurses, and diabetes educators, who can help you deal with living with diabetes.

MONITORING BLOOD SUGAR

People with diabetes can easily and quickly monitor blood-sugar levels with a simple finger stick or blood-glucose meter. By monitoring your blood-sugar levels daily, you can determine what effect your food choices and physical activity have on your levels. These results can help you modify your diet and make adjustments to help you achieve as close to normal blood-sugar levels as possible. If you have type 1 or type 2 diabetes and are taking insulin, it is best to monitor your blood sugar three or four times a day. If you have type 2 diabetes and are taking oral medications, it may be necessary to monitor your blood sugar only a few times a week.

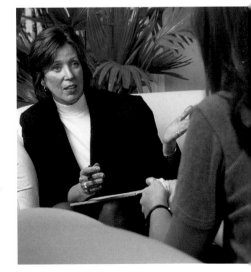

Meeting with a dietitian Your doctor can refer you to a dietitian who will help you manage your diabetes, suggest menu plans, and teach you how to count carbohydrates.

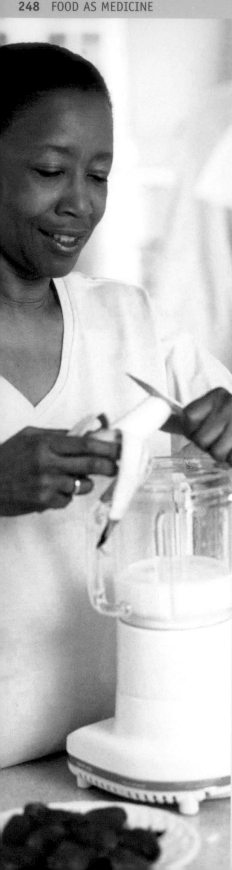

Nutrition for diabetes

Use food to maintain control of your blood-sugar levels, and lose weight if necessary.

If you have diabetes, the primary goal of medical nutrition therapy is to keep your blood-sugar levels in the normal range to prevent diabetes-related complications. Diet is therefore the cornerstone of treating your illness. You can manage blood-sugar levels, lower your blood pressure, and avoid hypoglycemia just by watching what you eat, when you eat, and learning to manage your condition.

Hyperglycemia
This term means "high glucose in the blood" and is what all people with diabetes are trying to control. Severe hyperglycemia can occur if you eat something very high in sugar, or if you have not produced enough insulin. The symptoms are similar to those you may have had before you were diagnosed with diabetes—fatigue, thirst, and excessive urination.

Treating your condition
Research shows that treating your diabetes through a combination of dietary changes, weight control, and exercise—implemented and supervised by a registered dietitian —can have a dramatic effect, and in some cases remove the need for medications that lower high blood-sugar levels.
   By managing your diabetes in this way you can effectively lower your hemoglobin A1c levels. Testing for this type of hemoglobin shows your average blood-sugar levels

over the last three months, and regular testing can help you track your blood-sugar levels over time.

Healthy eating
Having diabetes does not mean that you have to follow a strict nutritional regime, nor do you have to eat a carbohydrate-free or sugar-free diet (see p.250); it just means that what you eat must be healthy and well-balanced.

Weight control
Being overweight contributes to an increased risk of developing diabetes because the body cannot make enough insulin to keep blood-sugar levels normal.
   If you have a family history of type 2 diabetes and are overweight it is important to lose weight and maintain a healthy weight: even modest amounts of weight loss can improve insulin resistance and help correct high blood-sugar levels.

Cardiovascular disease
If you have diabetes, you are at increased risk of developing cardiovascular disease (see pp.214–215). Reducing saturated fat is one of the most important changes you can make to reduce your risk. If you have high blood pressure, you should limit your total sodium intake (see p.221).

Jargon buster

Hypoglycemia This is when blood sugar levels drop dangerously low. It is caused by too high a dose of insulin, missed meals, or being more active than usual. Symptoms are similar to drunkenness—unsteady movement, slurred speech, nausea, sweating, dizziness, headache, or weakness. Any carbohydrate-rich food will raise blood-sugar levels, including sugar tablets, sucrose, juice, regular soda, or a sports drink.

Make a delicious fruit smoothie Blend soft fruits, such as bananas and strawberries, with low-fat milk or yogurt to make a healthy drink.

What to eat

Knowing what you are eating will make it easier to control and maintain your blood-glucose levels. It is especially important for you to control your intake of carbohydrates if you have diabetes (*see p.250*). Eating a high-fiber diet can help lower your blood-glucose levels, reduce your insulin needs, and improve your blood-glucose control.

MAINTAIN PROTEIN LEVELS
There is no evidence to suggest that your usual intake of protein (15–20 percent of your total calories) should be changed if you have diabetes. Protein has a small effect on blood-sugar levels, so following a healthy diet should be sufficient for your needs. See page 45 for a list of healthy protein sources.

The long-term effects of diets high in protein and low in carbohydrate are unknown. Initially, blood-sugar levels may improve and you may lose weight, but it is not known whether long-term weight loss is maintained any better

When to eat

It is important to recognize when you need to eat or drink in order to balance the effect of any medication or insulin on your blood-sugar levels. People with diabetes need to eat at regular intervals throughout the day to maintain blood-sugar levels and ensure they do not drop to a point that may cause hypoglycemia.

with these diets than with other low-calorie diets. Since they are usually high in saturated fat, the long-term effect of such diets on LDL-cholesterol is also a concern (*see p.38*).

LIMIT DIETARY FAT
It is important to limit your intake of saturated fats, trans fatty acids, and dietary cholesterol, especially if you have elevated LDL levels greater than 100mg/dL. Fats have a limited effect on blood-sugar levels, but you should cut your fat intake to reduce calories,

If you only eat one large meal a day you run the risk of causing an imbalance in blood-glucose levels, as your body struggles to turn a large amount of food into energy quickly. It is better to eat regularly, with snacks in between your main meals, although watch that you do not overeat as a result.

especially if you have type 2 diabetes. For more information about fats and their role in your diet, see pages 38–43.

EAT LOW-FAT DAIRY PRODUCTS
Dairy products are a mix of fat, protein, and carbohydrate, and they do not directly affect your blood-sugar levels. If you have diabetes, make sure that you always choose low-fat or fat-free versions, and remember that your favorite ice cream or milkshake may be high in added sugar, so opt for a low-sugar version.

Sample day's menu

We have developed a low-fat, low-calorie one-day menu to help guide your food selection and enable you to make better choices. Remember to eat three small meals every day, and if you are taking insulin, try to eat at the same time each day, to keep sugar levels balanced. For breakfast, instead of oatmeal and banana, you could try low-sugar cereal with strawberries. If you would like a small glass of 100 percent juice, skip the fruit. Snacks are more important if you are on insulin. If you have type 2 diabetes and are not on insulin, then you may not need two snacks every day.

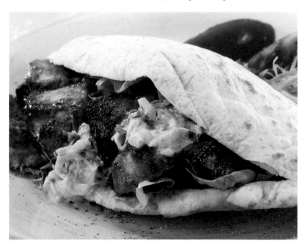

Pita pocket
Grilled chicken breast and salad in pita bread makes a tasty low-calorie lunch—perfect if you have diabetes. Make sure you use a low-fat dressing.

DIABETES MEAL PLANNER

Breakfast
- ½ medium banana
- 1 cup cooked oatmeal
- 4floz (120 ml) low-fat milk

Snack
- Fat-free yogurt with sucralose
- ½ cup unsalted mixed nuts

Lunch
- Pita bread with grilled chicken, salad, and low-fat ranch dressing
- Raw carrots with low-fat dip
- 1 medium apple

Snack
- 1 oz (28g) baked nacho chips
- ½ cup salsa

Dinner
- Baked salmon steak
- 1 cup steamed broccoli and zucchini and ⅔ cup brown rice
- Small crepe with fresh blueberries

Maintaining carbohydrate levels

It is important to remember that foods containing carbohydrate are important components of a healthy diet and should be included in a meal plan even if you have diabetes. Carbohydrates provide your body with fuel and help prevent

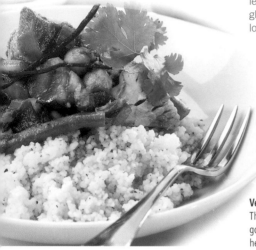

sharp increases or decreases in blood sugar levels. There is a great deal of discussion around rating carbohydrates into low and high categories (*see p.47*).

Different carbohydrates do cause different responses in blood-sugar levels—there is some evidence that low-glycemic index (GI) diets have a greater long-term benefit than high-glycemic diets. The glycemic index is best used for fine-tuning post-meal responses after first focusing on total carbohydrate intake (*see p.47*).

BLOOD SUGAR LEVELS

For those with type 1 diabetes, the amount of carbohydrate to eat is the key component that

Vegetables and chick peas with couscous
This meal is low in fat, high in fiber, and a good source of slow-release carbohydrate to help keep blood-sugar levels balanced.

affects your blood-sugar levels and the amount of insulin you need to control your levels. If you are receiving fixed insulin regimens rather than adjusting premeal doses, you should keep amounts of carbohydrate at meals consistent.

People with diabetes need to focus on eating low-glycemic-index carbohydrates, which take longer to break down in the body, thereby reducing the risk of high blood-sugar levels. These include oats, pasta, apples, tomatoes, and yogurt. By making sound food choices, and using carbohydrate counting, you will find it easier to control blood-sugar levels.

Carbohydrate counting, in which one serving of carbohydrate is equivalent to the amount of food providing 15g (or 80cal) of carbohydrate, is a way of assessing your carboydrate intake to calculate your insulin needs. You will soon learn how much carbohydrate you can or cannot eat and how to control your insulin requirements. Consult your doctor or dietitian for more information.

Eating your favorite foods

The first thing that people with diabetes ask is "Can I still eat my favorite foods?" The answer is yes—no foods are banned, just try every day to reach a balance.

YOU CAN EAT SUGAR

If you have diabetes, it does not mean you have to cut sugar out of your diet completely, but you should limit your intake as much as possible. Sugary foods can cause your blood-sugar levels to rise steeply, especially if you eat them on an empty stomach. If you do want something sweet, have it as part of a meal. If you do choose to eat a food containing sugar, you need to adjust the total amount of carbohydrate you eat accordingly, because both contribute to raised blood sugar (hyperglycemia).

ADAPT YOUR FAVORITE MEALS

You do not need to forget your favorite meals if you have diabetes, you just need to learn how to adapt them. Opt for low-fat or fat-free dairy products, choose lean

cuts of meat or skinned poultry, and grill, steam, poach, or bake food rather than frying or roasting. You should also reduce the sugar content when baking. Use no-calorie sweeteners to cook with as well as sweeten food after cooking.

When eating out, ask what is in the dish, and request sauces on the side. Many airlines offer a meal option for those with diabetes—check before you travel.

ALCOHOL AND DIABETES

You should always avoid drinking alcohol on an empty stomach since it can cause blood sugar levels to rise dramatically. If you have type 1 diabetes and choose to drink, always have a snack or a meal with alcohol, and drink sensibly—limit your consumption to no more than two drinks per day for men and no more than one drink for women.

No-calorie sweeteners

Most no-calorie sweeteners contain carbohydrate bulking agents, which contribute a small amount of calories. The Food and Drug Administration (FDA) allows foods to be labeled no-calorie provided they contain less than five calories per serving. These sweeteners are safe for people with diabetes if they are consumed within the accepted daily intake levels established by the FDA.

The most widely used sweeteners are aspartame, sucralose, saccharin, and acesulfame-K. These are added to processed foods and are available for use at home in tablet, liquid, and sprinkle forms. Most "sugar-free" products contain artificial sweeteners and they are a valuable asset if you are trying to lose weight. Remember that you only need a small amount as they are very sweet (*see p.280*).

Exercise is important

Physical activity has many benefits for people with diabetes. Studies continue to show that exercise lowers after-meal glucose levels by increasing the body's uptake of insulin and helping improve insulin sensitivity. In addition, exercise reduces your risk of cardiovascular disease, for example by reducing high blood pressure, helps control weight, increases energy levels, and generally brings about a healthier outlook on life.

Remember that exercise can lower blood-sugar levels, as your muscles use up the glucose in your body for energy.

DELAY THE ONSET OF DIABETES

Regular physical activity in people with prediabetes has also been shown to prevent or delay the onset of diabetes.

Prediabetes is defined as blood-sugar levels between 110 and 125mg/dL. If you have a family history of diabetes, are overweight, have prediabetes, or any other risk factors, it is time to be more active. Prevention is the key.

MAKE AN EXERCISE PLAN

Your exercise plan will depend on your age, general health, and level of fitness, so check with your doctor before starting. Make sure that you start off gently and do not overexert yourself. Try walking, swimming, and cycling, which can all be carried out at a pace that you find comfortable, and increased as your level of fitness improves.

Wear a visible diabetes ID, carry some carbohydrate with you, and exercise with a friend who knows that you have diabetes in case your blood sugar drops and you become hypoglycemic.

ENERGY-BOOSTING SNACKS

You need enough carbohydrate in your system to sustain you during exercise. Good energy-boosting snacks include:
- Low-fat, sugar-free fruited yogurt
- Banana or apple
- Slice of whole-wheat toast or a bagel with peanut butter or low-fat spread
- Rice crackers with hummus

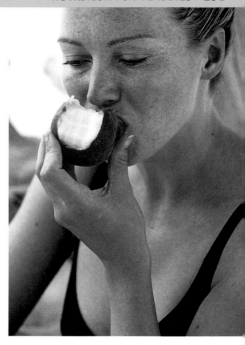

Have a snack to boost your energy It is important to regulate your blood-sugar level at all times, so make sure you have a snack before you start exercising to keep you going.

Case study Sedentary computer engineer with type 2 diabetes

Name David

Age 45 years

Problem David visited his doctor because he has felt tired for the past six months. He is 68in (172cm) tall and weighs 216lb (98kg) with a BMI of 33, making him clinically obese. He also has high blood pressure. From blood tests, David was diagnosed with type 2 diabetes. His 49-year-old brother also has this type of diabetes.

Lifestyle David is married with two children. He is an engineer and spends most of the day sitting at a computer. He occasionally plays tennis, he takes no medication, and has smoked a pack of 20 cigarettes every day for 25 years.

For breakfast, David has a large bagel with cream cheese and orange juice. He has a doughnut and coffee mid-morning. Lunch is usually a meat or cheese sandwich, potato chips, and cranberry juice. For dinner, he sometimes eats out with clients, or the family will get takeout Chinese or Indian food with large servings of rice. David usually drinks two bottles of beer with his evening meal.

Advice David's goals are to achieve and maintain normal or near-normal levels of blood glucose and blood pressure to prevent or reduce the complications of diabetes and risk for cardiovascular disease. In order to achieve this, he has to cut down on calories, saturated fat, cholesterol, and salt. Giving up smoking is very important, and exercising more will also be beneficial.

David can take medication for his blood pressure and diabetes, but to help him change his dietary habits and lose weight, he should see a dietitian who can help him focus on foods that he can eat. Involving David's wife in these discussions would also be helpful.

David should use the carbohydrate-counting approach (*opposite above*) to help manage his carbohydrate intake. Being made aware of low-calorie, low-fat, and low-salt alternatives to what David has been eating will also help him lose weight and reduce his blood pressure (*see pp.220–221*). For example, if he still wants Chinese for dinner, he can have one cup of steamed rice and vegetables with shrimp, scallops, or white-meat chicken, and an extra vegetable dish, such as green beans, with garlic sauce. David should realize that one-third of a cup of rice equals one serving of carbohydrate. Adding more fiber from whole grains, fruit, and vegetables is advisable.

David should also start an exercise program during his lunch break, which he could build up to walking for 30 minutes on most days.

Food allergies and intolerances

Some foods cause adverse reactions in susceptible people.

Food allergies occur when your body reacts to a food by triggering an immune response. Common foods that cause allergies are nuts, eggs, and shellfish (*opposite*). Food intolerances, on the other hand, do not trigger an allergic reaction but cause a response from the digestive system. The best-known example of a food intolerance is lactose (milk-sugar) intolerance (*see p.232*). In fact, up to 50 million North Americans suffer from lactose intolerance.

How reactions develop

The first time you eat a potentially allergenic food, you do not usually have symptoms, but your immune system mistakenly prepares to protect you against it. The next time you eat that food you release chemicals that cause symptoms such as eczema or life-threatening anaphylaxis (*see p.254*).

Food allergies usually begin in childhood and may be lifelong. However, some allergies, such as milk allergy, may be outgrown.

People with a food intolerance are not able to digest or process specific foods properly in the body, resulting in bloating, abdominal pain, gas, vomiting, or diarrhea. The problem usually involves a defect or deficiency in an enzyme necessary to digest some foods. Unlike food allergies, intolerances are usually not dangerous.

Symptoms of an allergy

These range from a tingling in the mouth, eczema, hives, vomiting, abdominal cramps, and diarrhea to swelling of the tongue and throat, breathing difficulties, and a drop in blood pressure. Symptoms typically appear within minutes to two hours after eating a suspect food.

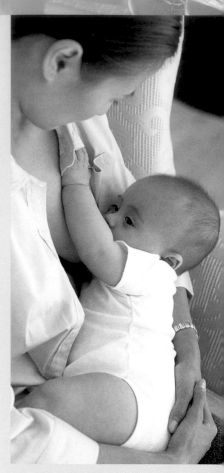

Preventing allergy problems Exclusively breast-feeding your baby for at least the first three months can help prevent allergies.

When do food allergies develop?

Food allergies are common in people who are susceptible to eczema, hay fever (allergic rhinitis), or asthma.

ALLERGY HISTORY

It is estimated that approximately six percent of all children may develop a food allergy by the age of two years, although studies suggest that babies with a family history of allergies may be two to four times more likely to develop an allergy or intolerance.

Since infancy is an especially vulnerable time for food allergies to develop, allergy prevention efforts must be started immediately after birth to be effective. Compared to babies fed cow's or soymilk formula, babies who are exclusively breast-fed for a prolonged period develop less eczema and wheezing in the first year of life.

ASSESS YOUR CHILD'S RISK

If you answer yes to any of these questions and are pregnant or breast-feeding, talk to your doctor about allergy prevention.

● Do you have a history of allergies (such as a food allergy, allergic eczema, hay fever, asthma, or allergy to furry animals, pollens, dust mites, or mold)?

● Does your spouse have a history of allergies?

● Do you have children have any allergies?

Skin-prick test

In this test for allergy, a drop of a common allergen (a substance that can cause an allergic reaction) is placed on the skin, which is then punctured with a small needle. If the skin reacts to the allergen by producing a weal, or hive, the test result is positive. A positive result should be followed with a diet that eliminates the suspected food and followed later by a food challenge, in which the food is reintroduced to see if symptoms return. Food-challenge tests must be medically supervised as they may trigger anaphylaxis (*see p.254*).

Avoiding foods that trigger allergies

Just eight foods account for 90 percent of all food allergies. These are peanuts, tree nuts (such as walnuts or almonds), eggs, milk, fish, shellfish, soy, and wheat. It is typically the protein component of a food that is responsible for the allergic response. However, even foods that we do not usually think of as containing protein, such as citrus fruits or potatoes, can actually contain enough protein to cause an allergic reaction.

TAKE CARE WHEN EATING OUT

It is very important to watch out for trigger foods when eating out. Some types of cuisines frequently serve foods that include peanut protein or oil or may contain wheat or soy products. Ask your waiter to check the ingredients in the dish you are ordering. You must make it clear that if you eat a particular food that you are allergic to, it could have serious implications; it is not just that you do not like something.

When traveling, you should learn how to say the name of any trigger foods, or get the name written down in the native language of the country you are visiting.

HIDDEN INGREDIENTS

If you have a food allergy or a food intolerance it is critical that you learn the different names of the substances that contain the food that affects you and look for them on labels. Dairy products and eggs are often hidden in a wide range of foods, as is wheat, which can be a hidden ingredient in deli meats, cheeses, sauces, gravies, yogurt, and even frozen vegetables. If you are allergic to corn, note that many processed foods contain corn starch or syrup and many products that are labeled with dextrose or fructose or even some food coloring may be made from corn.

The table below outlines foods that often contain peanuts, eggs, milk, wheat, or soy as ingredients.

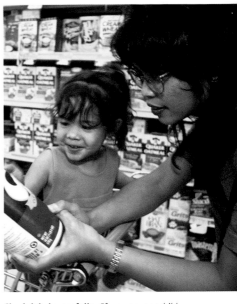

Check labels carefully If you or your child has a food allergy or intolerance, check food labels for hidden ingredients, and teach your child to be aware of ingredient labels, too.

FOOD	FOODS AND INGREDIENTS TO AVOID	WHERE FOODS MIGHT BE HIDDEN
Peanuts and tree nuts	• Peanuts are potentially life-threatening for anyone with an allergy to them. Avoid cold-pressured, expelled or extruded peanut oil or arachis oil; mandelonas; peanut butter; peanut flavor and nut butters • Allergies to tree nuts, such as walnuts, pecans, and almonds, are not as severe, but avoid all nuts	• Cereals, crackers, baked goods, cakes and pastries; marzipan; nougat; candies; ice cream • Barbecue sauces; chili powder; flavorings; sunflower seeds • African, Chinese, Mexican, Indonesian, Thai, and Vietnamese cuisine
Eggs and egg protein	• Eggnog, albumin, ovalbumin, lysozyme, mayonnaise, meringue or meringue powder, and surimi	• Pasta and noodles; soups; flavorings; lecithin • Cakes, pastries, and cookies; marzipan; nougat • Flu vaccine may contain egg protein
Milk and dairy	• All forms and types of milk, including goat's milk; all butter products and artificial butter flavorings; buttermilk; casein; all cheeses; curds; whey; custard; pudding; yogurt; ghee; half and half; all forms and types of cream; sour milk solids; lactoalbumin and lactoalbumin phosphate; lactulose	• Bread and baked goods; processed breakfast cereals; instant potato dishes; soups and sauces; salad dressings and dips; margarine; luncheon meats • Pancake, biscuit, and cookie mixes; mousses, puddings, and other desserts; protein shakes
Wheat	• Wheat, rye, oats, bran, and barley; bread and bread crumbs; bulgur wheat; couscous; durum; all types of flour; pasta; semolina • Wheat protein may be found in starch, hydrolyzed proteins, and natural and artificial flavorings	• Breads, muffins; cakes, cookies, and other baked goods; crackers; candy; cereals; luncheon meats; sauces; soups; catsup; soy sauce; surimi. • Pancakes; ice cream; chocolate
Soy	• Soy sauce; soybeans; soy oil; soy flour; tofu; tempeh; miso; textured vegetable protein (TVP) • Hydrolyzed plant and vegetable proteins	• Baked goods; canned tuna; cereals; crackers; infant formulas; sauces; soups; butter substitutes; peanut butter; frozen pizzas; meat substitutes

Preventing food allergies in babies

A food allergy develops when a baby's immune system creates antibodies to a specific food the first time that the food is eaten. The next time the food is eaten, the baby or young child may experience symptoms of a food allergy. Some babies with a family history of allergy may be made allergic to certain food allergens when they are ingested in minute amounts in their mothers' breast milk. Babies at risk for allergy may also become allergic to cow's milk and soy proteins in infant formulas.

BREAST-FEEDING AND NUTS
Based on recent research, the American Academy of Pediatrics recommends that breast-feeding mothers eliminate peanuts and tree nuts, such as walnuts and almonds, from their diets while breast-feeding. Apparently peanut

protein is secreted into breast milk, which may sensitize a baby who is at risk for developing a food allergy. Page 253 tells you where nuts may be hidden ingredients in foods.

HYPOALLERGENIC FORMULAS
If your child is at high risk for allergies, the American Academy of Pediatrics recommends using hypoallergenic infant formulas to supplement breast-feeding if necessary or if you are unable to breast-feed. This can reduce your baby's risk of developing a cow's-milk allergy and allergic eczema.

INTRODUCING SOLID FOODS
The introduction of solid foods to a food-allergic or allergy-prone baby should be delayed. Waiting until at least six months to introduce solid foods to a high-risk

Anaphylaxis

This is a severe, life-threatening allergic reaction. The symptoms of anaphylaxis include swelling of the tongue and throat, difficulty breathing, low blood pressure, and loss of consciousness. An injection of epinephrine can reverse the symptoms, but left untreated the condition can result in death.

baby is critical, with dairy products delayed until he or she is a year old, eggs until two, and peanuts, nuts, and fish until he or she is three years old. While this may seem to be overcautious, it is better to overstate the risk. If you are worried about introducing possibly allergenic foods to your child, it is a good idea to talk to your doctor or seek advice from a nutritionist or dietitian.

Treating food allergies and intolerances

For people with a true food allergy or food intolerance, even a tiny amount of a food that affects you can cause discomfort or, in the case of an allergy, potentially life-threatening anaphylaxis (*above*). Strict avoidance of the food is

the only way to prevent symptoms, but avoiding some common foods that cause allergy or intolerance can be difficult, particularly if you eat prepackaged food or dine out regularly.

RECOGNIZING PROBLEM FOODS
Since you can be allergic or intolerant to a complete food or to ingredients added during preparation or cooking, it is often difficult to recognize the foods that affect you. Therefore, your own observation is important in helping identify these foods. Keeping a food diary of what you or your child eats every day and any reaction to particular foods is very helpful. Over a period of four to six weeks, you may be able to recognize foods that cause symptoms, such as eczema or abdominal pain. It is then time to start eliminating specific foods from the diet to find the food that is responsible for these symptoms.

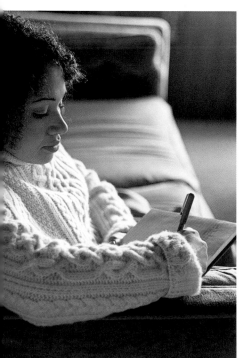

Keeping a food diary If you suspect that you have a food allergy or intolerance, keep a food diary to help you identify which foods may be the cause of your symptoms.

ELIMINATION DIET
Many studies have shown that the best dietary restrictions should start with elimination of foods suspected of causing the allergy or intolerance. Under a doctor's care, try eliminating possibly offending foods to see if there is any improvement in your symptoms.

If you then do a "food challenge," in which suspected foods are reintroduced one at a time, and one or more foods lead to the return of symptoms, the diagnosis is confirmed and you know which food or foods to avoid.

For example, studies in children who are allergic to cow's-milk protein have shown that the diagnostic procedure must begin with a diet that eliminates the suspected food component or with a diet containing a limited variety of foods for seven to 14 days or more. When the diagnosis is confirmed, the cow's milk is eliminated from the diet and substituted with a less harmful but nutritionally equivalent food. If more than one food is eliminated, you must make sure that important nutrients are not being left out and that you are getting a balanced diet (*see p.255*).

Getting a balanced diet

If you have a food allergy or intolerance, and avoid a whole food group, such as milk and dairy products, you may be missing out on key nutrients. This is especially important for those needing extra calories, vitamins, and minerals, such as growing children, pregnant and breast-feeding women, and older adults.

MILK ALLERGY OR INTOLERANCE

People who are allergic or intolerant to dairy products may fall short on the minerals calcium (*see p.62*) and phosphorus (*see p.63*), and vitamin D (*see p.57*), which is added to milk.

Many foods contain calcium, and good substitute sources of calcium for those avoiding milk and dairy products include calcium-fortified fruit juices, soymilk and rice milk, canned salmon with bones, tofu, and leafy greens, such as broccoli and spinach. Phosphorus is found in meat, poultry, fish, eggs, and whole-grain foods. Vitamin D is also made by the skin when exposed to sunlight, but growing children may also need a supplement (*see p.109*).

WHEAT ALLERGY

People who avoid eating wheat due to an allergy may not get sufficient B vitamins, especially thiamine (B_1), riboflavin (B_2), niacin (B_3), and folate (*see pp.53–56*) and the minerals magnesium (*see p.63*), potassium (*see p.63*), phosphorus (*see p.63*), and iron (*see p.66*).

You can get additional folate from orange juice, fruits, leafy greens, and legumes. Meat, poultry, and fish are good sources of iron, niacin, potassium, and phosphorus. Magnesium is found in many fruits, as well as in legumes and leafy green vegetables. Again, a multivitamin supplement (*see p.267*) may help fill some nutritional gaps.

CHECK FOOD LABELS

If you have a food allergy or intolerance, be sure to avoid the food that affects you by checking packages and labels and being extra careful when eating out in restaurants. You should also check labels to ensure that you are getting a balanced intake of the key nutrients, vitamins, and minerals.

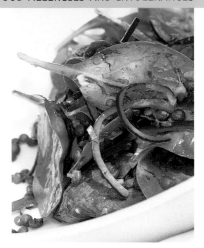

Leafy greens Spinach is a good source of nutrients that you may miss if you have to exclude milk or wheat products from your diet.

TALK TO A DIETITIAN

Anyone with multiple food allergies, or those who are allergic to difficult-to-avoid foods such as milk or wheat, may benefit from seeing a dietitian. A dietitian can analyze your diet to identify nutritional inadequacies and help you achieve a healthy, balanced diet.

Case study Active child with food allergies

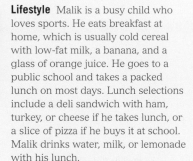

Name Malik

Age 10 years

Problem At age two and a half, Malik developed eczema and a runny nose. After repeated episodes, his doctor suggested that his mom keep a food and symptom diary. This helped identify eggs and chocolate as potential triggers of his symptoms. A skin-prick test (*see p.252*) gave positive results for walnuts, chocolate, watermelon, and eggs, but negative for peanuts, soy, citrus, wheat, and dairy. Since then, an elimination diet has kept Malik free of symptoms, but as he gets older he is exposed to more situations where he is at risk, and he has a lot of questions about what he can and cannot eat.

Lifestyle Malik is a busy child who loves sports. He eats breakfast at home, which is usually cold cereal with low-fat milk, a banana, and a glass of orange juice. He goes to a public school and takes a packed lunch on most days. Lunch selections include a deli sandwich with ham, turkey, or cheese if he takes lunch, or a slice of pizza if he buys it at school. Malik drinks water, milk, or lemonade with his lunch.

After school, Malik goes to either soccer or lacrosse practice for most of the year. He usually has some peanut-butter crackers or a piece of fruit and a sports drink for a snack after school, before practice.

For dinner, he eats whatever is prepared for the family, which may be pasta with sauce, steak, or chicken with green vegetables.

Advice Malik has continued to show signs of a food allergy when he has been tested by the doctor and has therefore not yet outgrown his food allergy, which happens with many children. Being allergic to chocolate, eggs, and walnuts can be a challenge for a child, as well as his parents, and reading labels for these ingredients is the best bet for preventing exposure to trigger foods. Homemade products such as cakes and cookies may also be a problem since they are likely to contain eggs. Now that Malik is more independent, he will need to make some decisions on his own. Because his symptoms are annoying but not dangerous, he can be allowed to make choices and may make some mistakes. He needs to learn to ask questions and to read food labels to avoid the foods that give him symptoms.

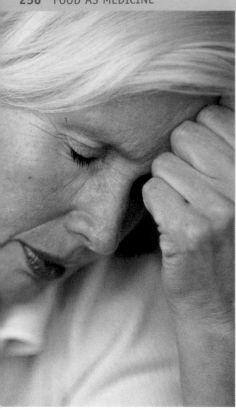

Migraine headache

Certain foods can trigger a migraine, while other foods may help prevent it.

Up to one in ten people regularly experience the misery of migraine. A migraine is a type of headache, but not all headaches are migraines; for example, a headache that occurs every day would not normally be described as a migraine. A migraine can occur as often as several times a week, or as seldom as once or

One-sided pain The symptoms of a migraine include a severe, throbbing headache that is usually felt on one side of the head, above one eye or around one temple.

twice a year. The condition can be so debilitating that it completely wipes you out for several days at a time. People usually have their first migraine attack before age 30. Initial attacks rarely occur in those over 40, but they can occur in children as young as 3 years old.

What are the symptoms?

The differences between migraine and other types of headaches are the characteristic symptoms. Up to half of people who suffer from migraines get a warning, known as an aura, that a migraine attack is coming on. The aura is a visual disturbance that occurs before the onset of the headache and can include flashing lights, zigzag lines, and blind spots. Other symptoms of a classic migraine aura include

Preventing and treating migraines

There are several things you can do to reduce your risk of geting a migraine. Eating regularly, drinking plenty of water or other caffeine-free drinks, and eating magnesium-rich foods can be beneficial.

EAT AT REGULAR INTERVALS

This is really important if you suffer from migraines or other types of headaches. Low blood sugar, caused by insufficient food, is a well-known trigger, especially when combined with fatigue and/or stress. Skipping meals, having fast-food snacks, and following drastic weight-loss diets can also cause attacks.

DRINK PLENTY OF WATER

Dehydration is another major cause of headache and migraine. If you don't drink enough during the day, the body takes fluid from the blood and other body tissues. The blood vessels constrict in an effort to conserve body fluids, and this can cause a headache. Drink plenty of water to avoid dehydration, especially when you are exercising or drinking

alcohol—alcohol consumption is a major contributor to dehydration, so drink plenty of water after you drink alcohol.

BOOST YOUR MAGNESIUM INTAKE

Eating foods rich in magnesium can help treat migraines. Magnesium deficiency may be due to reduced dietary intake, smoking, alcohol consumption, stress, or genetic problems, and can result in blood vessels in the brain constricting, which can cause a migraine. You should aim to boost your magnesium intake to 300mg per day (the Dietary Reference Intake for adults) to help increase the flow of blood to the brain.

Plant foods, such as grains, legumes, and vegetables, are rich in magnesium, whereas refined foods have a low content —processed grains, for example, lose up to 80 percent of their magnesium.

Add tofu to a vegetable stir fry Tofu is high in magnesium, which can help treat a migraine, so add it to your shopping list.

Boost your daily intake by eating bran and wheat cereals for breakfast and by substituting brown rice for white rice at dinner. All nuts and seeds are good sources of magnesium, too. Magnesium-rich vegetables include broccoli, spinach, and Swiss chard. Taking a magnesium supplement may also be helpful.

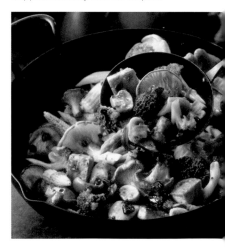

difficulty speaking, confusion, weakness of an arm or leg, or tingling of the face or hands. The symptoms of aura usually occur 10–30 minutes before the onset of the migraine headache.

Migraine headaches, both with or without an aura, are sometimes preceded by a group of symptoms, collectively known as prodrome. These symptoms tend to appear approximately one hour before the headache pain develops, and often include anxiety or mood changes, an altered sense of taste and smell, and either an excess of or a lack of energy.

Symptoms common to all types of migraines include a severe, throbbing headache that is made worse by movement, and usually felt on only one side of the head, over one eye, or around one temple; nausea or vomiting; or discomfort with bright light or loud noises.

Generally, if a headache and/or associated symptoms prevents you from continuing with normal activities, it could be a migraine.

What causes a migraine?

There appear to be many general triggers of a migraine, including stress, hunger, and dehydration. Many women often experience an attack around the time of menstrual periods, which might be why the condition occurs more commonly in women. In addition, migraine attacks usually run in families.

Migraines are sometimes linked to intolerance to particular foods, including cheese, chocolate, and red wine. Therefore, you may be able to reduce or even eliminate migraine attacks by identifying your particular trigger food and avoiding it in future. Magnesium deficiency may also contribute to a migraine (*opposite below*).

Trigger foods

Some foods, such as milk, cream, ice cream, hard cheeses, and alcohol contain amines, which migraine sufferers can find hard to process in the body. The result is that these substances remain in the body longer, and when detected by the nervous system can cause the brain to dilate or the blood vessels in the brain to constrict.

Research suggests that when people who suffer from migraines eat foods containing substances that cause blood vessels in the brain to constrict, this reduces the blood flow to the brain and causes a migraine. People can also have reactions to other foods, such as monosodium glutamate (MSG), nitrates and nitrites, and artificial sweeteners, so keep track of any reactions you may have.

Case study Busy legal assistant suffering from migraines

Name Julie

Age 30 years

Problem Julie is finding that she is suffering from more migraines than ever before. She eats breakfast, but often skips meals during the day because of her time schedule—Julie has a very stressful job. Her migraines occur more frequently at the end of the day, and for several days before and during her menstrual period, suggesting that hormonal changes could be the cause. She drinks in moderation, but after just a couple of glasses of wine, Julie often wakes up the next day with a severe migraine headache and nausea.

Lifestyle Julie works as a legal assistant, and is responsible for running a busy lawyers' office. She spends quite a lot of time in front of her computer screen. She rarely takes a lunch hour and keeps herself going with coffee and sugary snacks. She works full-time and takes pre-law classes two nights a week. She does not exercise regularly, although she has a free membership to the gym through work.

On Friday evenings, she unwinds with a couple of glasses of red wine, either at home, or out with friends. Sometimes, her whole weekend is ruined because of the migraine she suffers as a consequence. She often takes over-the-counter medication for her migraine headache.

Advice Since Julie is complaining about more and more migraines at the end of the day, the easiest and most realistic change that she can accomplish now is to make time to eat lunch. Julie could either plan to bring a frozen meal that can be microwaved quickly or prepare a sandwich at home such as peanut butter and jelly. Leftovers from dinner the night before could also be used. This would give her a break from staring at her computer screen, and would also help to reduce her stress levels. Rather than having coffee and sugary snacks, she could grab fresh fruit and a yogurt.

Although Julie does not drink excessive amounts of alcohol, she may not be drinking enough water with or after she has drunk alcohol. Alcohol can dehydrate the body and this can cause a headache. If drinking more water does not improve her condition, she may want to avoid red wine for a few weeks to see if her weekend migraines are reduced.

To further reduce her stress levels, she could try to exercise at least once a week, maybe after work on the days that she is not taking classes or even during her lunch break.

Cancer

The second leading cause of death, cancer is a major concern in the 21st century.

Cancer is a group of diseases characterized by the uncontrolled growth and spread of abnormal cells. Of the many different types of cancer, the majority form tumors in a specific part of the body, most commonly the skin, breast, lung, large intestine, or prostate gland. The disease may then spread within the body through the blood and lymphatic system (a system of glands that filters out infectious organisms from the body).

Because public knowledge and understanding of the disease has developed and increased over the last few decades, we have been able to implement lifestyle changes, adopt effective screening programs, and pursue new types of therapies in order to improve the prevention and treatment of cancer.

Different types of cancer

There are many different types of cancers, and the disease can affect organs (such as the colon, breast, or prostate) as well as tissues (such as the blood or bones). The most common types of cancer in North America are skin, lung, breast, prostate, and colorectal. About one in two men and one in three women in North America develops cancer at some point in their life.

Risk factors

Cancer risk is influenced by both external factors (tobacco smoke, chemicals, radiation, and infectious organisms) and internal factors (genes, mutations, hormones, and immune conditions). Exposure to the most common carcinogens (cancer-causing agents), such as tobacco smoke, ultraviolet light, and other types of radiation should be avoided when possible.

Your physical state, what you eat, your age, whether you are obese or not, and hereditary factors all influence whether you are more or less likely to get cancer.

Treating cancer

The treatment for cancer usually depends on the stage the disease has reached. Surgically removing tumors can be successful if the cancer has not yet spread to the lymph nodes or other sites in the body. For certain types of cancers, treatment with chemotherapy and radiation therapy may be used instead of or in combination with surgery. New therapies include inactivating damaged genes and

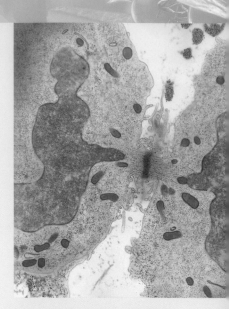

Cancerous cells multiply very quickly
In this magnified image, a cancerous cell is dividing to form two cells that contain damaged genetic material.

boosting the immune system's ability to destroy cancerous cells. However, the most effective way to lower the number of deaths is to prevent cancer from developing by eating healthy, exercising regularly, and screening to detect it early.

Nutrition and cancer

We deal primarily with three types of cancer in this section—breast, prostate, and colorectal cancer—because nutritional and lifestyle changes can be effective in their prevention and treatment. If you are undergoing chemotherapy or radiation therapy, nutrition can play an essential role in helping you feel better, giving you energy and increasing your well-being (*see p.262*).

Because some drugs used in chemotherapy can deplete vitamin and mineral levels in the body, your doctor may recommend a supplement. During treatment, however, you should not exceed the Dietary Reference Intake (DRI) for vitamins and minerals. High doses of certain micronutrients may interfere with the processing of some chemotherapy drugs.

Obesity and cancer

Scientific evidence suggests that about one-third of cancer deaths in North America each year are related to problems associated with poor nutrition and physical inactivity, particularly resulting from obesity.

According to a recent study by the American Cancer Society (ACS), about 90,000 people in the US die each year from cancers influenced primarily by being overweight. Obese people not only have a higher risk of developing cancer, but they also have a greater risk of dying from cancer—the ACS study showed that the death rates from all types of cancers combined were 52 percent higher in men and 62 percent higher in women who were overweight compared to men and women who were normal weight.

It is therefore very important that you maintain a healthy weight for your height to reduce your risk.

Who is most at risk of cancer?

The risk of developing any type of cancer generally increases with age. Older people are more likely to develop the disease, largely because their cells have had more time to accumulate genetic damage, but also because their immune system is not as efficient at finding and destroying abnormal cells and it takes a long while for some tumors to grow large enough to be diagnosed.

BREAST CANCER
This type of cancer is the leading cause of death in women between the ages of 40 and 55. Most cases of breast cancer develop in women over 50. At age 30, a woman's risk of developing breast cancer is about one in 2,500, but by age 50, her chances are one in 50, rising to one in 14 by age 70. Women who have a first-degree relative (mother, sister, or daughter) diagnosed with breast cancer are at increased risk of developing the disease, as are overweight or obese women, those who started having menstrual periods before age 12, and women who reach menopause after 55.

Women who have their first pregnancy after age 35 and those who have never had a full-term pregnancy also seem to have a higher risk of developing breast cancer. In addition, evidence shows that long-term use of hormone replacement therapy (HRT) may increase a woman's risk of breast cancer.

PROSTATE CANCER
The causes of prostate cancer are not well understood. Many studies have shown that certain factors may increase the risk of the disease. Age is the most important risk factor, as prostate cancer is found mainly in men over age 55. In fact, more than 50 percent of men in North America between the ages of 60 and 70 and as many as 90 percent between the ages of 70 and 90 have prostate cancer. Around 189,000 men in the US are diagnosed with prostate cancer each year. A family history of the disease also raises your risk. Finally, African–American men have a higher risk of developing prostate cancer compared to Caucasian men.

COLORECTAL CANCER
In 2003—according to the National Cancer Institute—there were about 105,500 cases of colon cancer and 42,000 cases of rectal cancer in the US. There appears to be a genetic component to the risk for developing colorectal cancer (cancer in either the colon or rectum), but the relationship is complex. About 25 percent of people with colorectal cancer have a family history of the cancer, and the risk of developing the disease increases substantially if two or more relatives have colorectal cancer. It is rare in people under age 40, and usually occurs in people over age 60.

Ways to reduce your risk

If you have a family history of cancer, it is important that you adapt your lifestyle to decrease your risk of getting cancer.

YOUR WEIGHT AND EXERCISE
Even a small weight gain can increase your risk, so maintain a stable weight right for your height. If you are currently overweight, exercise and reduce your caloric intake. Regular exercise is linked with a reduced risk of prostate, breast, and colorectal cancer.

SMOKING
If you smoke, it is very important to quit. A recent study looking at 3,000 smokers age 40 and over showed that female smokers are twice as likely as male smokers to develop lung cancer. The risk of lung cancer also increases with age and how much you smoke.

ALCOHOL
It is important to limit or avoid alcohol—many studies have shown that alcohol consumption increases the risk of some cancers, such as breast and colon cancer. People who drink alcohol should limit their intake to no more than two drinks per day for men and just one drink per day for women.

LIMIT FREE-RADICAL DAMAGE
Smoking, not washing fruits and vegetables (to remove harmful nitrates and fertilizers), and other environmental poisons can promote the production of free radicals in the body (*see p.58*). Free radicals can cause aging, cancer, and cardiovascular disease so adapt your lifestyle accordingly.

BREAST-FEED YOUR BABY
Recent studies have found that for every year that a woman breast-feeds, her risk of breast cancer goes down by just over four percent, on top of the seven percent reduction for each child she has. This may be because breast-feeding triggers a hormonal change in a woman's body that can make her cells more resistant to becoming cancerous.

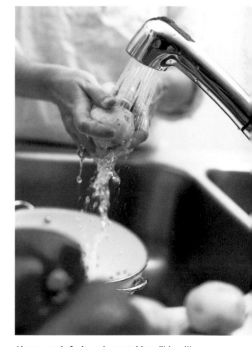

Always wash fruit and vegetables This will help reduce the risk of eating nitrates and fertilizers, which can promote free radicals.

Nutritional guidelines for preventing cancer

By eating a healthy, balanced diet emphasizing fruits, vegetables, whole grains, and legumes and maintaining a healthy weight, as many as one-third of all cancer deaths could be prevented. You should therefore try to include a least one of our "super" cancer-fighting foods in your diet each day (*below*). In addition, you should exercise regularly and limit your consumption of alcohol.

FIVE A DAY

Vegetables and fruits contain many vitamins, minerals, fiber, and hundreds of beneficial phytochemicals (*see p.59*), some of which have been proven to prevent and fight cancer. For example, some phytochemicals protect DNA (the substance that makes up our genes) from damage and promote DNA repair, which helps explain how these foods reduce the risk. A US study found that women who ate at least two servings of vegetables and fruits daily had a 17 percent lower risk of breast cancer than those who ate less than one. Therefore, make sure you eat at least five servings of fruits and vegetables a day.

CUT DOWN ON FATTY FOODS

Diets high in saturated fats are also high in calories and contribute to obesity, which is associated with an increased risk of many cancers, so make sure you eat a low-fat diet. Limit the amount of red meat you eat, especially any that is high in fat, and opt for white-meat poultry, fish, and shellfish instead.

EAT A HIGH FIBER DIET

Fiber can help eliminate cancer-related toxins and, like antioxidants, helps the body eradicate free radicals. In addition to fruits and vegetables, eating plenty of whole grains will boost your intake of dietary fiber. Whole grains are also a good source of several of the B vitamins and compounds called lignans—which are also found in flaxseed—that may have a protective role against breast, prostate, and colorectal cancers.

LOSE WEIGHT

By losing a little excess weight, you can make a big difference in reducing your risk for developing cancer. An increase in body weight of as little as five percent

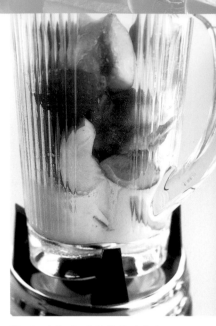

Blend or juice fresh fruit Fresh fruit contains essential vitamins, minerals, and phytochemcials that help prevent cancer.

in premenopausal women has been shown to significantly increase the risk of breast cancer after menopause, so you should lose weight if necessary. Once you have reached your target weight, work hard to maintain it.

"Super" cancer-fighting foods

No single food can protect you against cancer, but the right combination of foods can really help boost your immune system in the fight against cancer.

Cruciferous vegetables Broccoli, cabbage, cauliflower, and Brussels sprouts all contain substances that increase the antioxidant defenses of cells to fight cancer, and switch on enzymes that detoxify carcinogens.

Orange vegetables and fruits Carrots, pumpkins, mangoes, and squashes all contain antioxidants in the carotenoid family, including beta-carotene, which helps cells defend themselves against changes that can lead to cancer.

Tomatoes These are rich in lycopene—a potent antioxidant that may protect against prostate cancer. Lycopene levels are higher in cooked tomatoes.

Legumes These contain substances called saponins, which are thought to prevent cancer cells from multiplying.

Berries Strawberries and raspberries contain ellagic acid, a type of phenolic acid that reduces the damage to cells caused by smoke and air pollution.

Whole grains Wheat, rice, oats, and barley, and the foods made from them, are high in fiber and other nutrients and can reduce your risk of cancer.

Nuts and seeds These are rich in essential fatty acids and phenolic acids, which can help combat prostate cancer. Brazil nuts are also an especially good source of selenium, which studies suggest can help protect against prostate cancer.

Flaxseed This contains phytochemicals called lignans, which can help combat

cancer; this is possibly due to their high fiber content.

Green and black tea Both of these teas contain numerous active ingredients, including polyphenols, which may protect against stomach cancer, and flavonoids, which may protect against viral infections.

Antioxidants

These chemicals are mainly found in fruits and vegetables and have been shown to reduce the amount of free radicals in the body. They can neutralize free radicals and help repair their damage to body cells. A combination of antioxidants is most beneficial as they all have different protective roles.

Nutritional concerns and cancer

If you are suffering from cancer, there are likely to be times when you feel very weak, your energy levels are down, and you cannot face eating. This may be due to the cancer itself or the treatment you are receiving (*see p.262*).

MALABSORPTION
This may happen if your body is unable to properly absorb nutrients in the normal way. Malabsorption can lead to weight loss because the body does not get the nutrients it requires. Many disorders can cause malabsorption, and it can be treated. The most common symptoms include diarrhea, dehydration, fatigue, and weight loss. To avoid malnutrition, discuss your diet with your doctor and a nutritionist.

FEELING FULL
The feeling of being full after just a small amount of food is quite common. However, this will quickly lead to weight loss if you do not get enough calories to sustain you. You must make sure you do not become malnourished, so try to eat little but often. Choose small snacks that are packed with vital nutrients, vitamins, and minerals to boost your calorie intake, give you energy, and prevent weight loss (*right*).

LOSS OF APPETITE
As with feeling full after a small meal, loss of appetite is a common side effect among people with cancer. You may start to lose interest in food, or your appetite may decrease due to pain, nausea, or vomiting (*see p.262*), or because you are anxious or depressed about having cancer. Remember that for your body to be strong enough to fight against your condition you need energy. Even if you do not feel like eating, prepare something small that has an appetizing aroma to stimulate your appetite, such as homemade chicken noodle soup (*below*) or a high-protein snack (*see p.224 and right* for ideas).

Snacks when you are ill with cancer

If you are receiving chemotherapy or radiation treatment, your energy level may be low and foods may take on unpleasant tastes. For example, meats such as beef and pork may not appeal to you; substituting chicken or veal may be helpful because they have a milder flavor. The following high-protein, calorie-dense foods are good choices for meals or snacks to help you maintain your weight and keep your energy levels up:
- Cereal with fruit and whole milk
- Fruit yogurt with granola
- Instant oatmeal with raisins
- Soup with soda crackers
- Cream cheese and jelly on an English muffin
- Soft-flour tortilla filled with melted cheese
- Mixed nuts and crackers

Recipe Nutrient-dense chicken noodle soup

INGREDIENTS

14oz (400g) chicken breast

1 small onion

¼ stalk celery

1 clove garlic

Handful of fresh, flat-leaf parsley

2 pints (1 liter) chicken stock

½ tsp crushed thyme

1 cup dry egg noodles

Serves 4

1 Remove the skin and bone from the chicken breast and cut into fine strips. Peel and finely dice the onion and celery, and crush the garlic clove. Finely chop the parsley, reserving a few whole leaves for garnish.

2 Place the stock in a large saucepan and bring to a boil. Add the chicken breast, onion, celery, garlic, parsley, and thyme to the pan.

3 Return the soup to the boil, then reduce the heat, cover, and simmer for 30 minutes, or until the chicken breast is tender.

4 Add the egg noodles to the pan, bring the soup to a boil again, then reduce the heat and simmer, covered, for a further 10 minutes, or until the noodles are cooked.

5 Season the soup to taste with freshly ground black pepper. Serve, topped with grated Parmesan cheese and a garnish of a few leaves of flat-leaf parsley.

Each serving provides
Calories 152, Total fat 2.1g (Sat. 0.5g, Poly. 0.5g, Mono. 0.7g) Cholesterol 46mg, Protein 14g, Carbohydrate 19g, Fiber 1.3g, Sodium 730mg. Good source of—Vits: Fol; Mins: Ca, P, K, Se.

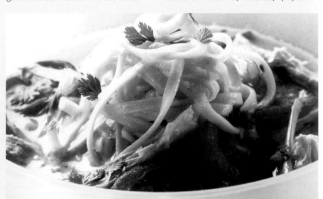

Dealing with the effects of chemotherapy and radiation

Although you may not feel much like eating due to the side effects of your treatment, you can adapt your eating to ensure you still get important nutrients.

SIDE EFFECTS OF TREATMENT

Chemotherapy drugs can damage both healthy and cancerous cells. The cells lining the entire gastrointestinal tract may be particularly affected, interfering with your ability to absorb food. You may experience changes in the way food tastes and smells or you may lose your appetite. The following are common side effects associated with these treatments.

LOSS OF APPETITE

To improve your appetite, try to eat by the clock. Make breakfast and lunch your main meals, since you may find that you have more energy at these times. If possible, have someone help you prepare meals. Try to avoid having treatment on an empty stomach, which might aggravate symptoms such as nausea, vomiting, and diarrhea. Eat small, frequent meals and choose high-calorie snacks, such as supplement drinks, desserts, shakes, avocados, nuts, and sandwiches.

NAUSEA

This is a common complaint among people undergoing cancer treatment. If you have nausea, try frequent small meals or snacks, such as crackers, toast, potato chips, and pretzels, and foods that are easy to digest, such as oatmeal, noodles, or boiled potatoes. Stick with low-fat protein sources, and avoid fried, greasy, and rich foods. Stay away from strong odors, and try to rest, sitting up, after eating. Try sipping apple juice, caffeine-free drinks, or ginger or peppermint teas throughout the day.

VOMITING

Do not eat or drink anything until you have stopped vomiting. When you feel better, try sipping small amounts of water, apple or cranberry juice, ginger ale, sports drinks, broths, and tea. Once these liquids are tolerated, move on to bland foods such as mashed potatoes, rice, and yogurt. Bananas, apricots, and juice can be added when you feel better.

DIARRHEA AND CONSTIPATION

When chemotherapy affects intestinal cells, it can cause diarrhea. Tips for treating diarrhea are on page 229.

Constipation can be caused by some anticancer drugs, pain relievers, and other medications. Tips for treating constipation are on page 229.

CHEWING AND SWALLOWING

Mouth sores are a common side effect of chemotherapy. To make foods easier to chew, cut them into bite-sized pieces or grind them up. Choose soft foods and add gravy, sauces, or butter to foods to make them easier to swallow. Avoid highly seasoned, spicy, tart, or acidic foods as they will aggravate the sores. In addition, you should add liquid nutritional supplements to your diet to ensure that it is balanced.

KIDNEY AND BLADDER

Some anticancer drugs can irritate the bladder or cause temporary or permanent damage to the bladder or kidneys. To treat irritation, drink plenty of fluids, such as water and diluted fruit juice, and choose liquid or soft foods, such as broth, soup, soft fruits, and fruit sorbet, to assure good urine flow and help prevent infection. Cranberry juice, in particular, may reduce your chances of getting a bladder infection.

Weight gain

This can result from medication given during cancer treatment, and is more common during the treatment of breast and prostate cancers. Weight gain may also result from overeating due to the stress of having cancer.

To avoid excessive weight gain, choose lean cuts of red meat, white-meat chicken and turkey, and fish; opt for low-fat dairy products; eat more vegetables and fruits; avoid high-fat, high-calorie snacks such as chips, candy, cookies, and ice cream; and make sure you exercise regularly. See pages 156–209 for more hints and tips.

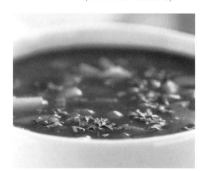

Dealing with nausea or difficulty swallowing A bowl of hot vegetable soup is easy to prepare and a good way to boost your nutrient intake if you do not feel like eating much.

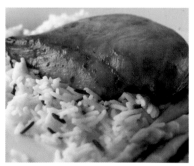

Loss of appetite Quick and easy to make, this broiled chicken and rice dish can be big or small. This dish contains a good low-fat protein, and rice is easy to digest.

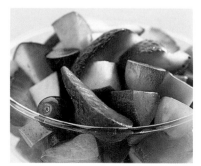

Difficulty chewing Cut food into small pieces, and choose soft fruit, such as berries. To make other fruits easier to eat, you can soften them by stewing or poaching.

Diets and cancer

Some people feel the need to go on a radical diet when diagnosed with cancer, but the body needs nutrients so a diet can be counter productive.

FAD DIETS

In the past, fad diets, such as eating only grapes, eliminating dairy products, just eating raw food, and other such radical approaches, have all been tried. In fact, eating raw food is not a good idea, because people undergoing radiation therapy are especially susceptible to infection and may be advised to follow a germ-free (neutropenic) diet (*below*).

MACROBIOTIC DIET

This vegetarian diet (*see p.101*) has been long promoted as an alternative cancer therapy, and has been proven to reduce rates of progression of prostate cancer and reduce the risk of colon cancer by 25 percent. However, the diet lacks certain vitamins and minerals, and supplements are often required.

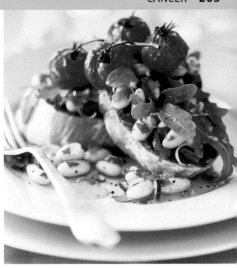

Crostini with protein-rich cannellini beans
If you follow a macrobiotic diet, which is vegetarian, make sure that you get enough protein—for example from legumes.

Germ-free (neutropenic) diet

People who receive chemotherapy often have a suppressed immune system and are therefore more likely to develop infections. Such infections can be caused by bacteria found in foods. Do not keep perishable foods such as milk, yogurt, and sandwiches at room temperature for more than two hours. Hot food should be kept hot (above 165°F/74°C), and cold food must be kept cold (under 40°F/4°C). If necessary, buy a thermometer for your refrigerator, to keep a consistent temperature of 34–40°F (1–4°C). Proper food handling and food preparation are discussed in the next chapter (*see pp.284–293*). The table below shows high-risk foods that are likely to promote an infection and low-risk alternatives.

FOOD GROUP	HIGH-RISK FOODS	LOW-RISK ALTERNATIVES
Vegetables and fruits	Raw fresh fruits and vegetables, including from salad bars; unpasteurized fruit and vegetable juices; dried fruits; raw nuts	Thick-skinned raw fruits (such as oranges and bananas); canned or bottled pasteurized fruit juices; nuts in baked goods; peanut butter; cooked, frozen, or canned vegetables
Meat, poultry, and fish	Raw or rare-cooked meat, poultry, or fish; processed meats and meats and cold cuts from the deli (such as salami, ham, and bologna); cold smoked salmon and lox; raw eggs	Well-cooked or canned meat, poultry, and fish; ready-packaged salami, ham, and bologna; canned tuna; well-cooked pasteurized egg substitutes
Bread, grain, and cereal products	Raw-grain products; bakery-made products (such as breads, cakes, doughnuts, and muffins)	Cooked pasta, rice, and grains; frozen breads, bagels, waffles, and commercially-baked cookies; chips, popcorn, pretzels, and snack crackers
Dairy products	Unpasteurized or raw milk, cheese, yogurt, and other milk products; naturally-aged moldy cheeses (such as Stilton, blue, and gorgonzola); soft cheeses (such as brie and camembert)	All pasteurized milk products (including yogurt); commercially-produced cheese and cheese products; ice cream and frozen yogurt; chilled nondairy whips
Drinks	Fresh apple cider; homemade lemonade; spring water	Pasteurized apple juice; canned, bottled, and powdered beverages; tap water
Miscellaneous	Raw honey; herbal and nontraditional nutritional supplements; leftover food	Pasteurized honey, jam, jelly, and syrups; commercial liquid and powdered nutritional supplements; frozen dinners

Vitamin and mineral deficiencies

Make sure you get enough of the right vitamins and minerals.

A varied diet should provide you with all the vitamins and minerals you need, and in their necessary amounts. The people most at risk of vitamin and mineral deficiencies are those who, for one reason or another, exclude certain foods or food groups from their diet.

For example, vegetarians and vegans may not get enough vitamin B_{12}, which occurs naturally only in foods of animal origin, and people who avoid milk and dairy products may miss out on sufficient amounts of calcium and vitamin D.

In addition, at different stages of life, you may need extra vitamins; for example, extra folate is needed during pregnancy.

However, isolated vitamin and mineral deficiencies are rarely seen, and the symptoms listed below provide an indication that you may not be getting adequate amounts of many nutrients. The chart lists potential symptoms of deficiencies and indicates which particular nutrients may be deficient.

Do I need a supplement?
If you have any of the symptoms in the chart, see your doctor, who may suggest that you have a blood test. Only take a supplement on the advice of your doctor.

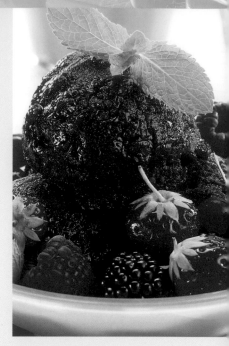

Fruit sorbet with fresh berries Jam-packed with essential vitamins, fruits can be presented in a number of ways, such as this refreshing mixed-fruit sorbet with fresh fruits.

Increase vitamin and mineral intake through your diet

This chart lists common signs and symptoms of vitamin or mineral deficiencies, together with suggestions of which particular nutrients may be deficient in your diet. However, it is rare to see an isolated vitamin deficiency, and the symptoms listed here may indicate that you are lacking in many nutrients. People who do not eat a wide variety of different foods are most likely be at risk of deficiencies. See page 296 for a key to the abbreviations used for vitamins and minerals in the chart.

BODY REGION	SIGNS AND SYMPTOMS	POSSIBLE VITAMIN / MINERAL DEFICIENCY
General	• Lack of energy • Weight loss • Poor appetite, or loss of appetite • Fatigue	• Vitamins B_1, Nia, B_6, B_{12}, Fol • Vitamins B_1, Nia • Vitamins B_1, Nia, Biotin, Fol / Minerals Mg, Fe, Zn • Vitamins B_6, C, D / Mineral Fe
Skin	• Easily bruised skin • Small red or purple spots on skin • Poor wound healing • Scaly, dry, flaky skin; eczema, or dermatitis; rash • Pale skin (pallor)	• Vitamins C, Vit K • Vitamin C • Vitamins A, C, E / Mineral Zn • Vitamins A, B_2, Nia, B_6, B_{12}, Biotin, Fol / Mineral Zn • Vitamins A, B_2, B_{12} / Mineral Fe
Hair and fingernails	• Hair loss • Poor hair condition • Dull or oily hair • Spoon-shaped (concave), brittle, and split fingernails	• Vitamins Biotin, D / Mineral Zn • Vitamins B_{12}, Biotin • Vitamin B_2 • Vitamin B_2 / Mineral Fe

BODY REGION	SIGN AND SYMPTOMS	POSSIBLE VITAMIN / MINERAL DEFICIENCY
Mouth	• Dry, cracked lips; inflamed mouth • Cracking at angles of mouth • Sore or bleeding gums • Sore and inflamed tongue • Dental cavities • Delayed tooth eruption in babies • Poor teeth enamel formation • Peridontal disease • Decline in sense of taste	• Vitamins B_2, Nia, B_6, Fol • Vitamins B2, Nia, B_6, Fol / Mineral Fe • Vitamins B2, C, Vit K • Vitamins B2, Nia, B_6, B_{12}, Fol • Mineral Fl • Vitamins C, D • Vitamin D / Minerals Ca, P, Fl • Vitamin C • Vitamin A / Mineral Zn
Abdomen and gastrointestinal tract	• Diarrhea • Nausea and/or vomiting • Abdominal pain • Blood in stool • Poor motility of the intestine • Constipation	• Vitamins Nia, B_6, B_{12}, Fol / Minerals Mg, Zn • Mineral Mg • Vitamin Nia • Mineral Fe • Minerals P, K • Mineral Mg
Respiratory system	• Frequent colds • Shortness of breath on exertion	• Vitamin C • Vitamin C
Eyes	• Blurred vision; blood-shot, itchy, watery eyes; sensitivity to bright light • Poor night vision; dry eyes	• Vitamin B2 • Vitamin A
Cardiovascular system	• Rapid heart beat • Irregular heart rhythm (arrhythmia) • Electrocardiogram abnormalities • Congestive heart failure	• Vitamin B1 / Mineral Mg • Minerals Ca, Mg, K • Vitamin K • Vitamin B1
Blood	• Microcytic (small-cell) anemia • Macrocyctic (large-cell) anemia • Prolonged blood-clotting time • Hemolytic anemia in babies • Hemorrhage in babies • Heavy menstrual periods or blood loss	• Mineral Fe • Vitamins B_6, B_{12}, Fol • Vitamin K • Vitamin E • Vitamin K • Mineral Fe
Bones, muscles, and joints	• Aching or weak bones • Muscle cramps • Sore, tender, or aching muscles • Joint pain • Muscle weakness • Swollen legs (fluid retention) • Growth retardation • Softening of bones • Abnormally curved spine	• Vitamins C, D / Minerals Ca, P • Vitamin B_6 / Minerals Ca, Mg, K, Na • Vitamins B_1, B_{12}, Biotin • Vitamins C, D / Mineral Ca • Vitamins B_6, C, D / Minerals Mg, P, K, Se • Vitamin B_1 • Vitamin D / Mineral Zn • Vitamin D / Minerals Ca, P • Vitamin D / Mineral Ca
Nervous system	• Spasms and twitching • Headaches • Tingling hands and feet • Irritability • Lack of concentration • Anxiety • Depression • Insomnia; sleeplessness	• Vitamin D / Minerals Ca, Mg • Vitamin Nia / Mineral Mg • Vitamins B_1, B_6, B_{12} / Mineral Ca • Vitamins B_1, Nia, B_6, B_{12} / Mineral Zn • Vitamin Nia / Minerals Mg, Fe • Vitamins Nia, B_{12}, Fol • Vitamins Nia, B_6, Fol, C / Mineral Zn • Vitamins Nia, B_6

Dietary supplements

Vitamin and mineral supplements can improve your health.

Public interest in vitamins and minerals for health has never been higher. Evidence continues to grow that certain supplements can improve health and possibly even prevent cardiovascular disease, cancer, and the bone disorder osteoporosis.

According to recent surveys, 18–40 percent of North Americans report that they take vitamin and mineral supplements as part of their routine health regime. In the US between 1994 and 2000, sales of supplements grew by nearly 80 percent, from $8.8 billion to an estimated $15.7 billion. In this section, we review the most

Supplements for health In the last decade, public interest in the benefits of supplements has increased and sales have skyrocketed.

popular vitamin and mineral supplements and tell you who may benefit from taking them and any precautions to be noted.

Safety of supplements
In 1990, the Nutrition Labeling and Education Act was passed in the US. This law means that the Food and Drug Administration (FDA) has to approve the safety and health claims made about supplements by the manufacturer before they can be marketed. Unlike medications, which are rigorously tested and their manufacturing processes monitored, the FDA does not examine the purity of supplements or determine their medical effectiveness. However, the FDA can prevent the sale of a supplement if they have proof that it is unsafe for consumption.

Manufacturers are allowed to make general health claims about their products as long as they do not contain reference to preventing or curing a specific disease.

Types of supplements
In 1994, the Dietary Supplement Health and Education Act (DSHEA) was passed in the US, defining a dietary supplement as a product that is taken orally and contains a dietary ingredient, such as a vitamin or a mineral. Other ingredients include herbs, botanicals, amino acids, enzymes, and fish oils. They can be extracts or concentrates of the particular ingredient and may be available as capsules, tablets, gel caps, liquids, or powders.

Buyer beware
Despite the form of the supplement, the DSHEA classifies supplements under the category of food, not medication, and it is important for companies to label their products accordingly. Unfortunately, this gives rise to a situation in which the buyer is at risk of purchasing supplements that have absolutely no benefit, such as shark cartilage, or that are potentially harmful, such as the herb ephedra.

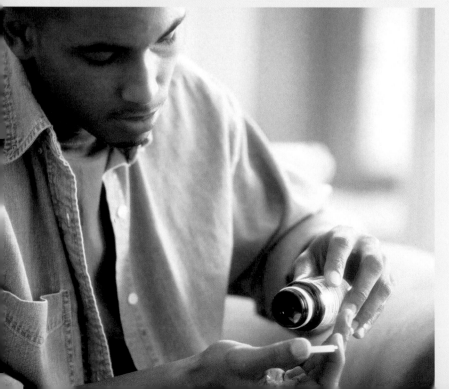

Chelated minerals

Minerals in supplements are often bound—or chelated—to another substance in order to improve their absorption and use by the body. Chelated minerals are also better tolerated and may be less harmful to the body than pure forms.

Substances to which a mineral can be chelated include amino acids, gluconates, citrates, and picolinates. If you read the labels on supplements, you will see different forms of minerals. For example, zinc as zinc picolinate, magnesium as magnesium oxide, iron as ferrous fumarate, and calcium as calcium carbonate.

Manufacturers of supplements choose a certain form of a mineral, depending on digestive factors and how well the intestine tolerates it.

Can you benefit from supplements?

A general multivitamin may provide some nutritional "insurance" against missing specific nutrients due to lack of variety in your diet or to make sure you get enough nutrients when you need extra, such as during pregnancy.

However, nutritionists are still trying to demonstrate a specific benefit for supplements with regard to prevention and treatment of chronic diseases. The use of vitamins and minerals in this way is different from correcting "classic" vitamin deficiencies, which are rare in North America. However, vitamin sales continue to climb and are a $15-billion-a-year business in the US.

NO PROVEN BENEFITS
The efficacy of vitamin E for treating and preventing cardiovascular disease has been studied for over 30 years, and tested in people with or at risk for the disease. However, it has not been shown to be effective, and recent trials have shown that it may even have a negative impact on cardiovascular health.

Chromium is needed by the body to process the hormone insulin and control levels of glucose in the blood, but supplements do not seem to help people with or at risk of developing diabetes. Beta-carotene is effective at blocking steps in cancer development when tested on cells in the laboratory, but when given to people at high risk of cancer it appears to have no effect.

GET PROFESSIONAL ADVICE
People who want to supplement their diet with any form of nutrient should consult a health-care professional. He or she can provide advice on which supplements you should or should not take if you have a preexisting disorder or are taking certain medications.

A general multivitamin and mineral supplement may be helpful as long as the contents are at the correct Dietary Reference Intake levels (see p.35). Data is lacking to support the benefits of taking isolated supplements of single nutrients or combinations, such as the antioxidant vitamins C and E, carotenes, and selenium. The charts on pages 268–271 show who would benefit from taking specific supplements. In fact, the body actually absorbs vitamins in food more easily than from supplements.

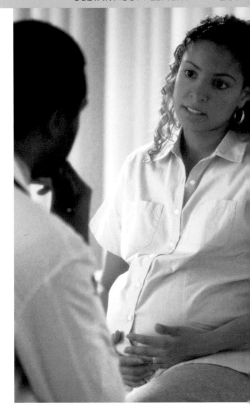

Taking a supplement You may need to take a vitamin or mineral supplement for various reasons, including pregnancy or illness.

Can you take too much?

Harmful effects of vitamins and minerals usually result from taking too much, misusing supplements, or dosage errors. If you are taking large doses of vitamins or minerals, your doctor should be closely monitoring you. The fat-soluble vitamins—vitamins A, D, E, and K—are stored in the liver, and if they are taken in excess may build up to harmful levels more quickly compared to the water-soluble vitamins—the B vitamins and vitamin C (see pp.268 271).

VITAMINS
Several of the vitamins can be harmful in excess. Too much vitamin A leads to cracked lips, headaches, blurred vision, and dry rough skin. Too much vitamin D causes poor appetite, nausea, vomiting, and deposits of calcium in body tissues. Large doses of B-complex vitamins can produce symptoms ranging from itching, flushing, nausea, lightheadedness, or tingling sensations in the fingers to progressive loss of balance and sensation in the legs. Symptoms usually disappear when the offending vitamin is withdrawn. Excessive doses of vitamin C can cause diarrhea and have also been reported to predispose those susceptible to oxalate kidney stones (see p.237).

MINERALS
Many minerals taken in excess can be harmful. In children, excessive intake of iron is dangerous and too much fluoride turns the teeth brown. People treated for ulcers may develop milk–alkali syndrome, due to excessive intake of calcium from medication, causing muscle pain and weakness. Excessive intake of vitamin D can cause overabsorption of calcium, and excessive zinc may suppress the immune system and interfere with the absorption of copper.

If you do take a supplement, select a sensible one with the levels of nutrients recognized as safe and avoid going over the tolerable upper limit (left).

Jargon buster

Tolerable upper intake level (UL)
This indicates the maximum safe amount of a nutrient to eat or take as a supplement without risk of side effects from poisoning. ULs have been determined for many of the vitamins and minerals, including the vitamins A, B_6, folate, C, D, and E and the minerals calcium, copper, zinc, magnesium, and selenium.

Vitamin and mineral supplements

This chart outlines who would benefit from taking a vitamin or mineral supplement and any relevant warnings. You are more likely to need a supplement if you are pregnant or breast-feeding; have had a recent severe injury or surgery; have a serious infection; are anemic; if you drink alcohol and/or smoke; or eat a restrictive or unusual diet. In general, it is best to first consult your doctor or dietitian before taking supplements, especially if you are taking any medication.

The amount of a vitamin and mineral supplement that the body absorbs depends on its needs. For example, women and growing children have a greater need for calcium and iron than adult males and therefore absorb more. How much the body absorbs depends on the chemical form of the vitamin or mineral and the acidity or alkalinity where absorption occurs in the digestive tract. For example, the acidic environment of the stomach increases the solubility of calcium and iron in food, resulting in increased absorption. In contrast, people suffering from achlorhydria, who have a reduced production of acid in the stomach, or those who take antacid medication, may be at risk of poorer absorption of calcium and iron.

SUPPLEMENT	WHO MIGHT BENEFIT FROM A SUPPLEMENT?	WARNINGS
Vitamin A (*see p.52*) Tolerable upper intake level: 3RE (retinol equivalents) per day	• People with skin problems such as acne and psoriasis • Those with infections such as measles or peritonitis, which is inflammation of the membrane lining the abdominal cavity (taken together with antibiotics) • People with osteoarthritis (*see p.241*) • Those with poor night vision	• Avoid if you are taking any vitamin A-derived medications for skin problems, if you are taking oral contraceptives, or if you are pregnant • High doses (over 7.5RE per day) can cause flaking, itching skin, blurred vision, and headache • Toxic levels can lead to enlarged spleen and liver and joint pain
Thiamine (B$_1$) (*see p.53*) Tolerable upper intake level not established	• People with a weakened immune system • Regular alcohol drinkers or smokers	• No known problems
Riboflavin (B$_2$) (*see p.53*) Tolerable upper intake level not established	• Vegetarians (*see pp.100–101*) • Athletes (*see pp.146–149*) • Those who suffer regularly from migraine headaches (*see pp.256–257*) • People with skin problems such as acne, eczema, and ulcers • Those with carpal tunnel syndrome (tingling and pain in hand and forearm)	• High doses may upset the stomach
Niacin (B$_3$) (*see p.53*) Tolerable upper intake level: 35mg per day	• People with high blood cholesterol	• Niacin is prescribed at up to 3g per day for treating high cholesterol • Pregnant women should not take more than the Dietary Reference Intake, which has been set at 18mg per day • Avoid if you have liver problems or a peptic ulcer • You should check first with your doctor before taking niacin if you have diabetes, gout, gallbladder disease, internal bleeding from weakened arteries, or the eye disorder glaucoma • Doses of 50mg per day can cause flushing, itching, headaches, cramps, and nausea • Very high doses can cause liver damage, high levels of glucose in the blood, and irregular heart rhythm (arrhythmia)

SUPPLEMENT	WHO MIGHT BENEFIT FROM A SUPPLEMENT?	WARNINGS
Vitamin B$_6$ (*see p.54*) Tolerable upper intake level: 100mg per day	• People who have a poor diet, such as heavy alcohol users or older people, who may have difficulties absorbing vitamin B$_6$ from food • Those sensitive to monosodium glutamate • Women taking oral contraceptives • People using the asthma medication theophylline or the tuberculosis medication isoniazide • Those with high blood levels of homocysteine (*see p.219*)—taken with vitamins B$_{12}$ and folate	• Do not take more than the Dietary Reference Intake if you are pregnant (1.9mg per day) or breast-feeding (2mg per day) • More than 100mg per day can cause numbness and tingling in fingers and toes • Very high doses can cause liver damage, and nerve damage, and affect your ability to walk • Check first with your doctor if you have intestinal problems, liver disease, an overactive thyroid gland, or sickle-cell disease, or if you are recovering from illness, injury, or surgery • Supplements may lead to kidney stones
Vitamin B$_{12}$ (*see p.55*) Tolerable upper intake level not established	• Vegetarians and vegans (*see pp.100–101*) • Those with problems absorbing it from food • People with anemia (*see p.55*) • Those who have had portions of their intestines removed or bypassed • Those with high blood levels of homocysteine (*see p.219*)—taken with vitamins B$_6$ and folate	• No known problems
Folate (*see p.56*) Tolerable upper intake level: 1 mg per day	• Pregnant women (*see pp.138–141*) • Those with problems absorbing folate from food • People with liver disease or on kidney dialysis (*see p.237*) • Those with high blood levels of homocysteine (*see p.219*)—taken with vitamins B$_6$ and B$_{12}$	• Can mask a vitamin B$_{12}$ deficiency • Consult your doctor if you have anemia • High doses may cause bright-yellow urine, fever, shortness of breath, rash, diarrhea, nausea, appetite loss, flatulence, and a swollen abdomen and interfere with the effectiveness of medications for epilepsy
Vitamin C (*see p.56*) Tolerable upper intake level: 2,000mg per day	• Regular drinkers or smokers • People with severe burns, fractures, pneumonia, rheumatic fever (in which there is inflammation of the joints and a high body temperature), or tuberculosis • Those preparing for surgery	• Do not take more than the Dietary Reference Intake if you are pregnant (85mg per day) or breast-feeding (120mg per day) • Consult your doctor if you have kidney problems, kidney stones, gout, sickle-cell disease, or iron-storage disease • High doses can cause nausea and vomiting, diarrhea, headache, and abdominal cramps
Vitamin D (*see p.57*) Tolerable upper intake level: 0.05mg per day	• People who do not drink milk, which is usually fortified with vitamin D • Those who do not get enough sunlight • People who cannot absorb fats from the intestine, such as those with cystic fibrosis • Those with a family history of osteoporosis (*see p.241*) • The elderly, who make less vitamin D in their bodies when skin exposed to sunlight	• Do not take more than the Dietary Reference Intake if you are pregnant or breast-feeding (5mg per day) • Consult your doctor if you have epilepsy, cardiovascular disease, persistent diarrhea, kidney, liver, or pancreas disease, intestinal problems, or the immune disorder sarcoidosis, or if you are planning to become pregnant • High doses can lead to kidney stones, irreversible hardening of tissues, nausea, headache, fatigue, lack of appetite, frequent urination, weight loss, irregular heart rhythm (arrhythmia), and weak bones and muscles • In babies and children, too much vitamin D can lead to retarded growth, rounding of the skull, and learning difficulties

SUPPLEMENT	WHO MIGHT BENEFIT FROM A SUPPLEMENT?	WARNINGS
Vitamin E (*see p.58*) Tolerable upper intake level: 1,000mg per day	• Pregnant women who smoke, as it can protect their babies from possible harm caused by the mothers' exposure to cigarette smoke • People at risk of Alzheimer's disease	• Do not take more than the Dietary Reference Intake if pregnant (15mg per day) or breast-feeding (19mg per day) • High doses may interfere with niacin's (B_3) ability to lower high blood-cholesterol levels, and increase the tendency to bleed and impair the function of white blood cells, cause dizziness, fatigue, headache, abdominal pain, diarrhea, flulike symptoms, nausea, blurred vision, and decrease libido • Avoid for two weeks before and after surgery • Consult your doctor if you are taking blood-thinning (anticoagulant) medications or have anemia, bleeding or problems with blood-clotting, cystic fibrosis, liver disease, or intestinal problems
Vitamin K (*see p.58*) Tolerable upper intake level not established	• Babies, given as an injection at birth to prevent bleeding • Women during and after menopause, to decrease bone loss • People with liver disease, jaundice, or problems absorbing nutrients, or with long-term use of aspirin or antibiotic medications	• Vitamin K reverses the effects of blood-thinning, or anticoagulant drugs (*see p.153*) • High doses may cause allergic reactions and brain damage in babies
Calcium (*see p.62*) Tolerable upper intake level: 2,500mg per day	• Pregnant (*see p.140*) and breast-feeding women (*see p.142*) • People at risk of osteoporosis (*see p.241*) • Those wanting to lose weight (*see p.62*) • People with diabetes (*see pp.246–247*)	• Calcium supplements are available in various forms, so consult your doctor for advice • Do not take more than 1,000mg if pregnant or breast-feeding • Do not take calcium and iron supplements together since calcium limits iron absorption. Calcium may also limit the absorption of the mineral zinc • Consult your doctor if you want to take more than 5,000mg per day or if you suffer from sarcoidosis, kidney disease, long-term constipation, colitis, diarrhea, stomach or intestinal bleeding, or heart problems • Supplements may cause gas, constipation, headache, confusion, muscle or bone pain, and nausea and vomiting, and affect heart rhythm • High doses may lead to kidney stones
Fluoride (*see p.65*) Tolerable upper intake level not established	• People who do not have fluoride added to their public drinking water (*see p.66*) • Some breast-fed babies, who do not get enough fluoride in breast milk (*see p.109*) • People with the bone disorder osteoporosis (*see p.241*)	• Various forms are available, so consult your doctor for advice on the best one for you • Do not swallow fluoridated tooth products • Children under the age of 6 years should use only a pea-sized amount of fluoridated toothpaste and be supervised by an adult when brushing • 20–40mg per day can interfere with how the body uses calcium • 40–70mg per day can cause heartburn and pains in the extremities

SUPPLEMENT	WHO MIGHT BENEFIT FROM A SUPPLEMENT?	WARNINGS
Iron (*see p.66*) Tolerable upper intake level: 45mg per day	• People with a low dietary intake of iron, such as vegetarians and vegans • Those with problems absorbing iron, with kidney disease, or who have lost a lot of blood, such as after an injury • People with iron-deficiency anemia • Pregnant and breast-feeding women • Women who have heavy menstrual periods	• Take only under the supervision of your doctor or health-care provider • Take vitamin C with iron supplements to aid absorption of the iron • People with hemochromatosis store too much iron and should avoid iron supplements • Prolonged high doses of iron supplements can cause bronzed skin, damage to the liver and pancreas, and diabetes
Magnesium (*see p.63*) Tolerable upper intake level: 350mg per day	• Athletes and those with muscle cramps • Pregnant women at risk of premature labor • People with high blood pressure or other cardiovascular diseases (*see pp.214–215*), or irregular heart rhythm (arrhythmia) • Those with asthma or frequent migraines • People with diabetes, to increase the production of the hormone insulin • Those with chronic constipation • People with excessive urinary loss of magnesium, very low blood levels of magnesium, long-term problems absorbing nutrients, severe diarrhea, or long-term vomiting	• Check with your doctor before taking magnesium supplements • High doses may cause diarrhea
Zinc (*see p.67*) Tolerable upper intake level: 40mg per day	• People with poor taste and smell • Those with a weakened immune system • People with a cold, influenza, or a sore throat	• Do not take more than the Dietary Reference Intake if pregnant (11mg) or breast-feeding (12mg) • Do not take with either calcium or iron supplements as these interfere with zinc absorption • Avoid if you have a peptic ulcer • Doses of over 15mg per day may weaken the immune system • Side effects include diarrhea, heartburn, nausea, vomiting, and abdominal pain • Long-term high doses can lower HDL cholesterol, which is protective, and cause copper deficiency, producing brittle nails
Multivitamin and mineral	• Pregnant (*see p.142*) or breast-feeding women (*see p.142*) • Those who are recovering from surgery or severe injury • People who have infections, such as HIV • Those who are anemic or have a low red blood cell count (hemoglobin) (*see p.55*) • Regular drinkers and smokers • People who avoid entire food groups, such as dairy products for lactose intolerance • Those who are following a low-calorie diet or have irregular eating habits and skip meals • Older people or anyone with a condition that affects their ability to absorb nutrients • Women taking oral contraceptives	• Those taking other supplements listed above may get too much of some nutrients • Those taking antiseizure or blood-thinning (anticoagulant) medications as listed above

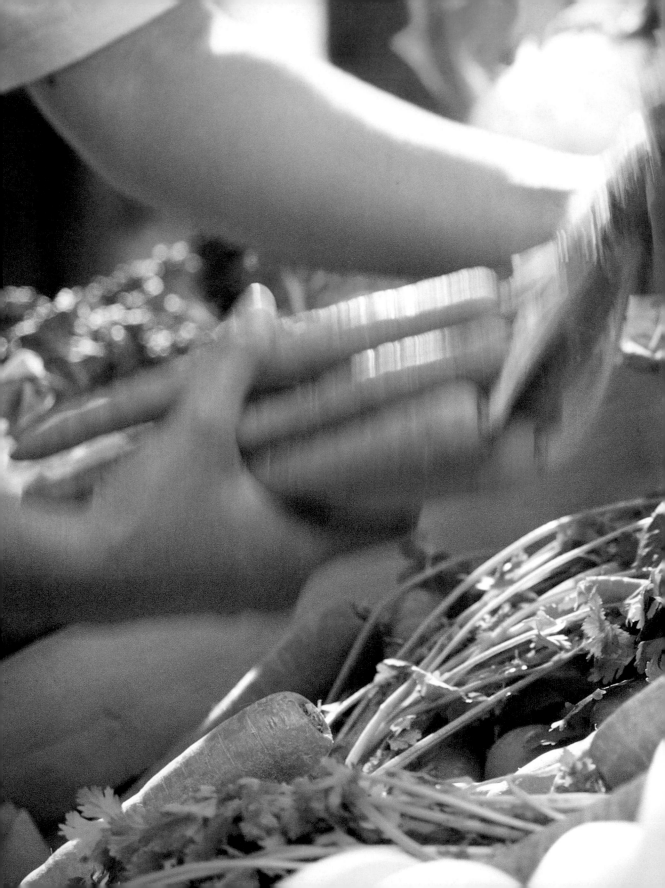

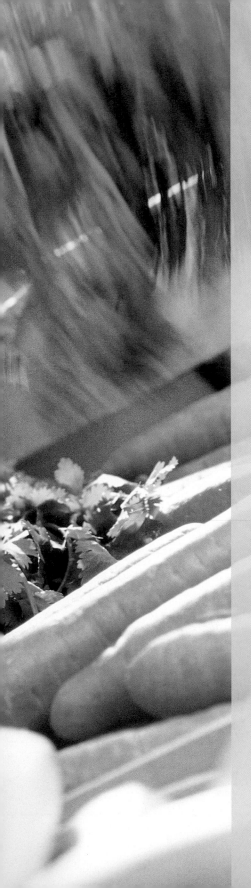

The food you buy

In this chapter, we explain nutritional theories and provide practical advice on how to make the best and healthiest choices when you go food shopping, hints on comparing products, and tips on storing, preparing, and cooking the food when you get it home.

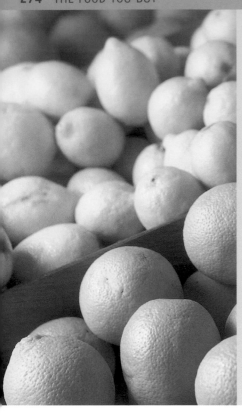

Nutrition and modern food production

Modern technology allows year-round availability of a vast array of foods.

From refrigerator–freezers to cans, jars, and bottles that let us keep food on our shelves for weeks or longer, the North American home is packed with appliances and products that have revolutionized

our way of eating. These results of modern technology save us a lot of time and energy, enabling us to assemble healthy meals whenever we want them, instead of having to make daily shopping trips for fresh produce. Food producers can now supply us all year round with perfect produce of uniform size, shape, color, and quality.

Mass food production Supermarket shelves, stacked with cans, jars, bottles, and frozen and chilled products as well as fresh produce, offer a year-round choice of affordable foods.

Impact on nutrition
The mass availability of food, at affordable prices, is made possible only by highly sophisticated food-production methods, some of which are now being questioned because of their impact on nutrition and health. For example, public concern

Is fresh food best?

There is no doubt that fresh food is best from a nutritional point of view: newly dug potatoes or freshly picked peas, taken straight from the garden to the kitchen, have more nutrients than either canned or frozen alternatives—not to mention being incomparably better in taste and texture. Not everyone has the luxury of growing and eating their own produce, however, and "fresh" produce on supermarket shelves may have been picked and kept in cold storage for a considerable time. Then, the distinction between "fresh" and canned or frozen becomes less clear-cut.

FRESH, FROZEN, OR CANNED?
Here are some guidelines to help you decide on the most nutritious food choices for your family.
• When buying fruits and vegetables, choose locally grown produce whenever possible, as this is likely to be almost as fresh as home-grown varieties.
• In supermarkets, if no locally grown produce is available, buy fruits and

vegetables in season, as they are least likely to have been in lengthy storage.
• Frozen fruits and vegetables are almost as nutritious as fresh varieties, if they were frozen immediately after picking.
• When choosing prepackaged foods, check the contents on the food label. It may include a long list of undesirable ingredients including additives, sugar, salt, and oil (*see pp.278–280*).
• Choose fresh meat, preferably low-fat varieties such as white-meat poultry and lean beef, over processed meats such as salami and cured beef, which are likely to contain high levels of saturated fat, salt, and additives.
• Buy freshly baked whole-grain bread, rather than sliced, packaged varieties, which often contain additives that give them a prolonged shelf life.

Choosing fresh foods While freshly picked fruits and vegetables are highest in nutritional content, remember that supermarket stock may have been in storage for several months.

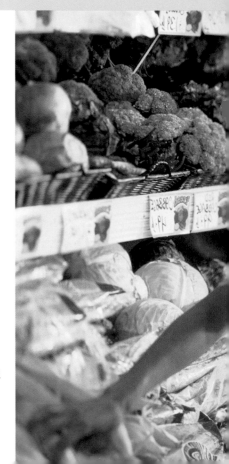

about the use of pesticides and herbicides, and the knowledge that most nonorganic cattle and chickens are infected with harmful bacteria, such as *Salmonella* and *E. coli* has led to a growing demand for organic foods produced by ecologically sensitive methods.

Research has shown that organic crops contain significantly higher levels of nutrients than crops that are grown conventionally. However, it is worth bearing in mind that organic products may spoil faster than nonorganic foods since they are not treated with preservatives. In addition, most organic products cost considerably more than foods produced by conventional means. This is because the production of organic foods necessitates more expensive farming practices, with tighter government regulations and lower crop yields. However, as the demand for organic foods

increases, they should become less expensive, making them a more viable option for a greater number of consumers.

Food and health claims

In addition to meeting the demand for an affordable variety of all-year-round products, the food industry now caters to a growing interest in nutrition and health, with consumer demand for foods that are lower in fat, salt, sugar, and cholesterol. More recently, products claiming additional health benefits, such as cholesterol-lowering margarines, have been launched.

In conclusion, while we may take for granted the convenience, abundance, and huge variety of affordable food that is available today, we must remain alert to the health implications of what we eat and strive to make the best choices from what is available.

Genetically modified food

Modern developments in genetics have been applied to agricultural crops, which can be modifed by transferring specific inherited traits from one species to another. This technique, known as genetic modification (GM), has been used to increase crop yields and improve pest resistance. Other benefits may also be possible in the future, such as improving crops' nutritional value and disease resistance and allowing them to survive flood, drought, or frost.

There is considerable concern, however, that GM crops may pose threats to human health and to the environment, such as allergic responses to substances in foods, inadvertent toxicity to wildlife, and herbicide tolerance. Therefore, the debate continues.

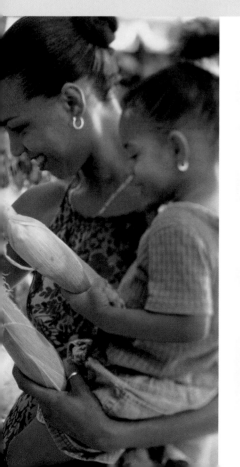

Tips on choosing organic foods

Before a product can be marketed as organic, strict conditions set by the US Department of Agriculture must be fulfilled. Organic fruit, vegetables, and grains must be grown without the use of any artificial fertilizers, pesticides, herbicides, or fungicides. Organic meat, poultry, eggs, and dairy products must come from animals that are not given growth hormones or antibiotics, are fed only on organic feed, and have access to the outdoors.

Organic foods are not treated with preservatives; therefore, you should always choose the freshest produce available to you.
● Select fruits and vegetables with care, avoiding those with blemishes or insect holes.
● Choose locally grown produce whenever possible.
● Ask your grocer on which day new produce is delivered, so you can buy it the day it arrives.

● Read labels carefully: remember that organic-food products are not necessarily "healthy" in every respect and can still be high in fat, sugar, or calories.
● Do not confuse foods labeled "natural" with organic products; only foods bearing the organic seal have met defined standards. Products bearing this seal will carry one of the following labels, which define and clarify its precise content:
"100 percent organic" contains only organically produced ingredients;
"Organic" contains at least 95 percent organic ingredients (excluding water and salt);
"Made with organic ingredients" contains at least 70 percent organic ingredients and has not been produced using nonorganic methods.

Note that small growers, such as those with an annual turnover of less than $5,000 in organic foods, are exempt from this certification.

How food is preserved

Various techniques are used to preserve the quality of food for long-term storage.

Since ancient times, food has been preserved by techniques such as curing, smoking, storing in salt or brine, and freezing: methods that ensure supplies will not run out when adverse conditions limit the availability of fresh products.

The commercial food producers of today use a variety of methods to prolong the life of their products, including canning, pasteurization, and irradiation, in addition to more traditional methods.

Preserving food not only helps maintain plenty of choices for the consumer throughout the year, but also saves time and energy, since fewer shopping trips are needed to stock up on the ingredients for daily meals.

Preservation methods

Freezing, which is one of the most common methods of preserving food, protects the flavor, color, moisture content, and nutritive value of food. Frozen vegetables, in particular, are often of excellent quality, since they are processed and packaged very quickly after harvesting, with the result that few of the nutrients are lost.

Canned foods are an excellent pantry standby, because they have a long shelf-life. Fruits, vegetables, soups, sauces, and basic meals are all available in this form, providing the basis for a quick meal at any time. All such products carry a food label listing ingredients and a detailed nutritional analysis of the contents (*opposite*).

To make milk and milk products safe for consumption, they usually undergo pasteurization, a process involving heating to a temperature high enough to eliminate bacteria. This process also extends the shelf-life of the product without affecting taste or nutritional value. A variety of other preservation methods are used with milk products, including evaporation, condensation, and UHT (*see p.82*).

One of the oldest forms of food preservation, smoking involves exposing foods such as fish, meat, or poultry to the smoke of burning aromatic woods. The process also imparts extra flavor to the food. Traditionally, fish and meats were salted before being smoked, giving a particularly strong taste.

Good and bad additives

A quick look at the food label on commercially produced food products reveals lengthy lists of substances that are added to the basic food ingredients to prolong the shelf-life of the contents and improve its color and taste. These substances are discussed on the following pages (*see pp.278–280*).

Well-stocked shelves Mass food-production methods ensure a plentiful, year-round supply of food products, preserved by a variety of methods, from canning to freezing.

Food irradiation

A relatively recent addition to the range of preservation techniques, irradiation involves the use of electromagnetic waves to eradicate the microorganisms that cause food spoilage and deterioration. Scientists believe it to be a useful, controlled, and predictable process that does not change the important characteristics of most products. Foods that have been irradiated must carry an international symbol in the form of a stylized flower, known as a "radura."

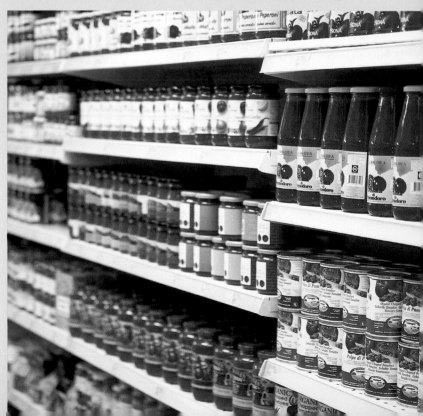

What do food labels mean?

Food manufacturers are required by law to supply a Nutrition Facts label on most of their products (*below*). This label includes 14 mandatory nutrients that must appear in a prescribed order. These particular nutrients were selected because they address current health concerns. The order in which they appear on the label reflects the priority of current dietary recommendations. The panel ends with a footnote explaining the basis of the Daily Values.

VOLUNTARY INFORMATION

In addition to the mandatory nutrients that must be listed are certain voluntary nutrients. These include the amount of monounsaturated and polyunsaturated fat, soluble and insoluble fiber, sugar alcohol, and other carbohydrates. The percentage of vitamin A present as beta-carotene and the amounts of other essential vitamins and minerals may also be listed. If a claim is made about any of these nutrients, or if a food is fortified or enriched with any of them, the label then has to give nutritional information about these nutrients. Particular claims relating to health issues are now allowed to be printed on food labels (*see p.280*).

INGREDIENTS LISTING

In addition to the mandatory Nutrition Facts panel, food labels must list all ingredients in the product. These are given in order of weight, starting with the greatest. Because some people may be allergic to certain additives,

Labeling exemptions

Foods that are exempt from labeling requirements include:
- Those for immediate consumption
- Bakery, deli, and also candy-store items
- Medical foods prepared for patients with nutritional needs
- Plain coffee and tea, some spices, and foods containing no significant amounts of any nutrients

the ingredient list must include the following, if appropriate:
- FDA-certified color additives
- Sources of protein hydrolysates, which are used in many foods as flavors and flavor enhancers
- Caseinate, which is a milk derivative used in foods claiming to be nondairy.

Serving size This information is based on consistent serving sizes that reflect the amounts most people eat.

Calories The amount of total energy (measured as calories) provided by one serving of the food is shown.

Total fat The total amount of fat provided by one serving of the food is shown in grams and as a percentage of Daily Value. This is followed by a similar analysis for saturated fat and trans fatty-acids content. Try to select foods with less than 3g total fat/1g saturated fat per 100 calories.

Cholesterol The total amount of cholesterol provided by one serving of the food is shown in milligrams and as a percentage of Daily Value. Try to select foods with less than 100mg cholesterol per serving.

Total carbohydrate The total weight of carbohydrate provided by one serving of the food is shown in grams and as a percentage of Daily Value. This is followed by a similar analysis for dietary fiber and sugars. Try to choose foods that are higher in starchy carbohydrates than in sugars, and increase total fiber intake to at least 24g per day.

Footnote The Daily Value figure is based on a diet of 2,000 calories per day. This section provides a comparison of values between a 2,000-calorie and a 2,500-calorie diet.

Calories per gram The last section indicates how many calories are provided by 1g of fat, carbohydrate, and protein.

Nutrition Facts

Serving Size ½ cup (114g)
Servings Per Container 4

Amount Per Serving

Calories 90   Calories from Fat 30

	%**Daily Value***
Total Fat 3g	**5%**
Saturated Fat 0mg	**0%**
Trans Fat 0mg	**0%**
Cholesterol 0mg	**0%**
Sodium 300mg	**13%**
Total Carbohydrate 13g	**4%**
Dietary Fiber 3g	**12%**
Sugars 3g	
Protein 3g	

Vitamin A 80%	•	Vitamin C 60%
Calcium 4%	•	Iron 4%

* Percent Daily Values are based on a 2,000 calorie diet. Your daily values may be higher or lower depending on your calorie needs:

		Calories:	2,000	2,500
Total Fat	Less than		65g	80g
Sat Fat	Less than		20g	25g
Cholesterol	Less than		300mg	300mg
Sodium	Less than		2,400mg	2,400mg
Total Carbohydrate			300g	375g
Dietary Fiber			25g	30g

Calories per gram:
Fat 9 • Carbohydrate 4 • Protein 4

Servings per container This is important, since the nutritional information that follows is given per serving, not for the entire contents of the container.

Calories from fat The amount of energy (measured as calories) provided by the fat in one serving of the food is shown.

% Daily Value This value indicates the percentage of Daily Value provided by one serving of the product. Nutrients that contain between 10 and 20 percent of Daily Value may be listed as good sources of that nutrient.

Sodium The total amount of sodium in one serving of the product is listed in milligrams. If you have high blood pressure, choose foods with less than 400mg of sodium per serving.

Protein The total amount of protein provided by one serving of the food is shown in grams.

Vitamins A and C Amounts per serving of these two vitamins are listed as a percentage of Daily Value.

Calcium and Iron Amounts per serving of these two minerals are listed as a percentage of Daily Value.

Nutrition facts label This part of the label is obligatory on most packaged foods and includes information on serving size, calorie content, and amounts of nutrients contained in the product.

Why are additives needed?

Food additives are substances that are added to processed foods in order to improve their flavor or appearance, maintain freshness, increase shelf life, and enhance their nutritional value. They can be either naturally occurring substances or synthetic.

Food manufacturers use at least 3,000 different additives, ranging from familiar substances, such as sugar and salt, to chemicals or preservatives, such as citric acid. The US Department of Agriculture (USDA) regulates additives in different categories. For example, additives can include coloring agents, natural and synthetic flavors, sweeteners, and flavor enhancers to make foods look more attractive and taste better, and stabilizers, thickeners, and emulsifiers to give body and texture to foods.

Additives can also protect foods from adverse conditions, such as variations in temperature and damage during the distribution process. Preservatives slow the spoilage of foods and help protect consumers from food-borne illness. They also help retain a food's natural color and freshness and keep oils and fats from turning rancid during storage and transportation. Acids, which help in the release of the gas carbon dioxide from yeast, may also have preservative effects in certain foods.

FORTIFIED AND ENRICHED FOODS

Many foods, such as bread and milk, are also fortified with vitamins and minerals that might otherwise be lacking in the diet, or enriched with nutrients that were lost in the refining process (*see p.50*). For example, milk is fortified with vitamins A and D, and salt is fortified with iodine, while orange juice contains added calcium and vitamin D. The vitamin folate is now added to cereals and grain products to help reduce the risk of babies being born with neural tube defects (*see p.140*).

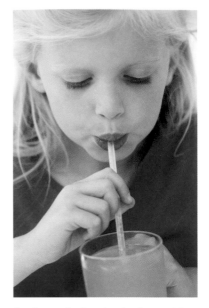

Growing needs Many brands of orange juice are fortified with calcium (*see p.62*) and vitamin D (*see p.57*), two nutrients that are important for growing children.

Case study Young boy with a soy allergy

Name Alexander

Age Four years

Problem This past winter, Alexander attended his cousin's birthday party at his aunt's house. A vegetarian, she decided to make pizza made with soy cheese, among other vegetarian alternatives. Alexander enjoyed the pizza, but soon began to sneeze, and had watery eyes with a stuffy nose for the remainder of the party. His parents thought he had a cold and treated him with over-the-counter cold medications.

Now it is summer, Alexander still has symptoms of what seems to be a persistent cold. He has developed an itchy rash that prompted a visit to the doctor. The doctor discovered that Alexander's parents had decided, soon after the birthday party, to incorporate his aunt's healthy lifestyle into their own. Since Alexander liked the pizza, they tried other soy products, such as soy nuggets and breakfast links, and tofu hot dogs, as well. The doctor referred Alexander to an allergist, who did a skin-prick test that came back positive only for soy. The test was negative for milk, chocolate, eggs, and peanuts—other common food allergens.

Lifestyle Alexander is a typical four-year-old who attends preschool five days a week, from 9a.m. to 1p.m. His mother prepares a packed lunch, and he enjoys staying with his friends until after lunch. His weekends are filled with playing in the backyard with his sister and outdoor birthday parties now that it is summer. He has just begun his first full day at camp, where lunch is provided. He eats breakfast and dinner at home, and usually has a snack in the afternoon when he returns home from camp at 3p.m.

Advice Since Alexander is allergic to the proteins found in soy, his parents must make sure he does not consume it in any form. They will need to read labels for soy and other ingredients that may contain soy. These include hydrolyzed vegetable or plant protein, vegetable broth, gums, and starches. Soy lecithin, which is made from fatty substances in soy beans, can be eaten safely by many people with soy allergy.

Alexander's parents should maintain their healthy eating, but with nonsoy products. The nuggets can be prepared with white-meat chicken and sautéed lightly in olive oil. They can buy fat-free hot dogs, low-fat turkey sausages, and pizza with low-fat mozzarella. When they eat out, they must be careful of hidden sources of soy, such as salad dressings, mayonnaise, soy cheese, and certain sauces, such as soy and teriyaki sauce. They should include more grains, vegetables, and fruits as Alexander gets older.

Understanding food additives

The following are some of the additives or groups of additives approved by the Food and Drug Administration (FDA) for inclusion in foods.

Agar Vegetable gum used as a stabilizer or thickener in many foods.

Alginate Seaweed product used as a thickener in salad dressings.

Ammonium chloride Chemical used to help yeast grow in bread products.

Annatto Product used to color yogurt, margarine, and smoked fish.

Anti-caking agent Additive used to absorb moisture and prevent caking or lumping in powdered products.

Antioxidant Protects food from breakdown on exposure to air.

Baking powder Mixture of baking soda, starch, and an acidifying agent, used to help baked goods rise.

Calcium chloride Chemical that helps bread rise. It is also used to keep fruits and vegetables firm during cooking.

Calcium propionate Used to prevent mold from growing in cheese and baked goods. It occurs naturally in Swiss cheese.

Calcium sulfate Used to boost calcium content in bread and keep tomato products and canned vegetables firm.

Caramel color Coloring agent made from toasted sugar.

Carob (locust bean) gum Thickener used to improve texture and to blend ingredients together.

Carrageenan (Irish moss) Seaweed product used in ice cream to stabilize the size of ice crystals and to keep cocoa from settling in milk.

Cellulose gum Plant additive used to improve texture and retain moisture in candy, pastry fillings, and jellies.

Citric acid Chemical derived from citrus fruits and used to maintain food color, increase tartness, and prevent foods from becoming rancid.

Dextrin A starch, commonly used as a thickener in gravies, sauces, and baking mixes.

Emulsifiers Substances that help prevent the separation of ingredients that would not normally mix, such as oil and water. Used in salad dressings and mayonnaise where they prevent oil separating from vinegar.

Guar gum Plant substance used as a thickening agent in sauces, milk products, and baking mixes.

Humectants Help maintain moisture in foods by absorbing water from the air. They may be listed as glycerol, propylene glycol, and sorbitol.

Hydrolyzed vegetable protein Derived from soybeans, wheat, or corn and used as a flavor enhancer.

Leavening agents Products such as yeast and baking powder that cause baked goods to increase in volume during cooking.

Lecithin Typically derived from eggs and soybeans and used to keep foods from separating. Also prevents loss of flavor and food becoming rancid.

Modified food starch Substance made from grains, potatoes, or tapioca that keeps ingredients from separating and prevents lumps in powdered foods.

MSG Monosodium glutamate (MSG) is used as a flavor enhancer in a variety of foods prepared at home, in restaurants, and by food manufacturers.

Pectin Fruit-derived additive used in jellies, jams, and soft candies as a thickener, to prevent separation of ingredients and give a gel-like texture.

Phosphoric acid Used to make food acidic and to give texture to soft drinks.

Polysorbates Blending agents used to keep oil and water from separating.

Potassium sorbate Used in cheese, margarine, and wine to prevent microbes from causing food spoilage.

Sequestrants Chemicals that prevent discoloration or rancidity in food.

Silicon dioxide Used to keep salt from clumping or foaming.

Sodium aluminum phosphate Used in cheese processing to aid congealing. Also used to keep processed fruits and vegetables firm.

Sodium benzoate Prevents microbes spoiling processed foods.

Sodium erythorbate Maintains flavor and color in cured meats.

Sodium hexametaphosphate Used to retain moisture, preserve beef and pork products, and prevent cheese and ice cream from becoming rancid.

Sodium stearoyl-2-lactylate Helps bread dough bake evenly and prevents spoilage. Prevents separation of oil and water in salad dressings and nondairy creamers.

Sulfur Used to prevent discoloration in dried fruits and inhibit bacterial growth in wine.

Tartrazine A coal-tar derivative used to color foods, especially dairy products.

Xanthan gum Used as a thickener, emulsifier, and stabilizer in dairy products, desserts, and dressings.

Sugar and no-calorie sweeteners

In addition to adding sweetness, sugar's distinctive properties enable it to play an important role in food preservation. For example, sugar (otherwise known as sucrose) absorbs and retains water very easily and is therefore included in breads and muffins to help keep them moist and tender. Sugar also helps prevent the growth of bacteria in jams and preserves, and retain the bright colors of canned fruits, when they are packed in a sugar solution. Sugar, however, is also a source of "empty calories" (see p.129) and, as such, contributes to a number of health risks, including overweight and tooth decay.

A diet rich in sugar can also blunt your appetite for more nutritious foods, such as those containing complex carbohydrates, vitamins, and minerals. Therefore, try to limit your intake of sugary foods.

SWEETENERS

A variety of sweeteners—no-calorie sweeteners and sugar alcohols (polyols)—are used by food manufacturers in their products. These are many times sweeter than sugar and much less is needed, with a corresponding decrease in the calorie content. The following are among the most commonly used sweeteners.

Acesulfame-K Commonly known as Ace-K, this is 200 times sweeter than table sugar, yet contains only four calories per teaspoon. It is safe and, since it is not absorbed by the body, is ideal for people who have diabetes.

Aspartame This synthetic sugar is 200 times sweeter than sugar, yet contains less than four calories per teaspoon. It is not suitable for baking or cooking.

Studies done by the Food and Drug Adminstration conclude that aspartame is safe and especially useful for those with diabetes. However, aspartame is potentially life-threatening for people who have the inherited condition phenylketonuria (PKU), in which the body cannot process the amino acid phenylalanine. Products containing aspartame are marked with a warning.

Saccharin This was the first substitute sweetener and remains one of the most popular. It is 300 times sweeter than sugar and is suitable for baking and cooking. Studies confirm that it is safe and poses no danger to humans.

Sucralose This is 600 times sweeter than regular sugar, and is the most versatile sweetener. It is available in granular form that, cup for cup, can replace sugar in drinks and recipes.

Sorbitol Used as a sweetener and to protect against moisture loss in food products, sorbitol is 60 percent as sweet as sugar, with one-third fewer calories. It provides a cool, pleasant taste and withstands high temperatures.

Manitol This sweetener is also used in food products as a stabilizer, bulking agent, and humectant. It is more than 70 percent as sweet as sugar and, like sorbitol, has a cool, sweet taste.

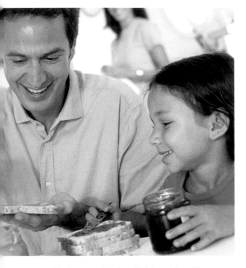

Limit sugar intake Children often like sweet things, but it is important to offer them reduced-sugar foods, such as low-sugar jelly.

Claims about fat

Increasing public awareness of the links between certain components of food, such as fat and sodium, and health have led manufacturers to market products with those concerns in mind. However, it is not always obvious what is meant by the various claims that are made.

The most confusing area of food labeling is with products that claim to be low- or reduced-fat. For example, a vegetable oil labeled "94 percent saturated-fat-free" may be mistakenly perceived as 94 percent fat-free and therefore much lower in calories than it actually is. If you take a second look at the nutritional information on the back of the bottle, you will see that 100 percent of the calories come from fat.

Understanding nutritional claims about fat content

The Food and Drug Administration has produced standard definitions for nutritional claims on food labels. Many of these relate to fat content per serving size, which is given on the food label. However, claims are also made about sodium, potassium, fiber, and calorie content. Here, we list the definitions relating to fat content:

Fat-free The product must contain less than 0.5g of fat per serving.

Low fat The product must contain less than 3g of fat per serving, or at least 50 percent less fat than a comparable product.

Low saturated fat The product must contain less than 1g of saturated fat per serving.

Lite The product must contain at least one-third fewer calories than a comparable product and must contain less than 50 percent of calories from fat.

Reduced fat The product must contain at least 25 percent less fat than a comparable product.

Low cholesterol Each serving must contain less than 20mg of cholesterol and 2g of total fat.

Smart shopping

Healthy eating starts with the choices you make when shopping.

With so many choices available, it is easier than ever to eat well. This section will help you develop some strategies to cope with the temptations that assail you each time you walk through the door of the supermarket, and to maintain control over what you buy. We give you strategies for supermarket shopping, tips for what to choose from each food group, and advice on buying healthier choices.

Maintaining control
One of the best ways of ensuring that your kitchen is stocked only with healthy foods and that you are always in a position to prepare a nutritious meal or snack for yourself and your family is to plan all the week's menus in advance. Compile your shopping list on this basis. Then, when you get to the supermarket, you will be less likely to be tempted by clever marketing promotions to buy items that were not on your list and you did not intend to purchase.

Making healthy choices
Shopping involves making choices —not just about which foods to buy, but between different brands and varieties. Health and nutrition should be the guiding factor in making choices—look at the list of ingredients, read the nutrition facts panel, consider what you know about nutrition and health, and choose appropriately. In this section, we help you do this.

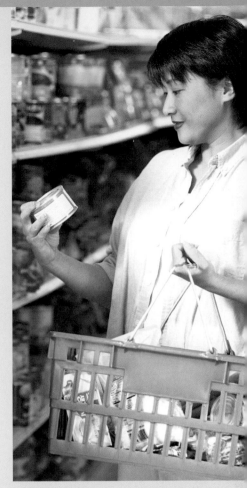

Check your choices Before putting anything in your basket, check that it has not passed its sell-by date, that packaging is intact, and you are happy with its nutritional contents.

Shopping on a budget
If you shop on a limited budget, it does not have to mean forfeiting nutritional quality, but it may mean adjusting your shopping habits.
- Compare prices and sizes to make the best-value purchases.
- Don't buy ready-made meals and prepared vegetables: it is healthier and cheaper to do it yourself.
- Remember you do not need meat every day: there are cheaper sources of protein (see pp.84–85).
- Keep money-off coupons and use them when you go shopping.
- Take advantage of special offers.
- Choose fruits and vegetables in-season, when they cost much less than they do out of season.

Supermarket strategies

There are always tantalizing sights and smells and unmissable offers to distract you in supermarkets. Here are some strategies to help you achieve your goal.

Plan your shopping Advance meal-planning is an effective way to manage your eating habits. Before you go out shopping, make a list and stick to it.

Eat before you go Shop after a meal, when you are less likely to find yourself buying cookies and pastries.

Start at the produce aisle These are the most nutritious foods you can buy, supplying a variety of valuable nutrients, so load up on fruits and vegetables when you first enter the store.

Shop the perimeter Most supermarkets display fruits, vegetables, bread, dairy products, meat, poultry, and fish around their perimeter. Since you want to buy mainly from those groups, shop the perimeter first and then go down only those aisles that contain other items that are on your shopping list.

Avoid impulse buys Supermarkets are designed to take advantage of impulse buyers. To avoid these distractions, stick to your menu-based shopping list.

Read food labels When comparing products, take time to read food labels, since this will help you make informed decisions. Make sure you pay special attention to total- and saturated-fat content, fat calories in relation to total calories, and serving sizes.

Use a delivery service Shopping on the Internet offers a great way of avoiding supermarket temptations, and such services are now widely available at low delivery charges. If your self-control is weak, this is an ideal way of avoiding impulse buys and unhealthy purchases.

Making choices from the food groups

When shopping for groceries, aim for a wide variety of foods in your cart, choosing products from all the major foods groups (*see pp. 70–71*).

Grains, cereals, and bread You should choose whole-grain varieties, which are naturally low in fat and high in B vitamins, minerals, and dietary fiber.
● Some refined foods, such as pasta, are enriched with calcium, iron, and B vitamins, making them healthy choices. Pasta is available in hundreds of forms. Although traditionally made from refined grain, whole-grain versions that boost fiber intake are your best choices.
● Brown rice is best nutritionally, since it has not had its bran coating removed.

Vegetables Buy firm, brightly colored, blemish-free vegetables. Discard any damaged specimens, since bruises and nicks attract mold, which can lead to spoilage of an entire bagful.
● Leaves or greens should be crisp and free of wilting.
● Buy only what you can use within a few days, since long storage times diminish nutrient levels and taste.
● Some frozen vegetables such as corn, green peas, and lima beans, which are processed quickly after picking, offer more nutrients than fresh varieties that have been on the store shelves too long. Canned vegetables are a useful standby: select those without added salt.

Healthy treats

Totally avoiding junk foods can be counter-productive, leading to over-indulgence when the perceived deprivation becomes too great to bear. Instead, include a few "treats" in your weekly shopping, so you do not feel deprived. For example:
● Sherbet or sorbet
● Angel food cake
● Gingersnaps
● Popsicles with 100 percent juice
● Vanilla wafers
● Fig bars
● Baked tortilla chips
● Low-fat popcorn
● Pretzels
● Nuts (unsalted or dry roasted)

Fruit For the best flavor and price, buy fruits in season. Some fruits, such as bananas and pears, should be bought before they are completely ripe, so that they do not spoil quickly.
● Choose fruits with a good color and smooth skin, and avoid any that have blemishes or insect holes.
● Bear in mind that dried fruits are a concentrated source of dietary fiber, but higher in calories than fresh fruit.

Dairy Wherever possible, choose low- or fat-free dairy products. Note that the labeling on milk has recently changed:
● 2 percent milk is now labeled reduced-fat.
● 1 percent milk is labeled low-fat.
● Skim milk is labeled fat-free or skim.
● Cheese is milk in concentrated form, so it has far more fat than milk, and the fat is highly saturated. Avoid full-fat cheese. Choose cheeses such as low-fat ricotta, part-skim mozzarella, or the many varieties of reduced-fat and fat-free cheese on the market today.

Eggs Available in many different sizes and types. Check expiration dates and always open the container to check for broken or cracked eggs.

Poultry Select poultry that looks moist and supple: the younger the bird, the more tender. Avoid poultry with signs of drying, discoloration, blemishes, or bruising. Check the packaging is intact.
● The leanest choice is white meat from the breast of chicken or turkey.
● Although skinless dark meat is also lean, it has almost twice the fat calories of white meat.
● When buying ground chicken or turkey, choose ground breast meat, rather than a mixture of dark and white.

Fish and shellfish You should always purchase the freshest fish possible: scales, skin, or shell should be moist, bright, and lustrous, with a clean smell and free of dry spots and discoloration. Eyes should be bright, clear, and bulging, and the skin should be firm and bounce back when pressed.
● If you are buying fillets or steaks, they should not have brown edges.
● Frozen fish should be completely frozen rather than partially defrosted, be odorless, and show no discoloration.

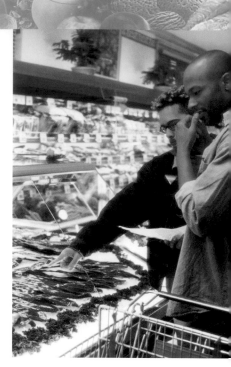

Fresh fish For the best flavor and nutritional value, buy the freshest fish possible, and cook it on the day you buy. Look for fish with a fresh odor, firm flesh, and bright eyes.

Meat Choose lean cuts (from the round or loin), and avoid meat that is heavily marbed with fat.
● Look for moistness and bright color— a pink color shows freshness, although vacuum-packed meats may look purplish due to lack of exposure to air.
● Check labels on ground meat for fat content, bearing in mind that "fat-free percentages" do not tell the whole story about fat content. Look for extra-lean.
● When choosing deli meats, turkey breast (homestyle varieties), lean ham (low salt), and roast beef are best. Some mixed deli meats (such as turkey salami and turkey pastrami) are marketed as healthy, but most are high in fat unless labeled fat-free or low-fat.

Legumes Look for legumes of a bright color and uniform size, clear of defects such as cracked seed coats, foreign matter, or pinholes made by insects. Buying in bulk is the cheapest option, but to ensure freshness buy from a source with a rapid turnover of produce. For convenience, you can use canned or frozen legumes. It is important to rinse them to reduce the salt.

Buying healthier alternatives

Shopping is often a routine activity, when purchases are made by habit rather than by considered choice. If you are serious about improving your health and well-being, then you must also change your approach to buying food. You are what you eat—and what you eat is what you buy—so your choices in the supermarket are vitally important for you and your family. To help you make better choices and save thousands of calories, check out the list below.

FOOD GROUP	HIGH-CALORIE CHOICE	LOWER-CALORIE CHOICE
Grains, cereals, and bread	• Sweetened breakfast cereal • White bread • Chocolate or fruit muffin • Croissant • Stromboli or cheese bread • Chocolate or carrot cake • Chocolate-chip or nut cookies	• Bran cereal, oatmeal, or grits • Whole-wheat bread • English muffin • Bagel or baguette • Ciabatta or tomato pie • Angel food cake with berries • Fig bars or graham crackers
Dairy	• Reduced-fat (2%) or whole milk • Half-and-half • Whole-milk yogurt • Full-fat cheese • Sour cream • Butter • Mayonnaise • Cheese sauce • Creamy salad dressing	• Low-fat (1%) or fat-free milk • Low-fat (1%) or fat-free milk • Low-fat, low-sugar, or sugar-free yogurt • Low-fat cheese and cottage cheese • Fat-free sour cream or low-fat plain yogurt • Low-fat margarine, apple butter, or olive or canola oil • Low-fat mayonnaise or mustard • Salsa • Vinegar, olive oil, and lemon dressing
Meat, poultry, and fish	• Beef on the bone • Pork spareribs • Bacon • Dark chicken or turkey meat • Breaded chicken fillet or nuggets • Breaded fish fillet	• Lean beef off the bone • Pork tenderloin • Canadian bacon, lean ham, or turkey bacon • White-meat chicken or turkey • White-meat chicken • Fish steak and filets and shellfish
Delicatessen	• Bologna, salami, or liverwurst • Corned beef or pastrami • Full-fat cheese (American, Muenster, Brie, or Swiss) • Potato salad or coleslaw	• Home-style turkey or low-salt ham • Lean roast beef or turkey breast • Fat-free or part-skim cheese, Swiss Lorraine, Farmer's cheese, low-fat and fat-free Feta cheese • Roasted peppers or carrot and raisin salad
Frozen	• Pizza topped with salami or meat • Breakfast biscuits • Vegetables with butter or cheese sauce • Meat or sausage patty • Breaded chicken fillet or nuggets • Whole-milk ice cream • Regular TV dinner	• Pizza topped with vegetables • Bagels or waffles • Frozen vegetables with no sauce added • Vegetable burger • White-meat chicken cutlet • Low-fat ice cream, frozen yogurt, or sorbet • Low-fat TV dinner
Canned food	• Tuna in oil or brine • Fruit packed in heavy syrup • Beans or refried beans • Regular chicken broth • Cream soup (New England clam)	• Tuna in water • Fruit packed in own juice • Baked beans or fat-free refried beans in tomato sauce • Fat-free and low-sodium chicken broth • Broth-based soup (Manhattan clam)
Snacks	• Fried potato chips or tortilla chips • Microwave popcorn with butter	• Baked potato chips or tortilla chips • Fat-free air-popped popcorn

How to store food

Food storage is easy and convenient with modern appliances.

Having bought the freshest and healthiest food, you must handle it carefully and store it correctly when you get it home in order to maintain the quality and taste.

Refrigerators and freezers

Indispensable for storing fresh food, refrigerators are the modern-day equivalent of the pantry. Invest in the most capacious model that you can fit in your home, since over-crowding the appliance will reduce its efficiency and may also shorten its life.

Freezing is a convenient way of storing food that also avoids loss of nutrients or taste. Some foods can be kept in the freezer for up to a year. Provided the freezer is kept at -20ºF (-23ºC), food will keep for

more longer but it is inefficient use of a freezer. For information about your appliance, refer to the manufacturer's handbook.

To help you keep a check on freezer contents, always label containers with the date of freezing as well as a brief description of their contents.

Keep them in the dark

Grains can be stored for up to a year in a cool, dark cupboard, as can canned vegetables, fruits, fish, and soups, and bottles of sauce, vinegar, and oil. Be sure to check the contents of your cabinet on a regular basis and discard any out-of-date products. Potatoes should also be kept in the dark, to prevent them from sprouting.

Well-stocked cabinet Keep pasta, grains, and legumes in a cool, dark cabinet. Once opened transfer into jars with close-fitting lids.

Refrigerator storage tips

To ensure that your food does not become contaminated while it is stored in the refrigerator, bear these points in mind. (Note that the coldest part of the refrigerator is against the back wall.)
- Allow warm food or beverages to cool down before placing them in the refrigerator.
- Wrap or cover food to be stored.
- Place wrapped uncooked meat, poultry, fish, and shellfish on a tray on the bottom shelf.
- Place dairy products, pastries, and ready-cooked meals on the upper shelves.
- Keep all fruits and vegetables (except potatoes) in the bin at the bottom of the refrigerator.
- Store bottles and cartons upright in the door compartments.
- Once a month, you should unplug your appliance and clean the inside with tepid water that has a mild antibacteria liquid soap added. Finally, rinse thoroughly.

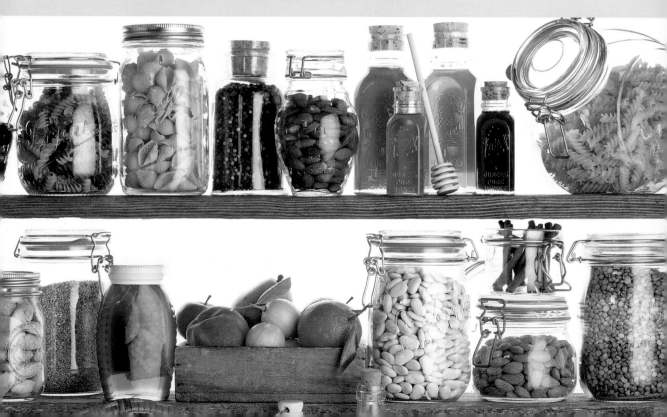

How to store the food you buy

Having chosen your purchases carefully, and brought them home safely, it is important to store foods correctly, so that they remain fresh and maintain their flavor and nutritional value. Different types of foods have to be stored in different ways—some require refrigeration, while others keep best in a cool, dark pantry. Yet others can be frozen and defrosted as required (see p.287). Keep an eye on expiration dates and make sure that you discard out-of-date foods.

FOOD TYPE	STORAGE HINTS
Grains and cereals	Store whole grains and cereals at room temperature in a dark cabinet. After opening, tightly reseal the original packaging or transfer the contents to containers with tightly fitting lids. Whole grains should be used within a year of purchase; alternatively, freeze for up to a year.
Pasta and noodles	Dried pasta and noodles are stored in the same way as grains. Keep fresh varieties in the refrigerator and use within two days, or freeze for up to two months.
Bread	Keep bread in the pantry, in a sealed bag or container, for two to four days, in the refrigerator for seven to 14 days, or in the freezer for six months.
Vegetables	Before storing vegetables, check and discard any that are damaged or blemished. Keep potatoes and other root vegetables in a cool, dark place, and store all other vegetables and salad leaves in the refrigerator. Store frozen vegetables in the freezer for 12 months.
Fruit	Discard any damaged or blemished fruits to prevent further spoilage. Make sure that all produce is dry, and do not wash before storing. Canned fruits, once opened and transferred to a glass or plastic container, can be stored in the refrigerator for one week. Many fruits are also suitable for freezing (see p.287). Keep unopened packages of dried fruit in the refrigerator or pantry for six months; once opened, keep in the refrigerator for one month.
Dairy	Refrigerate dairy products immediately after purchase, except those that have been irradiated, such as long-life milk in cartons. Store fresh milk in the refrigerator for five days. Hard cheeses, once opened, can be kept in the refrigerator for three to four weeks. Keep all cheese tightly packaged in moisture-proof wrap. Soft cheeses can be refrigerated for one to two weeks; shredded Parmesan will keep for at least one month in the refrigerator or three months in the freezer.
Fish and shellfish	Store in the coldest part of the refrigerator, wrapped in a plastic bag or moisture-proof paper, and use within two days of purchase. Alternatively, wrap tightly in air- and moisture-proof wrapping and store in the freezer for up to six months. Cook shellfish as soon as possible after purchase; once cooked it can be stored in the refrigerator for three to four days, or in the freezer for up to three months.
Poultry	Use fresh poultry within two days of purchase. Store, loosely wrapped, in the coldest part of the refrigerator. Alternatively wrap in an airtight freezer bags and store in the freezer for up to eight months. Never leave poultry at room temperature, since this encourages the growth of bacteria.
Meat	Keep meat, in its original packaging, in the coldest part of the refrigerator. Use whole cuts within three to four days, and ground meat within two days of purchase. Before freezing meat, wrap in an airtight freezer bag in addition to its original packaging and label with date of purchase.
Eggs	Store fresh eggs, in their carton (large end up), in the refrigerator for up to one month. Do not store eggs near strong-smelling foods, since they easily absorb unwanted flavors. Freeze egg whites for up to six months. Egg yolks can be frozen only if mixed first with $\frac{1}{8}$ tsp salt or $1\frac{1}{2}$ tsp sugar or corn syrup per four yolks. Defrost frozen egg yolks and whites overnight in the refrigerator before use.
Legumes	Store peas, beans, and lentils for up to one year in tightly covered containers, in a dry, cool place. Do not mix legumes bought at different times, since older ones are drier and will take longer to cook. Sort legumes before use and discard stones, fibers, and misshapen or discolored beans.

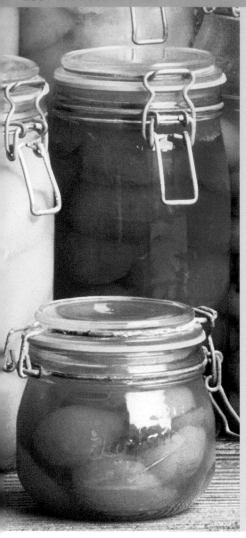

Preserving food at home

Freezing and home preserving enables you to store fresh foods for extended use.

Whether you grow your own fruits and vegetables, or wish to take advantage of buying in bulk, home-preserving is an effective way of storing food for later use. Freezing can also be a great time saver if you prepare batches of food and store until required—or even freeze whole meals for times when you are too busy to cook.

Traditional and modern
In the past, before home freezers became widely available, various preservation techniques were

Home preserves There is something deeply satisfying about stocking your pantry with jars of homemade jams, jellies, and relishes, and home-preserved fruits and vegetables.

employed. These methods included drying, salting, smoking, pickling, and canning. While the use of such methods has become less common, due to the year-round availability of supermarket foods, they provide a satisfying and healthy way of preserving home-grown produce.

Traditionally freezing involved packing food in ice, but modern freezers have streamlined the process with carefully regulated temperatures. How long you can keep food in your home freezer depends on the food; some foods can be kept for up to a year, others only a few weeks (*see opposite*).

Maintaining quality control
Whichever method you choose, home preserving allows you to provide a constant supply of healthy food, rather than relying on convenience meals, which are likely to contain more salt, sugar, and other additives than their homemade equivalents.

Canning your own produce

If you have a garden and grow your own fruits and vegetables, you may find yourself at certain times of the year with more produce than you can possibly eat. Canning is a traditional technique for preserving seasonal produce so that you can continue to enjoy it at any time during the year in the form of appetizing preserves and pickles.

PRESERVING FRUITS
Unlike store-bought varieties, home preserves are free of additives and you can be certain that they contain only the best of ingredients. For the best results, try these tips.
• Use only freshly picked, barely ripe fruits, which are highest in the setting agent pectin.
• Prepare fruit by washing and removing the peel, pith, any damaged flesh, stems, and pits or seeds.
• To avoid contamination, sterilize containers before filling by boiling or using a sterilizing unit.

• Seal containers tightly to make sure germs do not get in; if you use jars with self-sealing lids, use new rubber seals each time to ensure a close fit.

PICKLING VEGETABLES
Choose firm young vegetables. For specific information, follow your favorite recipe. The following tips for pickling will help you.
• Cauliflower florets, shredded cabbage, cucumbers, beets, and gherkins are ideal for pickling.
• Wash and drain selected vegetables and prepare for pickling by dry-salting or packing in brine: this draws moisture from the vegetables, making them more receptive to the pickling vinegar. Remove the vegetables from the brine, rinse well, and then pack in the sterilized jars.
• Add whole spices such as allspice, black peppercorns, cloves, mustard seeds, and coriander seeds.
• Fill the jars with vinegar and seal tightly.

Tips for freezing

The easiest, most effective technique for preserving the flavor, color, moisture content, and nutritive value of food is freezing. For the best results, wrap the food first in specialist freezer paper and then in a sealable plastic bag or container. This helps prevent freezer burn, which occurs when frost forms on the outside of the food and can alter the taste and quality.
- Cool all foods and liquids completely before placing in the freezer container or bag. Depositing warm foods in the freezer raises the temperature and may defrost neighboring foods.
- Pack food in quantities that will be used for a single serving, so you need defrost only the amount that you require.
- When placing food to be frozen in plastic bags, exclude all air before sealing tightly with a wire tie.

- Ensure that lids on rigid freezer containers are properly sealed to prevent spillages.
- Before freezing, label each package with the name of the product, any added ingredients, and the packaging date.
- Avoid overloading your freezer with unfrozen food, which slows the freezing rate: some freezers offer a "super-freeze" mode that ensures rapid freezing.
- While food is freezing, leave space between the packages so that air can circulate; once it is is frozen, you can store the packages close together.
- To save space in the freezer, freeze liquids in shallow, rectangular trays; transfer the frozen slabs to plastic bags that can then be stacked up.

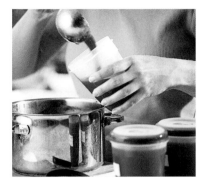

Batch freezing Make batches of soup, stew, or baby's meals when you have time, and freeze in individual-size portions for later use.

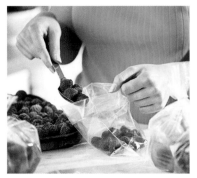

Seasonal fruits Most fruits freeze well. Soft fruits, such as raspberries, should be tray-frozen then transferred to bags or containers.

Defrosting frozen food

Apart from vegetables, most of which can be cooked from frozen by placing straight into boiling water, frozen foods should be defrosted before cooking. This may be done in the refrigerator, at room temperature, or in a microwave oven. Which method you use depends mainly on how soon you wish to cook the food. Room-temperature defrosting times are given below; defrosting in a refrigerator takes longer.

Which foods can be frozen?

Most foods, including bread, pizza crusts, fruits, vegetables, meat, poultry, fish, and ready-prepared soups and stews, are suitable for freezing.

In general, any vegetable that is eaten steamed or boiled can be frozen, while those that are eaten raw, for example scallions, lettuce, and radishes, are not suitable. In order to retain the aroma and vitamin content of vegetables, it is advisable to blanch them first, before freezing. This involves immersing the prepared vegetables in boiling water for a few minutes.

Eggs cannot be frozen in their shells, but the yolk and white can be frozen separately or stirred together and frozen in plastic containers or ice-cube trays.

FOOD	FREEZER STORAGE	DEFROSTING
Bread	6 months	2–3 hours
Pizza	2–3 months	2–4 hours
Broccoli	9–12 months	Cook from frozen
Carrots	12 months	Cook from frozen
Corn-on-the-cob	12 months	3–4 hours
Plums	10–12 months	5–10 hours
Raspberries	10–12 months	3–7 hours
Beef	6–12 months	10–12 hours
Chicken (2–3lb/0.9–1.35kg)	8 months	10–12 hours
Fish fillets	2–3 months	6–8 hours
Part-skim ricotta cheese	1 month	3–4 hours
Soup	3–6 months	Reheat from frozen

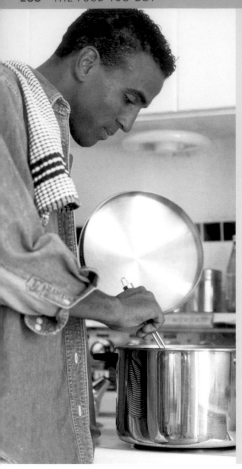

Food preparation and cooking

Make the most of nutritious ingredients by adopting healthy cooking methods.

Cooking food in a healthy way does not take extra time, effort, or special cookware. A few simple adjustments to your usual cooking methods may be all you need to improve the nutritional quality of the food you cook, without losing flavor or appeal. In many cases, the food will taste even better.

Reducing the amount of saturated fat in your diet is one of the most important changes that you can

make to benefit your health (*see pp.42–43*). This means choosing ingredients carefully, removing all visible fat, adding as little extra fat as possible while cooking, and discarding any excess. The cooking techniques listed opposite are all healthy and retain the nutritional content of food as well as enhance natural flavors and textures.

Reducing added salt is another dietary change that will benefit your health, especially if you have a tendency for high blood pressure (*see p.221*). This requires a gradual reduction in the amount of salt you add to your food and becoming accustomed, instead, to healthier flavorings, such as seasonings, herbs, and spices.

On the following pages, we give you a few ideas to help you find healthier ways of preparing and cooking food at home.

Home-cooking Preparing meals at home allows you to choose the best ingredients and to use the healthiest cooking methods.

Experiment with seasoning

Healthy food need not taste bland or uninteresting; it does, however, require an adjustment in your sense of taste if you are used to seasoning everything you eat with salt and enjoy the flavor that fat gives to meat, poultry, breads, and pastries. You can try using different herbs and spices, or marinating foods in juices before cooking.

HEALTHY SEASONING
By experimenting with different ways of flavoring food you will soon begin to appreciate the lighter, fresher flavors of herbs and other natural seasonings.
• For the best flavor, dry roast and grind your own spices.
• Lemon or lime juice squeezed over food during and after cooking imparts a fresh, tangy taste; grated lemon zest can also be added during cooking.
• A dash of balsamic, wine, herb, or

fruit vinegar added toward the end of cooking time adds a zesty flavor.
• Sprinkle some toasted nuts or seeds over a dish for a crunchy topping.
• Garnish a dish with roasted bell peppers for a sweet, smoky taste.

BENEFITS OF MARINATING
In addition to flavoring poultry, meat, fish, and vegetables, marinating tenderizes meat, reducing the need to add fat during cooking. Studies have shown that marinating foods prior to cooking reduces the harmful hydrocarbons that are produced during grilling. Marinades containing herbs such as sage, oregano, or marjoram also provide antioxidants that may help protect against cancer.

Use any combination of citrus juice and fresh herbs; pour the marinade over the raw ingredients, cover and refrigerate for a few hours before cooking.

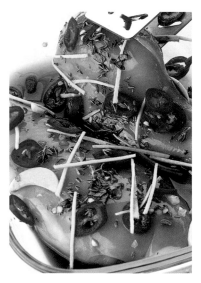

Adding flavor Marinades help tenderize meat, poultry, and fish as well as adding healthy flavoring. Here chilis, garlic, and ginger add a Chinese flavor to chicken.

Healthy cooking methods

All cooking destroys nutrients to some extent, but some methods are better than others in both this respect and in minimizing other unhealthy factors, such as fat and salt content.
- Nonstick cookware is a healthy investment, since it reduces the need for added fat during cooking.
- A light spray of vegetable oil should be enough to avoid food sticking to the pan.
- Sauté vegetables and meat in wine, water, or broth instead of using butter.
- Remove fat from soups, stews, sauces, and gravies by chilling after cooking and skimming fat off the surface.
- Substitute healthy oils such as olive or canola for butter or dripping.

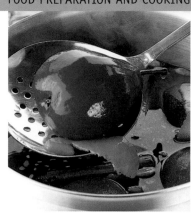

Poaching This is a healthy, low-fat method of cooking fruits, fish, eggs, or meat in a suitably flavored liquid.

METHOD	HOW IT WORKS
Braising	Also known as simmering, braising cooks food in liquid in an open or covered pan, either on top of the stove or in the oven. There is no need for any fat to be added, since the cooking liquid keeps the food moist. The juices from the food add flavor to the cooking liquid, which may be reduced by rapid boiling to provide an intensely flavorful, nutrient-rich sauce of thickened consistency.
Broiling	Ideal for cooking thin cuts of poultry, meat, and fish, broiling cooks food quickly on the outside while sealing the flavor inside. The food is cooked on a broiler rack, directly under a heat element, allowing the fat to drip into a tray and be discarded. It may be necessary to brush the food first with a little oil to prevent it from sticking to the rack and drying out.
Grilling	This quick method of cooking fish, meat, or poultry, without added fat infuses food with a smoky flavor. The food is cooked on a rack above hot coals. Marinating before grilling will enhance flavor (*opposite below*), as will burning aromatic herbs or wood below the food.
Microwaving	Microwave ovens cook food by emitting high-frequency radio waves that cause food molecules to vibrate. This creates friction that heats and cooks food very quickly. No added fat and very little liquid is required, so microwaving is a healthy cooking method that retains nutrients well. It is particularly suitable for vegetables, which retain all their color, taste, and texture.
Poaching	In this low-fat method, fruit, fish, eggs, and meat are gently simmered in water, broth, tomato or fruit juice, or wine until tender. Food can be poached in a pan on the stove-top, with enough liquid to cover, or it can be cooked in the oven.
Roasting	For healthy roasting of large cuts of meat, poultry, place the food on a rack in a roasting pan in the oven. The rack allows the fat to drain into the pan and be discarded. Use a meat thermometer to ensure that meat and poultry are thoroughly cooked (*see p.292*).
Sautéing	Also known as pan-frying and similar to stir-frying, sautéing involves cooking food quickly in a sauté pan or skillet over direct heat. Use a good quality nonstick pan to minimize the need for added oil. If necessary, use just a light spray of oil to prevent the food from sticking to the bottom of the pan. Sautéing is a healthy alternative to frying, which generally uses more fat.
Steaming	Ideal for cooking fish, poultry, and vegetables, this quick cooking method retains nutrients and does not require any added fat. Place a steamer basket with the food to be cooked over a pan of boiling water, cover, and cook over a low heat. Electric steamers are also available; these may incorporate several separate baskets so that a variety of foods can be steamed at the same time.
Stir-frying	This is a fast and healthy method of cooking, particularly if you use a nonstick wok. Cut ingredients into similarly sized small pieces and use just a small amount of oil or fat-free cooking spray to prevent them from sticking to the pan. Fry quickly over a high heat, constantly moving the food around.

Stock up on pantry basics

Keep a stock of pantry basics—cans, jars, and basic ingredients (including frozen foods)—that can be transformed into healthy meals, either alone, or with the addition of other fresh products. If you choose wisely, these basic items can form the foundation of a healthy diet: for example, if you have whole-grain pasta and brown rice—rather than regular pasta and white rice—in your cabinet, then you are already halfway to a nutritious meal.

Copy our healthy shopping list (*right*), amending it to fit your food preferences, and stick it to the refrigerator door. Have your family add to it, and bring it with you to the supermarket every week.

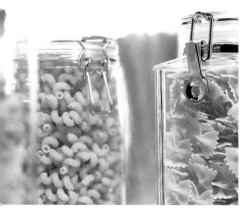

Satisfying pasta Pasta is cheap, filling, and quick to prepare. Whole-wheat pasta is an excellent source of B vitamins and folate.

Healthy shopping list

Stock up on these healthy basics, then you can prepare a nutritious meal at any time.

Cans, jars, and cartons
- Apple sauce (no added sugar)
- Beans
- Egg whites or substitutes
- Fat-free evaporated milk
- Fat-free refried beans
- Fruit in own juice
- Fruit juice (no added sugar)
- Lentils
- Low-salt chicken broth
- Low-salt crushed tomatoes
- Low-salt soy sauce
- Low-salt tomato paste
- Low-salt tomato sauce
- Low-salt vegetable juice
- Peeled whole or crushed tomatoes
- Salsa
- Sardines in olive oil
- Tuna in water
- UHT (long-life) fat-free milk

Frozen foods
- Chicken and turkey breasts
- Low-calorie dinners
- Low-fat frozen yogurt
- Low-fat waffles
- Mini whole-wheat bagels
- Pizza crusts
- Popsicles (made with fruit juice)
- Salmon steaks
- Sherbet and sorbet
- Vegetable burgers
- Vegetables (no added salt)

Grains and cereals
- Brown rice
- Buckwheat (kasha)
- Couscous
- Low-sugar granola
- Oatmeal
- Whole-grain cereal
- Whole-grain pasta

Desserts
- Gingersnaps
- Graham crackers
- Jello
- Pudding (made with low-fat milk)
- Vanilla wafers

Snacks
- Baked potato chips
- Baked tortilla chips
- Dried fruit
- Fat-free crackers
- Fig bars
- Low-fat or fat-free popcorn
- Pretzels
- Rice cakes
- Unsalted nuts (almonds, walnuts)

Oils and spreads
- Apple butter
- Canola oil
- Fat-free or low-fat margarine
- Low-sugar preserves
- Nonstick vegetable oil spray
- Olive oil

Drinks
- Bottled water and diet soda

Tips on safe microwave cooking

The speed and convenience of microwave cooking has ensured the popularity of these appliances, which can be used for defrosting, reheating, and cooking. However, it is important to be aware of the potential hazards of this form of cooking in order to avoid health risks. Microwaves do not enter the oven uniformly and cold spots can occur in food being cooked, allowing bacteria to survive and possibly leading to food poisoning.
- To minimize uneven cooking, stir the food once or twice during microwaving, arrange foods uniformly, and turn large items upside down halfway through cooking.
- Remove plastic wraps and foam trays from store-bought food before defrosting, since these may melt and allow chemicals to be absorbed by the food.
- Frozen meat and poultry may begin to cook during microwave-defrosting and should be cooked immediately.
- Never use any metal or foil utensils or wraps in the microwave oven; this includes brown grocery bags, colored paper towel, and newspapers, which may contain metal.
- If microwaves are used to heat baby food, always stir well to ensure even cooking and no hot spots.
- Use a meat thermometer or probe (*see p.292*) to check that food has reached a safe temperature. Check in several places when cooking large pieces of meat.

Fast, homecooked healthy food

If you have followed our suggestions on pantry basics (*opposite*), you will be in a position to create quick, nutritious meals for yourself and your family at short notice and at any time. Here are some suggestions:

Pasta Serve with store-bought, fat-free sauce—or make your own sauce and freeze in serving-size portions until required. If there is any leftover pasta, use it in a salad, adding chopped raw vegetables and a little low-fat dressing.

Rice Brown rice forms the basis of a satisfying meal. For a spicy pilaf, add chopped cooked vegetables, shredded chicken breast, or tofu, and season with cumin, coriander, and ginger.

Pizza Top a store-bought pizza crust with chopped tomatoes, mushrooms, onions, and bell peppers, finishing with grated low-fat cheese.

Omelet An omelet takes just a few minutes to prepare and cook, but can make a satisfying light meal. Add lightly steamed vegetables to the eggs before cooking. For a low-fat cheese omelet, you can blend ricotta cheese in a food processor until smooth then mix with egg whites only (no yolks).

Broiled chicken or salmon steak Rub ground spices or herbs over a chicken breast or salmon steak then broil until cooked through; serve with steamed vegetables and steamed rice.

Stir-fry Buy a commercially prepared mixture of beansprouts, carrots, onions, and mushrooms, and stir-fry with tofu cubes, shrimp, or chicken breast for a satisfying dish. Season the meal with a little low-salt soy sauce.

Baked potato Bake a medium-sized potato in the microwave for about 12 minutes and then place it under the broiler. Serve with store-bought salsa, vegetarian chili, grated low-fat cheese, or refried beans.

Vegetable couscous This is a type of pasta that is quick and simple to prepare. While the couscous absorbs water, stir-fry cubes of tofu and some sliced vegetables and add a little vegetable broth. Top the couscous with the vegetable–tofu mixture (*below*).

Vegetarian burgers For a quick and nutritious meal, grill a vegetable burger and serve in toasted ciabatta with sliced tomato, salsa, and a green salad.

Cottage-cheese dip For a simple dip to serve with vegetable crudités, or as a quick pasta sauce or salad dressing, purée fat-free cottage cheese in a food processor, then add garlic powder and dill, basil, or Italian seasoning to taste.

Grilled vegetables Brush vegetables with a little olive oil and grill for between 3 and 5 minutes on each side. Serve with French bread, as an appetizer, as a side dish to accompany an entrée, or with rice or pasta as a satisfying meal. Vegetables that are ideal for grilling include broccoli florets, baby carrots, slices of eggplant, mushrooms, slices of onion, quartered bell peppers, asparagus tips, strips of summer squash, sweet potato rounds, and tomato wedges.

Recipe Quick vegetable couscous

INGREDIENTS
1 bouillon cube
1 cup uncooked couscous
2 zucchini
1-in (2.5-cm) cube of ginger root
6 scallions
2 bell peppers
12oz (350g) tofu
2 garlic cloves

Serves 4

1 Dissolve the bouillon cube in 12floz (360ml) boiling water.

2 Place the couscous in a medium-sized bowl. Pour over the bouillon. Leave until the couscous has absorbed all the liquid.

3 Spray a wok with a little oil and place over a medium heat. Slice the zucchini crosswise, add to the wok, and stir-fry for 5 minutes, moving it around constantly to prevent it from sticking to the pan.

4 Grate the ginger, slice the scallions, deseed and slice the bell peppers, cube the tofu, crush the garlic, and add to the wok. Stir-fry for a further 5 minutes, constantly moving the vegetables around the wok to prevent sticking.

5 Remove the vegetables and tofu from the wok and stir into the couscous, taking care not to break up the vegetables.

Variation You can replace the tofu with cubes of chicken breast, flavor with cumin and coriander, and garnish with sliced almonds.

Each serving provides
Calories 300, Total fat 6g (Sat. 0.7g, Poly. 2.1g, Mono. 0.9g), Cholesterol 0.2mg, Protein 15g, Carbohydrate 46g, Fiber 5g, Sodium 301mg. Good source of—Vits: A, Fol, C, K; Mins: Ca, Mg, P, K.

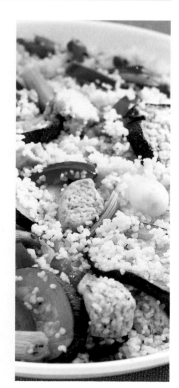

Food hygiene

Prevent food-borne illnesses by adopting safe food practices.

According to the World Health Organization, every year about 5,000 people die in the US from food poisoning. Bacteria such as *E.coli*, *Salmonella*, and *Listeria* can cause life-threatening illnesses, especially in the young, in older adults, and in pregnant women.

Food contamination may occur during the storage, handling, or cooking of food, at home and in stores and restaurants, and it is important that you bear this issue in mind whenever you are dealing with food. For example, when you are shopping, always check the condition of food packages and reject those that are damaged in any way, such as dented cans and torn plastic wrapping. Keep frozen and chilled foods cold with ice blocks on the journey home, and transfer them to your refrigerator or freezer as soon as possible.

Keeping food separate
Because cooked foods can become contaminated through contact with raw foods, make sure that you keep them separate in your shopping cart at the supermarket, pack them separately, and keep them apart in the refrigerator. You should always use separate cutting boards for preparing raw and cooked foods, and wash utensils and surfaces thoroughly after use.

Cook thoroughly
Most food-borne illnesses occur after eating raw or inadequately cooked meat, poultry, or fish, since animals sometimes carry bacteria that are killed only by thorough cooking. Until recently, the advice was to cook meat and poultry for a specified time per weight until their juices run clear. Now, the US Department of Agriculture advises that the only way to ensure that any bacteria is destroyed, is to use a meat thermometer. Safe cooked temperatures vary for different kinds of meat (*see below*).

Safe refrigeration
Refrigerated foods should be kept at temperatures below 40°F (4°C). Check the temperature in

Using a food thermometer

The US Department of Agriculture recommends checking the temperature of meat with a thermometer to ensure that it is cooked to a high enough temperature to destroy bacteria. There are two types of food thermometers: one is inserted into the meat at the start of cooking and left in throughout; the other gives an instant reading and is inserted toward the end of cooking. The dials on meat thermometers often indicate the temperatures at which different meats should be done. Always insert a thermometer near the center of the meat, avoiding bone. There are also thermometers for microwave cooking.

FOOD	TEMPERATURE
Ground beef, pork, veal, and lamb	● 160°F (71°C)
Whole cuts of beef, veal, and lamb	● Medium-rare 145°F (63°C) ● Medium 160°F (71°C) ● Well-done 170°F (77°C)
Poultry	● Whole birds 180°F (82°C) ● Breasts, legs, thighs, and wings 170°F (77°C) ● Ground 165°F (74°C)
Pork	● Medium 160°F (71°C) ● Well-done 170°F (77°C)
Ham	● Fresh 160°F (71°C) ● Precooked 140°F (60°C)
Fish	● 145°F (63°C)
Egg dishes	● 160°F (71°C)
Casseroles, stews, combination dishes, leftovers, and stuffings	● 165°F (74°C)

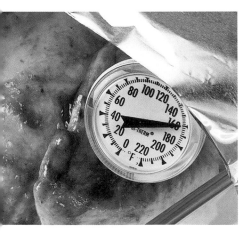

Is it done? The best way to check whether meat and poultry have been cooked long enough to destroy bacteria is to use a food thermometer. Some, like the one shown, are left in the food throughout cooking; others are inserted toward the end.

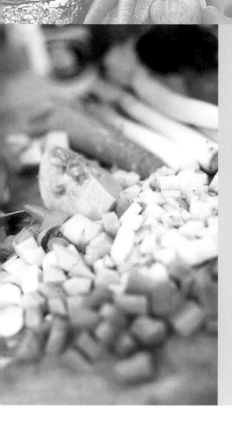

your refrigerator regularly, and always adjust the temperature as you fill and empty the appliance. You can keep a refrigerator thermometer in the appliance.

Keep food hygiene in mind

Plastic cutting boards should be washed daily in the dishwasher, and replaced regularly. Wooden boards and kitchen sponges can be microwaved to kill bacteria. Wash dishes or utensils in very hot water. Disinfect work surfaces daily.

By taking sensible precautions, you will protect yourself and your family from the health dangers posed by food-borne illnesses.

Cutting-board hygiene To prevent cross-contamination, use separate boards for raw and cooked food. Keep them scrupulously clean and replace them regularly.

Kitchen hygiene

Scrupulous cleanliness is essential in the handling of food to prevent the risk of food-borne illnesses.
• Wash your hands every time you handle, prepare, or cook food. Use warm, soapy water and wash your hands, front and back, up to the wrists, between your fingers, and under fingernails and rings.
• Dry your hands thoroughly using disposable paper towels or hand-dryers. Do not use fabric towels, which can harbor bacteria.
• Wash your hands after using the telephone or bathroom, sneezing or blowing your nose, touching your pet, or changing diapers.
• Keep your fingernails clean and trimmed, and cover any cuts or abrasions on your hands with a waterproof dressing.

Keeping food safe at picnics

Ensuring that cold food remains cold and hot food stays hot are major safety concerns when planning a picnic. This will affect not just the food you choose to take, but also how you pack it and store it before you sit down to eat.

Hot food that has been allowed to cool in a picnic basket provides an ideal environment for bacteria to grow, so take hot food with you only if you can keep it piping hot until you are ready to eat. This means keeping it in a vacuum flask or bottle. Similarly, cold food that is allowed to become tepid also becomes potentially hazardous to consume.
• Pack salads and deli meats with ice packs in a cooler box or bag, and keep food in the cooler until required.
• Discard any uneaten food that has been left out in the hot sun.
• Keep the cooler in the passenger compartment rather than in the trunk.
• Your body needs plenty of water in the summer months, especially when it is very hot, so take a cooler box filled with bottles of water and juice boxes to keep you refreshed.

FOOD IDEAS FOR PICNICS
Here are some tips on what to take on your picnic, bearing in mind both food safety and nutritional factors.
• Pack chilled, refreshing salads, such as shredded carrot and raisin or tomato and onion drizzled with olive oil.
• Pasta, rice, and couscous salads are perfect for picnics. Try different kinds of pasta, adding canned tuna chunks, vegetables, olives, and low-fat dressing.
• Pack a selection of sliced deli meats, such as turkey, ham, or lean roast beef, and crunchy bread and rolls.
• Snack on pretzels rather than chips.
• Chilled fruit makes a refreshing snack. Pack soft fruits such as grapes, cherries, and slices of cantaloupe or honeydew melon in zip-top plastic bags.
• Take a portable, disposable grill and a selection of vegetables, including corn-on-the-cob and skewered peppers, red onions, zucchini, and eggplant.
• If you plan to grill meat or fish, store them in a cooler bag with ice packs until required, and then grill until piping hot and cooked thoroughly.

Food safety while traveling abroad

When traveling in regions where the water supply and food hygiene are less than ideal, take sensible precautions to avoid becoming ill.
• Give your body time to adjust by moderating your intake of unfamiliar foods.
• Eat in busy restaurants, where there is a rapid turnover of food.
• Make sure that food is piping hot and cooked thoroughly before you sit down to eat it.
• Drink only pasteurized or boiled milk, dairy products, and juice.
• Wash raw fruits and vegetables in bottled water if you have any doubts about the local water.
• Avoid salads (including fruit salads) in areas where they might have been washed in unsafe water.
• If the local tap water is unsafe to drink, boil it, use sterilizing tablets, or drink only bottled water; check that bottle seals are unbroken.

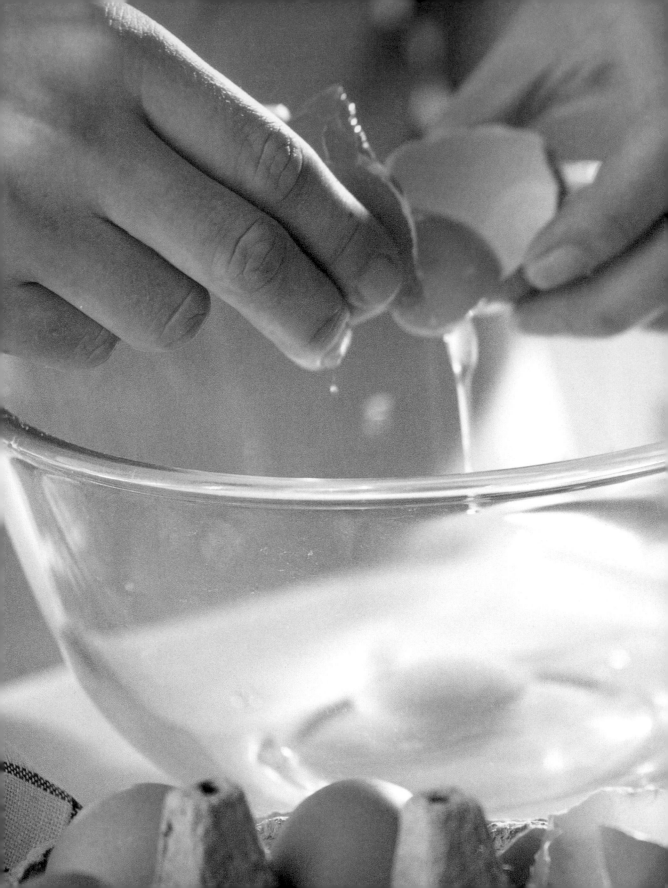

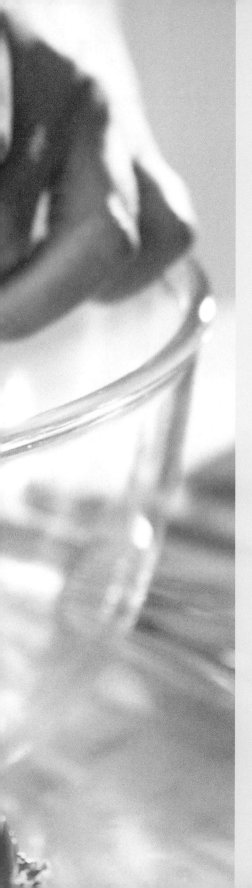

Food analysis

Knowing which nutrients the food you eat contains will help you make healthy choices and ensure that you have a balanced diet. In this chapter, we offer you a reference that provides you with the nutritional breakdown (fat, protein, carbohydrate, fiber, and vitamin and mineral content) of almost 500 different foods from the various food groups.

What is in the food you eat?

Understanding what food contains is the key to healthy eating.

A basic knowledge of what is in the food you eat and how many calories it provides is vital to ensure that you eat a balanced diet. This chapter is an important resource that you can use as a reference guide now and in the future. We have also used the information in this chapter as the basis for all the charts and menus that we have given throughout the book.

Macronutrients

Knowing which foods are high in protein or carbohydrate is the best way to get enough of these key macronutrients. Understanding

which foods to avoid because of high saturated-fat content and which to choose for unsaturated fats or fiber will help you plan a diet that optimizes health and reduces your risk of disease.

Micronutrients

In these tables, we also list many of the vitamins and minerals that are found in the foods we eat. We have included this information so you can compare different foods as good sources of specific nutrients.

Including a variety of foods that are good sources of these nutrients in your diet is the sensible way to ensure optimum health. Scientific studies have shown that the more vitamins and minerals you have in your diet, the healthier you are likely to be. While many people

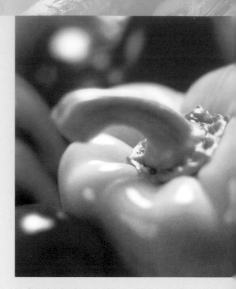

Variety is the key Eating a wide range of healthy foods—including fresh vegetables and fruits—every day is the best way to get all of the nutrients your body needs to stay healthy.

chose to take a multivitamin to ensure that they get all of the nutrients they need each day, the best way to get these nutrients is clearly from the foods you eat.

Understanding the charts

On the following pages, we detail the caloric, fats, protein, carbohydrate, and fiber content of almost 500 foods. We have also identified those foods that contain at least 20 percent of the Dietary Reference Intake (*see p.35*) for a particular vitamin or mineral and designated these as a good source. You will find some blank entries, mainly for types of fats and fiber, in the charts. These indicate that we do not at present have measurements for these nutrients.

Foods are listed in categories that, for the most part, follow the basic groups covered in the book (*see Elements of a healthy diet, pp.68–103*).

Grains and grain products We have divided these into the following categories in the food-analysis charts: Grains; Cereals, breakfast; Pasta and noodles; and Breads.

Vegetables Unless stated, vegetables are raw.

Fruits Unless stated, fruits are raw.

Dairy products Eggs have been included with dairy.

Protein sources These have been subdivided into Meat and poultry; Meat and poultry products; Fish and shellfish; Legumes and soy products; and Nuts and seeds.

Fluids and foods to eat sparingly The remaining items in the charts are grouped as Fats, oils, and spreads; Drinks; Frozen and chilled desserts; and Cakes, cookies, and snacks.

Abbreviations used in the book

In the following charts, and throughout the book, the names of vitamins and minerals have been abbreviated. Those that may not appear obvious are explained below.

Vitamins
B_1 Known as thiamine
B_2 Known as riboflavin
Nia Niacin, sometimes known as nicotinic acid, nicotinamide, or B_3
Pant Pantothenic acid. Sometimes called B_5
B_6 Also known as pyridoxine
B_{12} Also known as cyanocobalamin or cobalamin
Fol Folate. Also known as folic acid or folacin
C Sometimes known as ascorbic acid
Vit K Vitamin K

Minerals
Macrominerals (*see p.60*):
Ca Calcium
Mg Magnesium
P Phosphorus
K Potassium
Na Sodium
S Sulfur
Microminerals (*see p.60*):
Cr Chromium
Cu Copper
F Fluoride
I Iodine
Fe Iron
Se Selenium
Zn Zinc

	Cal (kcal)	Total fat (g)	Sat. fat (g)	Mono. fat (g)	Poly. fat (g)	Protein (g)	Carb. (g)	Fiber (g)	Good source Vitamins/Minerals
GRAINS									
Barley, pearled 1 cup cooked	193	0.7	0.1	0.1	0.3	3.5	44.3	6.0	Nia / Cu, Fe
Buckwheat groats, roasted 1 cup cooked	182	1.2	0.3	0.4	0.4	6.7	39.5	5.3	B_1, B_2, Nia / Ca, Mg, P, K, Fe, Zn
Bulgar 1 cup cooked	151	0.4	0.1	0.1	0.2	5.6	33.8	8.2	B_1, Nia / Fe, Zn,
Couscous 1 cup cooked	200	0.3	0.1	0.0	0.1	6.8	41.6	2.5	B_1, Nia
Millet 1 cup cooked	286	2.4	0.4	0.4	1.2	8.4	56.8	3.1	B_1, B_2, Nia / Mg, P, K, Fe, Zn
Quinoa ½ cup cooked	318	4.9	0.5	1.3	2.0	11.1	58.6	5.0	B_1, B_2, Nia, Pant, Fol / Mg, P, K, Fe, Zn
Rice, brown, long-grain 1 cup cooked	216	1.8	0.4	0.6	0.6	5.0	44.8	3.5	B_1, Nia / Mg, P, Zn
Rice, wild, cooked 1 cup cooked	166	0.6	0.1	0.1	0.3	6.5	35.0	3.0	B_2, Nia, Fol / Mg, K, Zn
Rice, white, long-grain 1 cup cooked	205	0.4	0.1	0.1	0.1	4.3	44.5	0.6	B_1, Nia / Fe
Wheat germ ¼ cup	104	2.8	0.5	0.4	1.7	6.7	15.0	3.8	B_1, B_2, Nia, Fol / Mg, P, K, Cu, Fe
CEREALS, BREAKFAST									
All-bran ½ cup	81	1.1	0.2	0.2	0.7	3.9	23.0	10.0	A, B vitamins, C / Mg, P, K, Zn
Bran flakes ⅔ cup	90	0.5	0.0			3.0	22.0	6.0	A, most B vitamins / Mg, P, K, Fe, Zn
Cornflakes 1 cup	120	0.5	0.0	0.0	0.0	2.0	26.0	0.0	A, B_1, B_2, Nia, B_6, Fol C / Fe, Zn
Corn grits, quick dry ¼ cup	140	0.5	0.0			3.0	31.0	1.0	B_1, B_2, Nia
Cream of rice, dry ¼ cup	170	0.0	0.0	0.0	0.0	3.0	38.0		
Cream of wheat, dry 3 tbsp	120	0.0	0.0	0.0	0.0	3.0	25.0	1.0	
Crispy rice 1 cup	111	0.1	0.0	0.0	0.0	1.8	24.8	0.3	A, B_1, B_2, Nia, B_6, Fol

	Cal (kcal)	Total fat (g)	Sat. fat (g)	Mono. fat (g)	Poly. fat (g)	Protein (g)	Carb. (g)	Fiber (g)	Good source Vitamins/Minerals
Granola, low-fat ½ cup	190	2.9	0.5	0.6	1.9	4.1	39.3	2.9	A, B_1, B_2, Nia, B_6, B_{12} / Fe, Zn
Muesli ⅔ cup	206	1.9	0.3			5.3	41.9	3.8	A, B_1, B_2, Nia / Fe
Oatmeal, dry ½ cup	148	3.0	0.4	0.8	0.9	5.5	27.3	3.7	A, B_1, B_2, Nia / Ca, Fe
Oats, bran ¾ cup	109	1.2	0.3	0.6	0.3	3.9	23.2	4.0	A, B_1, B_2, Nia, B_6, B_{12}, Fol / P, Fe, Zn
Oats, circles 1 cup	110	2.0	0.0	0.5	0.5	3.0	23.0	3.0	A, B_1, B_2, Nia, B_6, Fol / Fe, Zn
Puffed rice 1 cup	56	0.1	0.0			0.9	12.6	0.2	B_1, B_2, Nia / Fe
Puffed wheat 1 cup	51	0.2	0.0			2.1	11.1	0.6	B_1, B_2, Nia / Fe
Raisin bran 1 cup	197	1.5	0.0	0.5	1.0	6.0	47.1	8.2	A, B_1, B_2, Nia, B_6, B_{12}, Fol / P, K, Fe, Zn
Shredded wheat 1 biscuit	86	0.4	0.1	0.1	0.2	2.6	19.3	2.4	B_1, Nia / P, K, Fe, Zn
PASTA AND NOODLES									
Egg noodles, enriched 1 cup cooked	160	2.4	0.5	0.7	0.7	7.6	39.7	1.8	B_1, B_2, Nia / Cu, Zn
Lasagne 2oz (55g) dry	210	1.3				8.0	41.8		B_1, B_2, Nia / Fe
Macaroni, enriched 1 cup cooked	197	0.9	0.1	0.1	0.4	6.7	39.7	1.8	B_1, B_2, Nia / Fe
Rice noodles ½ cup dry	121	3.0	0.6			2.3	21.4	0.4	
Spaghetti, enriched 1 cup cooked	197	0.9	0.1	0.1	0.4	6.7	39.7	2.4	B_1, B_2, Nia / Fe
Spaghetti, whole-wheat 1 cup cooked	174	0.8	0.1	0.1	0.3	7.5	37.2	6.3	B_1, Nia / Mg, Zn
BREADS									
Bagel, oat bran 1 bagel	181	0.9	0.1	0.2	0.3	7.6	37.8	2.6	B_1, B_2, Nia / Fe, Zn
Bagel, plain 1 bagel	195	1.1	0.2	0.1	0.5	7.5	37.9	1.6	B_1, B_2, Nia, B_6, Fol / Fe, Zn

	Cal (kcal)	Total fat (g)	Sat. fat (g)	Mono. fat (g)	Poly. fat (g)	Protein (g)	Carb. (g)	Fiber (g)	Good source Vitamins/Minerals
Breadsticks, plain 2 breadsticks	82	1.9	0.3	0.7	0.7	2.4	13.7	0.6	B_1, B_2, Nia
Croutons 1 cup	122	2.0	0.5	1.0	0.3	3.6	22.1	1.5	B_1, Nia / Fe
English muffin 1 muffin	134	1.0	0.1	0.2	0.5	4.4	26.2	1.5	B_1, B_2, Nia / Fe
French bread 1 slice	81	1.1				2.7	14.8	0.6	B_1, Nia
French toast, frozen 1 slice	126	3.6	1.1	1.2	0.7	4.4	18.9	0.7	B_1, Nia / Fe
Irish soda bread, homemade 1 slice	174	3.0	0.7	1.2	0.9	4.0	33.6	1.6	B_1, B_2, Nia / K, Fe
Matzo 1 matzo	112	0.4	0.1	0.0	0.2	2.8	23.7	0.9	B_1, Nia
Melba toast 1 slice	20	0.2	0.0	0.0	0.1	0.6	3.8	0.3	
Mixed-grain bread 1 slice	65	1.0	0.2	0.4	0.2	2.6	12.1	1.7	B_1, B_2, Nia
Multi-grain bread 1 slice	71	1.6				3.1	12.6	1.6	B_1, B_2, Nia / K, Fe
Oatmeal bread 1 slice	73	1.2	0.2	0.4	0.5	2.3	13.1	1.1	B_1
Pita, white 1 pita	165	0.7	0.1	0.1	0.3	5.5	33.4	1.3	B_1, B_2, Nia
Pita, whole-wheat 1 pita	170	1.7	0.3	0.2	0.7	6.3	35.2	4.7	B_1, Nia / Fe
Pizza crust, homemade ⅛ of 9in (23cm) crust	121	8.0	2.0	3.5	2.1	1.5	10.9	0.4	B_1, B_2, Nia
Pumpernickel bread 1 slice	80	1.0	0.1	0.3	0.4	2.8	15.2	2.1	B_1, B_2, Nia
Raisin bread 1 slice	71	1.1	0.3	0.6	0.2	2.1	13.6	1.1	B_1, B_2, Nia
Roll, dinner 1 roll	85	2.1	0.5	1.1	0.3	2.4	14.3	0.9	B_1, B_2, Nia
Roll, hamburger 1 roll	123	2.2	0.5	1.1	0.4	3.7	21.6	1.2	B_1, B_2, Nia
Roll, hotdog 1 roll	110	2.0	0.0			4.0	21.0	1.0	B_1, B_2, Nia

	Cal (kcal)	Total fat (g)	Sat. fat (g)	Mono. fat (g)	Poly. fat (g)	Protein (g)	Carb. (g)	Fiber (g)	Good source Vitamins/Minerals
Roll, kaiser 1 roll	167	2.5	0.3	0.6	1.0	5.6	30.0	1.3	Fe
Roll, oat-bran 1 roll	78	1.5	0.2	0.5	0.5	3.1	13.3	1.4	B_1, B_2, Nia / Fe
Roll, rye 1 roll	81	1.0	0.2	0.4	0.2	2.9	15.1	1.4	B_1, Nia
Roll, whole-wheat 1 roll	75	1.3	0.2	0.3	0.6	2.5	14.5	2.1	Nia
Rye bread 1 slice	83	1.1	0.2	0.4	0.3	2.7	15.5	1.9	B_1, B_2, Nia
Rye crispbread 1 cracker	37	0.1	0.0	0.0	0.1	0.8	8.2	1.7	
Seven-grain bread 1 slice	65	1.0	0.2	0.4	0.2	2.6	12.1	1.7	
Sourdough bread 1 slice	70	0.5	0.0			2.0	14.0	1.0	Fe
White bread 1 slice	67	0.9	0.2	0.4	0.2	2.0	12.4	0.6	Fe
Whole-grain bread 1 slice	65	1.0	0.2	0.4	0.2	2.6	12.1	1.7	Fe
Whole-wheat bread 1 slice	69	1.2	0.3	0.5	0.3	2.7	12.9	1.9	B_1, Nia
VEGETABLES									
Alfalfa sprouts 1 cup	10	0.2	0.0	0.0	0.1	0.0	0.0	0	
Artichoke, boiled 1 medium	150	0.5	0.1	0.0	0.2	10.4	33.5	16.2	A, B_1, B_2, Nia, Pant, C / Ca, Mg, P, K, Fe, Zn
Arugula ½ cup	3	0.1	0.0	0.0	0.0	0.3	0.4	0.2	
Asparagus, boiled ½ cup	22	0.3	0.1	0.0	0.1	2.3	3.8	1.4	A, B_1, B_2, Nia, C, Vit K / K
Avocado 1 medium	306	30.0	4.5	19.4	3.5	3.7	12.0	8.5	A, E
Bamboo shoots, boiled 1 cup	14	0.3	0.1	0.0	0.1	1.8	2.3	1.2	K
Bean sprouts, canned 1 cup	11	0.1	0.0			1.3	1.2	1.1	C

	Cal (kcal)	Total fat (g)	Sat. fat (g)	Mono. fat (g)	Poly. fat (g)	Protein (g)	Carb. (g)	Fiber (g)	Good source Vitamins/Minerals
Beets, boiled ½ cup sliced	37	0.2	0.0	0.0	0.1	1.4	8.5	1.7	K
Beets, pickled ½ cup sliced	74	0.1	0.0	0.0	0.0	0.9	18.6		K
Broccoli, boiled ½ cup	22	0.3	0.0	0.0	0.1	2.3	3.9	2.3	A, B₂, C, Vit K / K, Cr
Brussels sprouts, boiled ½ cup	30	0.4	0.1	0.0	0.2	2.0	6.8	2.0	A, Vit K / K
Cabbage, green ½ cup shredded	9	0.1	0.0	0.0	0.0	0.5	1.9	0.8	C, Vit K / S
Cabbage, green, boiled ½ cup shredded	17	0.3	0.0	0.0	0.1	0.8	3.3	1.7	C / S
Cabbage, red ½ cup shredded	9	0.1	0.0	0.0	0.0	0.5	2.1	0.7	C / S
Cabbage, red, boiled ½ cup shredded	16	0.2	0.0	0.0	0.1	0.8	3.5	1.5	C / S
Cabbage, savoy ½ cup shredded	9	0.0	0.0	0.0	0.0	0.7	2.1	1.1	C / S
Cabbage, savoy, boiled ½ cup shredded	18	0.1	0.0	0.0	0.0	1.3	3.9	2.0	A, C / K, S
Carrots 1 medium	31	0.1	0.0	0.0	0.1	0.7	7.3	2.2	A, Vit K / K
Carrots, boiled ½ cup sliced	35	0.1	0.0	0.0	0.1	0.9	8.2	2.6	A / K
Cassava ½ cup chopped	120	0.4	0.1	0.1	0.1	3.1	26.9	1.6	B₁, B₂, Nia, C / K, Fe
Cauliflower ½ cup pieces	13	0.1	0.0	0.0	0.0	1.0	2.6	1.3	C, Vit K / K
Cauliflower, boiled ½ cup pieces	14	0.3	0.0	0.0	0.1	1.1	2.5	1.7	C
Celeriac ½ cup chopped	39	0.3	0.1	0.1	0.1	1.5	9.2	1.8	Vit K / K
Celeriac, boiled ½ cup chopped	25	0.2				1.0	5.9	1.2	K
Celery 1 stalk	6	0.1	0.0	0.0	0.0	0.3	1.5	0.7	
Chicory greens ½ cup chopped	21	0.3	0.1	0.0	0.1	1.5	4.2	3.6	A, Pant, C / K

	Cal (kcal)	Total fat (g)	Sat. fat (g)	Mono. fat (g)	Poly. fat (g)	Protein (g)	Carb. (g)	Fiber (g)	Good source Vits / Mins
Chili 1 pepper	18	0.1	0.0	0.0	0.0	0.9	4.3	0.7	C
Chilis, green, canned ¼ cup sliced	4	0.1	0.0			0.2	1.1	0.5	
Chilis, jalapeno, canned 2 tbsp	5	0.2	0.0			0.4	0.8	0.6	Fe
Chinese cabbage, boiled ½ cup shredded	10	0.1	0.0	0.0	0.1	1.3	1.5	1.4	C
Coleslaw, homemade ½ cup	41	1.6	0.2	0.4	0.8	0.8	7.4	0.9	A, C
Collard greens, boiled 1 cup chopped	35	0.2	0.0	0.0	0.1	1.7	7.8	3.6	A, C / K
Corn, canned ½ cup	66	0.8	0.1	0.2	0.4	2.1	15.2	1.6	Nia / K
Corn, creamed, canned	59	0.3	0.1	0.1	0.2	1.4	14.9	1.0	
Corn-on-the-cob, boiled 1 medium ear	183	0.9	0.2	0.3	0.6	5.1	38.7		K
Cucumber ½ cup sliced	7	0.1	0.0	0.0	0.0	0.4	1.1	0.4	
Eggplant, boiled ½ cup	13	0.1	0.0	0.0	0.0	0.4	3.2	1.2	
Endive ½ cup chopped	4	0.1	0.0	0.0	0.0	0.3	0.8	0.8	A
Fennel bulb 1 cup sliced	27	0.2				1.1	6.3	2.7	C / K
French beans, boiled 1 cup	228	1.3	0.1	0.1	0.8	12.5	42.5	16.6	A / K
Garden cress ½ cup	8	0.2	0.0	0.1	0.1	0.7	1.4	0.3	A, C, B$_2$ / K
Garlic 3 cloves	13	0.0	0.0	0.0	0.0	0.6	3.0	0.2	
Gourd, calabash, boiled ½ cup cubed	11	0.0	0.0	0.0	0.0	0.4	2.7		K
Green beans, boiled ½ cup	22	0.2	0.0	0.0	0.1	1.2	4.9	2.0	A / K
Green peas, frozen, boiled ½ cup	62	0.2	0.0	0.0	0.1	4.1	11.4	4.4	

	Cal (kcal)	Total fat (g)	Sat. fat (g)	Mono. fat (g)	Poly. fat (g)	Protein (g)	Carb. (g)	Fiber (g)	Good source Vits / Mins
Jerusalem artichoke ½ cup sliced	57	0.0	0.0	0.0	0.0	1.5	13.1	1.2	B_1, Nia / K, Fe
Kale, boiled ½ cup chopped	21	0.3	0.0	0.0	0.1	1.2	3.7	1.3	A, C / S
Leeks, boiled ¼ cup chopped	8	0.1	0.0	0.0	0.0	0.2	2.0	0.3	
Lettuce, iceberg 1 leaf	2	0.0	0.0	0.0	0.0	0.2	0.4	0.3	
Lettuce, romaine ½ cup shredded	4	0.1	0.0	0.0	0.0	0.5	0.7	0.5	A
Mushrooms, boiled ½ cup slices	21	0.4	0.0	0.0	0.1	1.7	4.0	1.7	B_2, Nia, Pant / K, Fe
Mushrooms, enoki 1 large	2	0.0	0.0	0.0	0.0	0.1	0.4	0.1	
Mushrooms, shitake, cooked 4 mushrooms	40	0.2	0.0	0.0	0.0	1.1	10.3	1.5	B_2, Nia, Pant
Mustard greens, boiled ½ cup chopped	11	0.2	0.0	0.1	0.0	1.7	2.3	2.1	A, C
Okra, boiled ½ cup sliced	30	0.2	0.1	0.0	0.1	1.7	4.6	2.2	A, B_2, C / Mg, K
Olives, black 1 medium	5	0.4	0.1	0.3	0.0	0.0	0.3	0.1	
Onion ½ cup chopped	16	0.1	0.0	0.0	0.0	0.9	3.7	1.3	
Pak choi, boiled ½ cup shredded	10	0.1	0.0	0.0	0.1	1.3	1.5	1.4	A, C
Parsley, freeze-dried ¼ cup	4	0.1				0.4	0.6	0.5	A
Parsnip, boiled ½ cup sliced	63	0.2	0.0	0.1	0.0	1.0	15.2	3.1	C / K
Pepper, bell ½ cup chopped	16	0.4	0.0	0.0	0.5	0.5	3.3	1.3	C
Pepper, jalopeno, canned ½ cup chopped	16	0.4	0.0	0.0	0.2	0.5	3.3	1.3	A / Fe
Potato, baked 1 potato	212	0.2	0.1	0.0	0.1	4.9	48.7	4.6	B_1, Nia, B_6, C / P, K, Cr, Fe
Potato, boiled without skin 1 potato	117	0.1	0.0	0.0	0.1	2.5	27.2	2.4	B_1, Nia, C / K

	Cal (kcal)	Total fat (g)	Sat. fat (g)	Mono. fat (g)	Poly. fat (g)	Protein (g)	Carb. (g)	Fiber (g)	Good source Vitamins/Minerals
Potato, mashed ½ cup	111	4.4	1.1	1.9	1.3	2.0	17.5	2.1	C / K
Pumpkin, boiled ½ cup mashed	24	0.1	0.0	0.0	0.0	0.9	6.0	1.3	A, B_2 / K
Radicchio ½ cup shredded	5	0.1	0.0	0.0	0.0	0.3	0.9	0.2	
Radish ½ cup sliced	8	0.0	0.0	0.0	0.0	0.3	1.8	0.7	C
Rutabaga, boiled ½ cup cubed	33	0.2	0.0	0.0	0.1	1.1	7.4	1.5	A, C / K
Salsify, boiled ½ cup sliced	46	0.1	0.0	0.0	0.1	1.9	10.5	2.1	B_2 / K
Seaweed, spirulina ½ cup	26	0.4	0.1	0.0	0.1	5.9	2.4		B_2, Pant, Fol / Ca, Mg, K, Fe, Zn
Seaweed, wakame ½ cup	45	0.6	0.1	0.1	0.2	3.0	9.1	0.5	B_2, Nia, Fol / Ca, Mg, Fe
Shallots 1 tbsp chopped	7	0.0	0.0	0.0	0.0	0.3	1.7		A
Spinach, boiled ½ cup	21	0.2	0.0	0.0	0.1	2.7	3.4	2.2	A, B_2, Fol, C, Vit K / K, Ca, Mg, Fe
Spring onion ½ cup chopped	16	0.1	0.0	0.0	0.0	0.9	3.7	1.3	
Squash, acorn, baked ½ cup cubed	57	0.1	0.0	0.0	0.1	1.1	14.9	4.5	A, B_1, C / K
Squash, butternut, baked ½ cup cubed	41	0.1	0.0	0.0	0.0	0.9	10.7		A, Nia, C / K
Sweet potato, baked with skin 1 sweet potato	117	0.1	0.0	0.0	0.1	2.0	27.7	3.4	A, B_2, C / K
Swiss chard, boiled ½ cup chopped	18	0.1	0.0	0.0	0.0	1.7	3.6	1.8	A, C / Mg, K, Fe
Tomato 1 tomato	26	0.4	0.1	0.1	0.2	1.0	5.7	1.4	A, C / K, Cr
Tomato, canned ½ cup	36	0.2	0.0	0.0	0.1	1.2	8.7	1.3	A, C / K
Tomato, sundried 1 cup	139	1.6	0.2	0.3	0.6	7.6	30.1	6.6	A, B_1, B_2, Nia, Pant, Fol, C / Mg, P, K, Fe, Zn
Turnip, boiled ½ cup chopped	14	0.1	0.0	0.0	0.0	0.6	3.8	1.6	C / S

	Cal (kcal)	Total fat (g)	Sat. fat (g)	Mono. fat (g)	Poly. fat (g)	Protein (g)	Carb. (g)	Fiber (g)	Good source Vitamins/Minerals
Turnip greens, boiled ½ cup chopped	14	0.2	0.0	0.0	0.1	0.8	3.1	2.5	A, C / Mg
Water chestnuts, canned ½ cup sliced	35	0.0	0.0	0.0	0.0	0.6	8.7	1.8	
Watercress ½ cup chopped	2	0.0	0.0	0.0	0.0	0.4	0.2	0.3	A
Zucchini, boiled ½ cup sliced	14	0.0	0.0	0.0	0.0	0.6	3.5	1.3	K

FRUITS

	Cal (kcal)	Total fat (g)	Sat. fat (g)	Mono. fat (g)	Poly. fat (g)	Protein (g)	Carb. (g)	Fiber (g)	Good source Vitamins/Minerals
Apple with skin 1 medium	81	0.5	0.1	0.0	0.1	0.3	21.0	3.7	K, Cr
Applesauce, unsweetened ½ cup	52	0.1	0.0	0.0	0.0	0.2	13.8	1.5	
Apricots 3 medium	51	0.4	0.0	0.2	0.1	1.5	11.8	2.5	A, C, Vit K / K
Apricots, canned in own juice 3 halves	40	0.0	0.0	0.0	0.0	0.5	10.4	1.3	A
Apricots, dried, sulfured 10 halves	83	0.2	0.0	0.1	0.0	1.3	21.6	3.1	A, Nia / K, Fe
Banana 1 medium	105	0.5	0.2	0.0	0.1	1.2	17.8	2.7	B_2, B_6, C / K, Cr
Blackberries ½ cup	37	0.3	0.0	0.0	0.2	0.5	9.2	3.8	C
Blueberries 1 cup	81	0.6	0.0	0.1	0.2	1.0	20.5	3.9	C
Cantaloupe 1 cup pieces	56	0.4	0.1	0.0	0.2	1.4	13.4	1.3	A, Nia, C / K
Cherries 10 cherries	34	0.2	0.0	0.1	0.1	0.7	8.3	1.1	A
Cherries, canned in water ½ cup	44	0.1	0.0	0.0	0.0	0.9	10.9	1.3	A / Fe
Crabapples 1 cup sliced	84	0.3	0.1	0.0	0.1	0.1	21.9		C / K
Cranberries 1 cup	47	0.2	0.0	0.0	0.1	0.4	12.0	4.0	C
Currants, red and white ½ cup	31	0.1	0.0	0.0	0.0	0.8	7.7	2.4	C

	Cal (kcal)	Total fat (g)	Sat. fat (g)	Mono. fat (g)	Poly. fat (g)	Protein (g)	Carb. (g)	Fiber (g)	Good source Vitamins/Minerals
Dates, dried 10 dates	228	0.4	0.2	0.1	0.0	1.6	61.0	6.2	Nia / K
Figs 1 medium	37	0.1	0.0	0.0	0.1	0.1	9.6	1.6	
Figs, dried 10 figs	477	2.2	0.1	0.5	1.0	5.7	122.2	17.4	B_1, B_2, Nia, B_6 / Ca, Mg, P, K, Fe, Zn
Fruit cocktail, canned in juice ½ cup	57	0.0	0.0	0.0	0.0	0.6	14.7	1.2	
Gooseberries 1 cup	66	0.9	0.1	0.1	0.5	1.3	15.3	6.4	A, C / K
Grapefruit, pink and red ½ medium	39	0.1	0.0	0.0	0.0	0.8	9.9	1.4	C / K
Grapes, american 1 cup	58	0.3	0.1	0.0	0.1	0.6	15.8	0.9	Vit K / K, Cr
Groundcherries 1 cup	74	1.0				2.7	15.7		A, B_1, Nia, C / Fe
Guava 1 medium	46	0.5	0.2	0.0	0.2	0.7	10.7	4.9	A, Nia, C / K
Honeydew melon 1 cup cubed	60	0.2	0.0	0.0	0.1	0.8	15.6	1.0	B_1, Nia, C / K
Kiwifruit 1 medium	46	0.3	0.0	0.0	0.2	0.8	11.3	2.6	Fol, C / K
Kumquats 1 medium	12	0.0	0.0	0.0	0.0	0.2	3.1	1.3	
Lemon 1 medium	17	0.2	0.0	0.0	0.1	0.6	5.4	1.6	C
Lime 1 medium	20	0.1	0.0	0.0	0.0	0.5	7.1	1.9	C
Loganberries, frozen 1 cup	81	0.5	0.0	0.0	0.3	2.2	19.1	7.2	Nia, C / K
Loquats 6 medium	47	0.2	0.0	0.0	0.1	0.4	12.1	1.7	A / K
Lychees 10 medium	66	0.4	0.1	0.1	0.1	0.8	16.5	1.3	Nia, C / K
Mandarin, canned in juice ½ cup	46	0.0	0.0	0.0	0.0	0.8	11.9	0.9	A, C
Mango 1 medium	135	0.6	0.1	0.2	0.1	1.1	35.2	3.7	A, B_1, B_2, Nia, C / K

	Cal (kcal)	Total fat (g)	Sat. fat (g)	Mono. fat (g)	Poly. fat (g)	Protein (g)	Carb. (g)	Fiber (g)	Good source Vitamins/Minerals
Melon 1 cup balls	57	0.4	0.1	0.0	0.2	1.5	13.7	1.2	A, C, B1, Nia / K
Mulberries 1 cup	60	0.5	0.0	0.1	0.3	2.0	13.7	2.4	C / K, Fe
Nectarine 1 medium	67	0.6	0.1	0.2	0.3	1.3	16.0	2.2	A, Nia / K
Orange, navel 1 fruit	60	0.1	0.0	0.0	0.0	1.3	15.2	3.1	B_1, Fol, C / K
Papaya 1 medium	119	0.4	0.1	0.1	0.1	1.9	29.8	5.5	A, B_2, Nia, Fol, C / K
Passion fruit (granadilla) 1 medium	17	0.1	0.0	0.0	0.1	0.4	4.2	1.9	
Peach 1 medium	37	0.1	0.0	0.0	0.0	0.6	9.7	1.7	A, Nia / K
Peach, canned in own juice 1 cup	109	0.1	0.0	0.0	0.0	1.6	28.7	3.2	A, Nia, C / K
Pear 1 medium	98	0.7	0.0	0.1	0.2	0.6	25.1	4.0	Vit K / K
Pears, canned in own juice 1 cup	124	0.2	0.0	0.0	0.0	0.8	32.1	4.0	K
Pineapple 1 cup pieces	76	0.7	0.0	0.1	0.2	0.6	18.4	1.9	B_1, C / K
Pineapple, canned in own juice 1 cup pieces	150	0.2	0.0	0.0	0.1	1.1	39.3	2.0	C / K
Plantain, cooked 1 cup sliced	179	0.3	0.1	0.0	0.1	1.2	48.0	3.5	A, Nia, Fol, C / Mg, K
Plum 1 medium	36	0.4	0.0	0.3	0.1	0.5	8.6	1.0	Vit K
Pomegranate 1 medium	105	0.5	0.1	0.1	0.1	1.5	26.4	0.9	K
Prunes, dried 10 prunes	201	0.4	0.0	0.3	0.1	2.2	52.7	6.0	A, B_2, Nia / K
Prunes, in own juice 5 prunes	90	0.2	0.0	0.3	0.0	0.7	23.9	3.3	A, B_2 / K
Pummelo 1 cup pieces	72	0.1				1.4	18.3	1.9	C / K
Quince 1 medium	52	0.1	0.0	0.0	0.0	0.4	14.1	1.7	C / K

	Cal (kcal)	Total fat (g)	Sat. fat (g)	Mono. fat (g)	Poly. fat (g)	Protein (g)	Carb. (g)	Fiber (g)	Good source Vitamins/Minerals
Raisins, seedless 2/3 cup	300	0.5	0.1	0.0	0.1	3.2	79.1	4.0	B_1, B_2 / K, Fe
Raspberries 1 cup	60	0.7	0.0	0.1	0.4	1.1	14.2	8.4	B_2, Nia, Fol, C / K
Raspberries, canned in syrup 1/2 cup	116	0.2	0.0	0.0	0.1	1.1	29.9	4.2	C
Raspberries, frozen 2/5 cup	103	0.2	0.0	0.0	0.1	0.7	26.2	4.4	C
Rhubarb, frozen 1 cup	29	0.2	0.0	0.0	0.1	0.8	7.0	2.5	Ca
Sapodilla 1 medium	141	1.9	0.3	0.9	0.0	0.7	33.9	9.0	C / K, Fe
Strawberries 1 cup	45	0.6	0.0	0.1	0.3	0.9	10.5	3.4	B_2, C / K
Tangerine 1 medium	37	0.2	0.0	0.0	0.0	0.5	9.4	1.9	A, C
Watermelon 1 cup	51	0.7	0.1	0.2	0.2	1.0	11.5	0.8	A, B_1, C, / K
DAIRY PRODUCTS AND EGGS									
American cheese 1oz (28g)	106	8.9	5.6	2.5	0.3	6.3	0.5	0.0	A / Ca, P
Blue cheese 1oz (28g)	100	8.1	5.3	2.2	0.2	6.1	0.7	0.0	A, B_2, Pant / Ca
Brie 1oz (28g)	95	7.8	4.9	2.3	0.2	5.9	0.1	0.0	A, B_2
Buttermilk, cultured 8floz (240ml)	99	2.2	1.3	0.6	0.1	8.1	11.7	0.0	B_2, B_{12} / Ca, P, K, Zn
Camembert 1oz (28g)	85	6.9	4.3	2.0	0.2	5.6	0.1	0.0	A, B_2 / Ca, P
Caraway cheese 1oz (28g)	107	8.3	5.3	2.3	0.2	7.1	0.9	0.0	A, B_2 / Ca
Cheddar cheese 1oz (28g)	114	9.4	6.0	2.7	0.3	7.1	0.4	0.0	A, B_2 / Ca, P
Cheddar cheese, low-fat 1oz (28g)	49	2.0	1.2	0.6	0.1	6.9	0.5	0.0	Ca
Cheshire cheese 1oz (28g)	110	8.7	5.5	2.5	0.2	6.6	1.4	0.0	A / Ca

	Cal (kcal)	Total fat (g)	Sat. fat (g)	Mono. fat (g)	Poly. fat (g)	Protein (g)	Carb. (g)	Fiber (g)	Good source Vitamins/Minerals
Chocolate milk, low-fat (1%) 8floz (240ml)	158	2.5	1.5	0.8	0.1	8.1	26.1	1.3	A, B_2, Nia, Pant, B_{12}, D / Ca, P, K, Zn
Chocolate milk, reduced-fat (2%) 8floz (240ml)	180	5.0	3.0	1.5	0.2	8.0	26.1	1.3	A, B_2, Nia / Ca, P, K, Zn
Chocolate milk, sugar-free 8floz (240ml)	70	1.1	0.5			4.5	12	0.0	A, B_2, Nia, Pant, Fol / Ca, Mg, P, K, Cu, Fe
Colby cheese 1oz (28g)	112	9.1	5.7	2.6	0.3	6.7	0.7	0.0	A, B_2 / Ca
Cottage cheese, creamed 1 round tbsp	117	5.1	3.2	1.5	0.2	14.1	3.0	0.0	A, B_{12} / P
Cottage cheese, low-fat (1%) 1 cup	164	2.3	1.5	0.7	0.1	28.0	6.1	0.0	A, B_2, Pant, B_{12}, / Ca, P, K
Cottage cheese, reduced-fat (2%) 1 cup	203	4.4	2.8	1.2	0.1	31.1	8.2	0.0	A, B_2, Pant, B_{12} / Ca, P, K
Cream cheese 2 tbsp	99	9.9	6.2	2.8	0.4	2.1	0.8	0.0	A
Cream cheese, light 2 tbsp	70	5.0	3.5			2.0	2.0	0.0	A
Edam cheese 1oz (28g)	101	7.9	5.0	2.3	0.2	7.1	0.4	0.0	A, B_2 / Ca, P
Egg, chicken 1 large	75	5.0	1.6	1.9	0.7	6.2	0.6	0.0	A, B_2, B_{12} / Ca, P, Zn
Egg, chicken, white white of 1 large egg	17	0.0	0.0	0.0	0.0	3.5	0.3	0.0	B_2
Egg, chicken, yolk yolk of 1 large egg	61	5.2	1.6	2.0	0.7	2.8	0.3	0.0	A, B_2 / S
Egg, duck 1 egg	130	9.6	2.6	4.6	0.9	9.0	1.0	0.0	A, B_1, B_2, Pant, B_{12}, / P, K, Fe, Zn
Egg, goose 1 egg	267	19.1	5.2	8.3	2.4	20.0	1.9	0.0	A, B_1, B_2, Pant, B_{12}, Fol / P, K, Fe, Zn
Egg, quail 1 egg	14	1.0	0.3	0.4	0.1	1.2	0.0	0.0.	
Egg substitute ¼ cup	44	1.3	0.4	0.5	0.2	5.6	2.2	0.0	
Egg, turkey 1 egg	135	9.4	2.9	3.6	1.3	10.8	0.9	0.0	A, B_2, Pant, B_{12} / Fe, Zn
Evaporated milk, low-fat 2 tbsp	25	0.5	0.0	0.0	0.0	2.0	3.0	0.0	B_1

	Cal (kcal)	Total fat (g)	Sat. fat (g)	Mono. fat (g)	Poly. fat (g)	Protein (g)	Carb. (g)	Fiber (g)	Good source Vitamins/Minerals
Evaporated milk, fat-free 1floz (30ml)	25	0.1	0.0	0.0	0.0	2.4	3.6	0.0	B_2, Pant
Evaporated milk, whole-milk 1floz (30ml)	43	2.4	1.5	0.7	0.1	2.2	3.2	0.0	B_2
Farmer's cheese 1oz (28g)	100	8.0	6.0			6.0	1.0	0.0	Ca, P
Feta cheese 1oz (28g)	75	6.0	4.2	1.3	0.2	4.0	1.2	0.0	B_2
Fontina cheese 1oz (28g)	110	8.8	5.4	2.5	0.5	7.3	0.4	0.0	A / Ca
Gjetost 1oz (28g)	132	8.4	5.4	2.2	0.3	2.7	12.1	0.0	A, B_2, Pant / K
Goat's milk 8floz (240ml)	168	10.1	6.5	2.7	0.4	8.7	10.9	0.0	A, B_2 / Ca, P, K
Goat's cheese, hard 1oz (28g)	128	10.1	7.0	2.3	0.2	837	0.6	0.0	A, B_2 / Ca, P
Goat's cheese, semi-soft 1oz (28g)	103	8.5	5.9	1.9	0.2	6.1	0.7	0.0	A, B_2
Goat's Cheese, soft 1oz (28g)	76	6.0	4.1	1.4	0.1	5.3	0.3	0.0	A, B_2
Gouda 1oz (28g)	101	7.8	5.0	2.2	0.2	7.1	0.6	0.0	A / Ca, P, Zn
Gruyere 1oz (28g)	117	9.2	5.4	2.8	0.5	8.5	0.1	0.0	A / Ca, P, Zn
Half-and-half 1 tbsp	20	1.7	1.1	0.5	0.1	0.4	0.6	0.0	
Lactose-reduced low-fat (1%) milk 8floz (240ml)	102	2.6	1.6	0.8	0.1	8.1	11.8	0.0	A, Nia / Ca, P, K
Limburger 1oz (28g)	93	7.7	4.7	2.4	0.1	5.7	0.1	0.0	A, B_2 / Ca
Milk, fat-free 8floz (240ml)	86	0.4	0.3	0.1	0.0	8.4	11.9	0.0	A, B_1, B_2 / Ca, P, K
Milk, low-fat (1%) 8floz (240ml)	102	2.6	1.6	0.7	0.1	8.0	11.7	0.0	A, B_1, B_2, Pant / Ca, P, K
Milk, reduced-fat (2%) 8floz (240ml)	121	4.7	2.9	1.4	0.2	8.1	11.7	0.0	A, B_1, B_2, Pant / Ca, P, K
Milk, whole 8floz (240ml)	150	8.1	5.1	2.4	0.3	8.0	11.4	0.0	A, B_1, B_2 / Ca, P, K

	Cal (kcal)	Total fat (g)	Sat. fat (g)	Mono. fat (g)	Poly. fat (g)	Protein (g)	Carb. (g)	Fiber (g)	Good source Vitamins/Minerals
Monterey Jack 1oz (28g)	106	8.6	5.4	2.5	0.3	6.9	0.2	0.0	A, B_2 / Ca, P
Mozzarella, part-skim 1oz (28g)	72	4.5	2.9	1.3	0.1	6.9	0.8	0.0	A / Ca, P
Mozzarella, whole-milk 1oz (28g)	80	6.1	3.7	1.9	0.2	5.5	0.6	0.0	A / Ca
Muenster cheese 1oz (28g)	104	8.5	5.4	2.5	0.2	6.6	0.3	0.0	A, B_{12} / Ca
Neufchatel cheese 1oz (28g)	74	6.6	4.2	1.9	0.2	2.8	0.8	0.0	A / Ca
Parmesan, hard 1oz (28g)	111	7.3	4.7	2.1	0.2	10.1	0.9	0.0	Ca, P
Port du salut 1oz (28g)	100	8.0	4.7	2.6	0.2	6.7	0.2	0.0	A / Ca
Provolone cheese 1oz (28g)	100	7.5	4.8	2.1	0.2	7.3	0.6	0.0	A / Ca, P
Ricotta cheese, part-skim ½ cup	171	9.8	6.1	2.9	0.3	14.1	6.4	0.0	A / Ca, P, Zn
Ricotta cheese, whole-milk ½ cup	216	16.1	10.3	4.5	0.5	14.0	3.8	0.0	A, B_2 / Ca, P, Zn
Romano cheese 1oz (28g)	110	7.6	4.9	2.2	0.2	9.0	1.0	0.0	B_2 / Ca, P
Roquefort cheese 1oz (28g)	105	8.7	5.5	2.4	0.4	6.1	0.6	0.0	A, B_2 / Ca
Sour cream, fat-free 2 tbsp	35	0.0	0.0	0.0	0.0		6.0	0.0	
Sour cream, full-fat 2 tbsp	52	5.0	3.2	1.4	0.2	0.8	1.0	0.0	
Swiss cheese 1oz (28g)	107	7.8	5.0	2.1	0.3	8.1	1.0	0.0	A, B_2 / Ca, P, Zn
Tilsit cheese 1oz (28g)	96	7.4	4.8	2.0	0.2	6.9	0.5	0.0	A, B_2 / Ca
Yogurt, fat-free 8floz (240ml)	127	0.4	0.3	0.1	0.0	13.0	17.4	0.0	B_2 / Ca, P, K
Yogurt, low-fat 8floz (240ml)	130	3.0	2.0			11.0	15.0	0.0	B_2 / Ca, P, K
Yogurt, whole 8floz (240ml)	139	7.4	4.8	2.0	0.2	7.9	10.6	0.0	B_2, Pant / Ca, P, K

	Cal (kcal)	Total fat (g)	Sat. fat (g)	Mono. fat (g)	Poly. fat (g)	Protein (g)	Carb. (g)	Fiber (g)	Good source Vitamins/Minerals
MEAT AND POULTRY									
Beef, brisket, lean, braised 3½oz (100g)	218	10.1	3.6	4.7	0.3	29.8	0.0	0.0	B_2, Nia, B_{12} / P, K, Cr, Fe, Zn
Beef, ground, lean, broiled 3½oz (100g)	256	16.3	6.4	7.2	0.6	25.4	0.0	0.0	B_2, Nia, B_{12} / P, K, Cr, Fe, Zn, Cr
Beef, tenderloin, lean, broiled 3½oz (100g)	244	14.3	5.5	5.7	0.5	27.0	0.0	0.0	B_1, B_2, Nia, B_{12} / K, P, Cr, Fe, Zn, Cr
Beef, top sirloin, lean, broiled 3½oz (100g)	200	7.8	3.0	3.3	0.3	30.4	0.0	0.0	B_1, B_2, Nia, B_{12} / P, K, Cr, Fe, Zn
Bison, roasted 3½oz (100g)	143	2.4	0.9	0.9	0.2	28.4	0.0	0.0	B_1, B_2, Nia, B_{12} / P, K, Cr, Fe, Zn
Boar, wild, roasted 3½oz (100g)	160	4.4	1.3	1.7	0.6	28.3	0.0	0.0	B_1, B_2, Nia / K, Fe, Zn
Chicken, dark meat no skin, roasted 3½oz (100g)	205	9.7	2.7	3.6	2.3	27.4	0.0	0.0	B_2, Nia, Pant / P, K, Zn
Chicken, white meat no skin, roasted 3½oz (100g)	173	4.5	1.3	1.5	1.0	30.9	0.0	0.0	B_2, Nia, / P, K, Zn
Chicken, white meat with skin, roasted 3½oz (100g)	222	10.8	3.0	4.3	2.3	29.0	0.0	0.0	B_2, Nia, B_6 / P, K, Zn
Duck, no skin, roasted 3½oz (100g)	201	11.2	4.2	3.7	1.4	23.5	0.0	0.0	B_1, B_2, Nia, Pant / P, K, Fe, Zn
Goose, no skin, roasted 3½oz (100g)	238	12.7	4.6	4.3	1.5	29.0	0.0	0.0	B_2, Nia, Pant / P, K, Fe, Zn
Guinea hen, no skin, raw 3½oz (100g)	110	2.5	0.6	0.7	0.6	20.6	0.0	0.0	B_2, Nia / P, K, Zn
Kidney, lamb, braised 3½oz (100g)	137	3.6	1.2	0.8	0.7	23.6	1.0	0.0	A, B vitamins / Mg, P, K, S, Fe, Zn
Lamb, leg, whole, roasted 3½oz (100g)	258	16.5	6.9	7.0	1.2	25.6	0.0	0.0	B_2, Nia, B_{12} / P, K, Fe, Zn
Lamb, loin, roasted 3½oz (100g)	202	9.8	3.7	4.0	0.9	26.6	0.0	0.0	B_1, B_2, Nia, B_{12} / P, K, Fe, Zn
Lamb, shoulder, whole, lean, roasted 3½oz (100g)	204	10.8	4.1	4.4	0.9	24.9	0.0	0.0	B_2, Nia, B_{12} / P, K, Fe, Zn
Liver, beef, braised 3½oz (100g)	161	4.9	1.9	0.7	1.1	24.4	3.4	0.0	A, B vitamins C / P, K, S, Cu, Fe, Zn
Liver, chicken, simmered 3½oz (100g)	157	5.5	1.8	1.3	0.9	24.4	0.9	0.0	A, B vitamins C / P, K, S, Cu, Fe, Zn

	Cal (kcal)	Total fat (g)	Sat. fat (g)	Mono. fat (g)	Poly. fat (g)	Protein (g)	Carb. (g)	Fiber (g)	Good source Vitamins/Minerals
Liver, lamb, braised 3½oz (100g)	220	8.8	3.4	1.8	1.3	30.6	2.5	0.0	B_2, Nia, B_{12} / P, K, Fe, Zn
Pheasant, no skin, raw 3½oz (100g)	133	3.6	1.2	1.2	0.6	20.6	0.0	0.0	A, B_2, Nia / P, K, Fe
Pigeon, no skin, raw 3½oz (100g)	142	7.5	2.0	2.7	1.6	17.5	0.0	0.0	B_1, B_2, Nia, Pant / P, K, Fe, Zn
Pork, leg, lean, roasted 3½oz (100g)	211	9.4	3.3	4.5	0.8	29.4	0.0	0.0	B_1, B_2, Nia / P, K, Fe
Pork, loin, lean, broiled 3½oz (100g)	202	8.1	3.0	3.6	0.6	29.8	0.0	0.0	B_1, B_2, Nia / P, K, Zn
Quail, no skin, raw 3½oz (100g)	134	4.5	1.3	1.3	1.2	21.8	0.0	0.0	B_1, B_2, Nia / P, K, Fe, Zn
Rabbit, roasted 3½oz (100g)	197	8.1	2.4	2.2	1.6	29.1	0.0	0.0	B_1, B_2, Nia, B_{12} / P, K, Fe, Zn
Turkey, dark meat no skin, roasted 3½oz (100g)	187	7.2	2.4	1.6	2.2	28.6	0.0	0.0	B_2, Nia, Pant / P, K, Fe, Zn
Turkey, white meat no skin, roasted 3½oz (100g)	157	3.2	1.0	0.6	0.9	29.9	0.0	0.0	B_2, Nia / P, K, Fe, Zn
Venison (deer), roasted 3½oz (100g)	158	3.2	1.3	0.9	0.6	30.2	0.0	0.0	B_1, B_2, Nia / P, K, Fe, Zn
Water buffalo, roasted 3½oz (100g)	131	1.8	0.6	0.6	0.4	26.8	0.0	0.0	B_2, Nia, B_{12} / P, K, Fe, Zn
MEAT AND POULTRY PRODUCTS									
Bacon, Canadian, grilled 2 slices	87	4.0	1.3	1.9	0.4	11.4	0.6	0.0	B_1, Nia / P, K
Bacon, cured, broiled 3 slices	109	9.4	3.3	4.5	1.1	5.8	0.1	0.0	B_1, Nia
Corned beef, jellied 1oz (28g) slice	43	1.7	0.7	0.8	0.1	6.4	0.0	0.0	Zn
Frankfurter, beef 1 sausage	180	16.2	6.9	7.8	0.8	6.8	1.0	0.0	Nia / Zn
Frankfurter, chicken 1 sausage	116	8.8	2.5	3.8	1.8	5.8	3.1	0.0	Nia
Frankfurter, fat-free 1 sausage	54	1.8	1.0	0.6	0.2	6.3	3.2	0.0	K, Zn
Frankfurter, pork and turkey 1 sausage	184	17.0	5.8	8.5	2.6	6.2	1.7	0.0	

	Cal (kcal)	Total fat (g)	Sat. fat (g)	Mono. fat (g)	Poly. fat (g)	Protein (g)	Carb. (g)	Fiber (g)	Good source Vitamins/Minerals
Frankfurter, turkey 1 sausage	102	8.0	2.7	2.5	2.3	6.4	0.7	0.0	Nia / Zn
Ham, lean 1oz (28g) slice		1.4	0.5	0.7	0.1	5.4	0.3	0.0	B_1, B_2, Nia / P, K, Fe, Zn
Ham, honey 3 slices	69	2.2	0.8	1.2	0.2	10.5	1.8	0.0	P, K, Zn
Ham, smoked 2 slices	46	1.3	0.5	0.7	0.1	8.1	0.4	0.0	P, K, Zn
Pastrami, turkey 2 slices	80	3.5	1.0	1.2	0.9	10.5	0.9	0.0	B_2, Nia / Zn
Pepperoni, beef and pork 1 slice	30	2.6	1.0	1.3	0.3	1.3	0.2	0.0	
Salami, beef 1 slice	60	4.8	2.1	2.2	0.2	3.5	0.6	0.0	
Salami, pork, dry 1 slice	41	3.4	1.2	1.6	0.4	2.3	0.2	0.0	
Salami, turkey, cooked 2 slices	112	7.9	2.3	2.6	2.0	9.3	0.3	0.0	Zn
Sausage, Italian pork, cooked 1 link	216	17.2	6.1	8.0	2.2	13.4	1.0	0.0	B_1, B_2, Nia / P, K, Fe, Zn
Sausage, Polish 1oz (28g)	92	8.1	2.9	3.8	0.9	4.0	0.5	0.0	B_1, Nia
Sausage, pork, cooked 1 link	48	4.1	1.4	1.8	0.5	2.6	0.1	0.0	B_1
FISH AND SHELLFISH									
Abalone, fried 3oz (85g)	161	5.8	1.4	2.3	1.4	16.7	9.4	0.0	B_1, B_2, Nia, Pant / P, K, Fe
Anchovy, canned in olive oil 5 anchovies	42	1.9	0.4	0.8	0.5	5.8	0.0	0.0	Nia
Bass, cooked 3oz (85g)	105	2.5	0.6	0.7	0.9	19.3	0.0	0.0	B_1, Nia, B_{12}, Pant / P, K
Bluefish, cooked 3oz (85g)	135	4.6	1.0	2.0	1.2	21.8	0.0	0.0	A, Nia, Pant, B_{12} / P, K
Carp, cooked 3oz (85g)	138	6.1	1.2	2.5	1.6	19.4	0.0	0.0	B_1, Nia, Pant, B_{12} / P, K, Fe, Zn
Catfish, cooked 3oz (85g)	129	6.8	1.5	3.5	1.2	15.9	0.0	0.0	B_1, Nia, Pant, B_{12}, / P, K

	Cal (kcal)	Total fat (g)	Sat. fat (g)	Mono. fat (g)	Poly. fat (g)	Protein (g)	Carb. (g)	Fiber (g)	Good source Vitamins/Minerals
Caviar 1 tbsp	40	2.9	0.6	0.7	1.2	3.9	0.6	0.0	A, B_2, Pant, B_{12}, / S, Fe
Clams, cooked 3oz (85g) (19 small)	126	1.7	0.2	0.1	0.5	21.7	4.4	0.0	A, Nia, Pant, B_{12} / P, K, S, Fe, Zn
Cod 3oz (85g)	89	0.7	0.1	0.1	0.2	19.4	0.0	0.0	Nia / K
Crab, Alaska king, cooked 3oz (85g)	82	1.3	0.1	0.2	0.5	16.5	0.0	0.0	Nia, B_{12} / P, K, S, Cu
Crab, blue, cooked 3oz (85g)	87	1.5	0.2	0.2	0.6	17.2	0.0	0.0	Nia, B_{12} / P, K, S, Zn
Crayfish, cooked 3oz (85g)	75	1.0	0.2	0.2	0.3	14.3	0.0	0.0	Nia, B_{12} / P, K, S, Zn
Flounder, cooked 3oz (85g)	100	1.3	0.3	0.2	0.5	20.5	0.0	0.0	B_2, Nia, B_{12} / P, K, S
Grouper, cooked 3oz (85g)	100	1.1	0.3	0.2	0.3	21.1	0.0	0.0	A, Pant / K, S
Haddock, cooked 3oz (85g)	95	0.8	0.1	0.1	0.3	20.6	0.0	0.0	Nia, B_{12} / P, K, S, Fe
Halibut, cooked 3oz (85g)	119	2.5	0.4	0.8	0.8	22.7	0.0	0.0	A, Nia, Pant, B_{12}, / P, K, S
Herring, cooked 3oz (85g)	173	9.9	2.2	4.1	2.3	19.6	0.0	0.0	B_1, Nia, B_{12} / P, K, S, Fe, Zn
Herring, kippers 1 piece	87	4.9	1.1	2.0	1.2	9.8	0.0	0.0	B_2, Nia, B_{12} / K, S
Herring, pickled 1 piece	39	2.7	0.4	1.8	0.3	2.1	1.4	0.0	
Lobster, cooked 3oz (85g)	83	0.5	0.1	0.1	0.1	17.4	1.1	0.0	B_{12} / P, K, S, Cu, Zn
Mackerel, cooked 3oz (85g)	223	15.1	3.6	6.0	3.7	20.3	0.0	0.0	A, B_1, B_2, Nia, Pant, B_{12} / P, K, S, Fe
Monkfish, cooked 3oz (85g)	82	1.7				15.8	0.0	0.0	Nia, Pant / P, K, S
Mullet, cooked 3oz (85g)	128	4.1	1.2	1.2	0.8	21.1	0.0	0.0	Nia / P, K, S, Fe
Mussels, cooked 3oz (85g)	146	3.8	0.7	0.9	1.0	20.2	6.3	0.0	A, B_1, B_2, Nia, Pant, B_{12}, C / P, K, Fe, Zn
Octopus, cooked 3oz (85g)	139	1.8	0.4	0.3	0.4	25.4	3.7	0.0	A, Nia, Pant, B_{12} / P, K, S, Fe, Zn

	Cal (kcal)	Total fat (g)	Sat. fat (g)	Mono. fat (g)	Poly. fat (g)	Protein (g)	Carb. (g)	Fiber (g)	Good source Vitamins/Minerals
Oysters, cooked 3oz (85g)	139	3.9	0.9	0.6	1.5	16.1	8.4	0.0	A, Nia, Pant, B_{12}, C / P, K, S, Cu, Fe, Zn
Perch, cooked 3oz (85g)	100	1.0	0.2	0.2	0.4	21.1	0.0	0.0	Nia, Pant, B_{12} / P, K, S, Zn
Pike, cooked 3oz (85g)	96	0.7	0.1	0.2	0.2	21.0	0.0	0.0	Nia, Pant, B_{12} / P, K, S
Pollock, cooked 3oz (85g)	100	1.1	0.1	0.1	0.5	21.2	0.0	0.0	K
Roe, cooked 1oz (28g)	58	2.3	0.5	0.6	1.0	8.1	0.5	0.0	Nia, B_{12}
Salmon, atlantic, cooked 3oz (85g)	175	10.5	2.1	3.8	3.8	18.8	0.0	0.0	B_2, Nia, Pant, B_6, B_{12}, Fol / P, K, S
Salmon, chinook, cooked 3oz (85g)	196	11.4	2.7	4.9	2.3	21.9	0.0	0.0	A, B_2, Nia, B_{12}, Fol / P, K, S
Salmon, coho, cooked 3oz (85g)	151	7.0	1.7	3.1	1.7	20.7	0.0	0.0	B_2, Nia, Pant, B_{12} / P, K, S
Salmon, pink, boneless, canned 2½oz (75g)	70	2.0	0.0			14.0	0.0	0.0	
Salmon, sockeye, cooked 3oz (85g)	184	9.3	1.6	4.5	2.0	23.2	0.0	0.0	A, B_1, B_2, Nia, B_{12} / P, K, S
Sardines, canned in soybean oil 2 sardines	50	2.7	0.4	0.9	1.2	5.9	0.0	0.0	Nia, Pant, B_{12} / P, S
Scallops 3½oz (100g)	88	1.0	0.2	0.1	0.4	15.9	2.9		
Sea bass, cooked 3oz (85g)	105	2.2	0.6	0.5	0.8	20.1	0.0	0.0	A, B_1, B_2, Nia, Pant / P, K
Shark 3oz (85g)	111	3.8	0.8	1.5	1.0	17.8	0.0	0.0	Nia, B_{12} / P, S
Shrimp, cooked 3oz (85g)	102	1.7	0.3	0.2	0.6	19.6	0.9	0.0	Nia / P, K, S, Fe, Zn
Skate 3½oz (100g)	98	0.7				21.5	0.0	0.0	
Snapper, cooked 3oz (85g)	109	1.5	0.3	0.3	0.5	22.4	0.0	0.0	Pant, B_{12} / P, K, S
Sole, cooked 3oz (85g)	100	1.3	0.3	0.2	0.5	20.5	0.0	0.0	Nia, B_{12} / P, K, S
Squid 3oz (85g)	78	1.2	0.3	0.1	0.4	13.3	2.6	0.0	B_2, Nia, B_{12} / P, K, S, Cu, Zn

	Cal (kcal)	Total fat (g)	Sat. fat (g)	Mono. fat (g)	Poly. fat (g)	Protein (g)	Carb. (g)	Fiber (g)	Good source Vitamins/Minerals
Swordfish, cooked 3oz (85g)	132	4.4	1.2	1.7	1.0	21.6	0.0	0.0	Nia, B_{12} / P, K, S, Zn
Trout, cooked 3oz (85g)	144	6.1	1.8	1.8	2.0	20.6	0.0	0.0	A, Nia, Pant, B_{12} / P, K, S
Tuna, canned in water 3oz (85g)	109	2.5	0.7	0.7	0.9	20.1	0.0	0.0	Nia, B_{12} / P, K
Tuna steak, cooked 3oz (85g)	153	5.3	1.4	1.7	1.6	25.4	0.0	0.0	A, B_1, B_2, Nia, Pant, B_{12} / Mg, P, K, Fe
Turbot, cooked 3oz (85g)	104	3.2				17.5	0.0	0.0	Nia, B_{12} / K, S
Whelk, cooked 3oz (85g)	234	0.7	0.1	0.0	0.0	40.6	13.2	0.0	Nia, B_{12} / P, K, S, Cu, Zn
Whiting, cooked 3oz (85g)	99	1.4	0.3	0.4	0.5	20.0	0.0	0.0	Nia, B_{12} / P, K, S
LEGUMES AND SOY PRODUCTS									
Adzuki beans, boiled 1 cup	294	0.2	0.1			17.3	57.0		B_1, B_2, Nia / Mg, P, K, S, Fe, Zn
Baked beans, homemade 1 cup	382	13.0	4.9	5.4	1.9	14.0	54.1	13.9	B_1, B_2, Nia / Mg, P, K, S, Fe, Zn
Black beans, boiled 1 cup	227	0.9	0.2	0.1	0.4	15.2	40.8	15.0	B_1, B_2, Fol / Mg, P, K, S, Fe, Zn
Black-eyed peas, boiled 1 cup	160	0.6	0.2	0.1	0.3	5.2	33.5	8.3	A, B_1, B_2, Nia, Fol / Ca, K, S, Fe, Zn
Broad beans, boiled 1 cup	187	0.7	0.1	0.1	0.3	12.9	33.4	9.2	B_1, B_2, Nia, Fol / P, K, S, Fe, Zn
Broad beans, canned 1 cup	182	0.6	0.1	0.1	0.2	14.0	31.8	9.5	Nia / P, K, S, Fe, Zn
Chickpeas, boiled 1 cup	269	4.2	0.4	1.0	1.9	14.5	45.0	12.5	B_1, B_2, Fol / P, K, S, Fe, Zn
Chickpeas, hummus 1 cup	421	20.8	3.1	8.7	7.8	12.1	49.6	12.5	B_1, B_2, Nia, Fol, C / Ca, P, K, S, Fe, Zn
Great Northern beans, boiled 1 cup	209	0.8	0.2	0.0	0.3	14.7	37.3	12.4	B_1, B_2, Nia, Fol / Ca, P, K, S, Fe, Zn
Kidney beans, boiled 1 cup	225	0.9	0.1	0.1	0.5	15.3	40.4	13.1	B_1, B_2, Nia, Fol / P, K, S, Fe, Zn
Lentils, boiled 1 cup	230	0.8	0.1	0.1	0.3	17.9	39.9	15.6	A, B_1, B_2, Nia, Pant, Fol / P, K, S, Fe, Zn

	Cal (kcal)	Total fat (g)	Sat. fat (g)	Mono. fat (g)	Poly. fat (g)	Protein (g)	Carb. (g)	Fiber (g)	Good source Vitamins/Minerals
Lima beans, boiled 1 cup	216	0.7	0.2	0.1	0.2	14.7	39.3	13.2	B_1, B_2, Pant, Fol / P, K, S, Fe, Zn
Miso 4floz (120ml)	284	8.4	1.2	1.9	4.7	16.3	38.6	7.5	B_1, B_2, B_{12}, Fol / P, K, S, Fe, Zn
Navy beans, boiled 1 cup	258	1.0	0.3	0.1	0.4	15.8	47.9	11.6	B_1, B_2, Nia, Pant, Fol / P, K, S, Fe, Zn
Pinto beans, boiled 1 cup	234	0.9	0.2	0.2	0.3	14.0	43.9	14.7	B_1, B_2, Fol / P, K, S, Fe, Zn
Snow peas, frozen ½ cup	35	1.5	0.0			2.0	4.0	2.0	C / S
Soybeans, green, boiled ½ cup	127	5.8	0.7	1.1	2.7	11.1	9.9	3.8	B_1, B_2, Nia, Fol, C / P, K, Fe
Soybeans, mature, boiled 1 cup	298	15.4	2.2	3.4	8.7	28.6	17.1	10.3	B_1, B_2, Fol / Ca, Mg, P, K, Fe, Zn
Soymilk 8floz (240ml)	79	4.6	0.5	08	2.0	6.6	4.3	3.1	
Tempeh ½ cup	165	6.4	0.9	1.4	3.6	15.7	14.1		A, B_1, Nia, Fol / Mg, P, K, Fe, Zn
Tofu, raw, firm ½ cup chopped	183	11.0	1.6	2.4	6.2	19.9	5.4	2.9	Fe
NUTS AND SEEDS									
Almonds, dry roasted 3 tbsp	166	14.6	1.4	9.5	3.1	5.6	5.7	3.1	B_2 / Mg, P, K, S, Cu, Fe, Zn
Brazils, dried 3 tbsp	186	18.8	4.6	6.5	6.8	4.1	3.6	1.5	B_1 / Ca. Mg, P, K, S, Cu, Zn
Cashews, dry roasted 3 tbsp	163	13.1	2.6	7.7	2.2	4.3	9.3	0.9	Mg, P, K, S, Fe, Zn
Chestnuts, boiled 3 tbsp	37	0.4	0.1	0.1	0.2	0.6	7.9		K, S
Coconut, dried 1oz (28g)	187	18.3	16.2	0.8	0.2	2.0	6.9	4.6	K, S
Coconut, raw 1 piece	159	15.1	13.4	0.6	0.2	1.5	6.9	4.0	Mg, K, S, Fe
Flaxseeds, dried ½ cup	186	12.7				6.7	14	3.3	Nia / Ca, P, Fe
Hazelnuts, dry roasted 3 tbsp	188	18.8	1.4	14.7	1.8	2.8	5.1	2.0	Mg, S

	Cal (kcal)	Total fat (g)	Sat. fat (g)	Mono. fat (g)	Poly. fat (g)	Protein (g)	Carb. (g)	Fiber (g)	Good source Vitamins/Minerals
Macadamias, dry roasted 3 tbsp	200	21.1	2.5	16.3	0.6	2.5	3.2	1.9	
Peanut butter, crunchy 2 tbsp	188	16.0	3.1	7.5	4.5	7.7	6.9	2.1	Nia / Mg, K, S
Peanuts, dry roasted 3 tbsp	166	14.1	2.0	7.0	4.4	6.7	6.1	2.3	B_1, Nia, Fol / Mg, K, S
Peanuts, unsalted 3 tbsp	166	14.1	2.0	7.0	4.4	6.7	6.1	2.3	Nia / Ca, P, K, S
Pecans, dry roasted 3 tbsp	187	18.3	1.5	11.4	4.5	2.3	6.3	2.6	B_1 / S, Zn
Pine nuts (pignolia), dried 3 tbsp	160	14.4	2.2	5.4	6.1	6.8	4.0	1.3	B_1, Nia / K, S, Fe, Zn
Pistachios, dry roasted 3 tbsp	172	15.0	1.9	10.1	2.3	4.2	7.8	3.1	B_1 / K, S, Cu, Fe
Pumpkin seeds ⅓ cup	110	5.0	1.0	1.5	2.0	5.0	14.0	2.0	
Sesame seeds, kernels, toasted 3 tbsp	161	13.6	1.9	5.1	6.0	4.8	7.4	4.8	B_1, B_2, Nia / Mg, P, S, Cu, Fe, Zn
Soy nuts, dry roasted ½ cup	387	18.6	2.7	4.1	10.5	34.0	28.1	7.0	B_1, B_2, Fol / Ca, Mg, P, K, S, Fe, Zn
Sunflower seeds, dry roasted 3 tbsp	165	14.1	1.5	2.7	9.3	5.5	6.8	3.1	Nia, Pant / Mg, P, K, S, Fe, Zn
Walnuts, black, dried 3 tbsp	172	16.0	1.0	3.6	10.6	6.9	3.4	1.4	Mg, S

FATS, OILS, AND SPREADS

	Cal (kcal)	Total fat (g)	Sat. fat (g)	Mono. fat (g)	Poly. fat (g)	Protein (g)	Carb. (g)	Fiber (g)	Good source Vitamins/Minerals
Apple butter, low-fat 1 tbsp	33	0.1	0.0	0.0	0.0	0.0	8.6	0.2	
Butter 1 tbsp	36	4.1	2.5	1.2	0.2	0.0	0.0	0.0	A
Canola oil 1 tbsp	124	14.0	1.0	8.2	4.1	0.0	0.0	0.0	E
Chicken fat, raw 1 tbsp	117	13.0	3.9	5.8	2.7	0.0	0.0	0.0	
Cod liver oil 1 tbsp	126	14.0	3.2	6.5	3.2	0.0	0.0	0.0	
Corn oil 1 tbsp	124	14.0	1.8	3.4	8.2	0.0	0.0	0.0	E

	Cal (kcal)	Total fat (g)	Sat. fat (g)	Mono. fat (g)	Poly. fat (g)	Protein (g)	Carb. (g)	Fiber (g)	Good source Vitamins/Minerals
Honey 1 tbsp	64	0.0	0.0	0.0	0.0	0.1	17.3	0.0	
Jam (jelly), preserves 1 tbsp	48	0.0	0.0	0.0	0.0	0.1	12.9	0.2	
Lard 1 tbsp	117	13.0	5.1	5.9	1.5	0.0	0.0	0.0	
Maple syrup 1 tbsp	52	0.0	0.0	0.0	0.0	0.0	13.4	0.0	
Margarine, soft 1 tbsp	40	4.5	0.0	2.5	1.0	0.0	1.0	0.0	
Margarine, stick 1 tbsp	50	6.0	1.0	1.5	1.5	0.0	1.0	0.0	
Marmalade orange 1 tbsp	49	0.0	0.0	0.0	0.0	0.1	13.3	0.0	
Mayonnaise 1 tbsp	100	11.0	1.7	3.3	5.9	0.2	0.1		
Mayonnaise, lite 1 tbsp	50	5.0	1.0			0.0	1.0	0.0	
Olive oil 1 tbsp	124	14.0	1.9	10.3	1.2	0.0	0.0	0.0	E
Peanut oil 1 tbsp	124	14.0	2.4	6.5	4.5	0.0	0.0	0.0	E
Safflower oil 1 tbsp	124	14.0	1.3	1.7	10.4	0.0	0.0	0.0	E
Sesame oil 1 tbsp	124	14.0	2.0	5.6	5.8	0.0	0.0	0.0	
Shortening 1 tbsp	110	12.0	3.0	4.0	3.0	0.0	0.0	0.0	
Soybean oil 1 tbsp	124	14.0	2.0	3.3	8.1	0.0	0.0	0.0	
Stanol spread 1 tbsp	60	8.0	1.0	4.0	2.0				A, E
Stanol spread, lite 1 tbsp	45	5.0	0.5	2.5	2.0				A, E
Sunflower oil 1 tbsp	122	13.6	1.7	1.9	9.1	0.0	0.0	0.0	
Vegetable oil spray 1 spray	2	0.2	0.0	0.1	0.1	0.0	0.0	0.0	

	Cal (kcal)	Total fat (g)	Sat. fat (g)	Mono. fat (g)	Poly. fat (g)	Protein (g)	Carb. (g)	Fiber (g)	Good source Vitamins/Minerals
DRINKS									
Ale 12floz (360ml)	190	0.0	0.0	0.0	0.0	2.7	17.4		
Apple juice, canned/bottled 8floz (240ml)	117	0.3	0.0	0.0	0.1	0.1	29.0	0.2	K
Beer 12floz (360ml)	146	0.0	0.0	0.0	0.0	1.1	13.2	0.7	B_2, Nia
Beer, light 12floz (360ml)	99	0.0	0.0	0.0	0.0	0.7	4.6	0.0	B_2, Nia
Carrot juice, canned 6floz (180ml)	74	0.3	0.0	0.0	0.1	1.7	17.1	1.5	A, B_1, B_2, C / K
Coffee, brewed 6floz (180ml)	4	0.0	0.0	0.0	0.0	0.2	0.7	0.0	
Cola 12floz (360ml)	152	0.0	0.0	0.0	0.0	0.0	38.5	0.0	
Ginger ale 12floz (360ml)	124	0.0	0.0	0.0	0.0	0.0	31.8	0.0	
Grapefruit juice, canned 3½floz (100ml)	94	0.2	0.0	0.0	0.1	1.3	22.1	0.2	B_1, C / K
Grape juice, canned/bottled 8floz (240ml)	154	0.2	0.1	0.0	0.1	1.4	37.8	0.3	K
Green tea 8floz (240ml)	2	0.0	0.0	0.0	0.0	0.0	0.4	0.0	
Orange juice, canned 8floz (240ml)	105	0.3	0.0	0.1	0.1	1.5	24.5	0.5	A, B_1, C / K, Fe
Pineapple juice, canned 8floz (240ml)	140	0.2	0.0	0.0	0.1	0.8	34.4	0.5	B_1, Fol, C / K
Root beer 12floz (360ml)	152	0.0	0.0	0.0	0.0	0.0	39.2	0.0	
Scotch 1½floz (45ml)	105	0.0	0.0	0.0	0.0	0.0	0.0	0.0	
Soda, diet 12floz (360ml)	0	0.0	0.0	0.0	0.0.	0.0	0.0	0.0	
Tea, black 6floz (180ml)	2	0.0	0.0	0.0	0.0	0.0	0.5	0.0	
Tea, herb 6floz (180ml)	2	0.0	0.0	0.0	0.0	0.0	0.4	0.0	

	Cal (kcal)	Total fat (g)	Sat. fat (g)	Mono. fat (g)	Poly. fat (g)	Protein (g)	Carb. (g)	Fiber (g)	Good source Vitamins/Minerals
Tomato juice 6floz (180ml)	31	0.1	0.0	0.0	0.0	1.4	7.7	0.7	A, Nia, Fol, C / P, Fe
Tonic water 12floz (360ml)	124	0.0	0.0	0.0	0.0	0.0	32.2	0.0	
Vodka 1½floz (45ml)	105	0.0	0.0	0.0	0.0	0.0	0.0	0.0	
Water, bottled 8floz (240ml)	0	0.0	0.0	0.0	0.0	0.0	0.0	0.0	
Water, tap 8floz (240ml)	0	0.0	0.0	0.0	0.0	0.0	0.0	0.0	
Wine, red 3½floz (100ml)	74	0.0	0.0	0.0	0.0	0.2	1.8	0.0	
Wine, rosé 3½floz (100ml)	73	0.0	0.0	0.0	0.0	0.2	1.4	0.0	
Wine, white 3½floz (100ml)	70	0.0	0.0	0.0	0.0	0.1	0.8	0.0	

FROZEN AND CHILLED DESSERTS

	Cal (kcal)	Total fat (g)	Sat. fat (g)	Mono. fat (g)	Poly. fat (g)	Protein (g)	Carb. (g)	Fiber (g)	Good source Vitamins/Minerals
Frozen yogurt, soft serve ½ cup	115	4.3	2.6	1.3	0.2	2.9	17.9	1.6	B₂ / K
Fruit and juice bar, frozen 3floz (90ml) bar	75	0.1	0.0	0.0	0.0	1.1	18.6	0.0	C
Ice cream, chocolate ½ cup	143	7.3	4.5	2.1	0.3	2.5	18.6	0.8	A, B₂ / K
Ice cream, strawberry ½ cup	127	5.5	3.4			2.1	18.2	0.2	A, B₂
Ice cream, vanilla regular ½ cup	133	7.3	4.5	2.1	0.3	2.3	15.6	0.0	A, B₂
Ice pop 2floz (60ml) bar	42	0.0	0.0	0.0	0.0	0.0	11.2	0.0	
Jello 3oz (85g) package	324	0.0	0.0	0.0	0.0	6.6	77.0	0.0	
Jello, sugar-free ½ cup prepared	10	0.0	0.0	0.0	0.0	1.0	1.0	0.0	
Sorbet, orange ½ cup	132	1.9	1.1	0.5	0.1	1.1	29.2	0.5	
Sorbet, peach 1 cup	200	0.0	0.0	0.0	0.0	2.0	70	1.5	A

	Cal (kcal)	Total fat (g)	Sat. fat (g)	Mono. fat (g)	Poly. fat (g)	Protein (g)	Carb. (g)	Fiber (g)	Good source Vitamins/Minerals
CAKES, COOKIES, AND SNACKS									
Angel food cake 1/12 cake	73	0.2	0.0	0.0	0.1	1.7	16.4	0.4	B_2
Apple pie, homemade 1/8 of 9in (23cm) pie	411	19.4	4.7	8.4	5.2	3.7	57.5		B_1, B_2, Nia / Fe
Banana cream, homemade 1/8 of 9in (23cm) pie	398	20.1	5.6	8.5	4.9	6.5	48.7	1.0	A, B_1, B_2, Nia / K, Fe
Boston cream pie, homemade 1/12 of 9in (23cm) cake	293	12.3	3.9	5.0	2.6	4.3	43.0		A, B_1, B_2, Nia / Fe
Brownie, homemade 1 medium brownie	112	7.0	1.8	2.6	2.3	1.5	12.0		A
Carrot cake 1/12 of 9in (23cm) cake	239	11.0	1.8	3.4	5.0	3.6	32.7	1.4	A, B_1, B_2
Cheesecake, homemade 1/12 of 9in (23cm) cake	457	33.3	18.4	10.3	2.6	8.7	32.3		A, B_2 / Fe
Chocolate cake, homemade 1/12 of 9in (23cm) cake	340	14.3	5.2	5.7	2.6	5.0	50.7	1.5	B_1, B_2, Nia / Fe
Cinnamon and raisin bun 1 roll	223	9.8	2.5	5.5	1.3	3.7	30.5	1.4	B_1, B_2, Nia
Cookie, choc chip, homemade 1 cookie	78	4.5	2.3	1.3	0.7	0.9	9.3	0.4	
Cream puff, homemade 1 medium cream puff	335	20.2	4.8	8.5	5.4	8.7	29.8	0.5	A, B_1, B_2, Nia / Fe
Croissant 1 medium	231	12.0	6.7	3.3	0.7	4.7	26.1	1.5	A, B_1, B_2, Nia / Fe
Cupcake, homemade 1 cupcake	172	5.5				1.6	29.8		
Custard pudding, homemade 1/2 cup	209	6.6	3.3	2.1	0.5	7.2	15.1	0.0	A, B_2 / Ca, P, K
Danish pastry, fruit 1 pastry	263	13.1	3.3	7.3	1.7	3.8	33.9	1.3	B_1, B_2, Nia / Fe
Doughnuts, sugared 1 doughnut	198	10.8	1.8	4.5	3.8	2.3	23.4	0.7	B_1
Eclair, chocolate 1 eclair	96	9.2				2.6	25.5		
Fig bar 1 bar	56	1.2	0.2	0.6	0.2	0.6	11.3	0.7	

	Cal (kcal)	Total fat (g)	Sat. fat (g)	Mono. fat (g)	Poly. fat (g)	Protein (g)	Carb. (g)	Fiber (g)	Good source Vitamins/Minerals
Flan, homemade ½ cup	220	6.3	3.0	2.1	0.5	6.9	34.9	0.0	A, B_2 / Ca, P, K
Fortune cookie 1 cookie	30	0.2	0.1	0.1	0.0	0.3	6.7	0.1	
Fruit bar ⅘oz (22g) bar	81	1.2	0.9	0.1	0.0	0.4	18.1	0.8	C
Fruitcake, homemade ¹⁄₃₆ of 10in (25cm) cake	302	9.7	1.2	4.0	3.8	3.0	54.4		B_1, B_2, Nia / K, Fe
Gingerbread, homemade ⅑ of 8in (20cm) sq cake	263	12.1	3.1	5.3	3.1	2.9	36.4		B_1, B_2, Nia / K, Fe
Gingersnap 4 cookies	118	2.8	0.5	1.6	0.4	1.6	21.8	0.6	Nia / Fe
Graham crackers, plain/ honey 4 crackers	120	2.9	0.7	1.4	0.4	2.0	21.8	0.8	
Lemon meringue, homemade ⅛ of 9in (23cm) pie	362	16.4	4.0	7.1	4.2	4.8	49.7		A, B_1, B_2, Nia / Fe
Mince pie, homemade ⅛ of 9in (23cm) pie	477	17.8	4.4	7.7	4.7	4.3	79.2	4.3	A, B_1, B_2, Nia / K, Fe
Muffin, blueberry 1 muffin	158	3.7	0.7	1.4	1.2	3.1	27.4	1.5	
Muffin, corn 1 muffin	174	4.8	0.9	1.9	1.6	3.4	29.0	1.9	B_1, B_2, Nia / P, Fe
Muffin, oat bran 1 muffin	154	4.2	0.5	0.8	2.6	4.0	27.5	2.6	B_1 / P, K, Fe, Zn
Multigrain cracker 4 crackers	69	2.7	0.6			1.7	9.6	0.7	
Oatmeal cookie 1 cookie	67	2.7	0.5	1.2	0.8	1.0	10.0		
Pancake, buckwheat, from mix 4in (10cm) diam.	62	2.3	0.6	0.6	0.8	2.4	8.5	0.7	B_1, Nia / Ca, P, Fe
Pancake, buttermilk, homemade 4in (10cm) diam.	86	3.5	0.7	0.9	1.7	2.6	10.9		B_2
Pancake, plain, homemade 4in (10cm) diam.	86	3.7	0.8	0.9	1.7	2.4	10.8		B_1 / Fe
Pancake whole-wheat, homemade 4in (10cm) diam.	92	2.9	0.8	0.8	1.1	3.7	12.9	1.2	B_1, B_2, Nia / Ca, P, K, Fe
Peanut butter cookie 1 cookie	72	3.5	0.8	1.3	1.2	1.4	8.8	0.3	

	Cal (kcal)	Total fat (g)	Sat. fat (g)	Mono. fat (g)	Poly. fat (g)	Protein (g)	Carb. (g)	Fiber (g)	Good sources Vitamins/Minerals
Pecan pie, homemade 1/8 of 9in (23cm) pie	503	27.1	4.9	13.6	7.0	6.0	63.7		A, B_1, B_2, Nia / K, Fe, Zn
Popcorn, butter, frozen 3 cups	212	13.6				2.9	20.0	1.1	
Popcorn, plain 3½ cups	107	1.2	0.2	0.3	0.5	3.4	21.8	4.2	
Potato chips 1oz (28g)	152	9.8	3.1	2.8	3.5	2.0	15.0	1.3	Nia / K
Pretzel 1oz (28g)	108	1.0	0.2	0.4	0.3	2.6	22.5	0.9	B_1, B_2, Nia / Fe
Pumpkin pie 1/8 of 9in (23cm) pie	316	14.4	4.9	5.7	2.8	7.0	40.9		A, B_1, B_2, Nia / Ca, P, K, Fe
Rice cakes, unsalted 1 cake	34	0.3	0.1	0.1	0.1	0.9	7.3	0.3	
Rice pudding, homemade ½ cup	217	4.3	2.6	1.2	0.2	5.5	40.1	0.8	B_1, B_2 / Ca, K, Fe
Saltines 1 saltine	13	0.4	0.1	0.2	0.1	0.3	2.1	0.1	
Shortbread 1 cookie	40	1.9	0.5	1.1	0.2	0.5	5.2	0.1	
Shortcake, homemade 1 shortcake	225	9.2	2.5	3.9	2.4	4.0	31.5		B_1, B_2, Nia / Ca, Fe
Sponge, homemade 1/12 of 10in (25cm) cake	187	2.7	0.8	1.0	0.4	4.6	36.4		A, B_1, B_2 / Fe
Tapioca, homemade ½ cup	190	6.5	3.3	2.1	0.5	7.1	25.8	0.0	A, B_2 / Ca, P, K
Tortilla chips 1oz (28g)	142	7.4	1.4	4.4	1.0	2.0	17.8	1.8	
Trail mix 1oz (28g)	131	8.3	1.6	3.6	2.7	3.9	12.7		B_1, Nia / K
Wafer, vanilla 7 wafers	125	4.3	1.0	1.7	1.0	1.4	20.9	0.5	
Waffle, homemade 1 waffle	218	10.6	2.1	2.6	5.1	5.9	24.7		Ca, P, Fe
Waffle, oat-bran, frozen 2 waffles	196	7.2	1.5	4.5	1.0	5.8	27.0	2.7	A, B_1, B_2, Nia, B_{12} / Fe
Wheat thins 16 crackers	140	6.0	1.0	2.5	0.5	2.0	19.0	2.0	

Useful addresses

The following organizations and associations provide an additional source of information about the topics covered in this book. They are presented in two broad categories: the first lists organizations dealing with nutritional and fitness-related issues; the second lists organizations that offer information and advice on specific medical conditions.

Information on nutrition and fitness

NUTRITION ORGANIZATIONS AND NEWSLETTERS

American College of Nutrition
Online: www.am-coll-nutr.org
300 S. Duncan Avenue, Ste. 225,
Clearwater, FL 33755
Tel: 727-446-6086

American Dietetic Association
Online: www.eatright.org
120 South Riverside Plaza,
Chicago, IL 60606
Tel: 1-800-366-1655
or 312-899-0040

American School Food Service Association
Online: www.asfsa.org
700 South Washington Street, Suite 300,
Alexandria, VA 22314
Tel: 703-739-3900

Centers for Disease Control and Prevention
Online: www.cdc.gov/nccdphp/dnpa/nutrition.htm

Children's Nutrition Research Center
Online: www.bcm.tmc.edu/cnrc
Children's Nutrition Research Center,
1100 Bates Street, Houston, TX 77030

Council for Responsible Nutrition
Online: www.crnusa.org
1828 L Street NW, Suite 900,
Washington, DC 20036-5114
Tel: 202-776-7929

Food and Drug Administration Center for Food Safety and Applied Nutrition
Online: vm.cfsan.fda.gov
Office of Consumer Affairs,
5600 Fishers Lane
Rockville, MD 20857
Tel: 888-463-6332 or 800-FDA-4010

Healthy People 2010
Online: www.healthypeople.gov
Office of Disease Prevention and
Health Promotion
Hubert H. Humphrey Building,
Room 738G, 200 Independence Ave., SW,
Washington, DC 20201

National Association of Nutrition and Aging Services
Online: www.nanasp.org
2675 44th Street, SW, Suite 305,
Grand Rapids, MI 49509
Tel: 800-999-6262

National Women's Health Network
Online: www.womenshealthnetwork.org
514 10th Street, NW, Suite 400,
Washington, DC 20004
Tel: 202-347-1140

National Institutes of Health Office of Dietary Supplements
Online: ods.od.nih.gov/index.aspx
6100 Executive Blvd., Room 3B01,
MSC 7517, Bethesda,
MD 20892-7517
Tel: 301-435-2920

North American Association For The Study Of Obesity
Online: www.naaso.org
8630 Fenton Street, Suite 918,
Silver Spring, MD 20910
Tel: 301-563-6526

North American Vegetarian Society
Online: www.navs-online.org
P.O. Box 72, Dolgeville, NY 13329
Tel: 518-568-7970

President's Council on Physical Fitness and Sports
Online: www.fitness.gov/
200 Independence Avenue, SW,
Humphrey Building, Room 738H,
Washington, DC 20201
Tel: 202-690-9000

Shape Up America
Online: www.shapeup.org
6707 Democracy Blvd., Suite 306,
Bethesda, MD 20817
Tel: 301-493-5368

US Department of Agriculture
Online: www.usda.gov
Center for Nutrition Policy and Promotion
14th and Independence Avenue, SW,
Room 304-A, Whitten Building,
Washington, DC 20250
Tel: 202-720-4423

Weight-Control Information Network
Online: www.niddk.nih.gov/health/nutrit/win.htm
1 WIN Way, Bethesda, MD 20892-3665
Tel: 1-877-946-4627 or 202-828-1025

Information on disorders

ARTHRITIS
American College of Rheumatology
Online: www.rheumatology.org
1800 Century Place, Suite 250,
Atlanta, GA 30345
Tel: 404-633-3777

Arthritis Foundation
Online: www.arthritis.org/default.asp
P.O. Box 7669, Atlanta, GA 30357-0669
Tel: 404-872-7100

National Institute of Arthritis and Musculoskeletal and Skin Diseases
National Institute of Health
Online: www.niams.nih.gov/an/index.htm
Building 31, Room 4C02, 31 Center Drive,
MSC 2350, Bethesda, MD 20892-2350
Tel: 301-496-8190

CARDIOVASCULAR DISEASES
American Heart Association
Online: www.americanheart.org
7272 Greenville Avenue,
Dallas, TX 75231-4596
Tel: 800-242-1793 ext. 1179
Local Chapters: 800-242-8721

National Cholesterol Education Program
Online: www.nhlbi.nih.gov/ncep.htm
NHLBI Health Information Network,
P.O. Box 30105,
Bethesda, MD 20824-0105
Tel: 301-592-8573

National Heart, Lung & Blood Institute Information Center
Online: www.nhlbi.nih.gov
P.O. Box 30105,
Bethesda, MD 20824-0105
Tel: 301-592-8573

CANCER
American Cancer Society
Online: www.cancer.org
1599 Clifton Road, NE,
Atlanta, GA 30329-4251
Tel: 800-ACS-2345

National Cancer Institute
Online: www.nci.nih.gov
NCI Public Inquiries Office
Suite 3036A, 6116 Executive Blvd.,
MSC8322, Bethesda, MD 20892-8322
Tel: 1-800-4-CANCER (1-800-422-6237)

DIABETES
American Diabetes Association
Online: www.diabetes.org
1660 Duke Street, Alexandria, VA 22314
Tel: 800-342-2383

Juvenile Diabetes Research Foundation International
Online: www.jdrf.org
120 Will Street, New York, NY 10005
Tel: 800-533-CURE

National Institute of Diabetes and Digestive and Kidney Diseases
Online: www.niddk.nih.gov/health/nutrition.htm
National Institute of Health, Building 31,
Room 9A04, Center Drive, MSC 2560
Bethesda, MD 20892-2560
Tel: 301-654-3327 or 301-496-3583

DIGESTIVE DISORDERS
Celiac Sprue Association/USA Inc.
Online: www.csaceliacs.org
P.O. Box 31700, Omaha,
NE 68131-0700
Tel: 402-558-0600

Crohn's and Colitis Foundation of America Inc.
Online: www.ccfa.org
386 Park Avenue South, 17th floor,
New York, NY 10016-8804
Tel: 1-800-932-2423 or 212-685-3440

Gluten Intolerance Group of North America
Online: www.gluten.net
15110 10th Avenue, SW, Suite A,
Seattle, WA 98166-1820
Tel: 206- 246-6652

Intestinal Disease Foundation
Online: www.intestinalfoundation.org
Landmarks Building, Suite 525,
100 West Station Square Drive,
Pittsburgh, PA 15219
Tel: 1-877-587-9606

FOOD ALLERGIES
National Institute of Allergy and Infectious Diseases
Online: www.niaid.nih.gov
9000 Rockville Pike, Bethesda,
MD 20892
Tel: 301-496-5717

The Food Allergy and Anaphylaxis Network
Online: www.foodallergy.org
10400 Eaton Place, Suite 107,
Fairfax, VA 22030
Tel: 703-691-3179 or 703-691-2713

HEADACHE AND MIGRAINE
American Council for Headache Education
Online: www.achenet.org
19 Mantua Road, Mt. Royal,
NJ 08061
Tel: 856-423-0258

EATING DISORDERS
American Anorexia and Bulimia Association, Inc
165 West 46th Street, Suite 1198,
New York, NY 10036
Tel: 212-575-6200

KIDNEY DISEASES
American Foundation for Urologic Disease
Online: www.afud.org
1000 Corporate Boulevard, Suite 410,
Linthicum, MD 21090
Tel: 410-89-3990 or 800-828-7866

National Kidney Foundation
Online: www.kidney.org
30 East 33rd St., Suite 1100
New York, NY 10016
Tel: 800-622-9010 or 212-889-2210

OSTEOPOROSIS
National Institutes of Health Osteoporosis and Related Bone Disease National Resource Center
Online: www.osteo.org
2 AMS Circle, Bethesda,
MD 20892-3676
Tel: 1-800-624-BONE

National Osteoporosis Foundation
Online: www.nof.org
1232 22nd Street N.W.,
Washington, DC 20037-1292
Tel: 202-223-2226 or 800-223-9994

RESPIRATORY AND SLEEP DISORDERS
American Lung Association
Online: www.lungusa.org
61 Broadway, 6th Fl., New York,
NY 10006
Tel: 212-315-8700

American Sleep Apnea Association
Online: www.sleepapnea.org
1424 K Street, NW, Suite 302,
Washington, DC 20005
Tel: 202-293-3650

Asthma and Allergy Foundation of America
Online: www.aafa.org
1233 20th Street, NW Suite 402,
Washington, DC 20036
Tel: 1-800-7-Asthma or 202-466-7643

Family of COPD Support Lists and Programs
Online: www.copd-support.org
COPD-Support, Inc,
PMB 127, 1940 Kings Hwy, Suite 4,
Port Charlotte, FL 33980

Index

Picture credits

The publisher would like to thank the following for their kind permission to reproduce their photographs:

(Abbreviations key: t = top, b = bottom, r = right, l = left, c = centre, a = above)

12-13: Getty Images: Stewart Cohen (t); **13: Corbis:** John Henley (b); **14: Camera Press:** Richard Stonehouse (tl); **15: Getty Images:** Arthur Tilley; **17: Getty Images:** Jonelle Weaver (br); **18: Corbis:** Darama (tl); **19: Corbis:** Nancy A. Santullo; **20: Zefa Picture Library:** creasource; **22: Getty Images:** Paul Avis (b); **23: Getty Images:** Photodisc; **24: Getty Images:** Ebby May; **25: Getty Images:** Barry Yee (bl); **27: Corbis:** LWA-Dann Tardif; **28-29: Masterfile UK:** Kathleen Finlay (t); **29: Alamy Images:** Imagestate (cl); **30: Retna Pictures Ltd:** Andrew Carruth; **31: Corbis:** Getty Images; **34: Getty Images:** Photodisc Blue (br), Mel Yates (tl); **40: Robert Harding Picture Library; 50: Getty Images:** The Anthony Blake Photo Library; **61: Alamy Images:** Jeff Singer (cl); **70: Getty Images:** Harald Sund; **72: Getty Images:** Gerard Loucel; **79: Getty Images:** Yellow Dog Productions; **83: Rex Features:** Woman's Own; **95: Rex Features** (tr); **Getty Images:** Rita Maas (bc); **96: Getty Images:** Photodisc/Ryan McVay (br), Antony Nagelmann (tr); **102: Getty Images:** Romilly Lockyer (bl); **107: Corbis:** Ariel Skelley; **109: Corbis:** Norbert Schaefer; **110: Getty Images:** Photodisc Collection; **111: Mother & Baby Picture Library:** Ruth Jenkinson; **112: Getty Images:** Paul Thomas; **116: Getty Images:** Bruce Ayers; **117: Corbis:** Rick Gomez; **119: Corbis:** Jose Luis Pelaez, Inc.; **126: Getty Images:** Duncan Smith; **128-29: Corbis:** Charles Gupton; **132: Alamy Images:** David Young-Wolff; **137: Corbis:** David Raymer; **138: Retna Pictures Ltd:** John Powell; **139: Food Features; 141: Getty Images:** Mark Williams; **142: Rex Features:** PHN (br); **Getty Images:** Photodisc (tl); **143: Alamy Images:** Jackson Smith; **144-45: Getty Images:** David Madison; **146: Corbis:** Steve Thornton; **147: Corbis:** Tim McGuire; **148: Empics Ltd; 149: Corbis:** Ed Bock; **150: Alamy Images:** Dennis Hallinan; **151: Photolibrary.com:** IPS Photo Index; **153: Corbis:** Ariel Skelley; **154: Getty Images:** Marc Romanelli; **155: Alamy Images:** Elvele Images (cl); **Anthony Blake Photo Library:** Joy Skipper; **158: Corbis:** Rob & Sas; **159: Corbis:** David Woods; **160: Science Photo Library:** BSIP, Chassenet; **161: Alamy Images:** ImageState/Pictor International (cbl); **Getty Images:** Photodisc (tr); **162: Getty Images:** David Sacks; **198: Science Photo Library:** BSIP Laurent/Pat H.Amer; **199: Getty Images:** Jurgen Reisch; **200: Getty Images:** Yellow Dog Productions; **202: Masterfile UK:** Kevin Dodge (tr); **203: Corbis:** Tom & Dee McCarthy (br); **204: Corbis:** Ken Kaminesky; **205: Alamy Images:** BananaStock (tr); **Getty Images:** Edward Holub (b); **206: Getty Images:** Sean Murphy; **207: Getty Images:** V.C.L.; **208: Alamy Images:** Photofusion Picture Library; **209: Corbis:** George Disario; **212: Alamy Images:** Studio M; **215: Science Photo Library:** Eye of Science; **216: Corbis:** Norbert Schaefer; **217: Alamy Images:** Mick Broughton; **223: Powerstock:** Fichtl (b); **Science Photo Library:** CNRI (t); **224: Alamy Images:** Rex Argent (cl); **Anthony Blake Photo Library:** Amanda Heywood (ca), Roger Stowell (cl), Steve Lee (cra); **225: Bubbles:** Lucy Tizard; **227: Science Photo Library:** Gca; **228: Masterfile UK:** Rick Gomez; **229: Anthony Blake Photo Library:** Georgia Glynn Smith; **230: Alamy Images:** Jackson Smith (b); **231: Getty Images:** Paddy Eckersley; **232: Alamy Images:** David Young-Wolff (b); **237: Science Photo Library:** CNRI (t); Getty Images: Victoria Blackie (b); **238: Masterfile UK:** Kathleen Finlay; **241: Science Photo Library:** Zephyr; **243: Science Photo Library:** Sheila Terry; **244: Alamy Images:** Butch Martin (b); **Anthony Blake Photo Library:** Eaglemoss Consumer Publications (c); **245: Anthony Blake Photo Library:** Sian Irvine (b); **Getty Images:** Zigy Kaluzny (t); **246: Getty Images:** Donna Day; **247: Getty Images:** Photodisc Green/David Buffington; **248: Corbis:** Michael Keller; **251: Alamy Images:** Jackson Smith (b); **252: Getty Images:** Caren Alpert; **253: Alamy Images:** Myrleen Cate; **254: Getty Images:** Photodisc Red/Ryan McVay; **255: Alamy Images:** Imagestate/Pictor (bl); **256: Anthony Blake Photo Library:** Martin Brigdale (b); Getty Images: Laurence Monneret (t); **257: Alamy Images:** Jackson Smith; **258: Science Photo Library; 259: Masterfile UK:** John Lee; **262: Anthony Blake Photo Library:** Joff Lee (bl), Tim Hill (bc); **263: Anthony Blake Photo Library:** Iain Bagwell; **266: Corbis:** Jose Luis Pelaez, Inc.; **267: Corbis:** Jose Luis Pelaez, Inc.; **274-75: Getty Images:** PBJ Pictures; **278: Alamy Images:** Butch Martin (cbl); **Getty Images:** Philippe Gelot (tr); **280: Alamy Images:** BananaStock (cla); **281: Getty Images:** Michael Krasowitz (tr); **282: Getty Images:** Photodisc Green (tr); **284: Getty Images:** Photodisc/K; Ovregaard/Cole Group; **286: Corbis:** Michael Boys (tl); **288: Getty Images:** Alan Becker (tl); **290: Alamy Images:** BananaStock; **293: Rex Features:** OPL (tl).

Every effort has been made to trace the copyright holders. Dorling Kindersley apologizes for any unintentional omissions and would be pleased, if any such case should arise, to add an appropriate acknowledgment in future editions. All other images © Dorling Kindersley

For further information see **www.dkimages.com**

Authors' acknowledgments

We would like to thank our science editors, Gabriella Maldonado and Jamie Spencer, for their much appreciated assistance in all aspects of Nutrition for Life. Gabriella completed the majority of research for the book, developed the majority of tables and charts, the vitamin and mineral directory, in addition to the nutrient and recipe analysis information. Jamie Spencer has been very helpful at editing much of the clinical information we use to teach medical students and doctors into easy to understand text for consumers. We have learned a lot from her and very much appreciated the opportunity to work together.

We would also like to thank DK, our publisher, for recognizing the importance of nutrition to health and the prevention of so many chronic diseases. We thank the entire team for their brilliant editing and production job on *Nutrition for Life*. Jemima Dunne, Senior Managing Editor, provided the leadership needed to direct this immense project and always managed to know what the book needed. She deserves a great deal of credit for her vision and experience, which will help to make the book a success both in North America and abroad for many years to come.

Irene Lyford and Liz Coghill, Senior Editors, for being so diligent about everything and including us in all the decisions about the text, photographs, headings, and charts. We are grateful for your writing, editing, and computer expertise and the ability to manage all the information that was sent back and forth via email, without ever losing anything. Sara Kimmins, Project Art Editor, and Marianne Markham, Managing Art Editor, also deserve many thanks for designing the book and directing all photography and selecting visual images.

We would also like to thank Isabel De Cordova, designer, Iona Hoyle, design assistant, Julian Dams, DTP Designer, Wendy Penn, Production Controller, and Sarah Coltman, Production Manager, for making this book a reality. We would not have been able to publish *Nutrition for Life* without you. Thank you!

Finally, we would like to thank our medical students at the University of Pennsylvania School of Medicine for research and writing numerous sections of *Nutrition for Life*. These are Jeremy Brauer, Caitlin Carr, Rex Parker, and Kristen Vierregger. They will surely make great doctors and their patients will benefit from their knowledge and continued interest in nutrition.

Dedication From Lisa Hark, PhD, RD

To my children, Jamie Erica (10) and Brett Daniel (6), for their never-ending love for their mommy. They are glad that the book is finally finished and look forward to seeing me on television, which they have been asking me about for the past two years.

To my parents, Diane and Jerry, for their incredible support and constant stream of love and attention which they have given me over the years and especially while writing this book. They have been excellent role models by eating healthy and exercising every day for most of their adult life.

To my brothers and their families, David, Cinde, and Nicholas; Richard, Pam, Alexandra, Mitchell, and Samantha; and Jeffrey, Stacy, Rachel, Louis, and Joel, for their love and support forever and always and for sharing in my excitement for the completion of the book.

To my mentor and friend, Dr. Gail Morrison, Professor of Medicine and Vice Dean for Education at the University of Pennsylvania School of Medicine, for helping me reach my full potential during the past 15 years at Penn and for giving me the time and encouragement to complete this huge project.

To Dr. Darwin Deen, my Medical Editor and friend, for being so committed to the science of nutrition and always looking for the evidence to support what we have written in this book. I could not have done the book without you, and I thank you for everything!

Dedication from Darwin Deen, MD, MS

I would like to dedicate *Nutrition for Life* to my family, the crucible for all my ideas. To my mom, Ruth, who taught me that eating well was the path to health. To my dad, Darwin Sr., who stimulated my interest in nutrition. To my brother Anthony and my sister Irene who have always been my best audience, and to my children, Benjamin (17) and Jesse (14), who have challenged everything I ever learned about nutrition.

To my patients, whose demand for a single, easy-to-read, practical, and accurate nutrition book motivated me to write this book. My patients have always stimulated me to learn more so that I can take better care of them. They have always tolerated my exhortations to eat better and exercise more with patience and forbearance. For all of you who have asked your doctor for one comprehensive book about nutrition, we hope that *Nutrition for Life* will go beyond your expectations.

Publisher's acknowledgments

Dorling Kindersley would like to thank Ian O'Leary for new photography; Beth Heald for buying and preparing food; Francis Wong for additional design assistance; Gemma Casajuana Filella and Karen Constanti for DTP assistance; Salima Hirani and Kathryn Wilkinson for editorial assistance; Anna Bedewell for picture research; Romaine Werblow—Picture Library; Babita Bholah, Liz Coghill, Laura Forrester, Martin Gough, Marek Gwiazda, Beth Heald, Iona Hoyle, Crispin Lord and Francis Wong for modelling; Hilary Bird for the index; and Mary Lindsay for proofreading.